# CONTROL OF COMMUNICABLE DISEASES

**LABORATORY PRACTICE**



For access to digital chapters,
visit the APHA Press bookstore (www.apha.org).

# CONTROL OF COMMUNICABLE DISEASES

## LABORATORY PRACTICE

Editors
Burton W. Wilcke, Jr, PhD
David L. Heymann, MD

APHA PRESS
AN IMPRINT OF AMERICAN PUBLIC HEALTH ASSOCIATION

American Public Health Association
800 I Street, NW
Washington, DC 20001-3710
www.apha.org



Georges C. Benjamin, MD, Executive Director

Printed and bound in the United States of America
*Book Production Editor*: Maya Ribault
*Typesetting*: The Charlesworth Group
*Cover Design*: Alan Giarcanella
*Printing and Binding*: BR Printers

Library of Congress Cataloging-in-Publication Data

Names: Wilcke, Burton W., Jr., editor. | Heymann, David, L., editor. | American Public Health Association, issuing body.
Title: Control of communicable diseases: laboratory practice / editors, Burton W. Wilcke, Jr, and David L. Heymann.
Other titles: Control of communicable diseases manual (Wilcke) | Complemented by (work): Control of communicable diseases manual.
Description: Washington, DC : American Public Health Association, [2019] | This manual is designed as a complement to Control of communicable diseases manual. | Includes bibliographical references and index.
Identifiers: LCCN 2019017277 (print) | LCCN 2019017825 (ebook) | ISBN 9780875532868 (ebook) | ISBN 9780875532851 (softcover)
Subjects: | MESH: Communicable Disease Control--methods | Clinical Laboratory Techniques--methods | Clinical Laboratory Services--standards
Classification: LCC RA643 (ebook) | LCC RA643 (print) | NLM WA 110 | DDC 616.9--dc23
LC record available at https://lccn.loc.gov/2019017277

# EDITORS

**Burton W. Wilcke, Jr**, PhD
University of Vermont
United States

**David L. Heymann**, MD
London School of Hygiene & Tropical Medicine
United Kingdom

# MANAGING EDITORS

**Robert Ewers**
Chatham House
United Kingdom

**Yvonne Salfinger**, MS, MT(AAB)
Florida Department of Agriculture and Consumer Services, Retired
United States

# EDITORIAL BOARD MEMBERS

# CHAPTER AUTHORS

**Centers for Disease Control and Prevention, USA**
http://www.cdc.gov

Ali I. K. M.
Arrowood M. J.
Bellini W. J.
Benedict T.
Bishop H. S.
Blaney D. D.
Bowen M. D.
Bradbury R. S.
Chen C. Y.
Chen M.
de Almeida M.
Drobeniuc J.
Dykes J.
Erdman D.
Goodman C. H.
Handali S.
Heneine W.
Herwaldt B.
Hickman C. J.
Johnson B. W.
Kamili S.
Kines K. J.
Kosoy M.
Latner D. R.
Lúquez C.
Maslanka S. E.
McAuliffe I. T.
Molins C.
Montgomery S. P.
Nichol S.
Nicholson W. L.
Oberste M. S.
Olson V. A.
Orciari L. A.
Owen S. M.
Paddock C.
Papp J. R.
Perelygina L.
Petersen B.
Pillay A.
Qvarnstrom Y.
Ridderhof J.
Rivera H.
Rollin P. E.
Rota P. A.
Russell B.
Satheshkumar P. S.
Schmid D. S.
Schriefer M.
Secor W. E.
Switzer W. M.
Talundzic E.

**Public Health England, UK**
https://www.gov.uk/government/organisations/public-health-england

Aarons E. J.
Afshar B.
Brooks T.
Brown C. S.
Brown D. W.
Brown K. E.
Chalker V.
Chattaway M. A.
Duggan J.
Efstratiou A.
Grant K. A.
Jenkins C.
Johnson E. M.
Kearns A.
McLauchlin J.
Nabarro L. E. B.
Nair S.
Ready D.
Sheeley H.
Swift C.
Ward K. N.
Zambon M. C.

**Other**

Arthur I.
Beebe J. L.
Beeching N. J.
Beissner M.
Bennett A.
Blackmore C.
Bonifaz A.
Borman A. M.
Bretzel G.
Chen D.
Chomel B.
Chu M.
Costa A. G.
Cote B.
Denning D. W.
Downes F. P.
Dumler J. S.
Dunn J.
Egan C.
Farnsworth L.
Fingerle V.
Hardiman M.
Hearn S.
Hu J.
Ishida M.
Jones J. L.
Kidd S. E.
Lim W.
Liu L.
Mackenzie J. S.
Marks M.
Martin I.
Mathison B.
Mochon A. B.
Morgan M.
Pentella M. A.
Pritt B. S.
Rej R.
Rice D.
Richardson M. D.
Safar J.
Sapp S. G. H.
Salfinger M.
Salfinger Y.
Saubolle M. A.
Scollard D. M.
Smith D. W.
Soehnlen M.
Stempak L.
Taylor J.
van de Sande W.
Wilcke B. W.
Wojewoda C.
Woolley S. D.
Woron A. M.
Wreghitt T.
Yost-Daljev M. K.
Zarcone P.

# CHAPTER REVIEWERS

Ali I. K. M.
Belay E.
Bowman D.
Breckenridge K.
Brooks T.
Buss S.
Castillo-Salgado C.
Dance D.
Downes F. P.
Eberhard M.
Ellis D.
Hajduk S.
Jenkins C.
Jones T.
Kauffman C.
Koehler J. E.
Limberger R.
Mabey D.
McCartney A. C.
Ndao M.
Pandori M.
Rollin P. E.
Rudrik J.
Saubolle M. A.
Shaw J.
Shiff C.
Taylor J.
Teshil D.
Timms P.
Walker D. H.
Wilcke B. W.
Wilkins P.

# CONTENTS

# FOREWORD

Invention of the microscope in the late 1600s followed by the germ theory as advanced by Pasteur and Koch in the late 1800s were key to understanding the role microorganisms play in the pathogenesis of infectious disease. Microbial agents like bacteria, virus, and fungi, as well as infectious particles like prions, have all been discovered to cause disease in living organisms.

Diagnosing the specific pathogen that causes an infectious disease requires a solid understanding of the usual clinical presentations, as well as its usual mode of transmission. While this understanding is good enough to make a tentative diagnosis and initiate presumptive therapy, definitive diagnosis almost always requires laboratory diagnostic testing. Such testing allows for the definitive identification and categorization of susceptibilities to therapeutic agents for these pathogens.

In its infancy, laboratory testing was limited to bacteria and fungi and included growth on specially prepared media and microscopic viewing with and without special stains. Viral cultures required more specialized procedures. Over time, immunologic tests and improved methods for culturing of viruses, bacteria, and fungi dramatically improved our capacity for rapid identification of these organisms. This resulted in a vast expansion in our understanding and an expanded taxonomy of both infectious and non-infectious organisms. This has enhanced our understanding of the pathogenesis of infectious disease and enabled targeted treatment.

Today state-of-the-art laboratory testing has taken another quantum leap with the utilization of new molecular and genetic tools such as recombinant deoxyribonucleic and ribonucleic acid technologies and the widespread use of polymerase chain reaction techniques. Such tools allow the laboratory scientist and disease control specialist to identify the exact species, subspecies, or strain by its specific genetic footprint. Such specificity allows for the pinpointing of a disease's source and the ability to specifically track its infectious pathway resulting in vastly improved communicable disease control.

This is the first edition of *Control of Communicable Diseases: Laboratory Practice*. The book was conceived at a time of explosive growth in laboratory diagnostic testing, prompting a more detailed accounting of laboratory services than in *CCDM*. This manual is designed as a complement to *CCDM*, which has been the primary reference source for disease control specialists for over 100 years. *Laboratory Practice* provides an overview of the latest laboratory procedures for each disease, as well as information on laboratory safety practices, the critical role of quality assurance in all testing, and the importance of laboratory informatics and rapid reporting processes. Going into in-depth detail for each disease, this is a must-have for all laboratory scientists, epidemiologists, and others involved with communicable disease control. *Laboratory Practice* supports both planning and response for disease control and deserves to be dog-eared. It will be found on the bookshelf or downloaded on the electronic reader of all health practitioners charged with identifying and controlling infectious diseases.

Georges C. Benjamin, MD
Executive Director
American Public Health Association

# PREFACE

The Laboratory Section was the first member section of the American Public Health Association (APHA). Established prior to 1900, its creation was undoubtedly a reflection of the critical role laboratory science played at the time in supporting early public health actions and interventions, most notably ones related to the control of communicable diseases.

APHA Press has long produced high-quality, laboratory publications: *Standard Methods for the Examination of Water and Wastewater*, *Compendium of Methods for the Microbiological Examination of Foods*, and *Standard Methods for the Examination of Dairy Products*. *CCDM* has also been an important APHA Press publication, dating back over 100 years, and has always included information related to laboratory practice. Over the last decade, however, laboratory practice evolved at such a rate that creating a companion *CCDM* publication, one that focused specifically on the laboratory role as it relates to communicable disease control and prevention, seemed critical. This new resource will not only benefit laboratory scientists but also public health leaders, disease control specialists, epidemiologists, and others. It provides important information regarding the full range of laboratory services required to successfully control and prevent communicable diseases, which may be applied not only to developed country settings but also developing ones.

In 2005 when the International Health Regulations were revised, having core laboratory capability and capacity was recognized as a necessity for every country of the world, even if the capability only consisted of recognizing, detecting, and referring testing to other reference laboratories within the region. The revised regulations reflected the importance and critical nature of laboratory services in communicable disease control and prevention. *Control of Communicable Diseases: Laboratory Practice* provides laboratory scientists working in different settings with the means to review what their capability and capacity should be with respect to specific diseases. This volume also provides any laboratory, irrespective of its location, with ready tools to determine what type of response is warranted, even for rare and unusual communicable diseases.

With the guidance of *CCDM20* Editor David L. Heymann, the support of an editorial board of globally recognized laboratory experts, and the contributions of excellent laboratory scientists serving as authors and reviewers, we are now pleased to offer this companion to the original *CCDM*; the manuals can be used in conjunction with each other. As a note of acknowledgment, this volume drew upon the text of *CCDM20*.

Burton W. Wilcke, Jr, PhD

# READER'S GUIDE

Each disease chapter in *Control of Communicable Diseases: Laboratory Practice* is presented in a standardized format that includes the following information:

**Disease name:** each disease is identified by the numeric code assigned by WHO's *International Statistical Classification of Diseases and Related Health Problems*, 10th Revision (ICD-10). Common names are also listed and can be matched to the ICD names using the index.

1. **Clinical features:** presents the main signs and symptoms of the disease and differentiates the disease from others that may have a similar clinical picture. Case-fatality rates may also be included.
2. **Causative agents:** identifies the specific agent or agents that cause the disease; classifies the agent(s); describes variations, subtypes, and strains; and may indicate important characteristics.
3. **Laboratory diagnosis:** describes the laboratory methods most commonly used to diagnose the disease and provides information on how results should be interpreted.
4. **Laboratory capability:** describes the type of facility and personnel training required to test for the suspected agent or disease.
5. **Safety requirements:** identifies what biosafety level is required for handling the suspected agent or samples which might contain the agent.
6. **Nonhuman hosts:** describes the nonhuman hosts that may harbor the agent or contract the disease; identifies disease as a zoonotic disease where applicable.
7. **Sample/specimen requirements:** identifies the most appropriate types of samples (clinical and nonclinical) that are required for testing. Provides information and recommendations regarding the timing, transportation, holding, and processing of samples.
8. **Testing requirements:** describes the currently recommended laboratory practices (e.g., culture, antigen detection, serology) that are applicable to test for the disease or agent; outlines quality assurance requirements and describes the sensitivity and specificity of various testing methods; categorizes testing as screening, diagnostic, presumptive, or confirmatory.
9. **Reporting requirements:** provides information about laboratory-based reporting for the agent, including what might be required or recommended (e.g. submission of pure isolates) in addition to the report of findings.
10. **Referral network:** identifies what laboratory referral networks exist and should be used as circumstances and regulations dictate.

11. **Special considerations:** describes any special laboratory-related considerations relevant for the disease or agent. General information may be found in "Overview Quality Laboratory Systems," "Laboratory Referral Networks," "Animal, Food, and Environmental Testing in Support of Communicable Disease Control: A One Health Approach," "Laboratory Informatics," and "Communicable Disease Laboratory Methods."

# LABORATORY SAFETY PRACTICES: BUILDING A STRONG BIOSAFETY PROGRAM

## Introduction

The occurrence of several well-publicized events at high-profile US government laboratories in 2014[1] has refocused the clinical and public health laboratory community on the need to pay constant attention to "how we do our work," to both protect staff from exposure and to prevent accidental release of infectious organisms. We now live in a world in which there are additional influences shaping how we maintain preparedness to respond to infectious agents. A remote country is now just a plane ride away and laboratories, irrespective of where they are located in the world, need to be prepared to receive, handle, and safely test heretofore unexpected organisms carried by infected travelers. Similarly, bioterror events perpetrated by bad actors require that high levels of caution must be constantly maintained. And at the bench, while many of our classical microbiological tests were previously based on culture methods, requiring close handling and observation by laboratory staff, many tests are now molecular, often automated, and much more hands-free. Despite these technical advantages, limited safety studies have been performed using these new technologies, and procedures used to prepare a sample before it is applied to the instrument are not uniform; therefore, we do not have documented published data to draw on and define best practices. All these factors reinforce the importance of recognizing biosafety as an essential component of any laboratory working with infectious agents, be it a hospital microbiology laboratory, a public health laboratory, or a commercial reference laboratory. This chapter defines the components of an effective biosafety plan and program.

As a first step, before developing a biosafety program, it is useful for the laboratory to have some prior knowledge of what the highest risk procedures and pathogens are likely to be. Although there is no national or international reporting requirement for laboratory-acquired infections (LAIs), there is a small body of literature that is helpful. However, it should be kept in mind that different laboratory practices would have been used in the older publications because of the different technologies in use at that time.[2-7] The review by Coelho and Garcia Diez[8] indicates that the most common probable routes of infection are via inhalation of aerosols, percutaneous inoculation, and direct contact between contaminated surfaces and mucous membranes. In reviewing these studies, it is important to ask whether the exposure occurred from the human specimen where pathogen load is likely to be relatively low, or the cultured isolate, where it may be much higher. While the pathogens most often associated with LAIs may vary from region to region, the most commonly reported bacterial pathogens associated with LAIs are *Brucella* spp., *Mycobacterium tuberculosis, Francisella tularensis,* and Enterobacteriaceae, including *Salmonella* and *Shigella*.[8] Baron and Miller[5] and Singh[6] documented these and other less common bacterial agents and some fungal agents, namely those that cause psittacosis and coccidioidomycosis, associated with LAIs, in their reviews. Pedrosa and Cardoso[7] documented LAIs from a wide range of viral families that similarly occurred by the aerosol, percutaneous, and mucocutaneous routes. This historical documentation is important to keep in mind when developing a local biosafety program.

**Essential Elements of a Biosafety Program**

Every laboratory that works with infectious substances should establish a comprehensive biosafety program. This program helps to ensure the protection of laboratory staff and prevents the unintended release of infectious agents into the community. A strong biosafety program is essential to maintaining good laboratory practices. After a program has been developed, there should be a process by which it is reviewed on a continual basis, at least annually, and when adverse events or near misses occur. This is especially important in clinical and public health laboratories where testing needs are continually evolving and where the addition of new tests for emerging pathogens will require a reevaluation of procedures. The elements that are necessary for this comprehensive program are as follows:

***Use of risk assessments for all laboratory work being performed***

One of the most critical aspects of an effective biosafety program is the performance of a risk assessment on all the work or testing that is being performed in the laboratory. When planning to implement any new test or assay, a risk assessment should be completed before any work begins. A risk assessment is the process by which the potential for human exposure or pathogen release incurred by performing a particular procedure in the laboratory is determined. The risk assessment process must include this determination, but there should also be a risk management component that reviews both the facility and personnel performing the method. *Biosafety in Microbiological and Biomedical Laboratories*, 5th Edition (*BMBL*)[9] provides a basic outline of a 5-step process that laboratories can utilize to perform a risk assessment. These steps are as follows:

1) Performance of a comprehensive hazard evaluation to determine the initial biosafety level at which the test or work should be performed.
2) Identification of laboratory procedural hazards.
3) Determination of a final containment level with any additional enhancements.
4) Evaluation of staff proficiency and safety equipment integrity.
5) Review of the assessment with competent biosafety professionals.

It is important to remember that the risk assessment should include all steps of the testing process from specimen accessioning to removal of potentially contaminated waste from the laboratory. This risk assessment needs to be reviewed on a frequent basis and, most importantly, when there are changes to methods or tests or if new methods are going to be utilized within the laboratory. There are several excellent references available that provide additional guidance on how to perform risk assessments.[9-13] Additionally, there are also templates available for performing risk assessments that may be especially helpful to public health and clinical laboratories.[10] Templates have also been developed for testing methods for emerging diseases such as Ebola virus and Zika virus that can be utilized and/or modified for work being performed with other infectious agents.

***Presence of experienced individuals with biosafety expertise***

After the 2015 Ebola outbreak, the lack of biosafety expertise in clinical, reference, and public health laboratories was recognized as a major gap in diagnostic laboratories worldwide.[14] This gap has been acknowledged over the last few decades, but it became a critical issue during the Ebola outbreak. It was observed that there were many clinical laboratories that were not prepared to package or accept specimens for Ebola testing due to inadequate biosafety training, including and especially the basic packaging and shipping of infectious substances.[15] There are a number of programs that are designed to provide a higher level of biosafety training such as the NIH National Biosafety and Biocontainment Program and the CDC Laboratory Leadership Service fellowship. Many organizations provide extensive biosafety training such as the American Biological Safety Association International (http://www.absa.org), the Eagleson Institute (http://www.eagleson.org), and the International Federation of Biosafety Associations (http://www.internationalbiosafety.org). Having the expertise to assist laboratorians in performing biosafety-related work is essential for maintaining a high-quality biosafety program. Laboratorians have also received on-the-job biosafety training supplemented with external professional training. It is important that the laboratory directors, managers, and supervisors realize the need for providing this training to all staff and to make it a priority to have at least 1 individual who can serve in the role of a biosafety officer. This person should be provided the opportunity to participate in national and regional biosafety conferences and attend biosafety-related trainings to enhance their knowledge and communicate this information to the rest of the laboratory staff. Many laboratories have also established biosafety committees, which allow for communication and discussion of biosafety related topics and a continued review of the biosafety program. It is highly recommended that all laboratories develop an Institutional Biosafety Committee (IBC) that meets routinely to discuss biosafety issues that may affect the laboratory. NIH requires that any institution receiving federal funds establish an IBC, or a similar committee, and provides detailed instructions on the duties and composition of the committee in the NIH guidelines.[16]

***Appropriate PPE for work being performed in the laboratory***

Staff in laboratories that work with specimens that may contain infectious agents need to be provided with the basic personal protective equipment

(PPE) necessary for performing laboratory testing. This supply must include the minimum necessary, including laboratory coats or scrubs, disposable gloves, and protective eye wear. If cloth laboratory coats or scrubs are used, they need to be autoclaved before laundering. Based on the risk assessment performed in the laboratory, the use of additional PPE may be necessary. This PPE could include the use of a respirator, double gloving, Tyvek suit, hair bonnet, and/or booties. The use of additional PPE should be reviewed with the biosafety professional in the laboratory to determine if it is appropriate for the tasks being performed in the laboratory. It should be noted that street clothes worn by staff in the laboratory should also meet certain minimal standards, including closed-toe shoes and covered limbs. PPE must be selected carefully so that the appropriate equipment is chosen for a required task. Critical to protecting all laboratorians is the development of a training program so that all personnel are comfortable in donning and doffing, and PPE is being utilized in the correct manner.

***Use of equipment such as biosafety cabinets and appropriate physical infrastructure***

*BMBL* describes several different levels when working with microorganisms. These biosafety levels (BSLs) 1–4 include specific controls that are recommended with each level, including standard microbiological practices, primary barriers, and PPE, and any special practices needed. BSL-1 is the lowest level and describes work with well-characterized agents with low potential hazard to the laboratory personnel and environment. Most work in clinical and public health laboratories is performed at BSL-2 or BSL-3. When working with infectious agents where there is a risk of aerosol and splashing (e.g., at BSL-2 or BSL-3 level), one of the essential pieces of biosafety equipment is the biosafety cabinet (BSC). The BSC provides an enclosed ventilated space that will protect both the user and the samples and is easily cleaned and disinfected. Laboratories that are performing any testing on clinical specimens should have a correctly functioning and certified BSC. *BMBL* provides excellent information for choosing the appropriate BSC.[9] Not all microbiological testing needs to be performed within a BSC, but there are many different situations in which a BSC should be utilized. Some examples of the need for working in a BSC include processing primary specimens such as a cerebrospinal fluid suspected of containing *Neisseria meningitidis* or testing a blood specimen sent to the laboratory for testing for *Brucella* spp. The use of BSCs and other enhancements in infrastructure, such as an increase in biosafety containment, may also be necessary. Testing of certain environmental samples for agents such as *Yersinia pestis* or *F. tularensis* should be performed in a BSL-3 facility, as there is increased risk of aerosol generation with laboratory methods for these agents, as well as a low infectious dose of these pathogens. This type of information should be captured in the risk assessment. While the BSC offers protection to the laboratory worker when used correctly, appropriate practices must be utilized by all laboratorians. These practices include safe workflow in the BSC, utilization of appropriate disinfection during and after use, and proper waste disposal from the BSC to waste containers in the laboratory. A laboratory can use a certified BSC appropriately, but if laboratory staff do not properly disinfect infectious waste before removing it from a BSC and discard it appropriately, the laboratory may be greatly increasing the risk to all employees.

**Use of Documented Standard Operating Procedures and Protocols**
High-quality laboratory testing that is performed in clinical and public health laboratories relies on the use of established safe working methods captured in the standard operating procedure (SOP). This is not the case in many research or academic laboratories. Generation of these formal documents can help to ensure that all laboratory members are performing the same method in the same manner which helps to minimize risk in the laboratory. Standard operating procedures should include a step-by-step documentation of how to perform the test and any biosafety information such as what type of PPE should be worn and any biosafety equipment that should be utilized (e.g., a BSC). Not only should the testing methods be documented in a SOP, but there should also be SOPs for operating equipment such as autoclaves or centrifuges safely.

**Reporting of Accidents, Near Misses, and Exposures**
For many decades, there has been a lack of documentation of accidents, near misses, and exposures of infectious agents in laboratories in the USA. In 2008, a Blue Ribbon Panel for Clinical Laboratory Safety convened by CDC, and in 2009, a Trans-Federal Task Force on Optimizing Biosafety and Biocontainment Oversight called for the development of a national surveillance system. Illnesses that resulted from laboratory exposure are documented by local health departments, but there has been no national database established to document these events. Formal documentation and reporting of these events in an institution leads to a careful examination of who, what, where, why, and how the situation occurred and, ultimately, to the development of improvements and enhancements that can be used to prevent these incidents in the future. It is therefore important for clinical and public health laboratories to keep a careful record and to document these types of events. There could be a systemic problem occurring in different areas or sections of a large laboratory resulting from seemingly minor problems such as defects in a collection tube that can result in injury or exposure to infectious agents. Only upon documenting and reviewing these events can these incidents be quickly acted upon to prevent future mishaps.

The Federal Select Agent Program was first created in the USA in 1996 after Congress passed the Antiterrorism and Effective Death Penalty Act and the subsequent USA Patriot Act of 2001 significantly enhanced the requirements. Since the mid-2000s, there has been good documentation of accidents, near misses, and exposures to select agents. Documentation of these events[17] has led laboratories and public health agencies assisting in investigations to recommend new algorithms and safety measures associated with some procedures to minimize exposure of laboratory staff. Unfortunately, the Federal Select Agent Program only requires documentation for the infectious agents and toxins that the program regulates (i.e., biothreat related agents). Work performed with other infectious agents such as *M. tuberculosis*, *Neisseria meningitidis,* and other high-risk pathogens does not have such requirements, so it is critical that each laboratory document any near misses, accidents, and exposures to determine the root cause and take preventative measures.

**Strong Training and Competency Program for All Laboratorians**

At the core of a robust biosafety program is a well-trained laboratory staff that is confident in the methods that they are performing and in the facilities that support their work. Developing a strong training and competency program that includes biosafety is key to the protection of the laboratory staff. Training of all laboratory staff, including those who accession specimens and those who destroy specimens after testing has been completed, needs to be performed. This training should include a formal review of the written documentation, including biosafety measures, SOPs utilized in the laboratory, and the biosafety plan (see next section). Initial and repeated training should be provided to all personnel for as long as is needed for the personnel to be confident in their ability to perform the required tests. Training for operating laboratory equipment such as centrifuges safely should be provided, as well as for donning and doffing all PPE that is necessary for their work. In addition to reviewing documents, training should include a period of time for the new employee to watch other laboratorians performing the methods and then an observational period of time in which the new employee performs the laboratory method to the satisfaction of the observing individual. A competency program that includes at least annual retraining for each method being performed in the laboratory is an important piece of the program. It is essential to re-review and observe laboratory personnel performing the method to determine that there has been no lapse in the use of appropriate biosafety measures, PPE, or protocols. Typically, laboratories provide unknown specimens to laboratory staff and have them perform the method to determine if they can detect or not detect the pathogen of interest, but the competency assessment needs to include actual observation to ensure that proper biosafety measures and appropriate techniques are still being utilized by all laboratory staff.

**Development and Implementation of a Biosafety Plan That Describes the Biosafety Program**

Based on the information obtained during the risk assessment process, a detailed biosafety plan should be developed and implemented. The plan should include a comprehensive biosafety manual that includes safety policies; roles and responsibilities of laboratory staff, including the director, supervisor, and laboratory staff; local, state, and federal regulations requiring adherence; potential routes of exposure; the risk assessment; the process for reporting incidents; all biosafety practices utilized in the laboratory; standard precautions; and SOPs related to biosafety. A general biosafety plan can be developed for an institution that covers all general policies and procedures, but ideally each individual laboratory or unit should develop a specific biosafety plan that covers any unique aspects. In addition, the plan should include hazard communications, engineering controls, PPE, use of the BSC, specimen transport, emergency procedures, decontamination, training program, and medical surveillance.

**Creation of a Culture of Safety in the Laboratory From Laboratory Leadership to Laboratorians at the Bench**

The creation of a culture of safety within the laboratory is key to establishing an effective biosafety program. This culture must start with laboratory leadership who must show their commitment to biosafety in both word and deed (e.g., by making sure appropriate PPE and equipment are available and by having biosafety items addressed at laboratory staff meetings). Laboratory leadership should promote education in this area in the form of trainings such as online courses or webinars that are available through multiple sources. Equally important, laboratory staff must always be committed to operating with this mindset and paying attention to detail. It is important for all laboratory staff to be able to speak freely and honestly, without fear of recrimination, if they see a potential lapse in biosafety in the laboratory whether it be in problems with equipment/PPE or if they observe a fellow laboratory staff member not following an SOP. If staff either intentionally take shortcuts or unintentionally not follow the SOPs, it is important to correct immediately as it can cause a problem for the whole laboratory. For example, inappropriately processing a specimen on an open laboratory bench when the SOP states that the specimen should be processed in a BSC needs to be corrected immediately. Not only can the laboratorian put themselves at risk of infection and/or illness, but everyone in the vicinity of the work being performed may be put at risk. Laboratorians need to be comfortable to report these occurrences immediately to correct the problem, as a delay in reporting could lead to illness (rather than just remain an exposure) if appropriate prophylaxis is not made available quickly.

**The Iterative Risk Assessment Process**

Established safe working methods and experienced laboratory staff are the most appropriate protections for routine clinical specimen handling; taking into account throughput and disease prevalence in the community that the facility serves are also appropriate. However, there are situations in which the exposure risk from the specimens may be greater, such as in an outbreak, during pandemics, and with newly emergent diseases. Critical to the assessment of risk is the information provided with the specimen on the test requisition form such as recent travel history, contact with animals, or specific disease conditions that may alert the laboratorian to the sample presenting higher risk. There are documented cases of laboratory staff being inadvertently exposed to serious pathogens or even infected due to poor communication of patient data. In situations of suspicion of high risk from a specimen, additional precautions may be prudent, including use of a BSC, thus separating the specimen from others to prevent cross-contamination and consequent exposure.

*BMBL* and other manuals define the containment levels, but these guidelines are only part of the selection of appropriate measures. Characteristics of the pathogens which should be considered in the assessment of risk of an unknown and suspected high-risk sample are as follows: low infectious dose, transmission by inhalation, persistence in the environment, and whether it is exotic to that population. It is not only the pathogen or its mode of transmission that may change the risk but also the processes used in the testing process. There is strong evidence that suspensions and cultures present an enhanced risk of generating an infectious aerosol, use of sharps may bypass normal transmission barriers, and some equipment used has great potential for spread of pathogen. New equipment, such as cell sorters and sonicators, that are adopted into the clinical laboratory may present operational risks and require additional containment.

Changing diagnostic test methods also may require assessment of whether the risk has changed, and if additional measures may be needed. The increase in use of molecular techniques that need not be performed in specialist containment cabinets still needs assessment of the risk presented when moving material from the contained environment for molecular processing elsewhere. The inactivation methods used are usually taken from the literature without considering whether the conditions are appropriate for that sample type or that the specified conditions have been adequately met (e.g., the presence of salts, organic material, and also the sample size). The validation of the method and the verification of efficacy must be thoroughly performed in each laboratory. There may also be legal and licensing compliance issues if the material is incompletely inactivated.

**Safety in Resource-Challenged Areas**

The common safety practices adopted in many laboratories have evolved over many decades in response to concerns and actual incidents. This concern has a relationship with the incidence in the community, which make the laboratory the point source of the infection back into the community. There is a principle that the laboratory worker should not be at a greater risk at work than in the community. Using this principle has worked well in developed countries, which have been able to control common infections in the community and progressively raised the levels of protection in the laboratory to protect staff. Increasing complexity in technology used in protective equipment and techniques in the laboratory has also contributed to the ability to control the risk. However, this requires expensive equipment that must be maintained and provided with consumables and reagents, having suitably educated and trained staff, and continuity of utilities. In many parts of the world, these utilities and the supporting infrastructure are not available, and thus, the same standards are not achievable or sustainable. The conundrum is that these are the areas of the world with the greatest burden of infectious disease and have great need of suitable laboratory systems and services. Inadequately funded laboratories can be found in many places in developing countries; it is not possible for external and international donors to always provide long-term support for enough laboratories, however. The need for affordable local and effective laboratories is a challenge that cannot be met with the complex high cost of laboratories in better resourced settings; therefore, more affordable solutions are required. Those conducting field operations and responding to emergencies are often confronted with a stark contrast in standards. WHO has developed guidance on alternative systems for emergencies such as severe acute respiratory syndrome and Ebola,[18] as well as management and quality systems that are less onerous and stepwise improvement programs, including low-cost, easily maintainable solutions for waste and containment, such as solar powered sterilizers and burn pit incineration.[19] One technical solution is to use natural ventilation to ventilate health care and laboratory premises.[20] Molecular methods are a particular advantage, as the infrastructure and facilities are not so demanding, but the availability of trained staff and reliable power supplies may continue to be a challenge. Further, the availability of reagents, consumables, and technical support in a country may also be a problem. Laboratory staff need to be adequately protected and often this is by primary containment and/or reliance on PPE.[21] The protection of the environment and the community is a relative risk to the social benefit of responding to real and current disease levels. The recent Ebola crisis saw the deployment of several alternative containment solutions such as tent-based laboratories, portable BSCs, and mobile self-contained laboratories. These temporary responses left no legacy facilities and limited capability. A persistent problem remained not only in the logistics of supplies but also in the use of robust PPE clothing in such high ambient temperatures. The local culture, climate, and the perception of risk can be different from one country to another and sometimes even within a country. It is not possible to effectively import biosafety measures. In addition, it is important to manage the risk according to the conditions, limiting activities, and assessing for the actual location, especially conducting fieldwork when there is no physical laboratory.

### Safety and How to Assess Safety Risks With New Laboratory Methods

Adoption of new methods and equipment in the laboratory can be an exciting and rewarding endeavor for laboratory scientists. Utilization of new technologies that are designed to improve turnaround time, decrease costs of supplies and reagents, and increase capacity in the laboratory will help to reduce the burden on the staff in many laboratories. When determining if a new instrument or technology is appropriate for the laboratory, it is important to include a biosafety risk assessment of the instrument or technology as part of the decision of bringing the equipment to the laboratory. Often, biosafety is not a top consideration when designing an instrument or assay. Therefore, it is important for the laboratorians who will be utilizing these tools to understand how the equipment can be decontaminated or if there are additional biosafety considerations that are applicable to the new instrument. A careful risk assessment should be performed that takes into consideration the use of the instrument and any biohazards that may be inherent in the specimens being tested. The risk assessment should also include a review of the literature and discussion with the manufacturer of the technology or assay to determine what biosafety studies have been performed.

A recent example of the benefits of utilizing new technology in clinical and public health laboratories is the use of matrix-assisted laser desorption/ionization time-of-flight mass spectrometry for the identification of bacteria and fungi. This technology dramatically decreased the cost of identification and has removed many additional tests that the laboratories would have had to perform to identify a microbe. However, there have not been careful analyses performed of potential biosafety risks associated with the use of this technology in the microbiology laboratory. In the last few years, there have been reports that the utilization of this technology has led to exposures of laboratory staff to infectious agents such as *Brucella* spp. In New York State, several health alerts have been distributed to all clinical laboratories within the state due to biosafety concerns associated with the use of the instrument for the identification of bacteria. In the time period from April–July 2015, there were 4 different laboratories within New York State that have reported utilizing this technology to identify various *Brucella* spp. that were isolated from blood specimens submitted to the laboratory. Laboratory staff were performing procedures with the organism, such as plating the organism on a target plate that is placed in the mass spectrometer outside of a BSC. These plates are extremely small, and there is a risk of aerosol exposure to laboratorians who do not have appropriate respiratory protection, as laboratorians are often working in very close proximity to these plates. In addition, there has not been enough information available to determine if this technology causes aerosols to be released from the instrument nor whether plating the organism onto a surface to place in the instrument can result in exposure. Based on the incidents in New York State, the state public health laboratory has recommended that this technology should not be performed on slow growing organisms without performing additional biochemical tests to rule out agents such as *Brucella* and *F. tularensis*, and to perform work within a BSC to reduce risk, including plating of the organisms onto the surface that is placed within the instrument. Fortunately, based on the exposures from the laboratories (100+) within New York State, there have been no reported illnesses associated with the utilization of this new method. This example highlights the need for more applied biosafety research to be performed before instrumentation is placed and utilized in clinical and public health laboratories.

### National Regulations That Impact Safety

In the USA, there are several different national regulations that impact safety in the laboratory. The Occupational Safety and Health Administration Bloodborne Pathogen Standard (29 CFR 1910.1030) builds on the concept of universal/standard precautions which involves working at a BSL-2 cabinet and the use of appropriate facilities, PPE, and practices that are outlined in *BMBL*.[9] Universal precautions have become standard practice in clinical microbiology laboratories. The Bloodborne Pathogen Standard also provides the requirement for all laboratories to establish an exposure control plan (i. e., a written policy for use of procedures in the laboratory to control infectious disease hazards). This plan should be updated at least annually and whenever necessary to reflect new or modified tasks and procedures that affect occupational exposure. Another regulation established to prevent worker injury and illness was the Needlestick Safety and Prevention Act, which was enacted in 2000. This regulation amended the Bloodborne Pathogen Standard to promote the use of safer medical devices designed to eliminate or minimize occupational exposure and stressed that appropriate devices should be implemented in the laboratory. This process should be documented annually. In 2002, the Select Agent Rule was enacted, which regulates the transfer and use of agents that are thought to be most likely used in a bioterrorism event. The Select Agent Rule established the Federal Select Agent Program, which is jointly managed by CDC and USDA. This rule enabled the program to require any laboratory working with infectious agents or toxins on the select agent list to register with either agency and comply with a strict set of requirements. There are significant biosafety-related components that have been included since the establishment of the Select Agent Rule. Laboratories that work with these agents must perform risk assessments and comply with the numerous biosafety and biosecurity requirements that are outlined in *BMBL* and the Select Agent Rule 42 CFR Part 73 (https://www.ecfr.gov).

### Use of Reference Materials

The safety regulations discussed earlier do not specifically deal with work practices. There have been several guidelines developed that specify the appropriate work practices to be utilized in the clinical and public health laboratory. The most well-known biosafety one is in *BMBL*.[9] This guideline provides detailed information on specific practices, PPE, and engineering controls that should be followed at each biosafety level. It also provides detailed information on many infectious agents.

## Conclusions

As has been illustrated in this chapter, there are several critical aspects to be aware of when developing a biosafety plan for an institution. The plan's content and procedures must be structured to match the local physical infrastructure of the laboratory, the experience and competency of the staff, the risk characteristics of the pathogens likely to be encountered, and the hands-on nature of the testing required. As an example, if the resources are not available to purchase sophisticated safety equipment such as BSCs, other protective barriers such as enhanced PPE should be introduced or staff exposure to pathogens should be limited by using closed system, sample-in-result-out instruments. Consequently, the biosafety plan must be considered a living document that will change over time in response to new pathogens, accidents, and near misses. The plan must also incorporate multiple layers of protection so that if one level fails, others are still in place to provide protection. In designing the plan, while many excellent guidance documents exist and can be used as reference materials, the importance of utilizing local biosafety personnel who are well versed in infectious disease and safety practices and understand the local context cannot be overstated. Lastly, the senior leadership of the laboratory must be seen to place the safety of the staff as the highest priority and to set the tone for the institution. Clinical and public health laboratories are on the front lines when it comes to dealing with new and unexpected pathogens and they must be trained and ready.

## References

1. Monaco L, Holdren J. Enhancing biosafcty and biosecurity. The White House, President Barack Obama website. December 16, 2014. Available at: https://obamawhitehouse.archives.gov/blog/2014/12/16/enhancing-biosafety-and-biosecurity-united-states. Accessed June 26, 2018.
2. Pike RM. Laboratory-associated infections: summary and analysis of 3921 cases. *Health Lab Sci.* 1976;13(2):105–114.
3. Collins CH. Laboratory acquired infections. *Med Lab Sci.* 1980;37(3):291–298.
4. Harding AL, Byers KB. Epidemiology of laboratory acquired infections. In: Fleming DO, Hunt DL, eds. *Biological Safety, Principles, and Practices*. 4th ed. Washington, DC: ASM Press; 2006.
5. Baron EJ, Miller M. Bacterial and fungal infections among diagnostic laboratory workers: evaluating the risks. *Diagn Microbiol Infect Dis.* 2008;60(3):241–246.
6. Singh K. Laboratory-Acquired Infections. *Clin Infect Dis.* 2009;49(1):142–147.
7. Pedrosa PBS, Cardoso TAO. Viral infections in workers in hospital and research laboratory settings: a comparative review of infection modes and respective biosafety aspects. *Int J Infect Dis.* 2011;15(6):e366–e376.
8. Coelho AC, Garcia Diez J. Biological risks and laboratory-acquired infections: a reality that cannot be ignored in health biotechnology. *Front Bioeng Biotechnol.* 2015;3:56.

9. US Department of Health and Human Services, Centers for Disease Control and Prevention, National Institutes of Health. *Biosafety in Microbiological and Biomedical Laboratories*. 5th ed. December 2009. Available at: https://www.cdc.gov/labs/pdf/CDC-BiosafetyMicrobiologicalBiomedicalLaboratories-2009-P.PDF. Accessed January 15, 2019.
10. Association for Public Health Laboratories. Lab biosafety & biosecurity resources. Available at: https://www.aphl.org/programs/preparedness/Biosafety-and-Biosecurity/Pages/BB-Resources.aspx. Accessed June 26, 2018.
11. Sandia National Laboratories. Biorisk assessment models (BioRAMs). Available at: http://www.biosecurity.sandia.gov/BioRAM. Accessed June 26, 2018.
12. Fleming DO. Risk assessment of biological hazards. In: Fleming DO, Hunt DL, eds. *Biological Safety, Principles, and Practices*. 4th ed. Washington, DC: ASM Press; 2006.
13. World Health Organization. *Laboratory Biosafety Manual*. 3rd ed. 2004. Available at: http://www.who.int/csr/resources/publications/biosafety/WHO_CDS_CSR_LYO_2004_11/en. Accessed June 26, 2018.
14. Sealy TK, Erickson BR, Taboy CH, et al. Laboratory response to Ebola—West Africa and United States. *MMWR Suppl.* 2016;65(3):44–49.
15. Association of Public Health Laboratories. Biosafety and biosecurity. Available at: https://www.aphl.org/policy/factsheet_Documents/Biosafety-2016.pdf. Accessed June 26, 2018.
16. National Institutes of Health. NIH guidelines for research involving recombinant or synthetic nucleic acid molecules (NIH guidelines). Available at: https://osp.od.nih.gov/wp-content/uploads/2013/06/NIH_Guidelines.pdf. Accessed January 15, 2019.
17. Centers for Disease Control and Prevention. Incident notification and reporting, APHIS/CDC form 3 (theft/loss/release). Available at: https://www.selectagents.gov/resources/APHIS-CDC_Form_3_English_PrintOnly.pdf. Accessed January 15, 2019.
18. World Health Organization. Guidance on regulations for the transport of infectious substances 2015–2016. Available at: https://www.who.int/ihr/publications/who_hse_ihr_2015.2/en. Accessed January 15, 2019.
19. World Health Organization. Managing medical waste in developing countries. 1994. Available at: http://whqlibdoc.who.int/hq/1994/WHO_PEP_RUD_94.1.pdf. Accessed June 26, 2018.
20. World Health Organization. Natural ventilation for infection control in health-care settings WHO guidelines 2009. Available at: http://www.who.int/water_sanitation_health/publications/natural_ventilation/en. Accessed June 26, 2018.
21. World Health Organization. WHO updates personal protective equipment guidelines for Ebola response. October 31, 2014. Available at: http://www.who.int/mediacentre/news/releases/2014/ebola-ppe-guidelines/en. Accessed June 26, 2018.

[C. Egan, J. Taylor, H. Sheeley]

# LABORATORY REFERRAL NETWORKS

## US Networks, Referral, and Processes for Testing Communicable Diseases

The test ordering process begins with the physician or authorized provider and is usually straightforward for ordering tests for common causes of disease. The process becomes slightly more complicated if specialized reference testing is required to help diagnose less frequent causes of infectious diseases that are usually not available at the hospital level. This chapter outlines the existing US-based and global networks of public and private laboratory testing services for accessing reference testing or when testing for specific communicable diseases requires mandatory referral to specialized state, local, or federal public health laboratories (PHLs).

The USA has extensive laboratory capabilities for detection of communicable diseases that rely on public and private laboratories, regional networks, and specialized referral centers. The public and private laboratories include thousands of hospital clinical microbiology laboratories, state and local PHLs, commercial laboratories with national reach, and federal laboratories, such as CDC. The challenge to the physician requesting reference level testing is both understanding the performance characteristics of specific laboratory tests in aiding diagnosis and knowing how to access the testing service that is needed. Reference testing is available through various private and public health laboratory networks, which extend often specialized PHL test services to all 50 states and the US territories. Hospital laboratories usually have standard test menus adapted to meet the needs of acute care medicine practices for sepsis, wounds, and pneumonia. Many microbiology testing services can also be accessed through ambulatory care clinics served by the commercial laboratories (e.g., LabCorp, Quest Diagnostics) that provide courier services and routine laboratory testing (e.g., clinical chemistry and hematology) in addition to infectious disease testing such as sexually transmitted infections (STIs), and for respiratory (e.g., influenza) and enteric pathogens.

Clinicians are advised to consult with infectious disease specialists who can help with test selection and provide guidance on navigating the myriad of public and private organizations and testing networks to access the appropriate tests. In addition to this manual, there are many manuals or guidebooks either for purchase or in the public domain that assist the clinician with test selection. One source of information is CDC, which provides information about appropriate testing for an extensive list of communicable diseases that can be accessed on the CDC website under A–Z list.[1] Within a hospital or health care system, specific testing services are usually directed to designated laboratory providers, many of which bundle multiple specialized testing services in contracts between commercial laboratories and the hospital. The exceptions to bundled service contracts are often tests linked to public health programs in which the hospital or provider is encouraged to refer testing to their local or state public health laboratory. Some of these tests, such as for enteric pathogens or tuberculosis (TB), involve local statutes which may require referral to PHLs within the jurisdiction. The referring clinical laboratory and many providers receive communications and instructions on test requests, packaging, and referral from the health department.

Testing for emerging infectious diseases, such as Ebola, Zika, or Middle East respiratory syndrome coronavirus, in addition to suspected biothreat agents, is initially accessed through the PHL system, which receives guidance, test technologies, and assistance from CDC. Although any company may seek emergency use authorization for these diagnostics from the FDA when a national public health emergency is declared, CDC or other national agencies often have access to specialized samples and materials, and therefore, the capability of rapidly developing and distributing test methods for newly emerging diseases. One key network that was developed to respond to both deliberate and emerging biothreats is the Laboratory Response Network (LRN), which was established in 1999 as a partnership of federal, state, and metropolitan laboratories. The LRN member laboratories have qualified staff, BSL-3 facilities, and information systems that allow states to rapidly adopt new technologies for emerging infectious diseases in addition to maintaining capacity for potential biothreat agents.

Specialized testing for rare or evolving communicable diseases of public health importance is accessed through the US system of local, state, and federal public health laboratories that represent multiple overlapping networks.[2] Many national disease control programs have established regions (e.g., for PulseNet, antimicrobial resistance) or designated referral centers (e.g., for TB, influenza, vaccine preventable diseases) to support enhanced reference testing capabilities in designated PHLs. Additionally, many states have come together to form state-directed networks that share technical information and training in addition to serving as collaborating networks to share selected testing services. Collectively, these different regional structures and referral centers provide a system to help ensure consistent access to specialized PHL testing services. The PHL is responsible and knowledgeable about which tests are referred to other states or CDC. Interstate referral represents either state-to-state agreements or procedures to refer to designated regional or referral laboratories for specific services. Although this may seem confusing to the provider, most states work to make the request and referral seamless, though the provider will receive the final report from whichever state PHL had the specific expertise and capabilities to perform the requested testing. An important component of encouraging sharing or referral of services is a national directory of PHL testing services. In the USA, the Association of Public Health Laboratories (APHL) has partially served this role through fielding multiple surveys and compiling PHL service profiles. APHL is now implementing the Public Health Laboratory System Database

(PHLSD), which aggregates all the state and local PHL testing services across the USA into a searchable national test directory. Clinical laboratories should contact their jurisdiction's state or local PHL for specific instructions and guidance for test requests and referral.

The USA publishes a list of national notifiable conditions every year that serves as consensus recommendations for implementing these requirements as law in each individual state or other jurisdiction, with health departments to monitor or intervene for specific conditions. Additionally, many states have statutes that require referral of isolates or specimens in the case of communicable diseases, such as foodborne pathogens (e.g., *Salmonella*, *Shigella*, *Listeria*). Clinical laboratories are usually knowledgeable of specific laboratory test results for notifiable conditions that must be reported to the health department in each jurisdiction; additionally, there is progress in the implementation of electronic laboratory reporting of results in the accepted health level 7 format that enables rapid reporting and response for surveillance and disease intervention.

Many communicable diseases in humans may also be zoonotic and involve animal diseases or have their origin in food or the environment. Most zoonotic diseases of concern are nationally notifiable diseases, with corresponding state-level statutes for case reporting and referral of specimens or isolates. Most of the animal diseases that are on the proposed list of reportable conditions are also potential zoonotic diseases. As outlined, the USA has different national and regional networks for animals, food, and environmental samples, such as the following:

- The *National Animal Health Laboratory Network (NAHLN)*, which is a cooperative effort by USDA Animal and Plant Health Inspection Service, USDA National Institute of Food and Agriculture, and the American Association of Veterinary Laboratory Diagnosticians (https://www.aavld.org). NAHLN consists of 62 state and university-associated veterinary diagnostic laboratories located in 40 states. Other federal members of NAHLN include USDA National Veterinary Services Laboratories in Iowa and New York and the US Geological Service National Wildlife Center Laboratory in Wisconsin (https://www.aphis.usda.gov).
- The *Environmental Response Laboratory Network (ERLN)*, which the US Environmental Protection Agency established to address chemical, biological, and radiological threats in environmental matrices by providing consistent analytical capabilities, capacities, and quality data in a systematic, coordinated response. ERLN integrates capabilities of existing public-sector laboratories with accredited private sector labs to support environmental responses (http://www.epa.gov).
- The *Food Emergency Response Network (FERN)*, which is an integrated, secure laboratory system for US federal, state, and local government agencies engaged in food safety and defense activities. Consisting

of 170 federal, state, and local laboratories, FERN is organized to ensure federal and state interagency participation and cooperation in the development and operation of the network, allowing participating government agencies to compare, share, and coordinate laboratory analysis findings and to strengthen the capacity of state laboratories. The system is jointly operated by the FDA and the USDA Food Safety and Inspection Service and can detect, identify, and respond to emergencies that involve biological, chemical, or radiological contamination of food. (For further information, see "Animal, Food, and Environmental Testing in Support of Communicable Disease Control: A One Health Approach.")

## Additional Regulatory Considerations

### *CLIA*

The Clinical Laboratory Improvement Amendments (CLIA) regulations is the law in the USA that requires all laboratories that handle patient testing to comply with quality management standards. CLIA laboratories must have written policies and procedures for collection, transport, and submission of specimens for testing. Within a health care system, this manual of services might be a directory of onsite and referred laboratory services. Most state PHLs will also publish this manual of services on their websites and usually have existing arrangements for transport of specimens to the PHL. A laboratory's manual of service should specify the appropriate specimen for specific tests in addition to the correct container. Ideally, the manual will also provide information on the interpretation and limitations of specific tests. The interpretation may also be included in the test report. In addition to paper-based test requisitions, tests are also ordered through many electronic formats either directly from the clinical laboratory or with the clinical laboratory using the test requisition of the referral laboratory.

Test requisitions require specific information, such as age, sex, date of birth, and other conditions that might be important to uniquely identify the patient and assist with test selection for specialized tests. Not following all the instructions or not including all the information may, in some cases, require the laboratory to reject the test request if this could interfere with accurately maintaining the identity of the patient or selecting the correct test (i.e, when the specimen source is not identified and tests are only approved for, or validated for, specific specimens). Similarly, the referring clinic or PHL within a jurisdiction should have written standard operating procedures (SOPs) with criteria and instructions for when and how to refer either samples, specimens, or culture isolates to reference laboratories. Each testing service has different requirements for when to refer specimens or isolates for additional testing; in many cases, these criteria reflect the priorities of individual disease programs, such as surveillance, rapid detection, and antimicrobial susceptibility testing. As an example, the state PHLs in the LRN focus significant efforts on maintaining training of a local system of sentinel clinical laboratories to rule out or refer suspected biothreat agents and promote specific SOPs for these methods.

### *Electronic test orders and results reporting between submitters and laboratories*

There are extensive national efforts to make the ordering of tests and receipt of patient results a seamless process between laboratories, providers, and the electronic medical record. This goal of interoperability has some success but is still challenging, especially between vendor-supported information systems in the health care arena and PHLs (state, local, and national), which often operate disparate systems or software. In many cases, the national commercial laboratories have the capacity for interoperability between the submitting provider or hospital laboratories and the regional or national commercial laboratory facility. This makes test ordering and results reporting more convenient, but providers may need to determine which test methods are more accurate for uncommon pathogens and how to access these methods within their designated laboratory networks. As an example, molecular diagnostic tests developed in reference laboratories for infrequent pathogens are often more accurate than the FDA-cleared tests preferred by many laboratories for ease of regulatory compliance and implementation.

### *Accessing specialized testing services from CDC*

CDC programs provide funding and technical support to promote availability of communicable disease testing in the state and local PHLs. There may be, however, situations where rare pathogens are suspected, and CDC is the only reliable source for specialized testing and consultation. CDC maintains a directory of specialized testing services for infectious diseases (http://www.cdc.gov/laboratory/specimen-submission/list.html). All specimen submissions to CDC must have the approval of the individual state health department unless participating in special studies or surveillance projects (https://www.cdc.gov/laboratory/specimen-submission/list.html).[1] The health department's role in screening requests for specialized CDC testing is an important component to ensure appropriate use of these national reference testing services.

## Global Communicable Diseases Networks and Their Function

### *Global laboratory networks: general description*

The reality that an epidemic is just an airplane flight away makes tracking and sharing information on communicable diseases a global responsibility. In addition, the adoption of rapid identification genomic-based laboratory diagnostics and increased international capability to access electronic data portend a shift in laboratory functionality and operations in the coming years. "Reporting of Communicable Diseases Under the International Health Regulations" is adapted from *CCDM20*. All countries share the need to strengthen their laboratory networks to detect infectious diseases for patient care, surveillance, and both domestic and global disease control. Laboratory capabilities are closely linked to fulfilling the requirements of the International Health Regulations (IHR). The monitoring of country compliance is now a formal process known as the Joint External Evaluation, which combines IHR and Global Health Security Agenda goals.[3]

Diseases with epidemic and pandemic potential that meet the requirements for notification to WHO and disease-eradication programs, including vaccine preventable diseases and those of humanitarian crises, bioterrorism, or emerging threats, are being monitored via global surveillance and laboratory networks on behalf of intergovernmental agencies, public health institutions, public-private consortiums, faith-based services, academic partnerships, philanthropic programs, and commercial interests. Information about these diseases comes from a broad and complex series of networks and individual programs. The information is collected and transmitted through a range of systems, from using highly organized linked systems to situation-related case-by-case reports. In general, disease networks are formed by entities with vested interest for surveillance or project purposes specific for a disease condition (e.g., malaria drug resistance, seasonal influenza, bioterrorism, cholera outbreak). The disease program sets the guidance, protocols, and surveillance methods, including collection of appropriate specimens for laboratory testing. Laboratories provide the evidence by examining collected specimens for agent detection/identification, immunological testing, and additional characterizations. Reference laboratories are often organized by the type of microbe they focus on: viruses, bacteria or parasites, and grouped by infective routes or disease expression (e.g., enteric, respiratory, vector-borne) and, within those groups, specialized for a specific agent or disease type (e.g., diarrheal, influenza, TB, dengue, malaria). The responsibility to collect data for these diseases and conditions usually falls under the public health domain as reportable conditions of a locality, region, country, and with potential to spread globally. The latter is where the IHR come into play; countries have the responsibility to investigate, confirm, and report events of international concern to WHO within 72 hours of its identification (see "Reporting of Communicable Diseases Under the International Health Regulations").

With the development of new technologies and the increased confirmation of diagnoses based on molecular testing, the trend for some laboratory testing is changing from collecting specimens and sending them to the laboratory to patient point-of-care testing for faster turnaround. This will likely not change the referral system but will change the type of laboratory services that will be provided. The increased number of point-of-care test settings will reduce the numbers of specimens that will be referred to the secondary or more advanced laboratories, many of which are PHLs with responsibilities to monitor infections of public health concern. This also means that physician office laboratories, clinics, hospitals, and other primary testing sites will perform less initial infectious agent recovery, and that referral sites such as PHLs will have to take up the recovery and confirmation of infectious agents. At the same time, the secondary and tertiary referral laboratories will be performing advanced molecular characterization, specialized services for identifying the specific genotype, or specific pathogenic feature.

***Global laboratory networks: how information is collected and reported***

WHO, the WHO regional offices, and WHO Collaborating Centers collectively guide and direct surveillance and laboratory networks associated with specific disease mandates.[4–8] WHO-associated surveillance and laboratory networks include polio (disease elimination), influenza (annual vaccine strain selection and emergence of viruses of pandemic potential), drug resistance (in TB, multidrug resistant bacteria), vectorborne diseases (monitoring transmission and spread), vaccine preventable diseases (covers measles, rubella, human papillomavirus, meningitis), malaria (control program efficacy and drug resistance), human immunodeficiency virus (HIV; treatment efficacy, transmission and drug resistance), emerging pathogens (covers viral hemorrhagic fevers and unknown diseases), outbreak response (deployment and training), and others. The list here is not exhaustive but intended to illustrate the various networks related to programmatic missions. The networks represent formal systems, such as the influenza surveillance network, which is the oldest of the WHO networks, with a formal structure consisting of over 170 contributing members. Country representation is organized with official designated national influenza centers (national and intra-country) and served by 6 WHO-designated collaborating centers. There is a Web-based reporting system that tracks influenza events in near real time, a system for reporting and sharing virus genotype and sequence data, reagent production system, and a global laboratory proficiency program. Another example is the Global Outbreak and Response Network (GOARN), where 220 institutional members volunteer their services to WHO to assist with epidemic response. Its members include most of the world's maximum containment (biosafety level 4 [BSL-4]) laboratories. Their role is to prepare and deploy, at the request of a country, to assist with response to an epidemic of a highly transmissible nature (e.g., Ebola, Marburg). In the USA, CDC, often as a WHO collaborating center, interacts and reports cases through these networks, serving as an important partner for the GOARN, influenza, polio, measles, and global networks of HIV, TB, vaccine preventable diseases, diarrheal diseases, foodborne infections, and other infectious diseases. CDC also supports and manages domestic and other non-WHO reportable disease networks aimed at preparedness to diagnose and respond to likely bioterrorism agents. The US system of local, state, and federal PHLs participate and contribute to sharing laboratory information, results for specific conditions that warrant surveillance, diagnoses of diseases with public health impact, emerging threats, and outbreaks. Some recent emergencies of international concern include pandemic influenza, polio, Ebola, and Zika.

### *Building global laboratory capacity with standard methods, shipping, and tiered technologies*

An important, beneficial aspect of laboratory networks is the building of laboratory capacity through technology transfer and facilitating and encouraging applied research to ensure quality laboratory performance.[2] Network members have to demonstrate their ability to perform the required tests correctly to ensure standardization across the network. These network members often receive training support, validated reagents and test kits, and standardized protocols so that they can perform the necessary tests on submitted specimens for each given program. Network members and partners are located throughout the world and they can become a vital link to first alert, identify, and investigate the appearance of an unusual case, or provide evidence of an outbreak. They also are pivotal in sending specimens to regional, national, or global laboratories for confirmation and additional analysis. Packaging and shipping specimens can be costly, especially if materials are deemed to be in the dangerous goods category. In order for a laboratory to ship specimens in the dangerous goods category, a laboratory or its institution has to have a certified shipper in compliance with international regulations. Only the certified shipper may be permitted to package materials and document the shipping. Laboratories often can receive training from partners in the infectious disease networks so that their staff can achieve certification to perform this task. Some of the more organized networks also supply shipping containers and assume the cost of shipping. Some countries have established regulatory restrictions on the shipping and sharing of specimens to another country, even if it is a part of a recognized network. Therefore, before shipping or referring specimens to another country, it is best to clarify what the requirements are from one location to another.

The USA has many networks that cross political jurisdictions and collectively provide reference level testing for the vast array of communicable diseases. Similar networks function at the global level and have similar requirements for packaging and shipping, referral agreements, and a focus on standardization of high quality laboratory testing. The existing US and global systems are continually evolving to provide consistent access to testing services, and this involves different responsibilities for communication, surveillance, and relationships from the initial clinical setting to established state and national referral networks to national agencies such as CDC.

### References

1. Centers for Disease Control and Prevention. Infectious disease laboratories test directory: submitting specimens to CDC. Available at: http://www.cdc.gov/laboratory/specimen-submission/list.html. Accessed June 26, 2018.
2. Association of Public Health Laboratories. APHL member laboratories. Available at: https://www.aphl.org/membership/Pages/memberlabs.aspx. Accessed June 26, 2018.

3. World Health Organization. *Joint External Evaluation Tool: International Health Regulations (2005)*. Available at: http://www.who.int/ihr/publications/WHO_HSE_GCR_2016_2/en. Accessed June 26, 2018.
4. World Health Organization. WHO HIV drug resistance laboratory strategy. Available at: http://www.who.int/hiv/topics/drugresistance/laboratory/en. Accessed June 26, 2018.
5. World Health Organization. WHO TB supranational reference laboratory network. Available at: http://www.who.int/tb/areas-of-work/laboratory/srl-network/en. Accessed June 26, 2018.
6. World Health Organization. WHO emerging and dangerous pathogens laboratory network (EDPLN). Available at: http://www.who.int/csr/bioriskreduction/laboratory network/en. Accessed June 26, 2018.
7. World Health Organization. Global influenza surveillance and response system (GISRS). Available at: http://www.who.int/influenza/gisrs_laboratory/en. Accessed June 26, 2018.
8. World Health Organization. The global polio laboratory network. Available at: http://polioeradication.org/polio-today/polio-now/surveillance-indicators/the-global-polio-laboratory-network-gpln. Accessed June 26, 2018.

[J. Ridderhof, M. Chu]

# LABORATORY INFORMATICS

## The Importance of Laboratory Informatics

As with other critical resources such as personnel, instruments, physical workspaces, and utilities (e.g., electricity, running water), the laboratory needs to manage data in a fashion that aligns with the mission of the laboratory. At its most fundamental level, a laboratory produces data. These data support analysis and decision-making related to surveillance, diagnosis, infection control, and threat detection among others. To be useful in vital public health decision-making, it is critical that these laboratory data meet the following criteria:

- Accurate: the laboratory data need to be valid and representative. The data need to be complete and consistent over time; changes to the data must be recorded and tracked.
- Unambiguous: the laboratory data should be interpreted the same way regardless of who is viewing it. For example, the date of May 10, 2017 can be represented as 5/10/2017 in the American data convention, or as 10/5/2017 in the European convention. This ambiguous representation may lead an observer to interpret this data as either May 10 or October 5. For the sake of clarity, the data should clearly indicate which value corresponds to the units of day, month, and year. By structuring the

data unambiguously, the laboratory can rely on multiple users interpreting it accurately.

- Readily available: data should be available to the data stakeholders in a timely and usable fashion. Health care and public health decision-makers in particular need to make rapid decisions on patient care and outbreak response, and so data availability is of utmost importance. Structured data allow for quick query and analysis as needed.

Applying these principles to laboratory data, whether that data exist currently as electronic or paper-based, requires a specific discipline called laboratory informatics, which is the "specialized application of information technology to optimize laboratory information management."[1] The practice of this discipline by laboratory informaticians is vital to laboratory operations. These specialized staff have an understanding of information technology, as well as the business of the laboratory and how laboratory data may be used. With this understanding, laboratory informaticians assist in data structure, development, and reporting. While informaticians specialize in information and data management, all laboratorians should have a basic understanding of laboratory informatics and its role in laboratory operations.[2]

There are laboratories, in the USA and internationally, that are still utilizing paper-based methods of documenting and communicating laboratory results. Whether this is due to lack of resources, both fiscally and human, underdeveloped national infrastructure or otherwise, the continued use of paper to maintain laboratory and patient records is quickly becoming a global health security risk and delays the implementation of early warning surveillance systems. With the emergence and reemergence of pandemic influenza, Ebola, and Zika virus, among others, it is critical to support laboratory informatics efforts and education on a global scale. This chapter provides a high level introduction to laboratory informatics, but there are a vast number of resources, and there are many higher level education opportunities available for those who want to learn more or even specialize in this domain.

It is important to point out for the proper perspective and understanding of this chapter that the information herein can be applied to laboratory informatics both in the USA and internationally. Where there is an important concept that is different between US-based informatics and international practice, a distinction will be made; however, the majority of these concepts are applicable worldwide, and therefore should be understood as such.

## Laboratory Information Management

Central to the ability to effectively manage the data in a laboratory is the use of a laboratory information management system (LIMS). LIMS is software that is designed specifically to handle laboratory workflow and supporting data, including sample test results, patient and sample metadata, and supporting data such as quality control, submitter lists, and inventory. Access to data within the LIMS can be controlled by individual role-based user accounts, providing the laboratory assurance that the data are accessed only by authorized users. A LIMS will also provide auditing capabilities for the data stored within it and can capture any changes made to the data and by whom. By using a LIMS that is implemented and configured correctly, the laboratory has a framework for data capture that is accurate, unambiguous, and readily available.

Historically, laboratory information management by electronic systems has been referred to as LIMS (described earlier) or as a laboratory information system (LIS). There is a distinction between the 2 terms. The term "LIMS" describes systems that are used to manage laboratory samples and are specimen centric. The term "LIS" is more clinical in nature and is intended to be more patient centric. Many laboratories in the international community use the term LIS, while in the USA, the term LIMS is used more frequently to describe an enterprise software program designed to handle the work flows internal to a laboratory. Within this chapter, we will use the term LIMS in this manner.

**LIMS Components**

LIMS captures data for laboratory workflows during the preanalytical, analytical, and postanalytical phases of testing.

- Preanalytical: preanalytical data captured by the LIMS include data about the sample and the patient from whom it was collected. The LIMS should also capture data on the staff entering the sample data and the intended recipient of the generated report. Importantly the LIMS will capture these data in a structured manner so that users can easily query standard values. For example, if the LIMS captures the patient name data unambiguously, it can easily aggregate a report of all the tests performed on that patient.
- Analytical: analytical data captured on a sample include the data associated with the test performed. These data include the raw data values of the experimental method, retests, calculations, and results. The LIMS can integrate directly with laboratory instrumentation to assist with capturing data in this testing phase. The LIMS capturing these data in a structured fashion allows laboratorians to review these data as needed and readily compare the results of multiple samples.
- Postanalytical: postanalytical data captured by the LIMS include the reported values, interpretation, and any flags used to alert the recipient to a value which is significantly outside of the norm. These data can be used for surveillance and diagnosis and can provide vital information to decision-makers concerned with patient and population health.

The functions available in any LIMS vary widely depending on needed capacity and audience. Although most LIMS capture the workflow data described earlier, they may also collect a variety of other data used for efficient laboratory functions[3]:

- Laboratory billing
- Laboratory staff training and competency

- Inventory
- Contracts and grant management
- Chain of custody
- Customer concerns
- Mutual assistance and disaster recovery
- Quality control charting
- Document management
- Laboratory safety
- Instrument integration
- Media, reagent controls manufacturing
- Laboratory certification and licensing
- Statistical analyses

**Automating Laboratory Functions**

One of the most important benefits of a LIMS is the efficiency gained by automating laboratory function and analytical processes. By digitizing the records associated with laboratory workflows, these data can be exchanged between systems. Using international data exchange standards, sample submitters can directly transfer sample and test order data from the patient record to the LIMS, and the LIMS can transfer the results data back to the submitting system. This exchange decreases time and labor associated with manually entering patient data and improves data integrity by reducing human error. Frequently, informaticians can configure the LIMS to integrate with laboratory instruments, directly transferring raw data to the LIMS for analysis and reporting.

Along with the efficiencies gained from data exchange capabilities, digital records can support laboratory plans for disaster recovery, outbreak response, and mutual assistance. The laboratory can easily back up digital records offsite and retrieve them in case of an emergency in the laboratory. The laboratory can also transfer the records to a partner if assistance is needed to meet a surge capacity or other circumstance.

**LIMS Policies**

Like other aspects of laboratory management, the LIMS requires specific policies for its maintenance. The laboratory should have a clear business case proposal written for the LIMS. This document should describe the proposed uses of the LIMS and the resulting quality improvement. The laboratory can use this business case for a variety of purposes: as a baseline document for a Request for Proposal, as substantiation for funding requests, and as an input for further project planning.

The business case will serve as a foundation of planning and budgeting for a LIMS. Not only will a LIMS require funding for its initial implementation and configuration, but also every year after for ongoing maintenance and support. The laboratory must budget for the software licensing, hardware, and personnel. This budget will vary considerably with the scope of the implementation, the use of the LIMS, and the size of the laboratory.

When implementing a LIMS, the laboratory will need to update its data use agreements to include digital records. A data use agreement is a legal document used for the transfer of data from any entity where the data are nonpublic, or where the use is restricted by law. The laboratory will need to update its data retention, sharing, and access policies as it moves from a paper-based to an electronic system. When updating data use agreements, laboratories should take into consideration the future need of exchanging data with other public health and personal health-related entities within and outside of its jurisdiction (e.g., state, district, province, or country).

## Stages of Implementing a LIMS

### *Choosing a LIMS*

The first consideration for implementation of a LIMS is selecting the right LIMS for the laboratory. The laboratory management should spend considerable time analyzing and documenting their current processes to identify the requirements for a LIMS. A subset of functions that should be considered includes

- Sample types
- Reporting requirements
- Business and fiscal requirements
- Analysis methods
- Quality assurance requirements
- Accreditation requirements
- User interface requirements

The laboratory should also determine any other information technology (IT) requirements of their respective agency or organization. For example, a state-funded laboratory may have to conform to the requirements laid out by a statewide IT agency. These requirements can have significant impact on the type of LIMS that can be installed and the infrastructure needed to support it. Before requesting bids on a LIMS, the laboratory must understand and be ready to comply with these policies; engaging with IT policy makers early will assist in understanding and meeting these requirements.

It is also important to mention that there are different types of LIMS that can be acquired by a laboratory based on the overall business requirements, laboratory staff, IT staff resources available internally, and hardware and software infrastructure capabilities. There are 2 major types of LIMS available:

1) Commercial off-the-shelf (COTS) LIMS: these types of LIMS are sold by different vendors as software packages that can either be installed locally on the laboratory IT infrastructure or can be sold as cloud-based (hosted) systems, also known as software as a service (SaaS). Some of these COTS LIMS are specific to a laboratory function, such as Newborn Screening, while some are enterprise-wide and have the functionality to manage

data generated across all public health laboratory functions. These types of LIMS are often installed and configured by a vendor.

2) Open source LIMS: these are LIMS whose software's source code is made available to the public through a special type of license for which the copyright holder provides the rights to study, change, and distribute the software freely. Often referred to as open source or collaborative development, this type of LIMS can eliminate the need to pay a vendor for licensing costs of a LIMS. This type of LIMS requires a very skilled, knowledgeable IT staff within the laboratory domain that understands laboratory workflows and also has expertise in the particular software language in which the LIMS is written. It is important to note that this type of software, although free to acquire, is not free to implement. The implementation of open source LIMS often shifts the costs from the vendor to a consulting firm that can help the laboratory implement the LIMS and customize the software to suit their workflows. Open source technology is used more widely outside the USA where resources are very limited and there are fewer commercial software options available.

***Working with the LIMS vendor***

Once a LIMS is chosen, the laboratory will need to form a strong relationship with the LIMS vendor, or in the case of an open source LIMS, the laboratory will need to identify internal staff capable of helping with the implementation and/or a technical consulting company that has the skills to do so. For the purposes of the rest of this chapter, the focus will be on the acquisition of a COTS LIMS. Depending on the LIMS and the implementation plan, the laboratory may work with the LIMS vendor directly; other options would be to work through a third-party contractor or in-house developers to implement and configure the LIMS. These relationships should be well established and contractually supported, if possible. The laboratory should understand the level of support it will receive and what the laboratory needs to do to support the vendor or developer. The laboratory should not expect that the LIMS vendor or developer will immediately comprehend their workflows and requirements, and laboratory staff should be prepared to spend considerable time with the vendors to convey their needs. As the liaison between these groups, the laboratory informatician should be able to assist with communication and information gathering for both teams.

***Implementing the LIMS***

After the laboratory has established a relationship with the vendor or developer, the implementation of the LIMS can begin. Note that a LIMS will not meet all of the laboratory's off-the-shelf needs. Depending on the requirements of the laboratory and the capabilities of the LIMS, important configuration or customization will be required. To ensure that the configuration addresses the needs and workflows of the laboratory, laboratorians should participate in this process, and the laboratory informatician should be almost completely dedicated to this effort. The laboratory can streamline the implementation by clearly conveying requirements to the vendor and/or developers. Laboratory staff should recognize that some processes cannot be readily configured in a LIMS and so some compromise might be necessary. Laboratory leaders need to manage the expectations of their staff, prepare the LIMS users for the impending workflow changes, and clearly communicate the benefits of the LIMS over the complications of changes to job function.

Implementation of a LIMS should not simply digitize the paper process. LIMS implementation provides the opportunity to review laboratory processes and business decisions. Paper-based processes that have evolved over time may have become disparate or convoluted, making cross-training, aggregate reporting, and laboratory management difficult. The laboratory can review and improve these processes during the LIMS implementation. For example, the laboratory may consider implementing centralized sample receiving, barcoding, standardized sample submission data, or other efficiencies along with the LIMS.

### *LIMS testing*

The laboratory must adequately test the LIMS before it can be fully accepted and moved into production. The laboratory should plan and perform the testing at several different levels:

- Unit and functional testing: this testing phase ensures that each functional requirement documented during the planning phases functions as expected.
- System and integration testing: during these tests, all the portions of the system(s) are tested together. Common and unusual scenarios should be identified and tested; some testers may think of this as a time to try to "break" the system.
- Performance and stress testing: the laboratory should perform stress testing to ensure that the LIMS has the capacity to support the volume of testing required. Stress testing should simulate the peak volume of users and samples in the system at one time.
- Parallel testing: during this phase, testers should process real samples through the previous and new systems. The legacy and new systems should generate identical reports, triggers, and flags.

The laboratory should document each of these testing phases with the performance of specific test cases. Before testing the system, the laboratory staff should document the expected behavior of the system so that, after performance of the test, the staff can determine whether the LIMS meets the expectation or not. Both laboratory and development staff will likely have to revisit implementation efforts to address issues that are found during the testing phase.

### *LIMS go-live*

Once the LIMS has been completely implemented and tested, the laboratory can begin using the system for routine daily operations, colloquially referred to as go-live. Prior to go-live, the laboratory must update the relevant standard operating procedures and arrange for all end users to receive training on the new LIMS. The laboratory should be prepared to respond to issues after the go-live event, as problems may arise that were not considered during the testing phase.

Once the system is in routine daily use, the laboratory will enter a maintenance and operations phase. The laboratory will need to plan for how issues are addressed during this phase and allocate staff appropriately. The laboratory may rely on the vendor support or have in-house IT staff provide support. The laboratory informatician can assist with ongoing training, issue validation, and general LIMS administration. As part of LIMS maintenance and operations, the LIMS administrator should monitor the data to reveal areas that can benefit from improved efficiencies. This information can contribute to the laboratory's continuous improvement efforts. For example, the laboratory may be able to more closely monitor turnaround time, unsatisfactory samples, and quality control failures by utilizing the LIMS' structured data.

## Core IT Infrastructure

The IT infrastructure required for managing laboratory data can vary depending on the requirements of the laboratory. At a minimum, the laboratory will need desktop computing hardware such as computers, printers, and a cabling infrastructure to connect these computers to each other and to a central database. The database is the central location where the laboratory data are stored and structured. Depending on the LIMS and IT capability of the laboratory, this database may be maintained locally, within the laboratory, or hosted externally by the LIMS vendor (i.e., SaaS) or other IT service provider; the LIMS and all associated data can be hosted in the cloud, or through a third-party server located in a data center off-site. (Cloud computing is discussed in more detail later in this chapter.) If the database is hosted externally, the laboratory will need a reliable Internet connection to access it for daily operations. Whether internally or externally hosted, the laboratory must put a backup procedure in place for the data. To avoid data loss as a result of hardware or software failure, regular copies of the data should be made and stored in an off-site location. The laboratory can then access these copies in case of a natural disaster or a failure of the central database. In addition, laboratory function and requirements may necessitate other hardware such as

- Barcode scanners
- Barcode printers
- Document scanners
- Fax machines

Along with IT hardware and the LIMS software, the laboratory may have additional software to support laboratory operations. In fact, many laboratories rely on a system of systems where data are exchanged between multiple software applications to meet the needs of the laboratory. For example, the laboratory may export aggregate data from the LIMS where patient data are held to a separate billing software for fiscal management. The laboratory will need to rely on desktop computing software such as e-mail, word processing, and spreadsheet software. Additional software used by the laboratory can be extensive and may include

- Quality control charting
- Instrument integration
- Inventory management
- Image analysis
- Billing
- Staff training and competency
- Environmental monitoring (e.g., temperature)

To support these hardware and software needs, the laboratory will have to engage specific services. The staff needed to support the infrastructure will vary as the infrastructure itself does. The IT support services can be centralized, decentralized, or a combination. Centralized IT service refers to staff, policies, infrastructure, and support that apply to multiple agencies. Decentralized IT refers to a service in which each agency supports its own IT requirements using internal resources. There are advantages and disadvantages to both models. Centralized IT consolidates the work required for support of the IT infrastructure (i.e., back-ups, security) but may not specifically address the needs of the laboratory. Decentralization puts the burden of support on the laboratory, which may meet the needs of the laboratory but does not take advantage of the support of a multiagency team. Managing the service needs of the laboratory may require balancing the needs of the laboratory with the policies and support of the central IT group.[1]

**Cloud Computing**

"Cloud computing" is a term that refers to computing hardware and software infrastructure (computer networks, servers, storage, and applications) that are maintained by a third-party. Access to rent or utilize a portion of 1 server or multiple servers within this infrastructure is granted for a predetermined fee, and the laboratory that rents that computing space can often choose among different services provided by that third-party. Examples of these services include long-term maintenance of their server space, routine data security monitoring, security patches and updates, utilization of different software applications, and routine updates to the software, sometimes even access to other databases hosted within that cloud infrastructure to enhance data analysis. Often these servers or shared services can be rapidly provisioned to a client with minimal effort. There are 3 main service models utilized when talking about cloud computing as defined by the National Institute of Standards and Technology (NIST):[4]

1) Software as a service (SaaS): defined as the capability to use a provider's applications running within their cloud infrastructure.
2) Platform as a service (PaaS): defined as the capability to deploy into the cloud infrastructure applications, services, databases, programming languages, and tools that can be supported by that provider. The client does not manage the underlying cloud platform, including network, servers, operating systems, or storage, but has control over its own applications, services, tools, etc., deployed into the environment.
3) Infrastructure as a service (IaaS): defined as the capability to provision processing, storage, networks, and other resources, where the client is able to deploy and run their own software, which can include operating systems and applications.

Cloud computing may help organizations save on infrastructure costs. By utilizing a cloud, there is no need to maintain any IT hardware on premise other than computers that have stable and reliable access to the Internet. Cloud computing can also help get applications up and running faster and can dynamically scale up or scale down based on fluctuating data flow or business demand.

There are many public and private laboratories in the USA that utilize the cloud in some capacity. There is much rhetoric about the security capabilities of large cloud providers and whether or not an organization's data are truly safe in such an environment. New regulations are being created to help provide guidance around the use of cloud computing especially by government agencies. One such program in the USA is called the Federal Risk and Authorization Management Program, a government-wide program that provides a standardized approach to security assessment, as well as authorization and continuous monitoring for cloud products and services. There are also companies that provide third-party, independent security audits for cloud providers. Audit services can range from going through the source code for a cloud environment line by line, to site visits where auditors go through a checklist and document that certain security policies and infrastructure are in place. Some cybersecurity firms also provide "hacking" services or penetration testing. This is when a prescheduled third-party tries to enter a private cloud environment in an effort to get to the data held or break the source code. These hacking exercises are invasive, but highlight where there are breaks or weaknesses in the source code or security of the environment so immediate remediation can occur.

Before using a cloud computing LIMS solution, the laboratory should review these security topics with their IT support team members and ensure local IT policy is being met or is properly in support of this option.

## Data Security and Privacy

Laboratory data will likely include information that is required to be kept secure. Examples of data security concerns in a laboratory include

- Patient information
- Outbreak tracking
- Biological or chemical threat information
- Trade secrets
- Billing information

The laboratory is responsible for meeting the data security needs of the information in their systems. In the USA, standards for patient identifiable information are outlined in the Healthcare Insurance Portability and Accountability Act of 1996 and should be completely understood and followed by the laboratory staff with access to these data. Additionally, CDC outlines the data security requirements for working with select agents of biological or chemical threat. The laboratory should understand the security requirements of the data for which it is responsible and document its compliance with these regulations. The software vendors for the LIMS or centralized IT services may be able to assist with meeting these requirements.

Internationally, every country has its own rules and regulations concerning data security and privacy. The EU has some of the strictest data protection laws, which were written to help member states standardize disparate legacy data use policies. The EU wrote the Data Protection Directive 95/46/EC of October 24,1995 to help countries harmonize around 1 set of regulations and to increase the ability to exchange data between member states.[5] To date, all EU member states have implemented this directive into national law. The directive provides some guidance specific to health data, and public health specifically. It defines, as a core principle, that any data which are capable of infringing fundamental freedoms or privacy should not be shared unless the data subject gives explicit consent to do so.

Not unlike the USA, the EU allows member states to deviate from the directive when it is justifiable by way of important public interests. In order to allow for the processing of sensitive categories of data, which are otherwise prohibited unless authorized by the individual, the data must be used for the purposes of combatting a public health emergency. In cases where data are required for prevention of illness, diagnosis, and the provision of care and treatment, member states may provide national exceptions to the directive.

## Data Standards and Interoperability

As a laboratory moves away from paper-based processes for recording and reporting results, it can take advantage of the efficiencies gained by implementing electronic test orders and results or electronic laboratory reporting. These electronic processes offer advantages to the laboratory by shortening the time needed to deliver the results to the submitter and increase data integrity by not requiring data entry into a receiver's system. The laboratory must implement data exchange standards to take advantage of electronic laboratory reporting and electronic test orders and results.

Structured, unambiguous, readily available data are essential to laboratory operations. Implementation of international standards assists laboratories in achieving these data attributes. Standards are the guidelines by which data are recorded, which ensures consistency and understanding for all data consumers. Standards provide a common method and vocabulary for conveying data between systems, allowing them to interoperate. There are many standards that can be used for laboratory data and are controlled by standards development organizations (SDOs), which develop, maintain, and update standards as needed within the industry.

- Logical observation identifiers names and codes (LOINC): LOINC codes identify health related observations, including codes for clinical test methods. These codes are commonly used to identify the method by which the sample was tested and provide sufficient detail for the data receiver to identify the test.
- Systemized nomenclature of medicine-clinical terms (SNOMED-CT): SNOMED-CT codes identify clinical terms related to health care. Frequently in laboratories these terms are used as an answer to the LOINC question.

For example, a LOINC of 10851-4 (*Escherichia coli* O157:H7 [presence] in stool by organism specific culture) asks the question, "Is there *E. coli* O157:H7 in this patient's stool?" Then, when paired with the SNOMED code 260373001 (detected), the data consumer understands the *E. coli* O157:H7 was found in this patient's sample.

In addition to LOINC and SNOMED-CT, there are a wide variety of standards for other data, including

- Unified code for units of measure (UCUM)
- Chemical abstract service (CAS)
- International classification of diseases (ICD)
- Object identifier (OID)
- Health level 7 (HL7)

In addition to coding the terms with which these data are conveyed, there are standards for the structure of the data presentation. HL7 provides standards for the exchange, integration, sharing, and retrieval of electronic health information. HL7 standards are the structure in which the data are conveyed, essentially providing the data consumer and receiving system with where to look for the data they need. This SDO provides the foundation of data exchange between clinical systems, including laboratories, pharmacies, patient records, and others. Specifically, for laboratories, HL7 provides standards for test orders and results in an electronic format. By complying with terminology and structural data standards, laboratories can interoperate between themselves and with their partners.

Federal and state governments, who surveil for diseases of public health importance, and laboratories can apply HL7 standards to report these notifiable disease findings. In conjunction with the LIMS, a laboratory can readily identify coded test results that meet the criteria for reporting and, using HL7, report these findings to the public health agency. This system provides a rapid and reliable method for reporting these diseases so that public health action can be taken. Implementation of these standards is the basis and the first step in implementing an electronic data exchange process.

### Areas of Concern

There are several common issues that laboratories should be aware of to implement and maintain a robust informatics program.

- Lack of preparation for LIMS implementations: laboratories frequently underestimate the amount of time and funding required for a full LIMs implementation. By not understanding the laboratories requirements and not adequately funding and staffing an implementation effort, the project will have a low chance of success.

  Laboratories should seek the assistance of other laboratories, nonprofit organizations, and/or consultants to assist in the planning and implementation of LIMS.
- Adopting standards does not automatically provide interoperability: standards such as HL7, LOINC, and SNOMED provide an excellent foundation for data exchange. However, there are many business, technical, and process requirements that make each data flow unique. Therefore, the standards must be constrained and tailored. Laboratories cannot always assume that since their data are coded and they can produce an HL7 message, that they can communicate with partners. It is critical for data exchange partners to come to an agreement on how the standards will be implemented for a specific data flow in order to achieve interoperability.

  Implementation of electronic data exchange should be viewed as a project in itself, engaging with stakeholders and subject matter experts as needed to meet the needs of all parties.
- Lack of understanding by agency/ministry leadership: the choice to implement a LIMS must be supported at all levels of the laboratory and throughout the health agency or ministry of health for the laboratory to be successful. Many times, laboratory leadership does not understand that the implementation of a LIMS is not a one-time funded project. The implementation of a LIMS is the cost of doing business as a laboratory in today's world, and there will need to be a line item every year after implementation in order to maintain and update the laboratory's LIMS.

There will be upgrades to the software that will need to be managed and implemented, as well as issues every so often with the IT hardware or the LIMS software itself that may require external help or LIMS vendor assistance. More broadly, the laboratory will need the support and understanding of its parent agency and partners to successfully implement and maintain a LIMS to allocate funding, resources, and time to its success.

- Insufficient resources or funding for proper training and continuing education for laboratorians in the area of informatics: it is fundamental for the viability of a LIMS that the laboratory staff using it be properly trained and knowledgeable about how to use the software. Training needs will continue as software is upgraded and new staff are hired into the laboratory. Additionally, there are many US- and international-based organizations that can provide training in many different LIMS and also general information technology subjects.

### References


1. Association of Public Health Laboratories. *The Brave New World of Laboratory Informatics II: Navigating in the Digital Age*. 2015. Available at: https://www.aphl.org/aboutaphl/publications/documents/informatics_bravenewworldii_updated102015.pdf. Accessed June 26, 2018.
2. Ned-Sykes R, Johnson C, Ridderhof JC, et al. Competency guidelines for public health laboratory professionals: CDC and the Association of Public Health Laboratories. *MMWR Suppl*. 2015;64(1):1–81.
3. Association of Public Health Laboratories. *Requirements for Public Health Laboratory Information Management Systems*. 2003. Available at: http://www.limsexpert.com/INF_2003Sept_Reqs-for-PHL-IMS.pdf. Accessed June 26, 2018.
4. Mell P, Grance T. *The NIST Definition of Cloud Computing*. 2011. Available at: https://csrc.nist.gov/publications/detail/sp/800-145/final. Accessed June 26, 2018.
5. EUR-Lex. Directive 95/46/EC of the European Parliament and of the Council of 24 October 1995. 2003. Available at: https://eur-lex.europa.eu/LexUriServ/LexUriServ.do?uri=CELEX%3A31995L0046%3Aen%3AHTML. Accessed March 15, 2019.


[P. Zarcone, M. K. Yost-Daljev]

# COMMUNICABLE DISEASE LABORATORY METHODS

Laboratory identification of the microbial cause of disease is not only essential for appropriate diagnosis and treatment of individual patients but it is also the cornerstone of community-based disease control efforts. This chapter is not intended to replace comprehensive microbial identification resources such as reference books and compendia. It does, however, direct the reader to reliable options for testing.

In selecting a laboratory identification method, it is first critical to determine the intended use of the test results. If testing is strictly for the purpose of individual patient diagnosis, a reliable identification to species or even only to genus level may be adequate. More advanced molecular testing, such as genotyping or whole genome sequencing methods that determine similarity between isolates, is usually reserved for public health or research investigations.

In either individual patient diagnosis or investigations, there may be no individual test that provides both sensitivity (i.e., lack of false-negative results) and specificity (i.e., lack of false-positive results). In these situations, testing algorithms are frequently recommended. A testing algorithm usually begins with a highly sensitive screening test. The screening test may be nonspecific. Therefore, before results of a screening test are acted upon, a highly specific confirmatory test is performed. This approach provides capture of all possible positive results and thus eliminates false positives. This tiered approach to testing is especially useful in areas of low disease endemicity where false positives may outnumber true positives in the population tested.

Laboratory methods should be selected based on the intended use of results and laboratory capacity, including equipment, reagents, and personnel expertise. In all testing situations, it is critical to support test result reliability through a comprehensive quality management program. In many areas, diagnostic laboratory quality is regulated through government and/or professional organizations. In areas where quality management is not legally required, it is still equally important for laboratories to participate in a voluntary quality program. Quality control and external quality assessment are important components of a quality management system, but a comprehensive quality system should address the 12 quality system essentials identified by WHO.

### Microscopy

The light microscope is the oldest and most prominent tool of the microbiologist. The light microscope provides the resolving power to visualize bacteria, parasites, and fungi in patient specimens and from culture growth. However, the extremely small size of viruses require resolution provided by electron microscopy.

Patient specimens and culture growth can be suspended in saline or broth media on a glass microscope slide in the direct wet mount examination. This wet mount is useful to visualize movement of live bacteria and parasites and shape. More information on the cellular components can be achieved by staining a heat-fixed specimen or growth. For example, the ubiquitous Gram stain provides not only bacterial shape but also reveals information about the cell wall structure and presence/absence of an outer membrane.

Gram-positive bacteria have a thick cell wall and no outer membrane. This information is used to direct culture conditions and identification schemes and provides rapid information that can be used immediately for treatment decisions. Other staining targets include flagella, capsule, and spore coats. Stains that do not specifically dye 1 cell component, like methylene blue and iodine, provide contrasts to all cellular components making morphology more easily determined.

Laboratories that utilize microscopy should have an active schedule of equipment cleaning and maintenance. A reliable power source should be available. Personnel should be trained and regularly assessed on technical competency to use the microscope and interpret images. If the microscope is to be used for wet mount examination of specimens to detect parasites, a calibrated ocular micrometer should be available.

All clinical specimens must be handled using universal/standard precautions. Residual specimens and cultures should be disposed of as infectious waste. Some stains and fixatives must be disposed of as hazardous chemical waste. The laboratory should assess all health and safety risks associated with all testing and develop appropriate practices to minimize risks to laboratory personnel, the facility in which the laboratory is located, and the larger community.

**Culture**

Microbial culture requires control of several critical processes and safety considerations. Without attention to quality essentials, the laboratory may produce results that are misleading, interfere with patient treatment and surveillance efforts, and put employees and the community at risk of infection.

Each laboratory should perform a risk assessment. Based on the risk assessment and guidance from reliable sources like *Biosafety in Microbiological and Biomedical Laboratories*, 5th Edition (https://www.cdc.gov/labs/pdf/CDC-BiosafetyMicrobiologicalBiomedicalLaboratories-2009-P.PDF), microbiology laboratories should develop a comprehensive safety program. This program should include appropriate safety practices, containment equipment, waste disposal practices, engineering design, a biosafety cabinet, other fixed equipment, and personal protective equipment. Personnel must be trained to use personal protective equipment and biosafety cabinets and be trained in universal/standard precautions and good laboratory practices.

Laboratories engaged in microbial culture and identification quality should operate within a robust quality assurance program. Refer to "Overview of Quality Laboratory Systems" for recommended components and practices of a comprehensive quality assurance program. Microbial culture requires attention to specimen collection and transport to assure that the appropriate specimen arrives at the laboratory in a condition suitable for recovery of viable pathogens. The laboratory must have access to sterile media, reagents, and supplies. Media must be appropriate for the recovery of the organism and within the expiration limit. The media lot should be tested with a quality control isolate strain to confirm that it is performing as intended. Selection of primary isolation media for inoculation of patient specimens and incubation conditions should be based on the best available media choice that will recover the most common pathogens for that specimen source and region. Refer to the disease-specific chapters in this manual for recommendations on the isolation of pathogens. Incubation conditions must be suitable for the recovery of specific microbes. For example, isolation of anaerobic bacterial requires incubators with an oxygen-free atmosphere, or media must be enclosed in sealed containers that are oxygen-free through chemical components of the container. Many bacteria and most live cell lines require elevated carbon dioxide atmosphere for optimal growth. Any attempt to isolate anaerobic bacteria requires specialized media and incubator space to accommodate a controlled anaerobic atmosphere or closed containers. A bacterium not only requires appropriately formulated media and atmosphere to grow, the incubation time needed to grow into a visible colony varies by species from just 8 hours to more than 6 weeks. The generation time of the species is a genetic trait that cannot be shortened.

Typical colonies of bacterial pathogens isolated on primary isolation media have traditionally required additional testing, including Gram stain, biochemical panels, antimicrobial susceptibility, and antigen detection tests. Biochemical testing often determines the presence of an enzyme, which is not common to all bacteria, by providing the substrate in the media and measuring the production of product through a color change in the media. Depending on the species, the number of biochemical tests required to reach species identification can vary from just a few to more than 30. Results of the identification test panels are compared with a reference scheme to determine species identification. The incubation time required for biochemical tests will again depend on the species and can extend to several days. Biochemical and other additional testing can be slow and resource intensive, and results can be ambiguous. As an alternative, molecular biology-based or matrix-assisted laser desorption/ionization time-of-flight (which relies on mass spectrometry to identify cellular composition) methods of species identification are increasingly used. These methods come at a high resource investment and require reliable infrastructure to maintain.

A major advantage of bacterial culture is the availability of an isolate for antimicrobial susceptibility testing and genotyping. Local antibiograms and reference materials (e.g., the Clinical and Laboratory Standards Institute), should be consulted to determine the best options to be included in the antimicrobial panel. Whichever method is selected for testing (e.g., solid agar-based methods, like the Kirby-Bauer disc diffusion, the gradient strip methods, or broth dilution), results are only reliable and useful in predicting treatment success if all quality control recommendations are strictly followed. Genotyping methods like pulsed field gel electrophoresis and 16S ribosomal typing also require viable bacteria growth. These methods provide support for outbreak identification and investigation but do not contribute to direct patient care.

Parasitology infrequently relies on culture; microscopy, immunodiagnostic and molecular testing are more common and reliable approaches. Culture is an acceptable approach for some protozoa.

While many yeast will grow on media designed to isolate bacteria, recovery of fungi requires special media and incubation conditions. Upon recovery of fungal growth, identification relies on microscopic determination of typical cellular morphology. Biochemical testing is useful in species identification of some yeast. Since some fungi require advanced biocontainment and safety practices to protect the laboratory worker, a risk assessment is essential.

Since viruses cannot replicate outside the host cell, viral isolation requires cell culture. Maintaining and propagating cell lines requires extreme attention to aseptic technique by laboratory personnel and availability of reliable cell culture media. A single cell line cannot support the growth of all viruses, so the laboratory may be required to maintain several cell lines. This poses additional complexity to avoid cross-contamination between cell lines. While cytopathic effect is predictably typical for a virus in a particular cell line, some viruses replicate without producing cytopathic effect, and cytopathic effect alone is not sufficiently specific to reliably identify viruses. Additional testing, usually direct fluorescent antibody testing with virus-specific antibodies is required for definitive identification. Known specific antibodies to the virus can be used to block viral replication and thus prevent cytopathic effect formation in virus identification by neutralization.

### Immunodiagnostics

Immunodiagnostics relies on the specific binding between an antigen and an antibody. Each microbe is composed of many antigens. A subset of antigens may be specific to an individual species or strain, while other antigens are common to other usually related species or strains. Antigens that are common to multiple microbes or stains produce cross-reactions that can complicate interpretation of results. Immunodiagnostic tests employ laboratory produced specific antibodies (polyclonal and/or monoclonal) and/or purified antigens, as well as a beacon that will indicate the presence of the antigen–antibody complex.

Polyclonal antibodies are produced by injecting whole microbes or crude cell components made up of multiple antigens into a laboratory animal. The diverse composition of antigenic sites on the injected material will produce a variety of antibodies, some of which will be specific and some of which will be nonspecific. Monoclonal antibodies are produced through a process of selection of a single antibody-producing cell and subsequent fusion of that cell to a cancer cell. The fusion results in a hybridoma that produces 1 antibody specific for a single antigen and can be maintained and reproduced in culture. Monoclonal antibodies are specific and can be produced in large quantities over a long time.

Immunodiagnostics can be designed to detect antigens in a specimen or culture or to detect antibodies produced in response to infection. In either case, antigen or antibody detection, detection of the antigen-antibody complex relies on a reporter system. Reporters can be cells or particles, like latex beads or red blood cells, to which the test reagent antigen or antibody is attached. Mixing the antibody-particle with the antigen results in a lattice of these complexes, which can be visualized. The test reagent antibody can be labeled with a fluorescent molecule. The fluorescent molecule will emit visual light when exposed to ultraviolet (UV) light. If the labeled antibody binds to its complementary antigen, the antigen-antibody complex can be visualized through use of a UV microscope. This test strategy is used in direct and indirect fluorescent antibody tests. The antibody may also be labeled with an enzyme that converts a substrate into a colored product. The enzyme labeled antibody is referred to as the conjugate. If the labeled antibody binds to its complementary antigen and the substrate is then introduced, a colored product develops. This test strategy is employed in the enzyme-linked immunosorbent assay, also known as the enzyme immunoassay (EIA). There are other examples of immunodiagnostic test formats, including those that rely on other reporter formats, including hemolysis of red blood cells by complement (i.e., complement fixation) and inhibition of red blood cell agglutination in the presence of antibody.

**Antigen Detection**

Microbial antigens can be detected by exposing culture material or specimen to a manufactured polyclonal or monoclonal antibody known to bind to that antigen. Examples of antigen detection assays include agglutination assays, in which known antibodies are fixed to latex beads, red blood cells, or other small particles. In the presence of antigen, the antigen-antibody complex will link the particles into a blanket, which is visible with the naked eye. Fluorescent-tagged antibodies produced with known specificity can be used to stain specimen or culture material. The antigen-antibody complex is visualized via the emission of light of the fluorescent reporter molecule when viewed with a UV microscope. EIA can be employed to detect antigen by first using a specific antibody to capture antigen and then using a second specific antibody to detect the initial antigen-antibody complex. In liquid-based EIA, the second antibody acts as the conjugate. In field assays, the first antibody is often labeled with colloidal gold or other reporter and the second antigen specific antibody binds and holds the antigen-conjugate in place, producing a visible color change at that site.

**Antibody Detection**

When exposed to a novel microbe or microbial antigen, humans require 10–14 days to develop antibodies. Antibodies assist in elimination of the current infection and are protective should the host be exposed to the microbe in the future. Antibodies are also a helpful laboratory analyte that can be used to diagnose current or past exposure to a pathogen by infection or vaccination. Since antibody production is delayed and may not be produced during symptomatic phase of disease, it is often necessary to collect

2 serum specimens. The initial, or acute serum specimen, should be collected as early as possible after exposure or onset of symptoms. This serves as the baseline prior to, or early in, antibody production. A second, or convalescent, serum specimen is collected 1–2 weeks later. In the case of recent infection, the convalescent serum specimen will contain significantly more antibody than the acute specimen. Detecting antibody in a single serum specimen is useful for establishing prior exposure to the microbe. In some tests an elevated antibody response is sufficient to confirm a recent infection. Since immunoglobulin class M (IgM) is the first antibody class produced in response to exposure to a foreign antigen, assays which employ antibodies that can detect IgM or isolate IgM antibodies from the specimen prior to testing are also useful in establishing recent infection.

Since antibodies are proteins, they can also serve as antigens. When injected into another species (e.g., goats, mice), the second species will recognize human-specific antigens as foreign and produce antibodies to those antigens. Host antibody can be detected by presenting a known antigen to antibody-containing serum or other body fluid in vitro. In a typical EIA to detect specific antibodies, antibodies from serum specimens are captured by binding to known antigen fixed to microtiter plates in liquid-based assays or fixed to paper in solid phase assays. Subsequently, an enzyme-labeled antihuman conjugate is added to bind to the antigen-host antibody complex. This sandwich is detected by adding the enzyme substrate or by collecting the sandwich in a reaction band.

### Molecular Testing

A successful approach to designing faster, more sensitive microbe detection assays is to target the deoxyribonucleic acid (DNA), ribonucleic acid (RNA), and enzymes that control genetic replication and maintenance. Molecular biology assays do not require lengthy incubation and cumbersome identification schemes of culture. Further, molecular techniques can detect microbes that cannot be cultured. These assays does not require the host to respond to infection and produce antibodies. Therefore, molecular tests can be used for diagnosis while the patient is still symptomatic and can detect pathogens that do not elicit antibody responses. Advances in molecular technology have brought this testing from the research laboratory into mainstream clinical and public health laboratories for a host of applications.

### Gene Probe Assay

Nucleic acid probes are sequences of DNA or RNA that are complementary to the nucleic sequences in a specimen or culture. Probes can be designed to hybridize to sequences shared by many microbes, specific to a single species or even to a strain. To detect the probe-target hybrid, the probe is labeled with a reporter molecule like an enzyme or chemiluminescent reporter. In liquid phase probe assays, free unhybridized probe must be eliminated prior to measurement. In solid phase or tissue-based probe assays, unbound probe can be removed by washing prior to measuring the probe-target signal.

Because of the 1 target sequence to 1 probe signal capacity of this technology, these assays are often insufficiently sensitive and have been largely replaced by nucleic acid amplification tests (NAAT).

**Nucleic Acid Amplification**

The diagnostic strategy of microbial culture is based on growth of entire cells or viruses to high numbers adequate for visual recognition and additional testing. Growth requires the cells or viruses to produce a full complement of structural, metabolic, and genetic macromolecules utilizing considerable external resources and time. Nucleic acid amplification tests rely on targeting only specific nucleic acid sequences within the pathogen to increase the number of the target sequence or a signal or probe that identifies the target sequence. Because of the specificity of NAAT, this has become the gold standard for laboratory diagnosis of many pathogens. NAAT are also faster than traditional cultures. Some NAAT have been formatted to detect several pathogens simultaneously. Although some NAAT are packaged to prevent contamination, other NAAT require dedicated work spaces and microbiological practices beyond sterile technique. The equipment and test reagents are generally more expensive than traditional diagnostic strategies. However, NAAT may be more cost effective when the delay in treatment or outbreak detection, laboratory labor, and other resources are included in the cost calculation.

A common NAAT format, target amplification, used in clinical and public health laboratories is the polymerase chain reaction (PCR). PCR is performed in a thermocycler, an instrument that cycles temperature changes of the reaction. The PCR reaction mixture (i.e., isolated DNA from the specimen [template DNA], heat-resistant DNA polymerase, nucleotides and ions) is first heated to a temperature sufficient for separating the DNA strands, (i.e., denature step). Next the temperature is lowered and 2 primers (one for the 5' DNA strand and one for the 3' DNA strand) hybridize to the sequence flanking the target DNA. The primer and source DNA complex serve as an initiation site for heat-tolerant DNA polymerase to replicate the target sequence resulting in 2 copies (or amplicons) of the target. Target DNA and amplified DNA serve as templates in subsequent cycles. This cycle of denaturation, hybridization, and extension is repeated approximately 30 times, resulting in the increase of the number of amplicons many thousand-fold. In the case of RNA viruses, reverse transcriptase is used to generate a DNA strand complementary to the viral RNA before initiating amplification cycling.

In traditional PCR, amplicons require an addition method of detection such as DNA gel electrophoresis, capillary electrophoresis, probe hybridization, or sequencing. In PCR, the results of amplification are not available until after the amplicon detection is complete. This two-tiered method of amplification and detection was improved in the real-time PCR assay. In addition to the amplification reagents of PCR, a probe is designed to hybridize with a sequence within the target DNA and contains a quencher and a reporter molecule. In the intact probe, light emission of the reporter molecule is interrupted by the proximity of the quencher. When DNA polymerase encounters the probe-target hybrid, it will degrade the probe, releasing the reporter molecule from the probe. When freed from the proximity of the quencher, the amplification instrument detects the signal emitted by the freed reporter molecule. Thus, amplification and detection of the amplicon are simultaneous or real time. Other types of reporter molecules can be incorporated into the probe, including dyes to accomplish detection as amplification occurs.

Variations on target amplification strategies include strand displacement amplification, which has 2 sets of primers. These primers are designed to hybridize target sequences to generate an amplification target that contains the target and sequences recognized by enzymes, endonucleases that cut at these DNA sites containing this special sequence. Restriction site-containing targets are then amplified exponentially. In loop-mediated isothermal amplification (LAMP), multiple primers are used to form loop structures flanking the target sequence. An additional set of primers facilitates development of compliment-ary amplicons. A byproduct of amplification can be measured with the naked eye or via turbidity measurements. Strand displacement amplification and LAMP do not rely on DNA denaturing and thus do not require thermocyclers.

In signal amplification assays, multiple probes with reporter molecules hybridize to target sequences to amply the strength of the signal. This NAAT format is temperature-cycle independent and can utilize longer target sequence probes. Signal amplification can also employ multiple probes that capture target DNA to a solid matrix and contain signal amplification probes with multiple reporter probe hybridization sites.

## Bibliography

Jorgenson JH, Pfaller MA, Carroll KC, et al., eds. *Manual of Clinical Microbiology*. 11th ed. Washington, DC: American Society for Microbiology; 2015.

Procop GW, Church DL, Hall GS, et al., eds. *Koneman's Color Atlas and Textbook of Diagnostic Microbiology*. 7th ed. Philadelphia, PA: Wolters Kluwer Publisher; 2017.

US Department of Health and Human Services, Centers for Disease Control and Prevention, National Institutes of Health. *Biosafety in Microbiological and Biomedical Laboratories*. 5th ed. 2009. Available at: https://www.cdc.gov/labs/pdf/CDC-BiosafetyMicrobiologicalBiomedicalLaboratories-2009-P.PDF. Accessed January 18, 2019.

Vandepette J, Verhaegen J, Engbaek K, Rohner P, Piot P. Basic laboratory procedures in clinical bacteriology. 2003. Available at: whqlibdoc.who.int/publications/2003/9241545453.pdf. Accessed January 18, 2019.

World Health Organization. *Laboratory Quality Management System: Handbook*. 2011. Available at: http://www.who.int/ihr/publications/lqms/en. Accessed January 18, 2019.

[F. P. Downes]

# REPORTING OF COMMUNICABLE DISEASES UNDER THE INTERNATIONAL HEALTH REGULATIONS

Compliance with the International Health Regulations (IHR) is core to a country's ability to prepare for identifying the cause of epidemics and tracking disease prevalence. Laboratories provide the evidence for identifying the cause and for conducting surveillance of the presence of specific diseases within a given country. Laboratories also provide the evidence for a country to report public health events of international concern as prescribed in the IHR Annex 1a and Annex 2. Thus, it is highly desirable that all countries share the need to strengthen their laboratory networks to detect infectious diseases for patient care, surveillance, and both domestic and global disease control. Laboratory capabilities are closely linked to fulfilling the requirements of the IHR, and the monitoring of country compliance is now a formal process called the Joint External Evaluation (JEE), which combines both IHR and Global Health Security Agenda goals (http://www.who.int/ihr/publications/WHO_HSE_GCR_2016_2/en). The JEE National Laboratory System section includes a series of questions and measures that are initially self-assessed by each country and then reviewed by WHO-sponsored teams of external reviewers. The JEE assesses the national and local laboratory networks and processes required for effective referral and testing. A key area for the JEE is the capacity to test for selected key pathogens, especially those with the potential for epidemics. Many countries do not have the extensive referral and reference testing capabilities found in the USA and must document processes and agreements to support the referral of specialized reference testing to other countries. Additionally, most countries do not have universal laboratory regulations and accreditation standards that require and monitor quality systems to ensure testing accuracy. The US model of jurisdictional public health laboratories, regional networks, specialized referral centers, and national test directories can serve as an example for efforts to strengthen national laboratory systems in other countries.

**Background**

The principal global agreement for addressing the risks of the international spread of infectious disease is the IHR, issued under the WHO constitution and adopted by its member states. The first version, then called the International Sanitary Regulations, was agreed to in 1951, and since then there have been a number of revisions, the most recent of which entered into force as a binding legal agreement in 2007. The current IHR (2005) has a much broader scope of application than that of earlier versions, which had focused on 3 infectious diseases after smallpox had been eradicated: cholera, plague, and yellow fever. In addition, the IHR was updated to take account of the new challenges presented by an increasingly globalized world and advances in information and communication technology. At time of writing in early 2013, the IHR has entered into force for 195 of the world's countries, including all the WHO member states.

The IHR provides broad newmandates and obligations both for participating countries and for WHO, with the following goal: to prevent, protect against, control, and provide a public health response to the international spread of disease in ways that are commensurate with, and restricted to, public health risks, and which avoid unnecessary interference with international traffic and trade.

The IHR depends heavily on global surveillance, alert, and response activities, which aim to support countries and the international community in identifying and responding to emerging public health risks. In this respect, the IHR now recognizes and mandates the use of information from a variety of sources, and not only the information officially reported by the country in which the health event may be occurring.

The IHR aims to avoid the stigmatization of particular diseases or of the countries in which they are occurring, factors that proved significant barriers to compliance with the previous regulations. In addition to the provisions dealing with the detection and response to emergency events, the IHR also mandates certain routine measures related to preventing the international spread of diseases (e.g., the use of the International Certificate of Vaccination or Prophylaxis in travelers from areas at risk of yellow fever transmission; see International Measures under Special Considerations section in "Yellow Fever" in *CCDM20*).

A new component of the IHR is commitment by the states parties to strengthen or reestablish the public health infrastructures designed to facilitate early recognition of, and rapid response to, emerging disease threats, which, for a variety of reasons, have either never been established or have declined in effectiveness in some parts of the world over recent decades.

The text of IHR consists of 66 articles and 9 annexes. This section addresses only those articles and annexes most directly relevant to the detection of, international reporting of, or notification of, and response to communicable disease outbreaks.

**Surveillance Under IHR**

The process of global surveillance involves the systematic collection of information from many different sources, its assessment, and taking prompt public health action based on the conclusion. When an event is assessed as a *potential* public health emergency of international concern (PHEIC), it shall then be notified to WHO while verification and further information are sought from the affected country. On the basis of the information thus obtained, events may be discarded from consideration or may undergo repeated risk assessment to monitor ongoing need for further information or response activities. The surveillance related provisions of the IHR provide a firm institutional mandate and legal framework for key elements of this process within WHO.

The provisions of the IHR do not of themselves create the basis for any international system of surveillance for specific diseases. Instead, the regulatory requirements include those for notification to WHO and obligations to respond to WHO requests for verification aimed at identifying any public health event that may constitute a PHEIC (see PHEIC section later in this chapter), as determined through a standard decision protocol.

### *National IHR focal points and WHO IHR contact points*

Under the IHR, urgent communications, including those concerning country reporting, are transmitted to WHO through specific National IHR Focal Points. Each of the 6 WHO regional offices has established an IHR Contact Point for the countries within its respective region; and as of early 2013, almost all WHO Member States have identified national IHR Focal Points.

### *Notification*

A central reporting obligation under the IHR is the mandatory duty for countries to carry out an assessment of public health events occurring within their territories, in accordance with the decision protocols and criteria found in Annex 2 of the regulations, and then to notify WHO of all qualifying events within 24 hours of the assessment. The events that are to be notified are effectively defined by 4 criteria in the decision protocol:

1) Whether the event has a serious public health impact
2) Whether the event is unusual or unexpected
3) Whether the event risks spreading internationally
4) Whether the event risks resulting in restrictions on international trade and/or travel

If an event within a country fulfills 2 of the 4 listed criteria, it qualifies as an event that *may* constitute an international emergency and so must be notified by that country to WHO through the National IHR Focal Point. In addition to these criteria, there are a number of subquestions and indicative examples of factual contexts to guide use of the decision protocol.

Consistent with the broad scope of the IHR, the decision protocol, and hence the notification, does not require that the event involve a particular disease or type of causative agent (i.e., biological, chemical, or nuclear). The decision protocol was designed to allow the assessment of events where the nature of any disease or agent is still undefined at the time of assessment and does not exclude events based upon whether they are or may be accidental, natural, or intentional in nature.

While the decision protocol and Annex 2 of IHR require that all events remain subject to assessment as indicated, they also specifically require that certain events, involving a limited number of specific diseases that have demonstrated the ability to cause serious public health impact and to spread rapidly internationally, must always be analyzed utilizing the decision protocol. These must be notified if the analysis indicates that they fulfill 2 of the 4 criteria. The diseases in this category are

- Cholera
- Pneumonic plague
- Yellow fever
- Viral hemorrhagic fevers (e.g., dengue hemorrhagic fever, Ebola, Marburg)
- West Nile fever
- Other diseases of special national or regional concern (e.g., dengue fever, Rift Valley fever, meningococcal disease)

Finally, the IHR identifies 4 specific disease entities that are always considered unusual or unexpected, which may have serious public health impact, and hence, which always may constitute a PHEIC. Accordingly, even 1 case of these diseases must be notified to WHO. These diseases are

- Smallpox
- Poliomyelitis due to wild type poliovirus
- Human influenza caused by a new subtype (e.g., H5N1 in humans)
- Severe acute respiratory syndrome (SARS)

WHO maintains the case definitions for the notification of cases of these diseases.

### *Other types of reporting under IHR*

As a complement to the obligation to notify, the IHR provides an option for countries to keep WHO informed, on a confidential basis, about events within their territories that are not notifiable as discussed earlier and to consult with WHO on the appropriate responsive health measures. This provision focuses in particular on those events for which there is insufficient available information to complete the decision protocol.

Countries are also required to inform WHO within 24 hours of receipt of evidence of a public health risk identified outside their territory that may cause international disease spread, as manifested by the following (exported or imported):

- Human cases
- Vectors carrying infection or contamination
- Goods that are contaminated

The IHR does not include any provision referring explicitly to reporting suspected intentional or deliberate releases of harmful agents. However, the IHR stipulates that where a country has evidence of an unexpected or unusual public health event within its territory, irrespective of origin or source, that may constitute a public health emergency of international concern, the country must provide to WHO all relevant public health information.

**Response Under IHR**

The IHR requires WHO to collaborate with countries in the risk assessment and response to public health events whenever they request WHO to do so. Such collaboration can include the provision of technical guidance, assessment of the effectiveness of control measures, and mobilization of international teams either for risk assessment or for control purposes. WHO event detection and verification activities provide risk assessment support needed by member states to protect the health of their populations during certain public health events. This support can take the form of different types of assistance to countries already affected by the event, as well as the provision of information regarding the event to countries as yet unaffected. This is so that the latter can take action to prevent their populations from becoming affected or prepare themselves to take effective response actions should they become affected.

WHO ensures that countries have rapid access to the most appropriate experts and resources for risk assessment and outbreak response through the Global Outbreak Alert and Response Network of institutions able to provide support and expertise. The Global Outbreak Alert and Response Network partnership was formalized in April 2000 to improve the coordination of international outbreak responses and to provide an operational framework to focus the delivery of support to countries. The network's primary aims are as follows:

- To support countries with disease control efforts by ensuring rapid and appropriate technical expertise to affected populations.
- To investigate and characterize events and assess risks of rapidly emerging epidemic disease threats.
- To support national outbreak preparedness by ensuring that responses contribute to sustained containment of epidemic threats.

Further information can be found at: http://www.who.int/csr/outbreak network/en.

***Provision of information***

Providing authoritative information on public health events that have particular international significance is an important part of an effective public health response. WHO manages the information provided by an affected country in ways that both protect that country from unjustified overreaction by other countries and ensures that other countries are provided with the information they need to protect their populations, including citizens who travel to the affected country/countries.

As part of an incentive to states parties to notify and report events to WHO, the IHR guarantees that information in notifications, reports, and consultations under the IHR is not made generally available to other countries unless circumstances arise that justify dissemination in order to address the risk of international spread. The contexts that justify communication of the information to other states parties are clearly specified and include situations where the director-general of WHO has declared a PHEIC (see PHEIC section later in this chapter), where international spread has been confirmed, where control measures are not likely to succeed, and/or where implementation of international control measures is required immediately.

When WHO intends to make such information available to other countries, it has an obligation to consult with the country experiencing the event. WHO may also make information available in the public domain if other information about the event is already public and if a need exists for public availability of information that is authoritative and independent.

### *PHEIC*

The experience gained during the international collaboration to respond to the emergence of severe acute respiratory syndrome (SARS) led to the inclusion within the IHR of specific provisions governing actions in response to rare and serious events, which are called PHEIC. The responsibility of determining whether a potential PHEIC falls into this category lies with the director-general of WHO, acting on the advice of the WHO secretariat, and requires the convening of a committee of health experts (the IHR Emergency Committee). If the director-general determines that the event constitutes a PHEIC, the IHR Emergency Committee advises the WHO director-general on appropriate temporary recommendations of health measures to be implemented by states parties. The emergency committee continues to advise the director-general throughout the period of the PHEIC, including advising on necessary changes to the recommended measures for control and on the termination of the PHEIC.

### Development and Maintenance of Core Surveillance Capacities

One of the most important elements of the IHR is the requirement for all participating countries to develop and maintain core public health capacities for surveillance and response, in accordance with the functions described in Annex 1 of the IHR. These core public health capacities had to be developed within 5 years of entry into force of the IHR for each country, but most countries requested a 2-year extension in June 2012, and some countries may require 2 more years, until June 2015, to develop the minimum core capacities. Through these requirements, the IHR seeks to ensure that all countries have the basic infrastructure, human resources, and procedures needed in order to undertake the timely identification and risk assessment of, and response to, outbreaks of disease and other public health events when and where they occur. This is key to avoid or minimize the international spread of such public health risks.

## National Reporting of Communicable Diseases

Surveillance is the cornerstone for effective disease prevention and control efforts, and disease reporting is 1 of the 3 legs of the surveillance platform, the others being timely and appropriate analysis, followed by the provision of the information needed to guide intervention. While the reporting of individual and aggregated data on disease occurrence is not the only input to the surveillance process, it is the most common and forms the bedrock on which public health surveillance is built.

The practice of, and the recommendations and requirements for, disease reporting vary widely between countries as a consequence of differences in epidemiological contexts, health care provision, role of national legislation, administrative structures, and available resources. The planned use to be made of the derived information will also influence the type of reporting needed; for example, reporting against very specific and detailed case definitions may be needed for clinical research purposes, while much broader and simpler definitions may suffice for the monitoring of health facility utilization. An increasing number of countries are supplementing case-based disease data reported from health information systems with event-based data from media reports or other informal sources to assist in the early detection of public health events requiring an urgent response.

Disease reporting usually takes the form of either a case or infection report (some countries only require aggregate reporting) or an outbreak or event report.

1) Case reports: case reporting provides diagnosis, age, sex, and date of onset for each person with the disease. Sometimes it includes identifying information, such as the name and address of the person with the disease. Further information, such as treatment provided and its duration, are required for certain case reports.

   National legislation or guidelines often indicate which diseases must be reported, who is responsible for reporting, the format for reporting, and how case reports are to be entered into and forwarded within the national system. If there is a requirement for international case reporting, national governments report to WHO.
2) Outbreak or event reports: outbreak reporting provides information about an increase in the number of cases above a certain threshold. However, the specific disease causing an outbreak may not be included in the list of diseases officially reportable, or it may be of unknown etiology if it is newly recognized or emerging. It would then lead to the report of an event of unknown etiology.

National legislation or guidelines may indicate which types of outbreak or event must be reported, who is responsible for reporting, the format for reporting, and how case reports are to be entered into and forwarded within the national system. In general, outbreak reporting is required by the most rapid means of communication available. When there is a requirement for outbreak or event reporting internationally, national governments report to WHO. General advice on the reporting of diseases listed in *CCDM20* is provided under the Special Considerations section for each disease. While the international legal requirement for disease reporting is described earlier in this chapter, it is important to note that, in addition to this, WHO has a number of diseases under routine international surveillance, including

- Louse-borne typhus fever
- Relapsing fever
- Meningococcal meningitis
- Paralytic poliomyelitis
- Malaria
- Tuberculosis
- Human immunodeficiency virus/acquired immunodeficiency syndrome
- Influenza
- SARS

Note: this chapter concentrates on those elements of the IHR that are of relevance to the control of communicable disease and particularly the recognition of and response to public health events such as disease outbreaks. The IHR also contains provisions for the routine application of health measures in the context of international travel and transportation in the absence of such events. Where these measures have relevance to a specific communicable disease (e.g., those pertaining to the international certificate of vaccination), they are mentioned in the relevant chapter of this book. Further IHR information can be found at: http://www.who.int/csr/ihr/en.

[M. Chu, M. Hardiman, J. Ridderhof]

# OVERVIEW OF QUALITY LABORATORY SYSTEMS

## Definitions

The following terms are defined as follows for use in this chapter. As indicated, the definitions are either derived from the respective International Organization for Standardization (ISO) standards, Clinical and Laboratory Standards Institute (CLSI) standards, College of American Pathologists (CAP) accreditation standards, or they reflect the common usage of the term as defined by the authors.

**Assessment:** systematic process of collecting and analyzing data to determine the current, historical, or projected status of an organization, person, process, or project. Note: when applied to an organization, may also be referred to as inspection or survey.[1]

**Competence:** demonstrated ability to apply knowledge and skills to achieve intended results.[1]

**Corrective action:** action(s) to eliminate the cause and prevent recurrence of a nonconformity or other undesirable situation. Note: there can be more than one cause for a nonconformity or undesirable situation.[1]

**Equipment:** single apparatus or set of devices or apparatuses needed to perform a specific task. Note: for the purpose of this guideline, equipment includes general purpose devices that do not independently produce results.[1]

**Examination:** set of operations having the object of determining the value or characteristics of a property. Note: (a) in some disciplines (e.g., microbiology) an examination is the total activity of a number of tests, observations, or measurements; (b) laboratory examinations that determine a value of a property are called quantitative examinations; those that determine the characteristics of a property are called qualitative examinations; (c) laboratory examinations are also often called analyses, assays, or tests.[1]

**Instrument:** mechanical device used to produce an analytical result.

**Postexamination:** processes following the analytical examination, including review and reporting of results, retention of examination records, storage of clinical material, and sample (and waste) disposal.

**Preexamination:** processes, in chronological order, from the request for examination, preparation and identification of the patient, collection of the primary specimen(s), transportation to and within the laboratory, preparation of the specimen for examination, and end at the beginning of the analytical examination.

**Preventive action:** action to eliminate the cause of a potential nonconformity or any other undesirable potential situation. Note: (a) there can be more than one cause for a potential nonconformity; (b) preventive action is taken to prevent occurrence, whereas corrective action is taken to prevent recurrence.

**Quality assurance (QA):** part of quality management focused on providing confidence that quality requirements will be fulfilled. Note: the practice encompassing all procedures and activities directed toward ensuring that a specified quality of product is achieved and maintained. In the testing environment, this process includes monitoring raw materials, supplies, instruments, and procedures; specimen collection/transport/storage/processing; recordkeeping; calibrating and maintaining equipment; conducting quality control procedures; proficiency testing; and training of personnel and all else involved in the production of the data reported.[2]

**Quality control (QC):** part of quality management focused on fulfilling quality requirements. Note: (a) in health care testing, the set of procedures designed to monitor the test method and the results to ensure appropriate test system performance; (b) includes testing QC materials, charting the results and analyzing them to identify sources of error, and evaluating and documenting any remedial action taken as a result of this analysis.[2]

**Quality indicators:** observations, statistics, or data defined by the organization or service that typify the performance of a given work process and provide evidence that the organization or service is meeting its quality intentions.

**Quality management:** coordinated activities to direct and control an organization with regard to quality.

**Quality policy:** overall intentions and direction of a laboratory related to quality as formally expressed by laboratory management. Note: generally, the quality policy is consistent with the overall policy of an organization and provides a framework for setting quality objectives.[3]

**Quality system:** the organizational structure, responsibilities, procedures, processes, and resources for implementing quality management.

**Quality system essential:** an essential building block of a quality management system that addresses, at a minimum, regulatory and accreditation requirements within a specific topic needed to fulfill those requirements and stated quality objectives.[1]

**Reagent:** any substance in a test system other than a solvent or support material that is required for the target analyte to be detected and its value measured in a sample.[4]

**Record:** evidence of results achieved, or activities performed. Note: (a) records can be used to demonstrate traceability and to provide evidence of verification, preventive action, and corrective action; (b) generally, records need not be under revision control.[5]

**Reference interval:** the range of test values expected for a designated population of individuals.[4]

**Remedial action:** the immediate action taken to correct an identified problem, usually to allow data to be reported to a customer; examples include making an adjustment, fixing a mistake, repeating analysis, calibrating equipment.

**Requirement:** need or expectation that is stated, generally implied, or obligatory. Note: (a) a specified requirement is one that is stated (e.g., in documented information); (b) "generally implied" means that it is custom or common practice for the organization and interested parties that the need or expectation under consideration is implied; (c) a qualifier can be used to denote a specific type of requirement (e.g., product requirement, quality management requirement, customer requirement, quality requirement); (d) requirements can be generated by different interested parties or by the organization itself; (e) it can be necessary for achieving high customer satisfaction to fulfil an expectation of a customer even if it is neither stated nor generally implied or obligatory.[1]

**Risk:** combination of the probability of occurrence of harm and the severity of that harm. Note: a potential hazard or quality deficiency associated with a process, product, or service.

**Root cause(s):** the bottom-line causal factor(s) underlying a nonconforming event.

**Root cause analysis:** process for identifying the causal factor(s) that underlies variation in performance, including the occurrence or possible occurrence of a nonconforming event.

**Traceability:** ability to trace the history, application, or location of that which is under consideration. Note: when considering a product, traceability can relate to the origin of materials and parts, the processing history, and the distribution and location of the product after delivery.[2]

### Quality Laboratory Systems

In the laboratory-based surveillance of human disease, the laboratory systems that contribute to the detection, control, and prevention of communicable diseases must adhere to established quality assurance practices in order to assure the quality of the information they generate. These quality assurance practices are related to the preexamination, examination, and postexamination aspects of laboratory practice. Different standard-setting entities exist in different regions of the world, but the basic elements of quality laboratory systems are similar. All laboratories, including those in resource-constrained settings, must adhere to basic quality standards of practice in order to assure that the information generated by laboratories worldwide is reliable.

### Organization/Personnel

Organizational structure, roles, responsibilities, and delegation of duties are the foundation of a quality management system. The organization may comprise 1 or 2 individuals or thousands. The written responsibilities of the person(s) within the laboratory covering all the topics listed in this chapter must be assigned or have written delegation to document and acknowledge roles within the quality management system. Keeping an up-to-date organizational chart for quick reference of personnel direct reports is recommended and visually supports organizational relationships. The educational requirements and professional experience of personnel hired at the laboratory must be clearly defined. The requirements for specific roles are frequently regulated by a governing body and must be adhered to in order to maintain certification or licensure. It is the responsibility of the organization to verify the credentials of staff prior to employment.

- Director: the laboratory director is responsible for deciding or approving changes to the laboratory that could impact any part of the laboratory system. The director has the authority and holds ultimate responsibility for every standard operating procedure (SOP), sample, assay, report, and the personnel delegated to perform the tasks.
- Quality assurance staff: if possible, it is best practice to have a staff member or a team assigned responsibility for the quality assurance role. The quality staff should be completely separate from laboratory processes, have direct access to the laboratory director, and the authority to ensure that the quality system is executed (e.g., direct access to all records). This separation and staffing organization assists in the removal of possible conflicts of interest that could include but are not limited to the following: review of personal work, fear of reporting nonconforming events due to potential personal penalty, personnel conflicts, financial interests, or inability to maintain objectivity.
- Training: Training new staff or providing training on new processes should be an organized and documented activity. Training plans should be developed that outline the training needs of the organization, position, and or specific tasks. A training plan could be in the form of a policy, procedure, or checklist. Delivery of the trainings should be appropriate for the complexity and associated risk of the information relayed or for activities performed if not implemented properly. A training that may only require documentation of a staff member reading a policy would be appropriate for low complexity and low-risk information or activity such as temperature monitoring. However, more in-depth training would be appropriate for a low complexity, high-risk activity, or conveying information such as safety topics. Whenever personnel resources allow, cross-training of activities should be implemented. Regardless of the delivery, each staff member should have completion records of the training performed.

  Organizational training plans are general trainings, which are evaluated based on needs or requirements. Generally, these trainings may include but are not limited to the following: orientation, safety, security (facility and data), computer systems/paper systems, overview of quality system, ethics, and human resources. These types of basic organizational trainings aid in consistent processes for all staff who support a strong quality management system. This also supports the need for every level of staff understanding their responsibility within these systems.

Training laboratory staff either based on position or task should heavily rely on risk-based evaluations. Application of universal/standard precautions towards potentially infectious materials is an example of an appropriate generalized risk-based safety practice. Knowing the complexity and risk of failures within the preexamination, examination, and postexamination processes will assist in the evaluation and identification of training needs, frequency of training, and frequency of competency assessments.

Technical competency: competency assessments provide an initial and ongoing mechanism to evaluate the effectiveness and proficiency of the organization's training plans and individual staff members ability to perform activities. At a minimum, competency assessments should cover preexamination, examination, and postexamination activities. The frequency of competency assessments may be defined by a governing body or determined within the organization. These activities may be performed by 1 or multiple individuals of a single process; however, each individual requires a record of competence for each of the activities.Best practice competency measures to document (if applicable) are as follows:

- SOP review
- Observation of trainer (this could be the documentation of the training, and only required for initial competency)
- Direct observation of sample collection, sample preparation, sample handling, and sample processing
- Direct observation of instrument operation, performance, and maintenance
- Direct observation of routine test performance (e.g., does the trainee understand the principles and process?)
- Review of intermediate test results, worksheets, QC records, and preventative maintenance records
- QC/QA (e.g., does the trainee perform appropriate QC and follow QA?)
- Recording and reporting of results
- Confirmed reproducibility; blind testing of known samples
- Assessment of problem solving skills
- Final acknowledgement of competence and authority to perform process independently.

Small organizations that do not have the cross-training personnel or financial resources to maintain process redundancies can determine nonobservational competence based on reproducibility of blinded samples. This practice is not recommended but may be the only option in certain settings.

### Customer Focus

Customer focus begins with the identification of customers. This is important for clinical testing in the context of where the samples are coming from, what the customers are requesting for services, and to whom specifically the customer is submitting samples.

1) Requisitions/test requests:

    - It is best practice to ensure that both the sample test requisition and sample have at least 2 unique identifiers to confidently match patient sample and test requisitions.
    - Examination(s) requested.
    - The minimal acceptance requirements of a sample should be determined during the verification/validation procedures and in turn the rejection criteria is then easily determined.

        - This may include acceptance of any external source (patient/guardian submitted), acceptance of samples only by authorized medical professionals (defined by local/governing regulation or independently), or acceptance of samples only from designated sites or officials with authority (e.g., *Yersinia pestis*).
        - Transport time, temperature, matrix, and volume are examples of sample requirements that can contribute to acceptance and rejection criteria.

2) Sample tracking: upon receipt of a sample, a unique tracking mechanism should be in place to allow traceability and identification of the sample throughout all phases of preexamination, examination, and postexamination processes.
3) Turnaround time: a realistic turnaround time from the laboratory receiving the specimen to reporting the test results should be established and communicated with customers. This may include considerations of hours of operation, staffing, and exclusions of these in outbreak or time/patient sensitive critical result reporting.
4) Test result reporting: reports generated should include all the necessary information to identify the following:

    - Laboratory name and location.
    - Patient name and unique identifier.
    - Date of collection and time, when applicable.
    - Sample received date.

- Report date.
- Type of sample tested or sample source.
- Test result with units of measure (with clearly identifying critical values).
- Identification of appropriate reference intervals.
- Submitting client (e.g., authorized person to receive results and submitting organization name, address, and phone).
- A dedicated area to include any qualifiers or comments needed for interpretation (when applicable to the test method and results being reported) to include any identified discrepancies.

**Facilities**

Laboratories should have a plan to evaluate and design the amount and type of space that will be required for testing and other related tasks. Laboratories should have space suitable for the performance of testing to allow for quality of testing as well as for the health and safety of laboratory personnel, patients, and visitors.

Access to specific areas may need to be controlled considering safety, confidentiality, quality, and local regulations. Required safety facilities and devices need to be provided and their functionality routinely verified.

- Storage: there should be adequate storage space and conditions that provide for the integrity of specimens, slides, documents, equipment, reagents, and supplies. Storage of clinical samples should be separate from reagents to minimize the potential for cross-contamination. Storage and disposal facilities for dangerous materials should be suitable for any known hazards and meet local regulatory requirements. Medical information should be stored to safeguard from unauthorized access and to meet applicable regulations that require protection of confidential patient medical records.
- Environmental controls: the laboratory premises should be maintained in a reliable condition with work areas clean and functional. Environmental conditions should be controlled and recorded where they may have an effect on the quality of the sample, reagents, and results. Attention should be given to conditions such as temperature, light, sterility, humidity, and electrical supply, as appropriate, so that these do not adversely affect the results and/or the quality of testing. Attention should be paid to separate laboratory sections with incompatible activities and to prevent cross-contamination where necessary.
- Patient sample collection facilities: patient sample collection facilities should have separate reception/waiting and collection areas. Patient privacy, comfort, and needs should be considered in organizing these areas. Sample collection should be made in a manner that does not adversely affect the quality of the results.

### Purchasing and Inventory Management

The laboratory should establish a system for tracking purchases and inventory to ensure that materials needed for analysis are available when needed, used within manufacturer defined specifications (i.e., expiration or stability), and not contribute to unnecessary waste. The laboratory should have a system to verify that the items requested on each purchase order are the same as the items received, especially in regard to reagents, media, and other supplies that may vary in grade or quality. Laboratories should also verify the condition of items received and exclude from use any items that are not of an acceptable quality, are damaged or opened. The environment where reagents and media are stored should be monitored to maintain appropriate temperature and humidity to maximize the shelf-life of stored items. Different environmental conditions may be required depending on the items being used and stored at the laboratory. The laboratory should utilize a "first in/first out" system to ensure that the items that have been stored the longest are easily accessible and used first by staff. Staff should verify that items with expiration dates are not used for testing patient samples after the expiration date.

### Instruments and Equipment

Instruments and equipment represent the tools utilized by testing personnel to perform testing activities and must be used as designed and maintained according to the manufacturer's requirements to avoid undermining the quality of test results.

1) Selection of instruments: when selecting instruments and equipment for purchase by the laboratory, management should consider the following:

    - Instrument performance capabilities and customer needs
    - Implementation cost (including validation cost)
    - Facility requirements (e.g., space, ventilation, electrical)

        - Ongoing reagent and supply costs
        - Ongoing maintenance costs
        - Equipment features, including ease of use, ability to interface with information management system, and alternative or future uses (value of investment)
        - Needs of staff (i.e., ergonomics or disability accommodations)

2) Performance verification: prior to being used for patient testing, new instruments and equipment should have their performance evaluated by an established procedure. This initial verification may be included as part of a method evaluation; however, if new equipment or instrument is procured to perform an established method, it must be verified before use.

    Procedures for performing verification for each instrument or equipment type should be established and may be used regularly by the laboratory. Some situations where a verification should be performed include following major maintenance or repair, following a move to a new location, or if the analyst questions the performance of the item. The procedure should detail the steps required to perform the verification and establish tolerance limits or acceptance criteria.

For instruments, the verification procedure typically involves analyzing controls and a panel of patient samples (at least 1 from each result type that is reported) both before the maintenance and again after it. It is possible to have this verification follow the same procedure as instrument comparisons discussed later in this chapter. This verification may be concurrent with patient samples, as long as the instrument is verified to be performing within the defined tolerance prior to releasing patient data.

For equipment, this verification procedure is confirmation that the equipment is conforming to defined standards or tolerance limits. Some examples of equipment verifications include checking that a centrifuge maintains the correct revolutions per minute, verifying that a pipette dispenses the correct volume, and checking that a balance reads the correct weight for a standard weight. It is important for a laboratory to continually verify the performance of instruments and equipment whenever the performance of the particular item may be compromised. By establishing a system to continually verify instruments and equipment, the laboratory will protect against reporting inaccurate data that may result from improper repair or unseen damage to instruments and equipment.

3) Calibration and calibration verification: instruments and equipment that require calibration should be recalibrated at least as often as recommended by the manufacturer following an established procedure. Often this calibration is performed by instrument or equipment service personnel during annual or semiannual preventive maintenance and involves adjusting the instrument or equipment to match defined expectations. For example, when a pipette is calibrated, it is adjusted to dispense more or less liquid to ensure that when it is set to dispense 1 mL, it actually dispenses 1 mL.

   Whenever a calibration is performed, the instrument or equipment should be verified to ensure that its performance meets defined expectations according to an established procedure. The calibration verification should utilize samples that test the range of results that will be reported by the instrument (or the range of use of the equipment) and focus on medical decision points or cutoffs, when applicable. Often manufacturers have sample panels for sale that can meet this need. Instrument and equipment verifications should be performed as often as deemed necessary by the laboratory to ensure that quality data is produced. For some assays, this may mean verifying the performance of equipment and instruments with each analysis.

4) Maintenance: laboratory equipment and instruments are the backbone of most examination procedures. The importance of performing regular maintenance and function checks cannot be overstated. Laboratories should review the manufacturer's instruction for each item of equipment and each instrument to establish a schedule for performing regular maintenance. If the laboratory opts to name the instruments, records will need to be created to link the name with the manufacturer assigned serial number. Ideally, these records should be maintained for the life of the instrument or equipment.

   The ability for staff to perform preventive maintenance correctly not only impacts the life of the equipment or instrument but also the quality of the results that are obtained while using the equipment. To protect the quality of laboratory test results, it is imperative that the laboratory establish a maintenance timeline and procedure, and that the performance of maintenance be assessed while performing competency assessments.
5) Monitoring performance of instruments: the performance of laboratory instruments should be continually monitored where instrument drift may impact the quality of patient results, as in quantitative and semi-quantitative methods. The performance can be monitored by tracking the performance of QC samples using a Levey-Jennings chart or by following the Westgard Rules if deemed appropriate for the method by laboratory management.

**Process Management**

Process management is the organized planning and monitoring of testing activities to ensure that quality results are produced at maximum efficiency. Process management requires investment by the laboratory in planning and monitoring activities to minimize the costs associated with failed analysis, improper experimentation, and inaccurate results. The processes described later in this chapter all serve to protect the quality of the data generated by the laboratory and minimize the risk of reporting an incorrect result that may lead to patient harm.

1) Method evaluation/validation: for procedures and test kits that are commercially available, the laboratory should verify that performance specifications of the test have been met for accuracy (trueness), precision (repeatability and reproducibility), and analytical measurable range. It should also verify that reference intervals are appropriate for the laboratory's population. The laboratory should document the procedures used and keep records for such verification. Commercially available test kits that are modified (including adjustments to specimen type or intended use) should include all additional performance specifications outlined later for laboratory developed tests.

For procedures developed by the laboratory, a documented plan should be followed to establish performance specifications for accuracy (trueness), precision (repeatability and reproducibility), reportable range of test results, reference interval(s), analytical sensitivity and specificity (including likely interfering substances), and other applicable performance characteristics. If the procedure is novel and without comparative methods, the diagnostic sensitivity and specificity should also be studied and confirmed.

2) Quality risk assessment and quality control: quality control samples can be positive controls, internal standard, blanks, or other examples of known analytical confirmation within every assay. Quantitative assays should have various levels of controls across the reportable range. When possible, established standard methods should be employed. Established standard methods generally have outlined frequency and acceptability of QC samples that have been either peer established or approved by governing agencies.

   Quality risk assessments identify, evaluate, and mitigate potential failures and sources of error within a process that have the potential to impact the accuracy and reliability of analytical results. Assessments can be performed on preexamination processes, examination processes, postexamination processes, safety practices, end-to-end processes, or any quality indicator. It is best practice to perform a quality risk assessment encompassing end-to-end (preexamination processes, examination processes, and postexamination processes) activities whenever a new method is being validated or verified. See the 2 tables in this section.

3) Reagent and media verification: reagents should be verified when a new lot is placed into service by comparing the new lot to the lot in use. This will help to rule out reagents as a potential source of laboratory error. Reagents can also be verified by performing an analysis with a known standard, including reference materials or previously tested samples.

   Culture media used to grow and characterize microbiological organisms should be checked prior to use for sterility, ability to support growth, and positive and negative reactivity when applicable.

**Example of Risk Assessment and Determination of Risk Level**

| Frequency of occurrence: | Severity of harm to patient: |
|---|---|
| • Unlikely (once every 2–3 years)<br>• Occasional (once per year)<br>• Probable (once per month)<br>• Frequent (once a week) | • Negligible (temporary discomfort)<br>• Minor (temporary injury; not requiring medical intervention)<br>• Serious (impairment requiring medical intervention)<br>• Critical (life threatening consequences) |
| Risk level:<br>• Risk level for any risk factor that is "not acceptable" *should* be addressed in the final assessment.<br>• Risk level for any risk factor that is "acceptable" may be included in the assessment at the discretion of the laboratory director. | |

**Example of Risk Acceptability Matrix**

| **Probability of Harm** | *Negligible* | *Minor* | *Serious* | *Critical* |
|---|---|---|---|---|
| *Frequent* | Not acceptable | Not acceptable | Not acceptable | Not acceptable |
| *Probable* | Acceptable | Not acceptable | Not acceptable | Not acceptable |
| *Occasional* | Acceptable | Acceptable | Acceptable | Not acceptable |
| *Unlikely* | Acceptable | Acceptable | Acceptable | Acceptable |

4) Instrument comparisons: if multiple instruments are used to perform an analysis, the instruments should be compared periodically to ensure that a specimen will have the same result regardless of which instrument performs the analysis. This comparison is typically performed by running the same batch of specimens and QC on both instruments. The reference instrument is the instrument that performed the most recent successful proficiency test for the assay. Both QC and patient specimens should be included in the instrument comparison to control for matrix effects. The laboratory should define the acceptable amount of variability allowed between instruments.
5) Repeatability and reproducibility: repeatability and reproducibility are the 2 components of precision in quantitative testing. Repeatability is used to describe the ability of a quantitative procedure to consistently repeat the same measurement under the same conditions. This is normally carried out over a short period of time by the same analyst; this was formerly referred to as "within assay precision" and is an estimate of the minimum value of precision.

   Reproducibility is used to describe the ability of a quantitative procedure to consistently repeat the same measurement under differing conditions. The changed conditions include performing measurements over many days, with different operators and using recalibrated equipment. The result is an estimate of the maximum value of precision.

## Document Control

Document control is a system to ensure that only current approved documents can be utilized. The control of documents should identify each document such that production, authorization (including identity and date), revision, retention, and disposal are easily identifiable and traceable. It is very important to note that all the documents listed later in this chapter must be integrated within the organization's document control system. Using outdated documents could lead to failures in preexamination, examination, and postexamination processes.

1) Documents:

   - Policies: a policy is an overall intention statement(s) of the organization. Policy documents can be as long or as short as needed and could be included with a procedure or developed as a stand-alone document.

- SOPs: consistent quality input and output of laboratories rely on standardization of processes. SOPs are step by step instructions that detail exactly how to execute an activity. The level of detail included in an SOP should accommodate the requirements of the process—regulation, validation/verification, flexibility of the process that could implicate outcome(s) of the activity, and amount of information required to ensure consistent, reliable output that personnel are accountable for. SOPs should include the following recommended minimum requirements (when applicable):

    - Requirements for patient preparation; sample collection, labeling, storage, preservation, transportation, processing, and referral; and criteria for sample acceptability and rejection
    - Step-by-step performance of the procedure, including test calculations and interpretation of results
    - Preparation of slides, solutions, calibrators, controls, reagents, stains, and other materials used in testing
    - Calibration and calibration verification procedures
    - The reportable range for test results for the test system as established or verified
    - Quality control sample procedures
    - Corrective action to take when calibration or control results fail to meet the laboratory's criteria for acceptability
    - Limitations in the test methodology, including interfering substances
    - Reference intervals (normal values)
    - The laboratory's system for entering results in the sample record and reporting sample results, including, when appropriate, the protocol for reporting imminently life-threatening results or critical values affecting patient safety.

      This section should be especially detailed depending on the analyst's involvement with result interpretation. Result interpretation should be consistent and detailed enough to execute minimal variation from interpretation by examination personnel.
    - Description of the course of action to take if a test system becomes inoperable
    - Pertinent literature references

- Work instructions/bench sheets/job aids: work instructions are usually a method of having a quick bench reference for procedures. Work instructions can be in the form of step-by-step instructions, bulleted reminders, flowcharts, or checklists. Use caution when posting work instructions on walls or keeping the documents at the bench; this practice can potentially lead to outdated instructions at the bench when official updates are made to the process.

- Instrument/equipment/kit user manuals package: instrument, equipment, and kit user manuals and package inserts may be used as an SOP if followed explicitly, controlled, and approved for use per the organization's document control procedure; however, when performing analysis using a manufacturer's kit package insert there are SOP components that will still require internal process documents (e.g., data entry of samples and reporting of results).
- Forms/worksheets: form and worksheet templates are documents that are intended to be filled with data, information, or acknowledgements when work is performed. It is best practice to have a form or worksheet for processes that include physical, visual, or verbal actions based on quality assurance, process risk assessments, or process improvements (examples of actions: verify balance daily, maintain chain of custody, weigh 20 mg, ensure calibrators and controls are within limit). Forms and worksheets may be paper or electronic. If electronic forms and worksheets are used, ensure document control practices and policies apply.

2) Record management: records are the evidence of actions and decisions that represent a vital asset to support daily functions and operations. They contain data, information, or acknowledgement that may be used to reconstruct the activities of a specific process. Once a form, worksheet, or any other document is completed, written upon, or changed, it is then considered a record.

The context of the record should be easily interpreted by the organization and should reliably represent the information and activities or events that have taken place at the time of the event. Best practice record keeping consistently includes the identity of the person(s) who recorded the information, the date when the information was recorded, and also, when applicable, the time of the recording (e.g., sample receipt time).

Records should be easily accessible and sufficient to reconstruct activities or events that have taken place and should be secure from unauthorized or inadvertent alteration or erasure. The use of indelible ink prevents the inadvertent loss of information or alterations. Ballpoint pens are suitable for this purpose, but pencils should be avoided. If a record needs to be corrected, it should be altered in a way that retains the original entry and identifies who made the correction. A single line strike-through is most often used with date and initials of individual making the correction.

Records should be retained, stored, and disposed of appropriately using a consistent and documented retention and disposal procedure. Retention and storage should be in a secure space and environment that is appropriate for the media. Records should be retained for a minimum period of time, for legal and operational reasons, either as required by law and/or determined by the organization. When applicable, disposal of records should be a recorded activity specific to the records (e.g., staff competencies, QC, QA, raw data, final test result reports), personnel responsible, and method of destruction.

**Information Management**

The laboratory should have access to the data and information needed to provide a service that meets the needs and requirements of the user and a documented procedure to ensure that the confidentiality of patient information is always maintained. The laboratory should describe the responsibilities of all personnel who use the system, in particular those who access, enter, modify, and/or authorize release of patient data and laboratory results (see "Laboratory Informatics"). The laboratory should verify that the laboratory results, associated information, and comments are accurately reproduced electronically and/or in hard copy where relevant. A documented contingency plan should be in place to maintain services in the event of failure or downtime in information systems that affects the laboratory.

**Nonconforming Event Management**

A nonconforming event management system is used to investigate the underlying causes of laboratory errors to prevent them from recurring. The system should include a process by which to report any instance of laboratory work that does not conform to defined standards. These standards may include regulatory requirements, quality control limits, analyst error, or a customer complaint. Management may also wish to include near-miss events in this system, as a near-miss may indicate that a problem with the system exists.

A nonconforming event management system must allow all employees to report identified nonconformance to management in a timely manner. This initial notification should be recorded, and all notifications should be tracked by management to identify recurring nonconformance. Since this system relies on the willingness of employees to report errors that occur to their management, it must be perceived as nonpunitive. A reporting system that allows for reporting nonconforming events anonymously may be more successful depending on the cultural norms of the laboratory staff.

When a nonconforming event is identified, it must be first corrected by remedial action. This immediate action corrects the primary cause of the nonconformance. This may mean reanalyzing samples after quality control does not meet defined acceptance criteria, remaking reagents, repairing equipment, or revising result reports. Remedial actions should be performed as soon as practical and only correct the primary cause of the nonconformance, without consideration for any underlying root causes.

After the primary cause of the nonconformance is corrected, management should decide if a formal root cause investigation is warranted. Not all nonconforming events are significant enough to justify the time and effort spent to mitigate a one-time error. A review of the tracking system should inform management if the error is significant (i.e., impacting multiple patients or with a negative impact to patient treatment) or if the error is recurrent (i.e., repeated nonconformance that may impact laboratory resources). Significant and recurrent nonconforming events must be investigated and have corrective actions implemented.

An investigation into the underlying cause(s) of a nonconformance (i.e., a root cause analysis) must be performed so that corrective actions that are implemented may mitigate any potential for the event to happen again. The investigation should focus primarily on the system (not the personnel) where the error occurred and include peripheral systems when appropriate. There are several formal methods for performing root cause analysis, including fish bone diagrams, five-whys, and cause-and-effect analysis. Laboratory management should identify and use the root cause analysis method that will best aid them in the discovery of the underlying causes of the nonconformance for each situation. It is best to include the input of laboratory staff who routinely perform the work being investigated, especially the employee who identified the nonconformance. There are also times when a formal root cause analysis is not needed to identify procedural changes that may prevent recurrence of an identified nonconformance.

Once the underlying causes of a nonconformance are identified, laboratory management should determine the corrective actions that may be implemented to prevent the laboratory error from recurring. These corrective actions may include adjustments to procedural steps, creation of new worksheets or job aids, or changes to the workflow or physical space. Following the implementation of these procedural changes, the laboratory should monitor the system for recurrence of the identified nonconformance, timeliness of resulting, or an increase in the burden to staff. Be aware that it is possible to implement a well-planned corrective action that has a negative impact on the test system.

### Assessments

The continual assessment of laboratory competence and proficiency is an important component of a quality management program. These processes are mechanisms to confirm that the laboratory has met its quality and scientific objectives on an ongoing basis.

### External Audits

External assessments may serve to fulfill several requirements. Two major types of assessments are for regulatory purposes (required by national, and/or local authorities) and for accreditation purposes (required by accreditation entities). Some common factors involved in determining whether mandatory external assessments are required include the physical location of the testing site, the test(s) offered, the complexity of the testing performed, and the environment under which the test results are reported. Such assessments are usually periodic (e.g., on a biennial basis) and may be carried out without advance notice to the laboratory. Nonroutine assessments may be conducted when there are allegations of noncompliance with accreditation and/or regulatory requirements or when there are changes to laboratory services, location, and/or ownership.

### Internal Audits

The role of internal audit is to provide assurance that the laboratory's SOPs are followed and that internal control and risk management processes are operating effectively. Laboratories should conduct internal audits at planned intervals to determine whether the quality management system is implemented and maintained.

- Audits are often conducted by laboratory personnel trained to assess the quality management system; auditors should be objective and impartial. Auditors normally should not audit their own activities; however, self-assessment often proves useful to prepare for a formal internal, or external, audit. Audit criteria, scope, frequency, and methods should be defined and documented.
- Personnel responsible for the area being audited should take prompt action when nonconformities are identified.
- The quality management system should be subject to regular internal audits; at least once each year is recommended.

### Proficiency Testing

Proficiency testing and external quality assessment programs usually utilize simulated patient specimens prepared from a common pool that are analyzed by the laboratories enrolled in the program. Results are returned to the organizer and are evaluated to determine the acceptability of each laboratory's performance. These programs have been integral to modern medical laboratories for the past 50 years, and most regulatory and voluntary accreditation programs require participation in such schemes for assessing laboratory performance and verifying the accuracy and reliability of test results. Furthermore, proficiency testing provides valuable information in addition to comparative laboratory performance such as in measurement uncertainty, traceability, reference materials, education, and national infrastructure. ISO 15189 requires participation in interlaboratory comparisons and recommends that programs be selected that provide clinically relevant challenges that mimic patient samples and have the effect of checking the entire examination process, including preexamination and postexamination procedures. Often the proficiency test programs available to laboratories are those deemed acceptable to the regulatory or accrediting body.

A great deal of information can be obtained by review of results from proficiency testing programs. Unfortunately, considerable time may have passed since the analyses and the return of the results so that nonconformities may be difficult to resolve unambiguously, so prompt review is beneficial.

When no external program exists, the laboratory may evaluate the accuracy of testing through an internal proficiency testing program that may include performance of split-sample comparisons (patient and/or QC samples) with another validated method, evaluation of clinical outcomes, blind testing of specimens with known results, or other equivalent system. For microscopic tests not included in a proficiency testing program, the laboratory supervisor or director may retest a random sample of specimens throughout the year while assessing all testing personnel.

**Continual Improvement**

The laboratory quality management system should establish a means to continually improve laboratory testing and quality assurance processes. This system should rely on objective data to analyze and improve processes. Laboratory management should be mindful that attempts to improve testing services may result in unforeseen harm to a test system. Changes in laboratory testing should be planned, analyzed, and monitored to ensure that improvements in testing services are being made.

1) Preventive actions: employees should have a system for identifying and reporting to management *potential* sources of error or opportunities to make improvements to laboratory procedures. The technical staff should be empowered by management to implement changes in a thoughtful way in cooperation with management to reduce the temptation for staff to not follow established procedures. Depending on the procedural change, a re-evaluation of the method may be required.
2) Quality monitoring: quality monitoring encompasses high level processes by which data is evaluated to monitor the overall performance of a given process. Quality monitors should be established for high-risk procedures or when quality improvement initiatives have recently been made. Some examples of common quality monitors are

   - Tracking the turnaround time of testing from specimen received to result reporting.
   - Tracking the positivity rate of molecular assays to detect contamination.
   - Tracking the number of unsatisfactory specimens and the reason.
   - Tracking the number and type of reporting errors.

   Quality monitors that are used to monitor high-risk processes should include a threshold at which some action will be taken to correct the deviation in performance.

3) Quality improvement projects: quality improvements should be made in a thoughtful manner. They should rely on objective data to quantify the problem to be addressed. Data monitors should be established before

any change in testing is made to ensure that a problem exists and is not just perceived to exist. The scope of the improvement project should be clearly stated.

After implementing a change to a procedure with the intention of making an improvement, the system should be monitored by gathering data as described earlier. In this way, you will be able to compare both before implementation and after implementation data to objectively determine the outcome of the improvement project. Management should also be mindful of any increased burden to staff and ensure that any improvements that increase the burden are worth it in the context of objective evidence.

## Conclusions

It has been estimated that 60%–70% of all clinical decisions are based at least in part on the results of laboratory testing. Patient outcomes rely heavily on the work performed in the laboratory, and work is only as reliable and accurate as the quality efforts described in this chapter. There is only 1 way to prove that these quality efforts (although they may be included in policies and procedures) were, in fact, implemented and executed, and that is through record-keeping.

Detailed records represent the scientific accountability required to recreate as best as possible the preexamination, examination, and post-examination processes for any specific sample that leads to a clinical result and impacts the patient outcome.

There are many resources, guidelines, and templates that can assist in the success of your organization such as, but not limited to, the resources from the following organizations: CLSI, American Society of Microbiology, and CAP.

## References

1. Clinical and Laboratory Standards Institute. Harmonized terminology database. Available at: https://clsi.org/standards-development/harmonized-terminology-database. Accessed February 6, 2019.
2. International Organization for Standardization. ISO 9000:2015. Available at: https://www.iso.org/standard/45481.html. Accessed February 6, 2019.
3. International Organization for Standardization. ISO 15189:2012. Available at: https://www.iso.org/standard/56115.html. Accessed February 6, 2019.
4. College of American Pathologists. Available at: https://www.cap.org. Accessed January 23, 2019.
5. International Organization for Standardization. ISO/IEC guide 51:2014. Available at: https://www.iso.org/standard/53940.html. Accessed February 6, 2019.

[L. Farnsworth, R. Rej, S. Hearn]

# ANIMAL, FOOD, AND ENVIRONMENTAL TESTING IN SUPPORT OF COMMUNICABLE DISEASE CONTROL: A ONE HEALTH APPROACH

The term "One Health" is used to describe the collaborative consideration of the human, animal, and environmental factors around optimal health. Human factors include behavioral and medical considerations, including cultural, political, and other socioeconomic drivers for disease. Food, as a requirement for human and animal health, plays a key role in providing nutrition and must be safe to prevent disease introduction. Changes in the environment have an impact on populations of disease carriers, such as rodents and insects, and our ability to control them. Animal exposure to contaminated food translates to potential human exposure and disease, especially with the increase in companion animals and pets. Animal ingestion of contaminated feed can contaminate the animals as a food supply and, if mishandled or improperly processed, can contaminate the human or animal that ingests them. Understanding the consequences of animal proximity to food sources and the use of fertilizers derived from animal matter is also an important consideration for this holistic approach.

Knowledge of this synergy can help prevent diseases in humans and animals and help with management of the environment. Several zoonotic or vector-borne diseases, such as human rabies transmitted via dog bites and yellow fever transmitted by mosquitoes, are now more controllable or manageable using One Health approaches. Control or prevention is best achieved through integrated public health, food and feed safety, veterinary medicine, animal management, and ecological approaches. The responsibility may shift not only to farmers and veterinarians ensuring the health of animals so that people do not become infected with a disease but also to public health practitioners, or even to the general public using improved kitchen hygiene and behavior, since not all premarket contamination is absolutely preventable. For example, farmers and veterinarians work to reduce infection of poultry by *Campylobacter* spp., public health services (such as USDA workers) reduce contamination of meat, and public health workers and the public increase preventive measures in the kitchen through proper hygiene and cooking to the correct internal temperature.

Laboratories play a role in supporting One Health by assuring that the laboratory diagnosis of zoonotic diseases occurs in a timely fashion. The incorporation of testing for rapidly emerging diseases is necessary, and the response to outbreaks using surveillance systems helps break the cycle of disease. The control and prevention of communicable diseases in humans is supported through laboratory practice and through the appropriate testing of human specimens; however, there are many circumstances for which the testing of animal specimens, environmental samples, and food samples is also required. This chapter describes these 3 areas (animals, environment, and foods ingested by humans and animals) of testing and their significance to health. Coordination of testing for these 3 realms and the communication of results contribute to more rapid diagnoses and better disease prevention.

## Food Analysis

### *Relevance of human and animal food analysis*

CDC estimates that 48 million people become ill, 128,000 are hospitalized, and 3,000 die from foodborne diseases each year in the USA. The global burden of foodborne disease is considerable and affects individuals of all ages, particularly children younger than 5 years of age and persons living in resource poor regions of the world. Societal impacts from lost lives, lost labor, lost wages, and lost revenue in the food industry, and its subsequent impact, are substantial. Molecular techniques and information management have transformed foodborne disease investigation. With the advent of molecular subtyping networks such as PulseNet in the USA, laboratory surveillance has become indispensable for the detection of multijurisdictional foodborne outbreaks. PulseNet is a system that links bacterial isolates that are dispersed in a wide geographic area and facilitates cluster analysis, faster outbreak investigations, timelier interventions, and prevention of illness and death.[1] This type of system can also demonstrate links between animals, the environment, and humans. Even the food eaten by animals can contaminate the humans that feed them if proper precautions are not taken.

Laboratories are part of a multidisciplinary team when performing food testing for regulatory action or for foodborne illness investigation. The success of government activities (federal, state, and local) to protect the public health often depends on the ability of laboratories to quickly and accurately analyze samples.

### *Laboratory types*

In the USA, when a food product has been found to be in violation of the Food, Drug, and Cosmetic Act,[2] FDA uses its field laboratories to analyze samples and report results for regulatory action. State and local laboratories, many within departments of agriculture or public health, also have the capability to analyze samples collected from within their respective jurisdictions.

### *Collaborators*

- FDA operates high-throughput field laboratories, located strategically across the continental USA and Puerto Rico, to support FDA's mission to protect the public health and to create new knowledge in the field of regulatory science.
- The USDA Food Safety and Inspection Service has a system consisting of regulatory laboratories that coordinate and conduct laboratory analytical services in support of the agency's farm-to-table strategies in

the disciplines of chemistry, microbiology, and pathology for food safety in meat, poultry, and egg products.

- CDC has branches responsible for tracking the occurrence of foodborne illnesses, managing the deoxyribonucleic acid (DNA) fingerprinting network (i.e., PulseNet) for foodborne illness-causing bacteria in all states to detect outbreaks, and collaborating with state and local health departments to develop new and better methods to detect, investigate, respond to, and control outbreaks. The CDC laboratories provide reference diagnostic services for unusual or difficult to identify bacteria and provide consultation and training to empower public health partners at local, national, and international levels.
- Many states and some local jurisdictions have laboratories that perform testing for human and animal foods. Often, this testing is performed in state departments of agriculture laboratories, but this testing may also reside in the state or local public health, animal health, or environmental laboratories. The capabilities vary, but some basic capabilities include testing for food safety concerns such as microbiological contamination, unapproved food components, chemical and heavy metal contaminants, pesticides residues, filth contamination, and other health and safety issues. During a human or animal outbreak investigation involving a suspected food, a state or local laboratory may also be involved by providing linkages of the contaminated food to the human or animal illness, or noninvolvement of a food item.

As governmental food safety partners move toward more preventive-based approaches to food safety, including widespread surveillance efforts, the demand for laboratories that meet recognized best practices of analytical competency has risen dramatically. Regulatory agencies must utilize laboratory data expeditiously to identify, prevent, and remove unsafe food products from the marketplace. Considering the rapid globalization of food markets and the growing pressure to ensure that all human and animal food is safe for consumption, it has never been more important to leverage the resources of the nation's governmental food laboratories and join forces to take a prevention-based approach to food safety.

US governmental food testing laboratories have been tasked with adopting a standardized quality management system to assure validity, reliability, and timeliness of reporting defensible test results. In addition to accredited federal laboratories, state laboratories have received federal funding to become accredited under the international standard ISO/IEC 17025 for human and animal food testing. By spring 2017, at least 35 state human and animal food testing laboratories were accredited to the ISO/IEC 17025 standard.[3]

### *Sampling practices*

It is imperative to communicate with the laboratory to ensure that appropriate samples are submitted and that the laboratory has the analytical capabilities needed to prevent testing delays. Transport to the laboratory should ensure the sample remains intact and is protected from environmental degradation (e.g., exposure to heat or cold). Considerations for sampling procedures for human and animal food include determination of sample quality criteria, determination of material properties, and application of sampling theory. The resulting sampling protocol will specify minimum mass or volume needed, minimum number of increments, selection of increment location, sample integrity requirements, sampling tools and equipment, and quality control, resulting in defensible measurement data.[4]

### *Analysis*

Food analysis occurs for various reasons, including assurance of quality, assurance of sterility, assurance of food processing procedure, and assurance of safety. There are many reasons samples are sent to a regulatory food testing laboratory (a) to document and expand the regulatory food inspection, (b) to follow up on previous laboratory or inspection findings, (c) to assist in monitoring the establishment (such as grocery store, manufacturer, or distributor) affected by contamination, (d) as part of the foodborne illness investigation, or (e) because of suspected tampering or bioterrorism threat. Meaningful laboratory results are a combination of sample quality criteria, ensuring chain of custody from sample collection to reporting and destruction, performing fit-for-purpose testing (i.e., performing the test that gives the best results for the question to be answered), ensuring turnaround time is optimum, providing actionable results based on quality testing, and sharing of data.

### *Safety*

When sampling human and animal food, knowledge of a potential microbial or chemical hazard is required to decide on personal protective equipment to be used. This may consist of gloves and items for personal hygiene. However, other hazards should not be ignored, especially if sampling in industrial areas such as grain towers or warehouses.

### *Methods*

The laboratory can provide testing results that are qualitative (i.e., presence or absence of contaminant) or quantitative (i.e., how much of specific component is present or how many microbial colonies grew from the contaminated food). Other types of laboratory results are as follows: presumptive, confirmatory, and investigatory. Presumptive results are the information a laboratory can release rapidly (usually within 48 hours) after sample testing has begun. These results are from rapid screening methods (i.e., rapid methods) such as DNA-based tests (i.e., polymerase chain reaction [PCR]). Regulatory actions cannot be taken based on presumptive results because false-positive results may occur. However, this may allow diversion of potentially contaminated raw products to be destroyed or to a process with a kill step to ensure no contamination can be spread. Many food processing steps are taken to kill pathogenic bacteria, leaving behind traces of nonviable cells and DNA, which may be detected in a screening test. Only after the laboratory releases confirmatory results can regulatory action be taken. Confirmatory results are provided by methods that consist of bacterial growth of the actual contaminant or chemical identification. Confirmation for a microbiological contaminant ensures that the bacteria are viable and could potentially cause disease. Investigatory results are available when a laboratory provides information that can help in foodborne illness investigation or traceback investigation. Details for some of the investigatory results are described later in this chapter. Laboratory results are reported to the relevant authorities to provide data for defensible decisions and necessary actions.

### *Interpreting laboratory test results*

The selection of methods for food testing is a crucial and complex process. Many factors must be considered before selecting a method, including, but not limited to, purpose of testing (i.e., regulatory or emergency investigation), method source, throughput, accuracy, validation, robustness, precision, and practicality. Methods used for routine regulatory testing are often well validated, verified that they work within the laboratory using them for testing, and consistent with the ISO/IEC 17025 standard.[3] However, testing used for outbreaks and emergency investigations may require some situational method development. Each food commodity has a physical or chemical characteristic that can influence how a food matrix is tested and, consequently, how accurate results are. For example, natural bacteria flora found in certain food products can cause difficulty in the detection of foodborne pathogens. They can either provide false-positive results or entirely overgrow any foodborne pathogens leading to nondetection of the target. If the laboratory has not validated that specific food matrix and is unaware of natural bacteria flora, it could provide an erroneous interpretation of the results. An ISO/IEC 17025–accredited laboratory follows best practices to determine if the method is fit for purpose such as method validation, method verification, and matrix extension to include different food types in the method. In routine situations, time between sample collections and laboratory results could range from 1 to 3 weeks for an official sample result to be released, particularly if it is a confirmed result and includes potential strain typing.

Pulsed field gel electrophoresis (PFGE): bacterial DNA fingerprinting is an example of additional information that a laboratory can provide to help an investigation. Laboratories submit the DNA fingerprint (i.e., PFGE pattern) of their bacterial isolates to the PulseNet team at CDC. The PulseNet team has the role of comparing fingerprint data submitted from across the USA and to monitor foodborne pathogen occurrence over time using the PulseNet database. CDC looks for groups of matching patterns (clusters) with higher than normal incidence. By monitoring trends in PFGE patterns using the clustering detection tool BioNumerics, the PulseNet team can rapidly identify increases in case submissions from across the USA in real-time and quickly launch investigations into the cause of reported illnesses. Locally, laboratories can compare PFGE patterns and inform state regulators about contamination reoccurrence from the same establishment. PFGE can be used to determine with more accuracy which illnesses are part of an outbreak and which are not; to determine which ingredient in a multi-ingredient food is responsible for an outbreak; to identify geographic regions from which a contaminated ingredient may have originated; to differentiate sources of contamination, even within the same outbreak; to link illnesses to a processing facility even before the food product vector has been identified; to link small numbers of illnesses that otherwise might not have been identified as common outbreak; and to identify unlikely routes of contamination. CDC has plans to phase out PFGE in 2019 and replace with whole genome sequencing (WGS).

Whole genome sequencing: WGS is considered the next generation of DNA fingerprinting. WGS reveals the complete DNA makeup of an organism, enabling better understanding of variations both within and between species. FDA has used this technology since 2008 to perform basic microbial identification during foodborne illness outbreaks. WGS provides the same function as PFGE but has the additional power to differentiate virtually all strains of foodborne pathogens, no matter what the species. Its ability to differentiate between even closely related microbial organisms allows outbreaks to be detected with fewer clinical cases and provides the opportunity to stop outbreaks sooner and avoid additional illnesses. The GenomeTrakr network[5] is the first distributed network of laboratories to utilize WGS for pathogen identification. It consists of public health, agricultural, and university laboratories that collect and share genomic and geographic data from foodborne pathogens. The data, which are housed in public databases at the US National Center for Biotechnology Information (NCBI), can be accessed by researchers and public health officials for real time comparison and analysis that promises to speed foodborne illness outbreak investigations and reduce foodborne illnesses and deaths.

### *Coordination*

When food contamination investigations are being carried out in cases in which regulatory actions may be considered, interdisciplinary/jurisdictional coordination is required. It is important to ensure connections are present prior to events occurring. Acceptance of data created by state or local jurisdictions by federal agencies is paramount and is critical when a contaminated food item is found in multiple states, especially when linked to human or animal illness. Assurance that the sample was collected, and the testing was performed so that the result is defensible, is critical for action to be taken and the food removed from sale. Intraorganizational collaboration is essential to ensure laboratory testing is valid and can support programs. Coordination among all entities, including management, sample collector, regulatory program, and laboratory is necessary before undertaking sampling activities. Governmental human and animal food testing laboratories in the USA may belong to several national networks, including, but not limited to, the Food Emergency Response Network (FERN), the Laboratory Response Network (LRN), and PulseNet. As part of these networks, the laboratory has access to information, such as methods and best practices, used among the cohort of laboratories performing similar testing for similar reasons. These networks help to increase capacity during a major event and help with ensuring the latest technologies and practices are utilized for this important testing.

- The FERN integrates the nation's food-testing laboratories at the local, state, and federal levels into a network able to respond to emergencies involving biological, chemical, or radiological contamination of food. The FERN structure is organized to ensure federal and state interagency participation and cooperation in the formation, development, and operation of the network.
- The LRN is charged with the task of maintaining an integrated network of state and local public health, federal, military, and international laboratories that can respond to bioterrorism, chemical terrorism, and other public health emergencies. The LRN is a unique asset in the nation's growing preparedness for biological and chemical terrorism; it links state and local public health laboratories, veterinary, agriculture, military, and water- and food-testing laboratories.
- FDA's rapid response teams (RRT) are an initiative consisting of multiagency (i.e., federal, state, and local) to respond to human and animal food emergencies. The laboratory provides evidence of food contamination and data for foodborne illness investigation.
- The Manufactured Food Regulatory Program Standards (MFRPS) are a critical component in establishing the national Integrated Food Safety System (IFSS). The goal of the MFRPS is to implement a nationally integrated, risk-based, food safety system focused on protecting public health. The MFRPS establishes a uniform basis for measuring and improving the performance of prevention, intervention, and response activities of manufactured food regulatory programs in the USA. The laboratory is included in the MFRPS Standard 10-Laboratory Services,[6] which includes the use of an ISO/IEC 17025-accredited laboratory.
- The Animal Feed Regulatory Program Standards (AFRPS) is similar to MFRPS, establishing animal food standards to uniform foundation for the design and management of State programs responsible for the regulation of animal food. The laboratory is included in the AFRPS Standard 10-Laboratory Services.[7]

- Other networks that a human and animal food testing laboratory may be part of include CaliciNet, CryptoNet, FoodNet, VetLIRN, PulseNet (see description of pulsed field gel electrophoresis earlier), GenomeTrakr (see description of whole genome sequencing earlier), and PETNet, among others.

Note that the coordination of food testing networks in this section makes specific reference to US-based networks. It is imperative that clinical and public health laboratories located in countries other than the USA familiarize themselves with the various food-testing networks, facilities, and regulations that exist within their jurisdictions. (For further information, see "Laboratory Referral Networks.")

### *Impact*

Results from the sampling is interpreted to assess the level of human and animal food contamination, what risk it poses to exposed people, and what remediation will be required to remove the source.

## Environmental Sampling

### *Relevance of environmental sampling*

While the majority of human infections are spread human-to-human, contracted from animal exposures, or ingested from food, there are infections that have a completely environmental source (e.g, legionellosis, melioidosis, aspergillosis, histoplasmosis) or can be contracted from water ingestion (e.g., giardiasis, Norovirus infection), animal products (e.g., anthrax), working environments (e.g., anthrax, legionellosis,), or air (e.g., tuberculosis, influenza). To elucidate the source of such infections and to implement preventative measures, environmental sampling for the presence of pathogenic microorganisms may be necessary. Locating the source of an environmental infection can be essential in preventing ongoing outbreaks of infection. For example, in the case of Legionnaires disease, the location of numerous water systems which have the potential to generate aerosols must be mapped and samples taken. To be effective, the sampling and analysis for environmental sampling must be done with understanding of the constraints and limitations of these processes. While standards are generally available for sampling water and food, for other matrices there will often be no standard methods available, and the detection limits of assays may be unknown. Expert opinion will be needed to interpret any results in terms of risk to the exposed. For example, a pathogen found at a concentration of 1 microorganism per liter of drinking water will not generally be an infection risk for a population.

### *Laboratory types*

Environmental sampling takes place outside the laboratory; however, the analysis of these samples occurs within laboratories. For certain sample types, such as water, there are normally specialized laboratories set up to deal with these samples. In larger countries, there may be specialist laboratories for a range of sample types either within the public health, government, academia, or commercial sectors. However, in many countries, environmental samples are analyzed within public health laboratories using routine analysis, but the results need to be analyzed and assessed by those who carried out the sampling.

### *Collaborators*

Environmental testing should be carried out in conjunction with epidemiologists, who will provide information about the likely source of infection, and with experts who understand the environment being tested. Both can provide input about locations where the sampling should be undertaken. Local environmental health officers may have insight into regulatory requirements of sampling.

### *Sampling practices*

Special sampling considerations are as follows:

- Water: sampling water for the presence of pathogens requires knowledge of the body of water or water system being sampled. Samples should be collected in sterile receptacles containing biostatic substances such as sodium thiosulfite to prevent further growth during transport and storage. Large volumes need to be taken to ensure that low concentrations of agents can be detected following filtration. For water systems samples, decisions may need to be made as to where and when samples should be taken (i.e., should samples be taken when the tap is opened or after a period of flow). The first sample type will give an indication of residual contamination within the tap, and the second will give a better indication of contamination in the water supply. Advice on sampling of water is often available on a national and international basis. For example, in the UK there is detailed guidance freely available for the sampling and analysis of recreational water, drinking water, and hospital water (see Standing Committee of Analysts, Public Health England, and Environment Agency guidelines).
- Surfaces: sampling of surfaces for the presence of microorganisms can be carried out using a variety of swabbing and sponging techniques, many of which are commercially available. The type of surfaces to be tested will guide the choice of the technique to be used. No method will be 100% efficient, and many may be significantly lower than 50% efficient especially from complex surfaces such as carpeting. Thus, technique validation is of utmost importance. For surface samples, that are loosely attached (i.e., dust), vacuum-based filtration samplers that may be used.[8]
- Air: contamination of the air with microorganisms can be transient and highly localized. Therefore, decisions on when and where to sample are

of utmost importance to ensuring that the data obtained is relevant. Sampling the air for microorganisms requires the use of specialized air sampling equipment. These include the following: impactors which collect microorganisms on a surface, normally an agar plate or a microscope slide; impingers that collect microorganisms into liquid; and filtration that collects microorganisms onto filters.[9] Each of these methods may damage and inactivate airborne microorganisms. Polymerase chain reaction and other methods can be used that do not rely on microorganisms surviving the collection process. The drawback of these methods is how to determine whether the aerosol detected is infectious. Before sampling is undertaken, a sampling strategy needs to be defined. The rationale for the sampling needs to be agreed upon. Is it an aerosol generating process (e.g., a fountain, a composting process), personnel exposure (i.e., dose over a working day), or the aerosol concentration in an environment that is of interest? The following factors must be taken account when sampling and they should be recorded:

- Environmental factors (wind direction, sunlight, temperature, relative humidity).
- Location (static, on-person).
- Sample duration (short to capture an event, long to ensure capture of an agent).
- Activities occurring during sampling.

### *Sampling strategy*

It is important for any environmental sampling activity to have confidence in the interpretation of a negative result. To give an example, when a large field thought to have been used for burial of anthrax contaminated cattle carcasses is to be sampled for the presence of *Bacillus anthracis* in the top soil, how is confidence in a negative result affirmed? It is unfeasible to sample all the soil in the field, as this would be prohibitively expensive. There are 2 approaches that could be taken. First, an intelligence-based approach could be used (i.e., information is gathered on the location of any known cattle burial sites and sampling is only undertaken in these areas). Second, if evidence of the area of the burial sites is unknown, then statistical methods can be used to determine the number of samples required to give confidence that the field is free of the agent.

### *Analysis*

Environmental samples will often be analyzed using standard laboratory techniques after transportation to laboratories. If there are no specialist laboratories available, samples can be analyzed using preexisting methodologies within clinical or public health laboratories. However, environmental samples will be in different forms, and this may require modification of existing protocols.

For samples taken using complex media, the agent may need to be isolated from a community of microorganisms, some which may be present at higher concentrations than the agent of interest. If recovery of the agent in a viable form is required, then a stratagem to preferentially recover will need to be developed. This could involve the use of selective media containing compounds toxic to competing agents, the use of an enrichment step to enable the selective growth of the agent of interest, or the use of a separation step normally using antibodies to concentrate the agent of interest. If using PCR, special extraction kits may be used that are developed for different matrices, such as soil or water. Whole genome sampling methods can be used to provide strong confirmation of a link between the environmental sample and the resulting infection.

### *Safety*

When sampling air, water, and other environments, knowledge of the potential microbial hazard will be required to decide on the personal protective equipment required. In normal circumstances this will consist of gloves and items for maintaining personal hygiene. For aerosol risks, the use of respiratory protective equipment may be needed. In many instances, the major risk of sampling will not be related to the agent but may be related to the area being sampled. Sampling in industrial areas and bodies of water will have their own hazards, and good communication with the site owner and safety staff will be required.

### *Coordination*

When there is a suspected environmental source of contamination leading to human or animal infection, it is possible that the person responsible for the environment in question may not have conformed to legislation and may be regarded as negligent; a criminal or civil prosecution may ensue. In these instances, coordination with law enforcement agencies or regulatory authorities will be required, and care must be taken in documenting sample methods analysis and ensuring chain of custody procedures are closely followed.

### *Impact*

Results from the sampling will need to be interpreted to assess the level of environmental contamination, what risk it poses to exposed people, and what remediation will be required to remove the source. Expert knowledge in disease transmission from the environment will be required to assess the results. Just because an agent is detected in an environment does not mean it poses a risk to the public or was the cause of an outbreak. Therefore, the sampling and analysis should be designed to allow a quantitative assessment of the concentration of the microorganism in the environment and not just presence/absence data. For negative results, a detection limit value should be established.

## Animal Sampling

### *Relevance of animal sampling*

Zoonoses, diseases transmitted from animals to people, have always impacted human health and represent a large proportion of emerging infections. Animal sampling is an important component of public health investigation and laboratory response efforts done for communicable disease control. Historically, animal testing has been an integral part of assessing rabies risk when humans or domestic animals have a suspect bite or nonbite exposure. This type of animal testing is conducted by state public health and other laboratories in the USA. Capacity for rabies testing is maintained by many public health laboratories as a core function. However, brucellosis, tuberculosis, and many vector borne diseases are also historically important diseases for which animal testing is routinely a component of public health testing and human case investigations. Many of these diseases are important in causing both human and animal health problems; therefore, testing may occur in both public and animal health laboratories.

Over time, it has become clear that there is more disease transmission between animals and people than was previously thought. We have learned this from both doing more testing and using more sophisticated tests. The interactions between animals and humans have also changed through the development of suburban communities that support sometimes large populations of wildlife (e.g., deer, raccoons, and ducks) and closer physical contact by family members with a wide variety of household pets. Additionally, the increasing number of immunocompromised persons are susceptible to infections from animals that do not affect healthy people. Exotic pets, possibly with exotic pathogens, are becoming ever more popular. Animal testing is needed to assist with the understanding of these zoonotic emerging diseases and their animal reservoirs or as part of the investigation of zoonotic disease outbreaks.

There are numerous examples of animal testing during zoonotic disease outbreak investigations. Zoonotic viral, bacterial, and parasitic microorganisms have caused illness in humans irrespective of whether clinical illness is seen in the animal carrying the organisms. Public health investigations may look for serologic evidence or attempt to isolate the outbreak organism from animals or the animal environment (also discussed in this chapter). Outbreak examples for different pathogens include Seoul virus in rats, *Escherichia coli* O157:H7 in ruminants, *Salmonella* linked to live poultry, and *Cryptosporidium* associated with dairy calves.

Broad considerations when conducting animal sampling and testing include the species, the individual animal versus herd or flock-level testing, the sample size to detect the organism or antibodies, as well as numerous other factors.

### *Laboratory types*

Animal testing for public health purposes is generally secondary to the human health investigation. The laboratory involved depends on the disease agent and animal species of concern. In general, USDA Veterinary Services and state agriculture laboratories oversee testing of diseases in food production animals, including bovine tuberculosis, brucellosis, and animal influenza. In some cases, these diseases are also a priority for the animal health agency and the focus of a program to control or eradicate pathogens from animals. The US National Wildlife Health Center performs diagnostic testing of wildlife diseases, including avian influenza, West Nile virus, and chronic wasting disease. USDA Wildlife Services conducts animal testing for rabies as part of the US National Rabies Control Program, which oversees the Oral Rabies Vaccination campaign.

Public health agencies perform testing of pets when they are implicated as a potential source of human illness (e.g., *Campylobacter* transmission from sick puppies to people). Public health agencies also do most animal rabies testing. Public health agencies may also be involved in animal testing when animals are asymptomatic carriers of human pathogens (e.g., Shiga toxin-producing *E. coli* (STEC), *Salmonella*, hantavirus, and lymphocytic choriomeningitis virus) or for diagnosis of exotic pathogens (e.g., monkey pox, Ebola) and pathogens of bioterrorism concern (e.g., plague and tularemia). Leprosy, which in the southern USA may be linked to exposure to infected armadillos, is diagnosed by the National Hansen's Disease Program at the Health Resources and Services Administration. Some public health agencies utilize animal sampling and testing for sentinel surveillance routinely. For example, some agencies use sentinel chicken flocks in addition to mosquito pool testing for situational awareness and public messaging when arboviruses are actively circulating in communities.

University laboratories may be valuable partners as well. Veterinary diagnostic laboratories may provide pet, food, and exotic and wildlife animal testing. The US National B Virus Resource Center is housed at Georgia State University; entomology laboratories at universities can perform laboratory identification and pathogen testing of vectors to help assess the risk for human disease from vector-borne diseases.

In addition to accepting diagnostic specimens, state agriculture and university-based animal diagnostic laboratories may offer gross and histopathology services.

### *Collaborators*

Animal testing for public health purposes generally should involve partnerships with animal health professionals. The partnerships may differ depending on the organism, the animal species involved, and by state. The state public health veterinarian and the state agriculture veterinarian's office can provide guidance on how animal specimens should best be collected and handled. Veterinarians in private practice, clinical faculty from veterinary schools, and animal health technicians have also assisted in animal sampling. These collaborators, in addition to wildlife agencies, biologists, and wildlife veterinarians, often have species-specific expertise and can serve as important resources.

***Sampling practices***

Special sampling considerations may be necessary for animal sampling. For some animals, anesthesia may be necessary and should be done in a humane manner. For some populations, sample size considerations and the objectives of animal testing should be discussed in advance. Various sampling designs should be evaluated depending on the herd or flock, whether the population of animals is domestic or wild, and the availability of experienced personnel to collect samples. Different sample types (e.g., whole blood, serum, stool, urine) require varying levels of expertise to collect, and considering in advance the restraint, sample handling, and other species-specific factors is critical. A critical element in animal sampling is to coordinate with the laboratory doing the testing to be sure samples are labeled correctly with all relevant and required information. Additionally, the testing laboratory should be consulted in advance regarding the testing capacity, sample handling, sample shipment, desired testing, and anticipated timeline for results. Coordination and communication regarding sampling, submission, and testing in advance are important for the testing laboratory. In addition, often environmental sampling, which is discussed elsewhere (e.g., swabs, manure, aquarium water), may accompany the live animal samples.

***Safety***

Safety is a major concern for animal testing. If the specimen is taken directly from the animal, it is always important to plan carefully. Animal handling and sampling are impacted greatly by the experience of persons handling the animals and by the facilities that are available. The risk for bites, scratches, and other injuries is high even when handling normally friendly animals. Animals can sense stress and can become nervous or even fractious with unfamiliar people and unfamiliar procedures. Involve an experienced animal handler whenever possible to limit the risk of injury to both persons and animals. Stressful situations can also impact the shedding of pathogens from animals. A carefully planned sampling strategy where the animal is sufficiently restrained not to cause harm for as short a time period as possible is important to get accurate samples. Special considerations should be given to sampling of large animal species, such as elephants suspected to be infected with tuberculosis, and proper facilities and restraints (including chemical restraints) should be utilized to minimize the risk of human injuries. Use of personal protective equipment such as gloves, gowns, masks and safety goggles should also be considered depending on the potential route of transmission of the agent of concern. Environmental contamination can occur from organisms shed in body fluids, such as enteric pathogens and herpes B virus. Care needs to be taken when doffing personal protective equipment to limit accidental exposures. When the doffing is complete, it is important to wash hands. Thorough handwashing with soap and water is always important after handling animals and animal specimens.

***Methods***

Diverse laboratory testing methods are used in public health and other reference laboratories. If the organism of concern is not known, then traditional culturing methodologies for bacteria and viruses are often used. Biochemical and serological techniques have historically been used to speciate and type organisms. *Salmonella*, for example, have more than 2,000 serotypes. Most human infections are caused by a subset of these (i.e., <100). *E. coli* O157:H7 and other Shiga toxin-producing organisms that can cause bloody diarrhea and kidney disease are also differentiated by serotyping. Typing is often done in public health laboratories, since the information is primarily used to characterize and contain outbreaks and is not for patient care. Automated techniques, which are faster, are continually being developed for organism identification, including mass spectrometry (e.g., matrix-assisted laser desorption/ionization time-of-flight or MALDI-TOF) and PCR. Polymerase chain reaction requires that the organism of concern is known or strongly suspected. The PCR test and other genetic tests involve probes with a known genetic code that bind to genetic materials from the organism and then get amplified into gene segments that can be detected. The gene segments can be further characterized by sequencing the amplified DNA product.

PFGE and more recently WGS are tests used to detect clusters of genetically related organisms. These methods have been used to identify and initiate outbreaks and outbreak response. These tests help further characterize (i.e., type) organisms, and are used to complement, or in lieu of, serotyping, which was discussed earlier. Both tests are designed to identify closely related organisms. During outbreak investigations involving animals, these methods help determine that bacteria from animals and infected persons are genetically similar or identical. This information is used by epidemiologists to assess transmission routes and aid in understanding zoonotic spread of pathogens.

PFGE data from public health and agriculture laboratories are gathered and analyzed nationally by PulseNet (see Food Analysis section in this chapter for a detailed description) to detect multistate outbreaks. When a series of identical or similar PFGE patterns indicate a suspect outbreak, CDC coordinates with public health department for detailed epidemiological interview, data and food sample collections, and with FDA for potential regulatory actions related to contaminated food sold for consumption. PulseNet has also been used to investigate zoonotic disease outbreaks from pets sold nationally, including dogs, turtles, chickens, hedgehogs, and snakes.

A similar model is being implemented for WGS data. These data sets are large, and scientists are still analyzing the data to determine what genetic variability is biologically meaningful. Not all genes produce proteins that are essential to the infectious process, and some changes in the genetic code have a greater impact on the pathogenicity of the organism than others.

States submit sequence data to the NCBI. The sequences can be analyzed and compared against a national library of strains. Currently, the interpretation of the results is an ongoing collaboration with CDC. Similar to PFGE, the genetic information is reported back to public health laboratory and shared with epidemiology staff. This is still an emerging resource that requires substantial information technology resources and genetic sequence analysis (i.e., bioinformatics) expertise. Many public health laboratories are partnering with universities to help build this diagnostic capacity.

Serology (i.e., immunoglobulin class M [IgM] and immunoglobulin class G [IgG] antibody tests) tests are also available for animals. However, these tests are generally not used for bacteria because of the microorganism's complex outer protein structure. The usefulness of serology (sensitivity and specificity) can vary greatly and is in part dependent on the cross reactivity among related organisms (e.g., influenza viruses). Enzyme-linked immunosorbent assay serologic tests can be specific for either IgM or IgG antibodies to detect acute infection or immunity. Culture-based serologic testing, such as the plaque reduction neutralization test, used for confirmatory arbovirus testing are total antibody tests.

For animal rabies, confirmatory testing is done by immunofluorescent assay. State public health laboratories follow CDC protocols and standardized methods. Testing involves testing brain tissue using anti-rabies virus antibodies labeled with a fluorescent dye. If the brain is infected, the anti-rabies antibodies bind to the tissue, which lights up under the microscope.

Gross and histopathology are also used routinely for animal diagnostic testing, especially in wildlife diagnostics and during animal mortality events. Pathology testing is an important animal disease diagnostic tool when the organism of concern is unknown or difficult to identify. These findings assist during investigations by providing important clues to further direct pathogen or serological testing on animal samples.

Note that the coordination of animal testing in this section makes specific reference to US-based laboratory systems. It is imperative that clinical and public health laboratories located in countries other than the USA familiarize themselves with the various animal-testing networks, facilities, and regulations that exist within their jurisdictions.

### *Impact*

Animal testing done as part of public health investigation is generally done with a clear scientific question in mind, and as a result, often impacts future public health guidance and policy. Sometimes legal actions also occur. Communication between stakeholders and testing laboratories is therefore critical, including attention to appropriate sample handling and documentation. Animal sampling is an important component of public health and is often complimentary to human and environmental sampling.

## Bibliography

### *Food analysis*

Association of Public Health Laboratories. Best Practices for Submission of Actionable Food and Feed Testing Data Generated in State and Local Laboratories. 2017. Available at: https://www.aphl.org/aboutAPHL/publications/Documents/FS-2017Jun-Best-Practices-Food-Feed-Data.pdf. Accessed June 28, 2018.

Association of American Feed Control Officials Laboratory Sampling Working Group. GOOD Test Portions. Available at: https://www.aafco.org/Publications/GOODTestPortions. Accessed June 28, 2018.

### *Environmental sampling*

Environment Agency. Microbiology of recreational and environmental waters: methods for the examination of waters and associated materials. 2000. Available at: http://standingcommitteeofanalysts.co.uk/library/The%20Microbiology%20of%20Recreational%20and%20Environmental%20Waters%20(2000).pdf. Accessed June 28, 2018.

Environmental Agency. The microbiology of drinking water. Part 2. Practices and procedures for sampling. 2010. Available at: https://www.gov.uk/government/uploads/system/uploads/attachment_data/file/316769/MoDW-2-232.pdf. Accessed June 28, 2018.

Public Health England. Examining food, water and environmental samples from healthcare environments: microbiological guidelines. 2013. Available at: https://www.gov.uk/government/uploads/system/uploads/attachment_data/file/446981/Hospital_F_W_E_Microbiology_Guidelines_PHE_format_June_2013.pdf. Accessed June 28, 2018.

### *Animal sampling*

American Association of Zoo Veterinarians. Diagnosis, treatment and management of tuberculosis in elephants in human care. 2017. Available at: http://www.aazv.org/news/370159/2017-Diagnosis-Treatment-and-Management-of-Tuberculosis-in-Elephants-in-Human-Care.htm. Accessed June 28, 2018.

Health Resources and Services Administration. National Hansen's Disease (Leprosy) Clinical Center, Baton Rouge, Louisiana. Available at: https://www.hrsa.gov/hansens-disease/clinical-center.html. Accessed June 28, 2018.

National Association of State Public Health Veterinarians Disease Control Compendia. Available at: http://www.nasphv.org/documentsCompendia.html. Accessed June 28, 2018.

National Association of Public Health Veterinarians. Designated and acting state public health veterinarians. Available at: http://www.nasphv.org/Documents/StatePublicHealthVeterinariansByState.pdf. Accessed June 28, 2018.

US Animal Health Association. State animal health officials. Available at: http://www.usaha.org/upload/STATE_ANIMAL_HEALTH_OFFICIALS.pdf. Accessed June 28, 2018.

US Department of Agriculture. Animal disease laboratory information and services. Available at: https://www.aphis.usda.gov/aphis/ourfocus/animalhealth/lab-info-services. Accessed June 28, 2018.

## References

1. Centers for Disease Control and Prevention. PulseNet. Available at: https://www.cdc.gov/pulsenet/index.html. Accessed February 04, 2019.

2. Food, Drug, and Cosmetic Act, 21 USC §301–399 (2018).
3. International Organization for Standardization. ISO/IEC 17025:2017. Available at: https://www.iso.org/standard/66912.html. Accessed January 23, 2019.
4. Association of American Feed Control Officials. GOODSamples. Available at: https://www.aafco.org/Publications/GOODSamples. Accessed February 4, 2019.
5. US Food and Drug Administration. GenomeTrakr Network. Available at: https://www.fda.gov/Food/FoodScienceResearch/WholeGenomeSequencingProgramWGS/ucm363134.htm. Accessed February 04, 2019.
6. US Food and Drug Administration. Manufactured Food Regulatory Program Standards. Laboratory Services. Standard 10. Available at: https://www.fda.gov/ForFederalStateandLocalOfficials/ProgramsInitiatives/RegulatoryPrgmStnds/ucm475064.htm. Accessed February 5, 2019.
7. US Food and Drug Administration. Animal Feed Regulatory Program Standards. Standard 10. Available at: https://www.fda.gov/ForFederalStateandLocalOfficials/ProgramsInitiatives/RegulatoryPrgmStnds/ucm475063.htm. Accessed February 5, 2019.
8. Estill CF, Baron PA, Beard JK, et al. Recovery efficiency and limit of detection of aerosolized Bacillus anthracis Sterne from environmental surface samples. *Appl Environ Microbiol*. 2009;75(13):4297–4306.
9. Grinshpun SA, Buttner MP, Mainelis G, Willeke K. Sampling for airborne microorganisms. In: Yates MV, Nakatsu CH, Miller RV, Pillai SD, eds. *Manual of Environmental Microbiology*. 4th ed. Washington DC: American Society of Microbiology; 2016.

[C. Blackmore, J. Dunn, M. Ishida, A. Bennett, Y. Salfinger]

# TRANSPORT OF INFECTIOUS SPECIMENS

The need to send specimens and samples to other locations within the same building or further afield for diagnosis, confirmation, and specialist processing or sharing is a regular part of a clinical or public health laboratory activity. The shipping of potentially infectious specimens must comply with national and international standards and regulations.[1] These are intended to give assurance to the shipping companies' operatives and to the general public that there is not significant biohazard risk from these packages when in transit.

Transporting specimens within a hospital also needs to be carried out properly to ensure that they get to the intended location in good condition and without risk to handlers or others who may come into contact with a damaged or leaking package. Common sense must prevail and distance, frequency, potential hazard, who will be handling the specimens, and the complexity of the route should all be taken into account. Normally, tubes that are in racks, or individually contained in plastic bags, within a rigid, closed, suitably marked container are adequate for transporting within a laboratory or facility. Procedures should be in place to respond to a potential incident during the transportation of specimens. The transfer on public roads, by air or other transport means, and across public spaces is regulated locally, nationally, and internationally. These regulations include classification of the infectious material, packaging, labeling, and training in shipping hazardous substances. There are exemptions, and these include the following:

- Dried blood spots, which can be sent in public postal systems.
- Where the material is a licensed medical product.
- Where the infectious material is in an animal or incidental to the shipment (i.e., not the focus or purpose or is not known).
- Where there is minimal risk from the material (e.g., where there is verified inactivation or are human patient specimens where there is no suspicion of infectiousness).
- Examples of specimens that may be transported under this include blood or urine tests to monitor cholesterol levels, blood glucose levels, hormone levels, or prostate specific antigen, and those required to monitor organ function such as heart, liver, or kidney function. These should be marked "exempt human specimen."

**Identification and Classification of the Infectious Specimens**

There are specific criteria for determining the proper shipping category:

- Is there a known or strongly suspected risk of infection from the sample?
- Is the sample infectious to animals?
- Is the sample infectious to humans?
- Is the sample infectious to humans and animals?

Within UN classification,[2] infectious substances are in division 6.2 and assigned to UN 2814, UN 2900, UN 3291, or UN 3373 as appropriate. High consequence pathogen-containing samples or cultures are assigned to category A; all others are category B.

**Packaging and Labeling**

Packaging of potentially infectious specimens normally requires a triple packaging system. All packaging including combinations should be certified (P650 or P620), although there are exemptions for low income countries where certified packaging may not be available, but the alternative must still meet triple packing requirements, including labeling and classification.[3,4] The packaging should meet the following conditions:

1) The packaging should consist of 3 components:

    - A leak-proof primary receptacle(s)
    - A leak-proof secondary packaging

- An outer packaging of adequate strength for its capacity, mass, and intended use, and with at least 1 surface having minimum dimensions of 100 mm x 100 mm

2) For liquids, absorbent material in sufficient quantity to absorb the entire contents must be placed between the primary receptacle(s) and the secondary packaging, so that, during transport, any release or leak of a liquid substance will not reach the outer packaging and will not compromise the integrity of the cushioning material.
3) When multiple fragile primary receptacles are placed in a single secondary packaging, they should be either individually wrapped or separated to prevent contact between them.

Specimen information must be included on the primary container, but a separate information sheet with the same information must be in a waterproof envelope and accessible without opening the secondary packaging. Other information may include consignment documentation and handling instruction on receipt. Labeling must be in English with approved international symbols. The correct UN number must be used if packaging is to pass through customs or border controls. See the next 2 figures for examples of packaging and labeling for category A and category B infectious substances.

**Mode of Transport**

The route of transport is an important consideration, whether by road, rail, air, inland waterways, or by sea, as each has internationally agreed upon

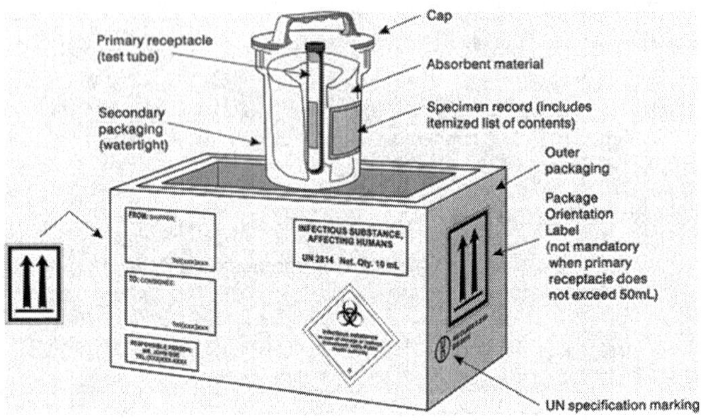


Source: Reprinted with permission. © 2019 International Air Transport Association. All rights reserved. Reproduced under license by the American Public Health Association.

**Example of Triple Packaging System for the Packaging and Labelling of Category A Infectious Substances**

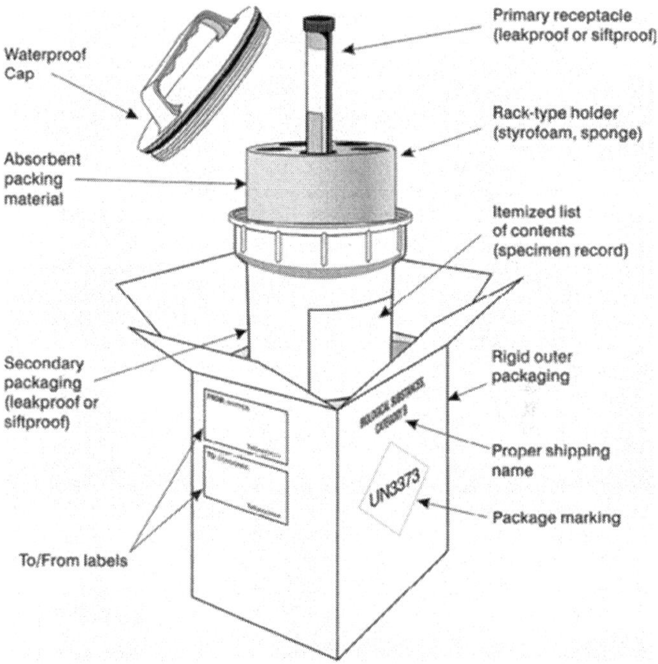


*Source:* Reprinted with permission. 

**Example of the Triple Packaging System for the Packing and Labelling of Category B Infectious Substances**

regulations. Some representative authorities include ADR (European Agreement concerning the International Carriage of Dangerous Goods by Road), RID (Regulations concerning the International Transport of Dangerous Goods by Rail), ADN (European Agreement concerning the International Carriage of Dangerous Goods by Inland Waterways), and IMO (International Maritime Organization).[2,5]

The international regulation for air transport is the International Air Transport Association,[6] which controls air transport of packages and is the most stringent because of the potential for conditions that could damage the package in handling or transport and have the greatest consequence.

The packaging and shipping of potentially biohazardous specimens and materials requires training and periodic certification. There are specialist courier companies and specialist training companies. The rules are complex and may change frequently, so it is necessary to consult with or employ these qualified organizations.

The risks from specimen packages may include the materials that are used to maintain temperature control, such as solid carbon dioxide (i.e., dry ice) or liquid nitrogen, which can cause asphyxiation or expand rapidly. Correct placement of these material is critical, and the hazard they pose must be clearly marked on package with the internationally accepted symbol and notation. Proper documentation must accompany the shipment; this includes the completion of the dangerous goods document for category A shipments. In addition to shipping regulations for hazardous substances, there may also be national prohibitions. Documentation must be country-specific, as required.

It is not permissible to transport specimens in the postal system, personal luggage, on public transport, or in private cars. All packages must be properly labeled and packed by persons who have been specifically trained in the class of hazard packaging. It is important to note that there are specific restrictions on the number of tubes, the volume, and the types of packing material.

### Biosecurity

Packages containing specimens while in transit may be at risk of loss or theft, thus having in place a tracking system and only using responsible and accredited couriers is essential. For the highest risk samples such as those classified as select agents or bioterrorism targets, there are requirements for using tamper-proof packaging and tracking. Best practices[7] dictate that all specimens be logged initially and through any transfers and never left unattended. If high-risk pathogens are suspected to be in the specimen, then prior special permissions to ship, additional security measures, and authorizations to receive are all required.

### Reuse of Packaging

The approved certified packaging is expensive, and some components could be reused if suitable safeguards are in place, such as relabeling and discarding any damaged or contaminated packages.

### Incidents

There are few published incidents of infection arising from specimen transport, but there are frequent examples of poorly packed, damaged, and leaking packages being received in clinical laboratories. It is best practice to record and implement measures to minimize all such incidents. Systems should be in place to record and report back to the original sender any occasions of insufficient information, poor quality samples, or damaged or poorly packed specimens. Safety measures that include the availability of spill kits must be in place to deal with the receipt of damaged, leaking packages.

### References


1. World Health Organization. Guidance on regulations for the transport of infectious substances. 2015. Available at: http://www.who.int/ihr/publications/who_hse_ihr_2015.2/en. Accessed June 27, 2018.
2. World Health Organization. UN recommendations on the transport of dangerous goods: model regulations. 2017. Available at: https://www.unece.org/trans/danger/publi/unrec/rev20/20files_e.html. Accessed June 27, 2018.
3. Centers for Disease Control and Prevention. Interim guidelines for collection, processing and transport of clinical specimens from patients under investigation for Middle East respiratory syndrome (MERS). 2017. Available at: https://www.cdc.gov/coronavirus/mers/guidelines-clinical-specimens.html. Accessed June 27, 2018.
4. World Health Organization. Guidelines for the collection of clinical specimens during field investigation of outbreaks. 2000. Available at: http://apps.who.int/iris/bitstream/handle/10665/66348/WHO_CDS_CSR_EDC_2000.4.pdf;jsessionid=5D2B928C5FC7BCF3769047B0E32F3540?sequence=1. Accessed June 27, 2018.
5. World Health Organization. Guidelines for the safe transport of infectious substances and diagnostic specimens. 1997. Available at: http://www.who.int/csr/emc97_3.pdf. Accessed June 27, 2018.
6. International Air Transport Association. Dangerous goods regulations. Available at: http://www.iata.org/publications/dgr/Pages/index.aspx. Accessed June 27, 2018.
7. World Health Organization. Biorisk management laboratory biosecurity guidance. 2006. Available at: http://www.who.int/ihr/publications/WHO_CDS_EPR_2006_6.pdf?ua=1. Accessed June 27, 2018.


[H. Sheeley]

# OUTBREAK RESPONSE IN CASE OF DELIBERATE USE OF BIOLOGICAL AGENTS TO CAUSE HARM: LABORATORY CONSIDERATIONS

Biological agents have been used to cause harm since ancient times, but large-scale deliberate releases of biological agents intended to cause harm have only been experienced in the last few decades. The potential for terrorist attacks (and the consequent public alarm) has led to greater awareness of the problem and resultant national-level planning and preparation to deal with such incidents. Ultimately, the identification and confirmation of a deliberately released biological threat agent falls on the laboratory system within a given country or jurisdiction. The individual laboratory that is potentially in a position to first detect a deliberately released biological threat agent could be at a hospital level, part of the public health system, or in some other setting within the laboratory system.

## Characteristics of Biothreat Agents

A wide variety of biological agents have been proposed, developed, and used as weapons or to cause harm to individuals or communities. These include bacteria, viruses, fungi, and toxins. WHO, CDC, NATO, and others have created lists of high-threat agents of concern, and restrictions on access to these organisms are embedded in laws and regulations such as the Select Agent Regulations (US)[1] and schedule 5 of the Antiterrorism and Security Act (UK).[2] In addition to national regulations, WHO has published guidance on biosecurity and management of potential threats for laboratories.[3]

Agents may be chosen to have a high mortality (e.g., smallpox) or a low mortality and cause incapacitation or long-term malaise (e.g., *Brucella*); agents can be used to affect a given population, high-profile individuals or groups, domestic animals, or crops. They may be delivered by bombs, missiles, through the food chain, water supply, or ventilation systems or disseminated locally through novel methods such as powder in envelopes. Whatever method is chosen, the perpetrator has to have access to the organism and the ability to produce it in large quantities and to purify specific hazardous products such as toxins. The chosen agent needs to be stable and retain its efficacy throughout these processes. Terrorists may not have scientific expertise and may choose a crude substance (e.g., raw sewage) or a delivery method that is unanticipated.

## Recognition of a Deliberate Event

The laboratory plays a key role in the recognition of a deliberately released biological threat agent.

When an unusual case presents at an emergency department or some primary care site, an alert health care provider may recognize the disease, but it is likely that the symptoms may be nonspecific, and it may take several cases with similar presentations to trigger suspicion. Some of the agents that are of concern as biothreat (BT) agents (e.g., *Francisella tularensis* and *Brucella* sp.) may be missed unless specific laboratory tests are ordered. For that reason, it is imperative that health care providers consult with their laboratory counterparts at the earliest point of suspicion.

## Laboratory Testing

Most agents likely to be used in a biological attack are high-hazard pathogens in hazard groups 3 or 4 and should normally be handled in laboratories operating to biosafety level 3 or 4. Under some circumstances, however, the primary isolation may take place in frontline clinical or hospital laboratories, especially when the cause of an illness or outbreak is unknown. When samples are transported to a reference facility for confirmation, both international and local legislation may require that specialist couriers and packaging are used. (For further information, see "Transport of Infectious Specimens"; also see: http://www.who.int/csr/emc97_3.pdf).

Some biological threat incidents could be detected with the first cases, and hence the diagnosis might be made at the local hospital laboratory as a result of positive cultures or serological tests. Recognition of both the causative organism and the link to a possible deliberate release relies both on the clinical acumen of the physician and the scientific expertise of the laboratory staff. Heightened awareness is key. Some classic bacterial agents such as *Bacillus anthracis* or *Burkholderia mallei* may be misinterpreted as contaminants in some settings and be discarded. Some matrix-assisted laser desorption/ionization time-of-flight mass spectrometry systems may misidentify isolates, especially *Francisella, Burkholderia*, and *Brucella* spp., either as harmless organisms or, conversely, flag environmental variants as pathogens. All positive samples from a primary diagnosis of suspected BT disease should be sent for confirmation. In addition, when the identification of a causative agent is inconsistent with the patient's condition or presenting circumstances, then confirmatory testing should be pursued. This further emphasizes the need for clinicians and laboratorians to be in close communication whenever a potential BT disease is suspected.

### *Polymerase chain reaction testing*

A number of commercial companies have developed assays for many of the Select Agents, which run on their proprietary equipment and allow hospital laboratories to undertake immediate testing. These are usually self-contained systems and do not require specialist know-how or containment as they will work directly from a primary sample. Examples are the BioFire and Cepheid GeneXpert systems, but many others are also on the market. Their availability is ultimately dependent on the economic viability in a given center of maintaining reagents and quality systems for the analytes involved. A number of other rapid tests are on the market based largely on solid phase enzyme-linked immunosorbent assay systems; again, their value depends on their sensitivity and specificity and the quality systems required to make them viable in the given regulatory environment.

### *Specialist services and confirmatory testing*

For cases in which the clinician thinks a particular disease is a strong possibility of being the result of a deliberate release, specialist and reference laboratories should be consulted and be able to advise as to the best samples to take. In general, these should include an ethylenediaminetetraacetic acid sample of blood as a minimum and ideally an aspirate or swab of any pus, fluid (e.g., pleural effusions), cerebrospinal fluid, or other types of specimens as appropriate. If appropriate, fresh tissue from biopsies should also be collected. Samples should be packaged appropriately and transported expeditiously. Depending on the proximity to the primary testing laboratory, results may be available as early as 4 hours from the time of receipt at the laboratory. In the USA, CDC has set up the Laboratory Response Network (LRN) to offer these services at the state level, and the local LRN facility should be contacted in the first instance (see. https://emergency.cdc.gov/lrn/index.asp for full details and contacts). In the UK, the Rare & Imported

Pathogens Laboratory (RIPL) offers a 24/7 advice and testing service (call +44-77890-31672). In other settings, national facilities may have similar capabilities, but it is the responsibility of all laboratories to know what response networks are in place within their respective jurisdictions. (For further information, see "Laboratory Referral Networks.")

Reference laboratories for BT agents will also provide confirmatory testing and assist with follow-up of cases, including any genetic analyses required for outbreak investigation. CDC and RIPL also offer support for testing environmental samples and confirmation of results from on-site testing systems, in conjunction with other national facilities as appropriate.

### First Responders and Environmental Detection

Many local police, ambulance, and fire departments have purchased rapid tests for use on site to detect various BT agents in powders or other materials. The quality and performance of these tests is quite variable, and any results should always be confirmed by an appropriate agency. Such rapid testing kits are of limited value for agents spread by the aerosol route or by injection or ingestion. Qualified laboratory scientists should always be consulted on the advisability of using field tests by nonlaboratorians for the detection of BT agents.

Air sampling through fixed detectors may be of value where they are installed to give a preliminary warning that an attack may have taken place. The final confirmatory steps for these types of detectors rely on polymerase chain reaction testing.

Testing of water and food may be relevant in some cases. Specialist teams will usually be deployed to deal with local sampling and detection; they are equipped with the necessary collection systems, protective clothing, analyzers, and expertise. They are normally activated through an incident command system, usually via the police, and should operate under established forensic procedures.

### Communications

Communications are a critical part of the overall response. Within the teams at each level there needs to be timely and accurate communication of data, and all discussions and electronic communications should be logged and recorded. While individual patient data may be subject to privacy laws, laboratories should agree with colleagues in the wider response team as to what information they will be able to provide to whom and in what time frame.

Communication specialists are needed to prepare briefs for the public, government and local officials, and the media. It is essential that individuals with laboratory expertise be involved in the public communication aspects of a BT threat event. The success and credibility of any given response depends heavily on the accuracy and quality of public information provided.

### Safety and Prophylaxis

Within the responding laboratory, normal best practices should always be observed. If an isolate is suspected of being a BT agent in hazard group 3 or 4, all material (e.g., samples, plates, culture bottles) should be transported to the facility at the appropriate containment level. If this is not possible, a designated area should be set aside for storing these items safely and securely until follow-up referrals can be safely undertaken. Records of the staff involved with handling risk agents and any potential exposure and the nature of it should be maintained. The risk of infection from normal laboratory work should be minimal provided normal precautions against aerosolization, spillage, and contamination of skin and mucous membranes are taken. If an individual has been exposed through contact or splash, prophylaxis may be required. Medical advice can be obtained from CDC or other national centers. Any further work should only be carried out at the correct containment level.

## The Laboratory Role in Biothreat Planning

Planning for the possibility of the deliberate release of a biological agent to cause harm is a large and important undertaking for any governmental body. The participants in such planning must include representatives of the public health, health care, public safety, first responders, agriculture, environment, and military communities. Given the important role of laboratories, the laboratory system including public health must be included in such planning. The planners must plan for the possibility of a threat being posed to humans, animals, or crops. In addition, the possibility that a threat could be biological, chemical, radiological, or some combination must also be considered. The most appropriate approach is to consider an all-hazards approach that will cover various targets, using various agents delivered in various ways. In addition to having written planning materials and agreements among all parties, it is also essential to carry out periodic exercises that simulate a BT event.

From the laboratory perspective, planning must consider the following:

- Writing policies, procedures, and protocols
- Obtaining all necessary permissions or certifications required
- Implementing training for testing personnel, including backup
- Establishing testing supply stockpiles and replenishment procedures
- Assuring that surge capacity and mutual aid plans are incorporated
- Creating a process for safe and secure sample chain of custody including secure storage

## Conclusion

A deliberate biological release is a major event. National, state, and regional governments plan for such eventualities. The response is a team effort between the emergency services and government, with the participation of the health services and other relevant bodies and experts. Hospital laboratories may be the first to identify an attack by isolating an unusual organism and should be aware of the possibility and how to react. National networks of reference laboratories can provide confirmation of the diagnosis. Safety and infection control are essential to protect personnel at all levels, and good communication is central to a successful outcome.

## General Information Links

These documents are mostly produced by individual nations, but the principles are applicable to many other situations or locations.

### *Response planning and control*

- https://www.fema.gov/national-incident-management-system
- https://www.gov.uk/government/uploads/system/uploads/attachment_data/file/253488/Emergency_Response_and_Recovery_5th_edition_October_2013.pdf
- http://www.who.int/csr/en

### *Safety, protection, and personal protective equipment*

- https://www.nist.gov/news-events/news/2002/09/nist-issues-guidelines-protect-first-responders-exposed-chemical-biological
- http://www.hse.gov.uk/pubns/clinical-laboratories.pdf

### *Decontamination*

- https://www.epa.gov/emergency-response/chemical-biological-radiological-and-nuclear-consequence-management (Source of advice on all aspects of contamination and control)
- https://www.gov.uk/government/groups/government-decontamination-service
- https://www.gov.uk/government/uploads/system/uploads/attachment_data/file/622617/SNG_5thEdition_Final_March_2017__1_.pdf
- https://www.ncjrs.gov/pdffiles1/nij/189724.pdf

### *Recovery after an incident*

- https://www.fema.gov/media-library-data/20130726-1910-25045-1918/20_rrkp_key_planning_factors_biological_incident.pdf
- https://www.gov.uk/government/uploads/system/uploads/attachment_data/file/253488/Emergency_Response_and_Recovery_5th_edition_October_2013.pdf

## References


1. US Department of Agriculture. Federal Select Agent Program. 2016. Available at: https://www.selectagents.gov. Accessed September 20, 2018.
2. The National Archives. Anti-terrorism, Crime and Security Act 2001. Schedule 5. Available at: http://www.legislation.gov.uk/ukpga/2001/24/schedule/5. Accessed September 30, 2018.
3. World Health Organization. Laboratory biosecurity guidance. 2006. Available at: http://www.who.int/csr/resources/publications/biosafety/WHO_CDS_EPR_2006_6.pdf. Accessed September 30, 2018.


[ T. Brooks, B. W. Wilcke]

# ACTINOMYCOSIS

| DISEASE | ICD-10 CODE |
|---|---|
| ACTINOMYCOSIS | ICD-10 A42 |

**1. Clinical features**—A chronic bacterial disease, most frequently localized in the orocervicofacial (55%), thoracic (15%), or abdominopelvic (20%) regions. The lesions, firmly indurated areas of purulence and fibrosis, spread slowly to contiguous tissues. Eventually, draining sinuses may appear and surface on the skin. In infected tissue, the organism grows in clusters, called sulfur granules.

**2. Causative agents**—The organisms identified as causing actinomycosis are part of a polymicrobial, commensal group that are commonly found in the oral cavity and intestinal tract of humans and other animals. They are nonspore-forming, anaerobic or micro-aerotolerant, Gram-positive rods. The primary causative agents of actinomycosis include *Actinomyces israelii, Actinomyces gerencseriae,* and *Actinomyces graevenitzii.* Actinomycosis may also be caused by an organism of a different genus, *Propionibacterium propionicum,* displaying growth and morphologic characteristics similar to *Actinomyces* spp. and also commonly found as a member of the human oral flora. Less frequently associated with human disease are *Actinomyces naeslundii, Actinomyces meyeri, Actinomyces odontolyticus,* and *Actinomycesviscosus. Actinomyces turicensis* has been associated with infections of the genital tract.

**3. Laboratory diagnosis**—The classic diagnosis of actinomycosis involves the direct examination of pus taken from suspect lesions or draining sinuses. The presence of sulfur granules is suggestive of actinomycosis. When the sulfur granules are crushed and Gram-stained, the presence of Gram-positive branching, filamentous bacteria provides additional presumptive diagnostic evidence. For definitive identification, isolation must be undertaken. Specimens collected from the lesions should be cultured using standard anaerobic isolation techniques (i.e., using an anaerobe chamber or anaerobe jars). Using pre-reduced selective agar, which contains colistin and nalidixic acid, can enhance the recovery rate of *Actinomyces* spp. Identification is further carried out using a battery of biochemical tests. Several commercially available kits have been used to identify the bacteria that cause actinomycosis; however, they have yielded results of mixed accuracy. Deoxyribonucleic acid (DNA) analysis is a useful tool available in some settings but is not widely available in resource-constrained settings. Serologic tests for actinomycosis have not proven to be useful.

**4. Laboratory capability**—Most clinical laboratories with experience in culturing anaerobic organisms can perform the laboratory tests necessary to diagnose actinomycosis. Laboratorians should be well trained in microscopy and anaerobic culture techniques. Those laboratories performing DNA sequence analysis require scientific staff with specialized training.

**5. Safety requirements**—*Actinomyces* spp. are classified as biosafety level 2 (BSL-2) agents. Therefore, any laboratory performing tests to diagnose actinomycosis must follow all BSL-2 standards, including, but not limited to, the use of biological safety cabinets, the use of personal protective equipment (e.g., laboratory coat, gloves, and eye protection), the adherence to all laboratory safety protocols, and adherence to proper infectious waste disposal practices.

**6. Nonhuman hosts**—Many *Actinomyces* spp. are found in the oral and genital tract of animals, and some can be pathogens (e.g., *Actinomyces bovis*, which causes bovine actinomycosis). *Actinomyces* spp. have been found to be part of the normal microbial flora in cattle, dogs, cats, and pigs. The species of *Actinomyces* that cause human disease are not commonly found in animals, and there is no evidence that actinomycosis is zoonotically spread.

**7. Sample/specimen requirements**—The collection of specimens for isolation and identification can be challenging since the causative organisms of actinomycosis are part of the normal flora in humans and only opportunistically pathogenic. Swabs are not suitable for specimen collection. Techniques that support the isolation of anaerobes are required. Appropriate specimens include biopsied tissue, aspirated pus, or fluid from the suspect lesion. Once collected in suitable anaerobic transport containers, the specimens should be protected from exposure to oxygen and transported to the laboratory promptly for testing.

**8. Testing requirements**—Testing for *Actinomyces* spp. should be carried out using standard anaerobic culture and identification methods. Biochemical testing is required to speciate any isolates. Commercial kits may be subject to both false negative and false positive findings with respect to *Actinomyces* and should be interpreted with caution. If available, DNA analysis can be performed and produces the most reliable identifications. Since the causative organisms of actinomycosis can also be found as members of the normal flora, it is important that the clinician and the laboratorian discuss the laboratory findings to assure the correct interpretation. In some cases, repeat testing with newly obtained specimens may be required to confirm the causative association.

**9. Reporting requirements**—The isolation and identification of *Actinomyces* or *Propionibacterium* should be reported at the species level. All isolations from normally sterile sites should be considered significant. Isolations from sites where normal flora contamination could have occurred must be interpreted with caution. The reporting of actinomycosis to public health authorities by laboratories is not regularly required.

**10. Referral network**—There are no specific referral networks for testing for the causative agents of actinomycosis. Laboratories that are not experienced in testing and identifying anaerobic organisms should contact their referral laboratory for guidance and assistance.

**11. Special considerations**—Individuals who have extensive dental caries or periodontitis are particularly at risk of developing actinomycosis. Also, women who use intrauterine devices for prolonged periods of time are at greater risk of contracting pelvic actinomycosis.

[B. W. Wilcke]

# AMEBIC INFECTIONS

| DISEASE | ICD-10 CODE |
|---|---|
| AMEBIASIS | ICD-10 A06 |
| INFECTIONS WITH FREE-LIVING AMEBA | ICD-10 B60.2, B60.1 |

## I. AMEBIASIS (amoebiasis)

**1. Clinical features**—Most infections are asymptomatic and commensal, but some may be invasive and give rise to intestinal or extra-intestinal disease. Intestinal disease varies from acute or fulminating dysentery with fever, chills, and bloody or mucoid diarrhea (amebic dysentery), to mild abdominal discomfort with diarrhea containing blood or mucus, alternating with periods of constipation or remission. Amebic granulomata (ameboma), sometimes mistaken for carcinoma, may occur in the wall of the large intestine in patients with intermittent dysentery or colitis of long duration. Dissemination through the bloodstream may occur and produce abscesses of the liver and less commonly of the lung or brain. Painful ulceration of the skin is a rare manifestation that can occur anywhere but most commonly in the perianal and genital regions, usually in association with amebic dysentery. Penile lesions may result from anal intercourse. The ameba reach the skin either directly through contact with contaminated feces or indirectly through hematogenous spread; amebic colitis is often confused with forms of inflammatory bowel disease, such as ulcerative colitis; care should be taken to distinguish them since corticosteroids may exacerbate amebic colitis. Amebiasis can also mimic numerous noninfectious and infectious diseases. Conversely, the presence of amebae may be misinterpreted as the cause of diarrhea in a person whose primary enteric illness is the result of another condition.

**2. Causative agents**—*Entamoeba histolytica*, a parasitic organism. Other similar organisms are *Entamoeba hartmanni*, *Entamoeba dispar*, *Entamoeba moshkovskii*, *Entamoeba bangladeshi*, *Entamoeba coli*, or other intestinal protozoa. Not all *E. histolytica* strains are equally virulent. Additionally, the morphologically identical *E. dispar*, present in many asymptomatic cyst passers and once thought to be nonpathogenic, has recently been associated with cases of amebic colitis and amebic liver abscess, putting into question its avirulent status. Immunological differences, isoenzyme patterns, and polymerase chain reaction (PCR) permit differentiation of *E. histolytica* from *E. dispar*.

**3. Laboratory diagnosis**—By microscopic demonstration of trophozoites or cysts in fresh or suitably preserved fecal specimens, smears of aspirates, scrapings obtained by proctoscopy, or aspirates of abscesses or sections of tissue. The presence of trophozoites containing red blood cells is indicative of invasive amebiasis. Examination should be done on fresh fecal specimens by a trained microscopist, as the organism must be differentiated from macrophages. However, even trained microscopists cannot differentiate *E. histolytica* from the morphologically identical *E. dispar* and *E. moshkovskii*. In patients with intestinal disease, examination of at least 3 specimens collected on 3 separate days will increase the yield of organisms from approximately 50% in a single specimen to 75%–95%, but the yield in stool from patients with amebic liver abscesses is only 8%–44%, even with repeated stool examinations. Only 1 commercially available stool antigen-detection test distinguishes *E. histolytica* from *E. dispar*. Other available assays specific for *E. histolytica*, such as enzyme immunoassay and PCR, may require reference laboratory services. Serological tests, particularly immunodiffusion and enzyme-linked immunosorbent assay (ELISA), are very useful in diagnosis of invasive disease in persons living in nonendemic areas. Scintillography, ultrasonography, and computerized axial tomography scanning are helpful in revealing the presence and location of an amebic liver abscess and can be considered diagnostic when associated with a specific antibody response to *E. histolytica* in persons from a non-endemic area.

**4. Laboratory capability**—Ideally, a laboratory should have at least 1 of the following 2 testing capabilities: (a) detection of *Entamoeba* species-specific deoxyribonucleic acid (DNA) in biological specimens such as stools, pus aspirates from abscesses, and tissues by PCR, and (b) detection of *E. histolytica*-specific antigens in biological specimens. Laboratory capability for serologic detection of *E. histolytica*-specific antibodies by ELISA is advantageous in certain circumstances. For example, serology is useful in nonendemic countries for amebiasis and for acute amebic liver abscess patients who generally have higher antibody titers compared with those seen in amebic colitis patients. The laboratory personnel should be appropriately trained in PCR and ELISA techniques prior to start of their work, and a competency assessment of laboratorians should be performed at least once annually. In resource-poor settings, if none of the mentioned testing capabilities are available, at least a trained microscopist should look for ingested red blood cells (RBCs) inside the ameba in an attempt to differentiate it from non-pathogenic species. However, ingested RBCs are not always detected in *E. histolytica*-positive patients, especially in individuals who are asymptomatically infected. Additionally, *E. moshkovskii* can have ingested RBCs, at least in animal model experiments. Therefore, microscopic observation of *Entamoeba* species should be reported with cautions, and the laboratory should seek to build molecular diagnostic capacity for detection of *Entamoeba* species.

5. **Safety requirements**—*E. histolytica* has been designated a biosafety level 2 (BSL-2) agent. It is also a category B agent of bioterrorism, because only 1–10 organisms are needed to establish an infection, and it forms environmentally stable cysts. Therefore, BSL-2 laboratory safety procedures are required to handle the suspected agent or specimens that might contain the agent. Specimens suspected for *E. histolytica* are handled and disposed of as infectious materials. Laboratories should follow universal/standard precautions for BSL-2 agents. Disinfectants such as 10% bleach or 70% ethanol should be used to clean bench surfaces after work is complete.

6. **Nonhuman hosts**—Monkeys, wild rats, and dogs have been reported to have been infected with *E. histolytica;* however, it is not clear whether these animals serve as true hosts or reservoirs for this pathogen.

7. **Sample/specimen requirements**—Fresh, unpreserved stools are the best specimens for clinical diagnosis of intestinal amebiasis. Since amebae are not excreted uniformly in the stools, 3 separate stools should be assessed, especially in asymptomatic individuals. A single stool may be sufficient to reach a definitive conclusion in acute diarrhea/dysentery cases. Since trophozoites disintegrate within 1–2 hours after production, the stool specimens should ideally be processed within an hour. Specimens without any preservatives should be kept refrigerated (4°C) or frozen (−20°C). PCR-compatible fixative (e.g., TotalFix, UniFix, EcoFix) and modified polyvinyl alcohol (zinc- or copper-based) can be used to keep stool specimens at room temperature prior to PCR testing. Alternatively, stool specimens in 2.5% potassium dichromate (1:1 dilution) or in absolute ethanol (1:1 dilution) can also be used prior to PCR testing. In general, specimens fixed in formalin-containing preservatives or low-viscosity polyvinyl alcohol are not suitable for PCR or ELISA testing. For extraintestinal amebiasis such as amebic liver abscess, pus aspirate is most useful for diagnosis by PCR or antigen detection ELISA tests. Specimens from the untreated patients are usually more sensitive than those treated with anti-amebic drugs. A fresh stool sample may be checked by wet

mount microscopy for trophozoites and cysts of *Entamoeba*. However, trophozoites with ingested RBCs will only be useful in species identification. The majority of the individuals infected with *E. histolytica* will not have trophozoites with ingested RBCs, especially in asymptomatic cases. Frozen samples are not suitable for microscopic examination.

At CDC, a duplex real-time PCR is available for simultaneous detection and differentiation of *E. histolytica* and *E. dispar.* This is a Clinical Laboratory Improvement Amendments-accredited test, which requires 0.5 g of formed stool or 0.5 ml of diarrheal stool or aspirated pus for testing. Additionally, it requires 2 patient identifiers on the specimen container and the test requisition.

**8. Testing requirements**—The recommended laboratory tests are PCR and antigen detection ELISA. Several *Entamoeba* species-specific conventional and real-time PCR tests based on the multicopy (>200 copies) 18S ribosomal DNA sequences exist. PCR tests are sensitive enough to detect 1–10 amebae per test. The FDA-approved TechLab *E. histolytica* II ELISA is sensitive enough to detect 0.2–0.4 ng of *E. histolytica*-specific Gal/GalNac lectin per test, and it does not cross-react with other *Entamoeba* species. For both PCR and ELISA tests, a positive and a negative control are run in parallel with each test and must give satisfactory results for a test to be considered valid. In the absence of species-specific PCRs or antigen detection ELISA tests, a trained microscopist may try to detect ameba structure in fresh stool samples; however, extreme cautions should be taken in the interpretation of microscopy results.

**9. Reporting requirements**—At CDC, *Entamoeba* PCR results are reported unequivocally at the species level using an electronic laboratory information system. Prior to reporting, the test results are reviewed and verified by 1 additional competent analyst. The antigen detection ELISA (not available at CDC) can report a specimen either as positive or negative for *E. histolytica*. Unlike PCR, ELISA cannot detect a mixed infection of *E. histolytica* with another *Entamoeba* species and only reports a specimen as positive for *E. histolytica*. Amebiasis is not a nationally notifiable disease in the USA. Laboratories outside of the USA should determine whether amebiasis is a reportable disease within their jurisdiction.

**10. Referral network**—None.

**11. Special considerations**—None.

## II. INFECTIONS WITH FREE-LIVING AMEBA (naegleriasis, acanthamoebiasis, balamuthiasis)

**1. Clinical features**—Naegleriasis causes a typical syndrome of fulminating pyogenic meningoencephalitis (primary amebic meningoencephalitis

[PAM]) with severe frontal headache, occasional olfactory hallucinations, nausea, vomiting, high fever, nuchal rigidity and somnolence, and death within an average of 5.3 days (range 1–12 days) of symptom onset. The mortality rate of PAM in the USA is greater than 99%. Acanthamoebiasis causes a granulomatous disease (granulomatous amebic encephalitis [GAE]) of insidious onset and lasting from weeks to several months. Balamuthiasis also causes GAE. The mortality rate of GAE in the USA is greater than 90%. In addition to causing GAE, several species of *Acanthamoeba* (*Acanthamoeba polyphaga*, *Acanthamoeba castellanii,* and *Acanthamoeba hatchetti*) have been associated with chronic granulomatous lesions of the skin, with or without secondary invasion of the central nervous system (CNS). *Balamuthia mandrillaris* has also been associated with skin lesions preceding CNS infections in some cases. Infections of the cornea (keratoconjunctivitis due to *Acanthamoeba*) have resulted in blindness.

**2. Causative agents**—*Naegleria fowleri*, multiple species of *Acanthamoeba* (*Acanthamoeba culbertsoni*, *A. polyphaga*, *A. castellanii*, *Acanthamoeba astronyxis*, *A. hatchetti*, *Acanthamoeba rhysodes*, and *Acanthamoaeba lenticulata*), and *B. mandrillaris*.

**3. Laboratory diagnosis**—Although free-living amebae (*N. fowleri*, *Acanthamoeba* spp., and *Balamuthia* spp.) have sometimes been misidentified as macrophages or *E. histolytica,* they can be differentiated morphologically through immunohistochemical staining and PCR testing of brain tissue in PAM and GAE cases. *N. fowleri* and *Acanthamoeba* spp. can also be cultured on non-nutrient agar seeded with *Escherichia coli*, *Enterobacter aerogenes*, or other suitable *Enterobacter* species; *Balamuthia* require mammalian cell cultures for isolation. These techniques can also be used with skin scrapings, swabs, and aspirates in suspected *Acanthamoeba* and *Balamuthia* infections involving the skin. Likewise, suspected *Acanthamoeba* eye infections can be diagnosed by histology, PCR, or culture of corneal scrapings; confocal microscopy can also be used. In addition, PAM can be diagnosed through microscopic examination of wet mount preparations of fresh cerebrospinal fluid (CSF) showing motile amebae and of stained smears of CSF.

**4. Laboratory capability**—The laboratories should be capable of performing (a) DNA extraction and PCR, and (b) immunofluorescence-based assays to detect intact amebae or ameba-specific antibodies. Additionally, laboratorians should be capable of identifying *N. fowleri* trophozoites in CSF by microscopy. This is important for a quick, and possibly early, diagnosis given the extraordinarily rapid nature of disease progression, but molecular testing is still required for confirmation purposes.

The laboratory personnel should be appropriately trained in PCR and immunofluorescence techniques prior to start of their work, and a competency assessment of laboratorians should be performed at least once annually. The laboratorians should also be trained to recognize the distinctive morphologic features of different free-living amebae (FLA).

**5. Safety requirements**—Laboratories with BSL-2 capabilities can perform testing. Laboratories should follow universal/standard precautions for BSL-2 agents. Testing personnel with any open wounds must be covered appropriately as *Acanthamoeba* spp. and *Balamuthia* spp. are thought to infect through wounds. Nasal ingestion or inhalation of FLA can be prevented by wearing appropriate facial masks. Safety glasses can also be worn to protect eyes from *Acanthamoeba* spp. Specimens suspected for FLA are handled and disposed of as infectious materials. Disinfectants such as 10% bleach or 70% ethanol should be used to clean the bench surfaces after work is complete.

**6. Nonhuman hosts**—Although a few sporadic animals such as cows, sheep, monkeys, tapirs, and ewes have been fatally infected with pathogenic FLA, they are not considered to normally harbor the agents or transmit the disease to humans.

**7. Sample/specimen requirements**—CSF is the most appropriate specimen for clinical diagnosis of *N. fowleri* infections. Although *B. mandrillaris* or *Acanthamoeba* spp. are occasionally detected in CSF, the most appropriate specimens for *Acanthamoeba* keratitis diagnosis are brain tissues (for GAE) or corneal scrapings. Formalin-fixed paraffin-embedded (FFPE) tissue slides are used for immunofluorescence-based diagnosis of suspected agents using FLA species-specific polyclonal sera. However, for PCR testing, fresh or frozen tissues are preferred over FFPE tissues since formalin treatment adversely affects DNA quality. Because FLA are thermophilic, specimens may be shipped at ambient temperature (i.e., without ice-packs). Serum samples should be shipped with ice-packs.

At the CDC, a triplex real-time PCR is available for simultaneous detection and differentiation of *N. fowleri, B. mandrillaris, and Acanthamoeba* spp. from CSF and tissue. This test requires 1.0 mL of CSF or a small piece (e.g., 0.1–0.2 g) of tissue specimen. Additionally, it requires 2 patient identifiers on the specimen container and the test requisition.

**8. Testing requirements**—Rapid diagnosis is crucial for FLA infections. For *N. fowleri*, a direct microscopic evaluation of CSF is the fastest way to reach a probable diagnosis, which may prove very useful in saving the life of a PAM patient. A trained laboratorian (or microscopist) should be able to differentiate between the *N. fowleri* trophozoites and host leukocytes by evaluating their nuclear architecture. CSF should also be subject to PCR testing for confirmation purposes. In early stage of PAM cases, however, trophozoites of *N. fowleri* may not be seen in CSF, but PCR can still detect *N. fowleri* DNA because of its higher sensitivity. The target of FLA real-time PCR is the 18S small subunit ribosomal DNA sequence, which is present in several thousand copies per genome. The FLA real-time PCR can detect a single ameba in the clinical specimen. The sensitivity of the immunofluorescence-based assays to detect intact FLAs in the tissue slides is unknown, but the assays are species-specific.

**9. Reporting requirements**—At CDC, the FLA real-time PCR and the immunofluorescence assay results are reported unequivocally at the species level using an electronic laboratory information system. Prior to reporting, the test results are reviewed and verified by an additional competent analyst. FLA infections are not nationally notifiable diseases in the US. Laboratories outside of the US should determine whether FLA infections are reportable within their jurisdiction.

**10. Referral network**—None.

**11. Special considerations**—None.

[I. K. M. Ali]

# ANGIOSTRONGYLIASIS

| DISEASE | ICD-10 Code |
|---|---|
| ANGIOSTRONGYLIASIS | ICD-10 B83.2 |
| INTESTINAL ANGIOSTRONGYLIASIS | ICD-10 B81.3 |

## I. ANGIOSTRONGYLIASIS (eosinophilic meningoencephalitis, eosinophilic meningitis)

**1. Clinical features**—Angiostrongyliasis affecting the central nervous system (CNS), also known as eosinophilic meningitis, may be asymptomatic or symptomatic; it is commonly characterized by severe headache, neck and back stiffness, and paresthesias. Temporary facial paralysis occurs in 5% of patients. Low-grade fever may be present. Illness is usually self-limiting and may last a few days to several months. Deaths have rarely been reported. Differential diagnosis includes cerebral cysticercosis, paragonimiasis, echinococcosis, gnathostomiasis, tuberculous, coccidioidal or aseptic meningitis, and neurosyphilis.

**2. Causative agents**—*Angiostrongylus (Parastrongylus) cantonensis*, a zoonotic nematode (lungworm of rats). The third-stage larvae in the intermediate host (terrestrial or aquatic mollusks) are infective for humans.

**3. Laboratory diagnosis**—Cerebrospinal fluid (CSF) usually exhibits pleocytosis with over 10% eosinophils; blood eosinophilia is not always present but can be quite elevated. Presence of eosinophils in the CSF and a history of eating raw mollusks or eating raw foods that may be contaminated by snails or slugs suggest the diagnosis, especially in endemic areas. Immature worms can be found in the CSF and in the eye, but such findings are rare. Serology by enzyme-linked immunosorbent assay (ELISA) or Western blot can be used to detect anti-*Angiostrongylus* antibodies.[1] However, currently available immunodiagnosis methods are based on native antigens, which can cross-react with other nematode infections, so results must be interpreted with care.[2] Polymerase chain reaction (PCR)–based molecular tests can be used on CSF and tissue to demonstrate presence of worm deoxyribonucleic acid (DNA).[3]

4. **Laboratory capability**—Most cases of angiostrongyliasis are diagnosed based on clinical features and exposure history. In the USA, a real-time PCR assay for detection of *A. cantonensis* DNA in CSF is available at CDC and at the Hawaii State Department of Health. A few reference diagnostic laboratories in other countries have the capacity to perform immunologic and molecular testing; for example in Australia, the Institute for Clinical Pathology and Medical Research at Westmead Hospital, Sydney, offers serology testing for angiostrongyliasis.

5. **Safety requirements**—Clinical specimens should always be collected and handled with universal/standard precautions. *A. cantonensis* is a biosafety level 2 (BSL-2) organism. Specimens should be disposed of as infectious waste.

6. **Nonhuman hosts**—The rat (*Rattus* and *Bandicota* spp.) is the definitive host. The infectious third stage larvae occur in mollusks (both snails and slugs). Many types of animals, such as amphibians and reptiles, can act as carrier hosts for the infectious larvae and can cause human disease if consumed raw or undercooked. Angiostrongyliasis is a zoonotic disease affecting other animals that may consume infected mollusks, including birds, nonhuman primates, dogs, and horses.

7. **Sample/specimen requirements**—CSF and tissue for PCR-based testing should be kept refrigerated or frozen during storage and shipping. Analysis of multiple CSF specimens, if available, is recommended since the concentration of worms in the CSF is likely to fluctuate as the infection progresses. Antibody detection can be performed on both serum and CSF, with serum being preferred.

8. **Testing requirements**—There is currently no widely available laboratory diagnostic test for angiostrongyliasis. Microscopic analysis of a CSF wet-mount may in rare cases reveal larva. Although PCR-based detection methods are highly specific, the diagnostic sensitivity of PCR-based detection is less than 80% and a negative PCR result does not rule out infection. Demonstration of worms or DNA from worms in CSF, eye, or brain tissue is confirmatory.

Antibody detection in serum or CSF is presumptive, but cross-reactivity with other nematode infections must be considered.

**9. Reporting requirements**—Angiostrongyliasis is a reportable disease in the state of Hawaii. Laboratories in other states and in countries other than the USA should determine whether positive laboratory findings for *A. cantonensis* are reportable.

**10. Referral network**—None.

**11. Special considerations**—Any grouping of cases in a particular geographic area or institution warrants prompt epidemiological investigation and appropriate control measures.

## II. INTESTINAL ANGIOSTRONGYLIASIS

**1. Clinical features**—Common findings of the intestinal form of angiostrongyliasis include abdominal pain and tenderness in the right iliac fossa and flank, fever, anorexia, vomiting, abdominal rigidity, a tumor-like mass in the right lower quadrant, and pain on rectal examination. Fever, anorexia, vomiting, constipation, or diarrhea are frequent in children. Leukocytosis is usually present, with eosinophils ranging from 20%–60%. Adult worms and eggs in the mesenteric arteries damage the endothelium, causing inflammation, thrombosis, and necrosis. On surgery, the whole wall of the intestine is thickened and hardened, with yellow granulomas in the subserosa of the intestinal wall; adult worms are found in the small arteries, generally in the ileocecal area, while eggs and larvae are found in lymph nodes, intestinal wall, and omentum. Intestinal obstruction and perforation can occur. Differential diagnosis includes malignant tumors, appendicitis, Crohn's disease, and Meckel's diverticulum.

**2. Causative agents**—*Angiostrongylus* (*Parastrongylus*) *costaricensis*, a nematode worm. The third-stage larvae in the intermediate host (mollusks) are infective for humans.

**3. Laboratory diagnosis**—High eosinophilia suggests the diagnosis, especially in children living in endemic areas. Clinical diagnosis may be aided by X-ray. Parasitological confirmation can be achieved by examination of tissue obtained by biopsy or at surgical resection. Investigative PCR-based molecular tests can be used to confirm presence of parasite DNA in tissue.[4] Serological diagnostic techniques, such as ELISA and immunofluorescence assay, are available in a few laboratories outside the USA but are not standardized and may produce false positive results due to cross-reactivity to other nematode infections.[5] In humans, eggs are not found in feces.

**4. Laboratory capability**—Laboratorians should be trained in the morphologic identification of worms in tissue sections and undergo regular proficiency testing. A few reference diagnostic laboratories have capacity to perform serologic and/or molecular testing to confirm the infection.

**5. Safety requirements**—Clinical specimens should always be collected and handled with standard precautions. *A. costaricensis* is a BSL-2 organism. Specimens should be disposed of as infectious waste.

**6. Nonhuman hosts**—The cotton rat (*Sigmodon hispidus*) is the definitive host, and various species of mollusks are intermediate hosts. Several species of other rodents and mammals, such as marmosets, dogs, and coatimundis, can be accidental hosts, as can humans.

**7. Sample/specimen requirements**—Hematoxylin and eosin stained histological sections of intestinal tissue should be examined for presence of worms.

**8. Testing requirements**—Identification of worms and/or eggs in tissue obtained from biopsy or surgical resection is confirmative. PCR- and antibody-based assays are available as research tools.

**9. Reporting requirements**—None.

**10. Referral network**—None.

**11. Special considerations**—Any grouping of cases in a particular geographic area or institution warrants prompt epidemiological investigation and appropriate control measures.

## References

1. Nuamtanong S. The evaluation of the 29 and 31 kDa antigens in female *Angiostrongylus cantonensis* for serodiagnosis of human angiostrongyliasis. *Southeast Asian J Trop Med Public Health*. 1996;27(2):291–296.
2. Morassutti AL, Rascoe LN, Handali S, Da Silva AJ, Wilkins PP, Graeff-Teixeira C. Cross-reactivity of the 31 kDa antigen of *Angiostrongylus cantonensis*—Dealing with the immunodiagnosis of meningoencephalitis. *Parasitology*. 2017;144(4): 459–463.
3. Qvarnstrom Y, Xayavong M, da Silva ACA, et al. Real-time polymerase chain reaction detection of *Angiostrongylus cantonensis* DNA in cerebrospinal fluid from patients with eosinophilic meningitis. *Am J Trop Med Hyg*. 2016;94(1):176–181.
4. Rodriguez R, Aramburú da Silva AC, Müller CA, Alves SL, Graeff-Teixeira C, Fornari F. PCR for the diagnosis of abdominal angiostrongyliasis in formalin-fixed paraffin-embedded human tissue. *PLOS One*. 2014;9(4):e93658.
5. Abrahams-Sandi E, Mesén-Ramírez P, Suarez-Chacón D, Fernández-Quesada K. An indirect immunofluorescence antibody test employing whole eggs as the antigen for the diagnosis of abdominal angiostrongyliasis. *Mem Inst Oswaldo Cruz*. 2011; 106(4):390–393.

[Y. Qvarnstrom]

# ANISAKIASIS

| DISEASE | ICD-10 CODE |
|---|---|
| ANISAKIASIS | ICD-10 B81.0 |

**1. Clinical features**—Symptoms vary according to the site of larval invasion into gastrointestinal mucosa. After eating uncooked/undercooked seafood, abdominal pain, nausea, vomiting, and occasionally hematemesis, starting within several hours, result from invasion in gastric mucosa (gastric anisakiasis). Subsequently, or alternatively, abdominal pain, distension, diarrhea (often with blood/mucus) and mild fever may occur about 1–2 weeks after eating seafood, and persist (granulomatous enteritis called enteric anisakiasis). In heavy infestation, larvae may lodge in the esophagus, causing esophagitis with pain and difficulty in swallowing. In some, allergic symptoms like skin rash including urticaria, itching, and, rarely, anaphylaxis may develop. Occasionally, only the allergic manifestations occur without larval infestation. Rarely, submucosal granulomas can cause intestinal obstruction; intestinal perforation may also occur, leading to peritonitis.

**2. Causative agents**—Third-instar larvae (L3) of *Anisakis*, *Pseudoterranova*, and *Contracaecum*, nematode parasites of marine mammals and fish-eating birds worldwide. Although the adult worms are found in marine mammals, the third stage larvae are found in fish and squid. Larvae do not develop further in humans.

**3. Laboratory diagnosis**—Diagnosis of anisakiasis is usually made by the identification of larvae expelled from the nose or mouth, less commonly passed in stools. Worms may also be discovered and removed via endoscopy. L3 larvae are 10–50 mm long, are cream to pink in color, and have 3 fleshy lips on the anterior end; members of the genus *Pseudoterranova* and some species of *Anisakis* possess a small spine-like process (mucron) at the posterior end. Worms in ectopic sites are usually identified incidentally during examination of biopsy specimens, often during the pursuit of other diagnoses. Diagnosis of allergic reactions is based on having compatible clinical manifestations following consumption of fish, a positive skin-prick test confirmed by specific immunoglobulin class E using additional assays (e.g., radioimmunoassay), and a lack of reaction to proteins from the host fish. Routine molecular and serologic assays, aside from detecting acute allergic reactions, are not available for anisakiasis. Because humans are a dead-end host for anisakid larvae, which do not develop to sexual maturity in humans, routine ova and parasites examinations of stool are not practical for the diagnosis of anisakiasis.

**4. Laboratory capability**—Microscopy/morphologic testing should be available. Laboratorians should be trained in the microscopic/morphologic detection of parasites and undergo regular proficiency testing. Confirmation at the genus level may require reference laboratory level skills.

**5. Safety requirements**—Clinical specimens should always be collected and handled with universal precautions. Anisakid nematodes are biosafety level 2 organisms. There is a low risk of infection from the worms themselves; however, they may be passed in bodily fluids containing other disease-causing agents. If used as a preservative, formalin should only be used in a well-ventilated area, preferably in a chemical fume hood. Specimens should be disposed of as infectious waste.

**6. Nonhuman hosts**—Anisakiasis is acquired from the ingestion of L3 larvae in undercooked fish and shellfish that serve as natural paratenic hosts. Over 100 species of fish and shellfish have been documented as paratenic hosts for *Anisakis* spp., and over 70 species of fish and shellfish for *Pseudoterranova* spp. Many species of common, commercial fish may serve as paratenic hosts, so the risk of acquiring anisakid nematodes from improperly prepared fish can be high. The definitive hosts in nature are fish-eating mammals (cetaceans and pinnipeds) and birds, and the first paratenic host is a marine planktonic crustacean. Ingestion of eggs excreted from the definitive host is not a risk factor for human disease.

**7. Sample/specimen requirements**—Whole, intact larvae, or pieces thereof, should be promptly placed in a liquid preservative, such as 10% buffered formalin or 70% laboratory grade ethanol, to prevent desiccation and alteration of morphologic features. Specimens in an appropriate preservative should remain intact indefinitely.

**8. Testing requirements**—Routine examination of whole/gross helminths. The genera may be separated by morphologic examination of the L3 larvae, but a species-level identification usually requires molecular sequencing analysis. Worms in ectopic sites are usually identified via microscopy in biopsy specimens processed for routine histologic work-up. Diagnosis is confirmatory in specimens meeting morphologic criteria.

**9. Reporting requirements**—Identification to the genus or species level is not needed for patient management but may be employed for epidemiologic purposes. Anisakiasis is not nationally reportable in the USA. Report to local health authority; official report is not ordinarily justifiable. International reporting is not required.

**10. Referral network**—None.

**11. Special considerations**—None.

[B. Mathison]

# ANTHRAX

(malignant pustule, malignant edema, woolsorter disease, ragpicker disease)

| DISEASE | ICD-10 CODE |
|---|---|
| ANTHRAX | ICD-10 A22 |

**1. Clinical features**—An acute bacterial zoonotic disease that historically has been described as occurring in 3 forms: cutaneous, inhalation or gastrointestinal, depending on the route of exposure. A fourth form, injection anthrax, has been described in recent outbreaks among heroin users in Northern Europe. Systemic illness, including fever, shock, and dissemination to other organs, can occur with any form of anthrax and may include meningitis that is usually fatal.

1) Cutaneous: more than 95% of naturally acquired human cases are cutaneous anthrax, manifested by initial itching of the affected site followed by a lesion that becomes papular, then vesicular, developing in 2–6 days into a depressed black eschar. Moderate to severe edema usually surrounds the eschar, sometimes with small secondary vesicles. Pain is unusual and, if present, is due to edema or secondary infection. The head, neck, forearms, and hands (exposed areas of the body) are the most common sites of infection. Differential diagnoses include arachnid bites such as brown recluse in North America and a variety of other infections (e.g., staphylococcal or streptococcal cellulitis, dermatomycoses, rickettsialpox, Orf virus, varicella zoster, herpes simplex, vaccinia). Untreated infections may spread to regional lymph nodes and the bloodstream with overwhelming septicemia. Edema associated with cutaneous lesions involving the head and neck can result in respiratory compromise due to compression of the trachea and require intubation. Untreated cutaneous anthrax has a case-fatality rate between 5% and 20%; with effective treatment, however, deaths from cutaneous anthrax are very rare. The lesion evolves through typical local changes even after the initiation of antimicrobial therapy.
2) Inhalation: initial symptoms of inhalation (also referred to as pulmonary) anthrax are mild and nonspecific and may include fever, malaise, and mild cough or chest pain. Symptoms progress to include respiratory distress, stridor, severe dyspnea, hypoxemia, diaphoresis, shock, and cyanosis over 3–4 days. X-ray evidence of mediastinal widening is present in the majority of cases, and pulmonary infiltrates or pleural effusions are usually observed. Maximum case-fatality

rate is estimated to be greater than 85%; however, early diagnosis and initiation of aggressive combination antimicrobial therapy and supportive care may considerably reduce mortality.

3) Gastrointestinal: gastrointestinal anthrax is rare and difficult to recognize; it tends to occur in outbreaks following consumption of contaminated meat from anthrax-infected animals. Symptoms include abdominal distress characterized by pain, nausea, and vomiting, followed by fever, signs of septicaemia, and death in typical cases. The case-fatality rate of gastrointestinal anthrax is estimated to be 40%. A rare oropharyngeal form of primary disease, characterized by edematous lesions, necrotic ulcers, and swelling in the oropharynx and neck, has been described.

4) Injection: patients with anthrax associated with heroin use have not presented with typical symptoms associated with the classic (cutaneous, inhalational, or gastrointestinal) forms of anthrax; however, presentation has been varied. Most patients have serious localized soft tissue infections accompanied by significant soft tissue edema. Fever is not a prominent feature, and pain is less severe than with other serious soft tissue infections. Compartment syndrome may be present. Not all cases have localized injection-related lesions; some cases presented with features more typical of systemic anthrax infection, including hemorrhagic meningitis and multiorgan failure. Differential diagnoses include necrotising fasciitis, cellulitis, or abscess. Injection anthrax has a case-fatality rate of 21% in confirmed and probable cases.

**2. Causative agents**—*Bacillus anthracis*, a Gram-positive, encapsulated, spore-forming, nonmotile rod. Specifically, the spores of *B. anthracis* are the infectious form; vegetative forms of *B. anthracis* rarely transmit disease. *B. anthracis* has 3 main virulence factors: a poly-D-glutamic acid capsule and 2 protein exotoxins—edema toxin (EF) and lethal toxin (LF).

**3. Laboratory diagnosis**—Laboratory confirmation is through demonstration of the causative bacilli in blood, lesion exudates or smears, or discharges by direct polychrome methylene blue (McFadyean)-stained smears; or by culture on sheep blood agar or selective media; or through detection of the bacterial deoxyribonucleic acid, antigens, toxins, or host immune response. Standard diagnosis remains culture of the organisms from clinical specimens, but this may be difficult to achieve after antimicrobial treatment is initiated. Rapid detection methods include polymerase chain reaction (PCR), antigen-detection methods including direct fluorescent assay and immunohistochemistry (IHC), and anthrax lethal toxin detection in serum by mass spectrometry. Sensitivity of these methods may also decline after antimicrobial treatment has been initiated. Serologic assays may be available at national reference laboratories, and a commercial enzyme-linked immunosorbent assay is available for antibody testing. Rapid assays such as real-time PCR are only available at testing laboratories and laboratories participating in the CDC Laboratory Response Network.

**4. Laboratory capability**—In general, biosafety level 2 (BSL-2) laboratory conditions are appropriate for laboratory diagnostic tests, but biosafety level 3 (BSL-3) conditions should be used for the following high-risk activities:

1) Producing quantities of the organism in culture
2) Activities that are likely to produce aerosols
3) Working with antibiotic-resistant strains

**5. Safety requirements**—Anthrax is not highly infectious, and humans tend to be moderately resistant to anthrax infection. In laboratories in countries with limited resources, good laboratory practice and use of appropriate personal protective equipment (e.g., laboratory gowns, gloves) should be worn. Manipulations of liquid cultures should be kept to a minimum and conducted in BSL-3 or as near to BSL-3 conditions as possible. Appropriate disinfectant, such as sodium hypochlorite at 10,000 parts per million, should be freshly prepared and used to mop up any spills. Cultures and specimens should be kept in sealed, leak-proof, nonbreakable containers, and contaminated items (e.g., pipette tips, tubes, loops, spreaders) should be fully immersed in disinfectant. All contaminated waste should be autoclaved.

**6. Nonhuman hosts**—Anthrax is a disease of domestic and wild animals, principally herbivores such as cattle, sheep, goats, antelope, and deer, and is found worldwide. In animals, it is acquired through contact with spores in the soil, on plants, and in water. Humans are infected through contact with dead animals and contaminated animal products such as meat, hides, fur, wool, and bone meal. Flies are thought to play a role in the spread of disease during large outbreaks in animals.

**7. Sample/specimen requirements**—Samples for diagnostic testing depend on the type of disease manifestation.

1) Cutaneous: swabs and biopsies of vesicles, lesions, and eschars for culture and PCR. Serum and plasma can be used to test for anthrax lethal toxin if taken 7 days or less following onset of symptoms. Acute and convalescent serum samples can be used for serology. Lesion biopsies and autopsy samples in the event of death can be used for histopathology, specialist staining such as McFadyean's stain, and IHC.
2) Inhalational: blood, pleural fluid, and cerebrospinal fluid (where meningitis is suspected) for PCR and culture. Acute (taken $\leq$7 days post onset of symptoms); serum and plasma for anthrax lethal toxin detection. Acute and convalescent sera for serology testing. Pleural/bronchial biopsies and autopsy tissue can be used for histopathology, specialist staining such as McFadyean's stain, IHC, and PCR.

3) Gastrointestinal: blood, ascites fluid, rectal swab, and oropharyngeal lesion swab (if lesions are present) for culture and PCR. Ascites fluid, plasma, and serum can be used for anthrax lethal toxin detection. Acute and convalescent sera for serology testing. If fatal, autopsy samples can be used for histopathology, specialist staining such as McFadyean's, stain, and IHC.
4) Injectional: blood and tissue biopsy (from localized tissue debridement) for culture and PCR. Plasma, tissue biopsy, and acute serum (taken ≤7 days post onset of symptoms) for anthrax lethal toxin detection. Acute and convalescent sera for serology. Autopsy samples for histopathology, specialist staining such as McFadyean's stain, and IHC.

Blood samples for culture and PCR should be collected in appropriate tubes (e.g., ethylenediaminetetraacetic acid [EDTA] or sodium citrate for PCR testing, blood tube [no coagulation] or blood culture bottles for culture) and should be shipped to the local laboratory providing anthrax diagnostic capability at 4°C–8°C. Serum and plasma should be taken according to local protocols and shipped to the nearest laboratory offering anthrax serology and/or anthrax lethal toxin testing at 4°C–8°C. For biopsies, lesions, and autopsy material, specimens can be fixed with 10% formalin and sent at ambient temperature, although it should be noted that fixing specimens in formalin may interfere with subsequent PCR analysis. Unfixed samples should be frozen and shipped to the laboratory on dry ice.

**8. Testing requirements—**

1) Culture and bacteriology: *B. anthracis* is a nonfastidious, facultative anaerobe that readily grows in culture. *B. anthracis* grows on a range of common agar media including 5% sheep or horse blood agar and nutrient agar. Specialist media such as polymyxin-lysozyme-EDTA-thallous (PLET) acetate can be used to distinguish *B. anthracis* from contaminated and mixed culture samples. Bicarbonate agar is used to confirm the isolation of *B. anthracis* due to the induction of capsule growth. Growth generally appears within 24 hours of incubation at 35°C–37°C. Cultures can be incubated at 5% $CO_2$; this is required for cultures on bicarbonate agar for capsule detection. *B. anthracis* colonies are generally grey and flat and can have a Medusa-head appearance with irregular edges and protrusions. *B. anthracis* is nonhemolytic on blood agar. Confirmatory testing includes gamma bacteriophage susceptibility, indirect hemagglutination, and the Ascoli test, which is a thermostable antigen precipitin test. *B. anthracis* can be identified following culture using traditional biochemical techniques such as catalase, oxidase, nitrate reduction, hemolysis, citrate utilization, and urease; commercially available biochemical assays such as API-ID can be used. Matrix-assisted laser desorption/ionization time-of-flight is also available in some specialist

clinical diagnostic laboratories, although not all databases are accurate enough to distinguish *B. anthracis* and can be misleading. Gamma phage testing can be used to confirm *B. anthracis* in culture. The phage will lyse *B. anthracis* grown aerobically on nutrient agar or sheep/horse blood agar; other Bacillus species are rarely lysed.

2) Microscopy and staining: *B. anthracis* is a spore-forming, Gram-positive rod easily visible using microscopy and staining such as Gram stain. More specialist stains can be used for identification of anthrax. McFadyean's stain uses polychrome methylene blue to determine cell morphology, particularly the capsule. For identification of anthrax, the stain identifies a pink capsule around a blue cell. McFadyean's stain can be used directly on a blood smear or a smear from a lesion, reducing the need for culture, and is suitable for use in low resource environments. Other stains, such as malachite green/safranin (or mal achite green/basic fuchsin) and modified Ziehl-Neelson stain can be used to identify anthrax using microscopy. Using malachite green/ safranin (or basic fuchsin) stain, the spores stain green, while the vegetative bacilli stain pink. Using modified Ziehl-Neelsen stain, spores will be stained red, and vegetative bacilli will be stained blue. These methods can be used as an initial screen for anthrax and are useful for use in first tier (e.g., local) laboratories and low resource settings, but other more sensitive methods such as PCR should be used for confirmation, and samples may need to be sent to reference laboratories for confirmation. Fluorescent antibody staining for capsule visualization is used by the CDC Laboratory Response Network.

3) Molecular methods: PCR for *B. anthracis* is widely available and primer sequences are widely published, including a number of real-time PCR assays such as TaqMan and SYBR Green. It is recommended that 3 targets are used: usually a conserved (housekeeping) gene on the chromosome, pXO1 (typically *pag*, encoding protective antigen or *lef* encoding LF toxin), and pXO2 plasmid (typically *capA, capB or capC,* encoding the capsule) to distinguish *B. anthracis* from environmental *Bacillus* isolates that can give a positive result with some PCR assays. Recently, a *Bacillus cereus* strain that closely mimics anthrax disease and contains the pXO2 plasmid and expresses capsule gene has been responsible for a number of human disease cases. Genotyping techniques such as single-nucleotide polymorphism analysis and whole genome sequencing are useful to track and investigate outbreaks but are generally confined to specialist laboratories.

4) Serology: serodiagnosis is important in areas where anthrax is highly endemic and can be used for surveillance and confirmation of infection. A number of enzyme-linked immunosorbent assays (ELISAs) have been developed to detect antibody responses to the

toxin components (LF, EF, and PA), the most common being PA. A number of commercial anti-PA ELISAs are available. Lateral flow assays, based on immunochromatography using colloidal gold particles, have been developed for rapid field-based detection of antibodies to PA in serum or whole blood. In animal studies, LF was found to evoke a higher immunoglobulin class G response, and studies of cutaneous anthrax suggests that the anti-LF antibody response is higher than that with PA or EF, and antibodies to LF appear faster than those to PA or EF. Some anti-LF ELISA assays have been developed. These ELISAs generally can distinguish between the immune response to infection and to anthrax vaccine, which is largely composed of PA. Antibody response to LF can also be detected using a toxin neutralizing assay, which looks at the ability of neutralizing antibodies in serum to neutralize LF on a cell layer. This test is generally used to measure antibody responses following vaccination and is only performed in specialist laboratories.

**9. Reporting requirements**—Anthrax is a notifiable disease in many countries and each country will have its own requirements for notification of suspected and confirmed cases. Anthrax is a notifiable animal disease and confirmed cases in livestock and wildlife should be notified to the World Organisation for Animal Health (see: http://www.oie.int for further details).

**10. Referral network**—The WHO collaborating laboratory for *Bacillus anthracis* is the Rare and Imported Pathogens Laboratory, Public Health England, Porton Down, Wiltshire, SP4 0JG. CDC runs a Laboratory Response Network that includes primary (i.e., local) laboratories, secondary (i.e., reference) laboratories, and tertiary (i.e., specialist) laboratories for the diagnosis and surveillance of anthrax and other pathogens on the select agent list. Each country will have its own referral networks, and these should be referred to individually.

**11. Special considerations**—*B. anthracis* is a tier-1 biothreat agent and is listed in the Select Agents and Toxins, 7 CFR Part 331, 9 CFR Part 121, and 42 CFR Part 73 (http://www.selectagents.gov). In the USA, confirmed isolates of select agents identified in a clinical or diagnostic laboratory must be reported. Each country may have specific registration requirements for laboratories working with *B. anthracis*, and these should be checked.

[J. Duggan]

# ARBOVIRAL DISEASES

(arthropod-borne viral diseases)

## Arboviruses of Medical or Unknown Significance

| I. ARBOVIRAL FEVERS | | | | | |
|---|---|---|---|---|---|
| **DISEASE** | **ICD-10 CODE** | **VECTOR** | **TAXONOMIC STATUS** | **BIOSAFETY LEVEL** | **OCCURRENCE** |
| BANZI | ICD-10 A92.8 | Mosquito: *Culex* spp. | *Flaviviridae* | 2 | Africa |
| BHANJA | ICD-10 A93.8 | Tick: *Haemaphysalis intermedia* in Asia, *Hyalomma* spp. in Africa, *Dermacentor* spp. in Europe | *Phenuiviridae* | 3 | Africa, Asia, Europe |
| BOURBON | ICD-10 A93.8 | Primary vector unknown, likely ticks | *Orthomyxoviridae* | 2 | USA |
| BUNYAMWERA | ICD-10 A92.8 | Mosquito: *Aedes* spp. | *Peribunyaviridae* | 2 | Africa |
| BWAMBA | ICD-10 A92.8 | Mosquito: primarily *Anopheles* spp., but also *Aedes* spp. | *Peribunyaviridae* | 2 | Africa |
| CHANDIPURA | ICD-10 A93.8 | Sandfly: *Phlebotomus* and *Sergentomyia* spp. and mosquito: *Aedes* spp., *Anopheles stephensi*, and *Culex tritaeniorhynchus* | *Rhabdoviridae* | 2 | Africa, India |
| CHANGUINOLA | ICD-10 A93.8 | Sandfly: *Lutzomyia* spp. | *Reoviridae* | 2 | Central and South America |
| COLORADO TICK FEVER | ICD-10 A93.2 | Tick: *Dermacentor andersoni* | *Reoviridae* | 2 | Western part of Canada and USA |
| DENGUE (1,2,3,4) | ICD-10 A90 | *Aedes* spp. | *Flaviviridae* | 2 | Pan distribution in tropical and subtropical regions |
| DUGBE | ICD-10 A93.8 | Tick: *Amblyomma* spp. | *Nairoviridae* | 3 | Africa |
| GROUP C VIRUSES (Apeu, Caraparu, Itaqui, Madrid, Marituba, Murutucu, Nepuyo, Oriboca, Ossa, and Restan) | ICD-10 A92.8 | Mosquito: *Culex* spp. | *Peribunyaviridae* | 2 | South America, Panama, Trinidad, Mexico |

*(Continued)*

| I. ARBOVIRAL FEVERS (Continued) | | | | | |
|---|---|---|---|---|---|
| **DISEASE** | **ICD-10 CODE** | **VECTOR** | **TAXONOMIC STATUS** | **BIOSAFETY LEVEL** | **OCCURRENCE** |
| HEARTLAND | ICD-10 A93.8 | Primary vector unknown, likely ticks | *Phenuiviridae* | 3 | North America |
| IQUITOS | ICD-10 A93.8 | Biting midge (primary vector unknown) | *Peribunyaviridae* | 2 | South America |
| NAIROBI SHEEP DISEASE | ICD-10 A93.8 | Tick: primarily *Rhipicephalus appendiculatus* | *Nairoviridae* | 3[a] | Africa, India |
| OROPOUCHE | ICD-10 A93.0 | Biting midge: *Culicoides paraensis* | *Peribunyaviridae* | 3 | South America, Panama, Trinidad |
| QUARANFIL | ICD-10 A93.8 | Tick: *Argas* spp. | *Orthomyxoviridae* | 2 | Africa, Middle East |
| RIFT VALLEY FEVER | ICD-10 A92.4 | *Aedes* spp. direct contact with the blood, body fluids, or abortion products of infected domestic ruminants | *Phenuiviridae* | 3[a,b] | Sub-Saharan Africa, Egypt, Madagascar, Arabian Peninsula (Yemen and Saudi Arabia) |
| SANDFLY FEVER NAPLES SICILY (Phlebotomus fever, Papatasi fever) | ICD-10 A93.1 | Sandfly: *Phlebotomus perniciosus, P. perfiliewi, P. papatasi*, primarily *P. papatasi* | *Phenuiviridae* | 2 | Europe, Asia, Africa |
| SEMLIKI FOREST | ICD-10 A92.8 | Mosquito: *Aedes* spp. | *Togaviridae* | 3 | Africa, Asia |
| SEPIK | ICD-10 A92.8 | Mosquito: *Mansonia* spp., *Ficalbia* spp., *Culex sitiens* | *Flaviviridae* | 2 | Papua New Guinea |
| SEVERE FEVER WITH THROMBOCYTOPENIA SYNDROME (Huaiyangshan) | ICD-10 A93.8 | Tick (primary vector unknown) | *Phenuiviridae* | 3 | Eastern Asia |
| SPONDWENI | ICD-10 A92.8 | Mosquito: Various species | *Flaviviridae* | 2 | Africa |
| TAHYÑA | ICD-10 B33.8 | Mosquito: *Aedes* and *Culex* spp. | *Peribunyaviridae* | 2 | Europe, Asia |
| THOGOTO | ICD-10 A93.8 | Tick: *Amblyomma, Boophilus, Hyalomma, Rhipicephalus* species | *Orthomyxoviridae* | 2 | Africa, Europe |

(Continued)

| I. ARBOVIRAL FEVERS (Continued) | | | | | |
|---|---|---|---|---|---|
| DISEASE | ICD-10 CODE | VECTOR | TAXONOMIC STATUS | BIOSAFETY LEVEL | OCCURRENCE |
| USUTU | ICD-10 A92.8 | Mosquito: *Culex* spp. | *Flaviviridae* | 2 | Africa, Europe |
| VESICULAR STOMATITIS | ICD-10 A93.8 | Sandfly: *Lutzomyia* spp. | *Rhabdoviridae* | 2[a] | Americas |
| WESSELSBRON | ICD-10 A92.8 | Mosquito: *Aedes* spp. | *Flaviviridae* | 3[a] | Africa |
| ZIKA | ICD-10 A92.8 | Mosquito: *Aedes* spp. | *Flaviviridae* | 2 | Africa, Asia, Federated States of Micronesia, Americas |

| II. ARBOVIRAL ARTHRITIS AND RASH | | | | | |
|---|---|---|---|---|---|
| DISEASE | ICD-10 CODE | VECTOR | TAXONOMIC STATUS | BIOSAFETY LEVEL | OCCURRENCE |
| BARMAH FOREST | ICD-10 A92.8 | Mosquito: *Culex annulirostris*, *Aedes vigilax*, and other *Aedes* spp. | *Togaviridae* | 2 | Australia |
| CHIKUNGUNYA | ICD-10 A92.0 | Mosquito: *Aedes aegypti, Aedes albopictus* in Asia; other *Aedes* spp. in Africa and Australia | *Togaviridae* | 3 | Africa, southeastern Asia, Pacific Islands, Middle East, Central and South America, Europe |
| MAYARO | ICD-10 A92.8 | Mosquito: *Haemagogus* spp. | *Togaviridae* | 2 | Central America, northern South America, Trinidad |
| O'NYONG-NYONG | ICD-10 A92.1 | Mosquito: *Anopheles* spp. | *Togaviridae* | 2 | Africa |
| ROSS RIVER | ICD-10 B33.1 | Mosquito: *Culex annulirostris*, *Aedes* spp. | *Togaviridae* | 2 | Australia. Sporadic in Papua New Guinea, Pacific Islands |
| SINDBIS | ICD-10 A92.8 | Mosquito: *Aedes* spp. and *Culex* spp. | *Togaviridae* | 2 | Africa, northern Europe. Rare in Asia, Australia |

| III. ARBOVIRAL ENCEPHALITIDES | | | | | |
|---|---|---|---|---|---|
| DISEASE | ICD-10 CODE | VECTOR | TAXONOMIC STATUS | BIOSAFETY LEVEL | OCCURRENCE |
| BANNA | ICD-10 A83.8 | Mosquito (primary vector unknown) | *Reoviridae* | 3 | Southeast Asia |
| CACHE VALLEY | ICD-10 A83.8 | Mosquito: *Anopheles*, *Culiseta*, and *Aedes* spp. | *Peribunyaviridae* | 2 | North America, Guyana |

(Continued)

| III. ARBOVIRAL ENCEPHALITIDES (Continued) | | | | | |
|---|---|---|---|---|---|
| **DISEASE** | **ICD-10 CODE** | **VECTOR** | **TAXONOMIC STATUS** | **BIOSAFETY LEVEL** | **OCCURRENCE** |
| CALIFORNIA ENCEPHALITIS | ICD-10 A83.5 | Mosquito: *Aedes* spp., primarily *A. melanimon* | *Peribunyaviridae* | 2 | USA, Canada |
| EASTERN EQUINE ENCEPHALITIS | ICD-10 A83.2 | Mosquito: *Culiseta melanura* (zoonotic cycle); some *Aedes, Coquillettidia*, and *Culex* spp. (human transmission) | *Togaviridae* | 3[a,b] | Americas |
| EYACH | ICD-10 A84.8 | Tick: *Ixodes* spp. | *Reoviridae* | 2 | Europe |
| ILHÉUS | ICD-10 A83.8 | Mosquito (primary vector unknown) | *Flaviviridae* | 2 | Central and South America |
| JAMESTOWN CANYON | ICD-10 A83.8 | Mosquito: *Aedes* and *Culiseta* spp. | *Peribunyaviridae* | 2 | North America |
| JAPANESE ENCEPHALITIS | ICD-10 A83.0 | Mosquito: Culex spp | *Flaviviridae* | 3 (in USA; 2 in endemic areas with high vaccine coverage)[a] | Asia, Western Pacific |
| KEMEROVO | ICD-10 A84.8 | Tick: *Ixodes persulcatus* | *Reoviridae* | 2 | Russia |
| LA CROSSE | ICD-10 A83.5 | Mosquito: *Aedes triseriatus* | *Peribunyaviridae* | 2 | USA |
| LIPOVNIK | ICD-10 A93.8 | Tick: *Ixodes ricinus* | *Reoviridae* | 2 | Russia |
| LOUPING ILL | ICD-10 A84.8 | Tick: *Ixodes ricinus* | *Flaviviridae* | 3[a] | UK, Ireland, Norway |
| SEMLIKI FOREST | ICD-10 A83.8 | Mosquito (primary vector unknown) | *Togaviridae* | 2 | Vietnam |
| MURRAY VALLEY ENCEPHALITIS | ICD-10 A83.4 | Mosquito: *Culex annulirostris* | *Flaviviridae* | 3 | Australia, Papua New Guinea, Indonesia |
| POWASSAN | ICD-10 A84.8 | Tick: *Ixodes* spp., primarily *Ixodes cookei* and *I. scapularis* in North America; *Ixodes persulcatus* and *Haemaphysalis longicornis* in Russia | *Flaviviridae* | 3 | Canada, USA, Russia |
| ROCIO | ICD-10 A83.6 | Mosquito (primary vector unknown) | *Flaviviridae* | 3 | Brazil |

*(Continued)*

| III. ARBOVIRAL ENCEPHALITIDES (Continued) | | | | | |
|---|---|---|---|---|---|
| **DISEASE** | **ICD-10 CODE** | **VECTOR** | **TAXONOMIC STATUS** | **BIOSAFETY LEVEL** | **OCCURRENCE** |
| SNOWSHOE HARE | ICD-10 A83.8 | Mosquito: *Aedes* and *Culiseta* spp. | *Peribunyaviridae* | 2 | USA, Canada, China, Russia |
| ST. LOUIS ENCEPHALITIS | ICD-10 A83.3 | Mosquito: *Culex* spp. | *Flaviviridae* | 3 | Americas |
| TICKBORNE ENCEPHALITIS | | | | | |
| EUROPEAN | ICD-10 A84.1 | Tick: *Ixodes ricinus* | *Flaviviridae* | 3 (if staff vaccinated)[b] | From Scandinavia down to the Adriatic region, and east to the Urals, Korea |
| FAR EASTERN | ICD-10 A84.0 | Tick: *Ixodes persulcatus* | *Flaviviridae* | 4[b] | Russia, China, northern Japan |
| SIBERIAN | ICD-10 A84.8 | Tick: *Ixodes persulcatus* | *Flaviviridae* | 4[b] | Siberia and the Baltic region |
| TOSCANA | ICD-10 A93.8 | Sandfly: *Phlebotomus* spp. | *Phenuiviridae* | 2 | Southern Europe |
| TRIVITTATUS | ICD-10 A83.8 | Mosquito: *Aedes* spp. | *Peribunyaviridae* | 2 | North America |
| VENEZUELAN EQUINE ENCEPHALITIS | ICD-10 A92.2 | Mosquito: Primarily *Culex (Melanoconion)* spp. (enzootic cycle); *Aedes* and *Psorophora* spp. (epizootic cycle) | *Togaviridae* | 3[a,b] | Americas |
| WESTERN EQUINE ENCEPHALITIS | ICD-10 A83.1 | Mosquito: *Culex tarsalis* | *Togaviridae* | 3 | North and South America |
| WEST NILE | ICD-10 A92.3 | Mosquito: *Culex* spp. | *Togaviridae* | 3 | All continents except Antarctica |

| IV. ARBOVIRAL HEMORRHAGIC FEVERS | | | | | |
|---|---|---|---|---|---|
| **DISEASE** | **ICD-10 CODE** | **VECTOR** | **TAXONOMIC STATUS** | **BIOSAFETY LEVEL** | **OCCURRENCE** |
| CRIMEAN-CONGO HEMORRHAGIC FEVER | ICD-10 A98.0 | *Hyalomma* spp., *Boophilus* and *Rhipicephalus* sp. | *Nairoviridae* | 4[b] | Eastern Europe, Middle East, Africa, Central and Southern Asia |
| DENGUE HEMORRHAGIC FEVER | ICD-10 A91 | *Aedes* spp. | *Flaviviridae* | 2 | Pan distribution in tropical and subtropical regions |
| KYASANUR FOREST DISEASE | ICD-10 A98.2 | *Haemaphysalis spinigera* | *Flaviviridae* | 4[b] | India (Karnataka and neighboring states) |
| ALKHURMA HEMORRHAGIC FEVER | ICD-10 A98.2 | *Ornithodoros savignyi*, *Hyalomma dromedarii* | *Flaviviridae* | 4 | Saudi Arabia, Egypt, Sudan |

(Continued)

| IV. ARBOVIRAL HEMORRHAGIC FEVERS (Continued) | | | | | |
|---|---|---|---|---|---|
| DISEASE | ICD-10 CODE | VECTOR | TAXONOMIC STATUS | BIOSAFETY LEVEL | OCCURRENCE |
| OMSK HEMORRHAGIC FEVER | ICD-10 A98.1 | *Dermacentor reticulatus (pictus)* and *D. marginatus* | *Flaviviridae* | 4[b] | Western Siberia, Russia |
| YELLOW FEVER | ICD-10 A95 | *Aedes* spp. | *Flaviviridae* | 3 | Africa, South America |

[a]Pathogens of significant agricultural importance by USDA and may require additional containment (up to and including BSL-3-Ag containment).
[b]Regulated as select agents under the US Bioterrorism Act of 2002.

Arthropod-borne viruses (arboviruses) are transmitted to humans primarily through the bite of infected arthropods (e.g., mosquitoes, ticks, sandflies, biting midges). There are more than 100 arboviruses known to cause human disease. Arboviruses of medical or unknown human significance are listed in the earlier table with the associated arthropod vector, geographical range, as well as the recommended laboratory biosafety level needed to work with the viruses. The arboviruses are grouped as in *CCDM20* by clinical features: arboviral fevers, arthritis, encephalitis, and hemorrhagic fevers.

Most arboviruses are maintained in zoonotic cycles between birds, or small mammals, and arthropods. Humans are infected incidentally and do not develop sustained or high-level viremia sufficient to infect arthropod vectors. Important exceptions, in which humans are the primary vertebrate amplifying host in the transmission cycle, are dengue, Zika, chikungunya, and yellow fever viruses. Arboviral disease is diagnosed in the laboratory by detection of virus-specific antibodies or viral ribonucleic acid (RNA), primarily in blood, cerebrospinal fluid (CSF), or tissue. Diagnostic testing algorithms have been developed based on the clinical symptoms, level of viremia, immune response, type of specimen, timing of specimen collection, travel history of the patient, and geographic range of the arbovirus, as well as the sensitivity and specificity of the diagnostic test. The prioritized diagnostic tests used for some of the most commonly tested arboviruses are listed in the later table.

**1. Clinical features**—For specific information on the clinical features of arboviral diseases (i.e., fevers, arthritis, encephalitides, and hemorrhagic fevers), see *CCDM20*.

**2. Causative agents**—There are approximately 100 arboviruses that can cause human disease. Arboviruses from the viral families *Flaviviridae*, *Reoviridae*, and *Togaviridae*, and the viral order *Bunyavirales* (bunyaviruses) cause the majority of arboviral infections in humans. The listing of specific arboviruses associated with each of the 4 arboviral disease clinical syndromes is included in the later table.

3. **Laboratory diagnosis**—The definitive diagnosis of arboviral disease requires laboratory testing (see later table). Arbovirus infections are diagnosed serologically by detection of virus-specific immunoglobulin class M (IgM), generally in serum and/or CSF. The IgM antibody capture enzyme-linked immunoassay (MAC-ELISA), or another immunoassay, is a sensitive test after the first few days following symptom onset. However, specificity may be low, particularly for flavivirus and bunyavirus diagnosis due to false positivity resulting from cross-reactivity in consensus regions of major immunogenic epitopes. IgM-positive results should be confirmed by plaque reduction neutralization test (PRNT). Detection of viral genome by quantitative reverse transcriptase (qRT)-polymerase chain reaction (PCR) or nucleotide sequencing are specific and sensitive methods for diagnosis of arboviruses in which humans are the amplifying vertebrate host, such as yellow fever, dengue, chikungunya, and Zika, because viremia can be of high titer and persist for 10–14 days postonset of illness. Specificity of conventional reverse transcription polymerase chain reaction (RT-PCR) can be low due to nonspecific amplification if primer sequences are in consensus regions with other closely related viruses. Sequencing of the RT-PCR product is needed for confirmation. RNA detection is not a sensitive method for those zoonotic arboviruses for which humans are incidental hosts (e.g., Japanese encephalitis, West Nile, St. Louis encephalitis) as viremia is brief and of low titer in humans and generally cleared by the onset of illness. Virus isolation is generally not recommended for arbovirus diagnosis due to the higher sensitivity of molecular assays, as well as the appropriate biosafety facilities required for virus isolation.

4. **Laboratory capability**—Personnel requirements and specialized equipment for performing ELISAs are dependent on the assay format chosen. Point of care (e.g., dipstick) or commercial ELISA kit formats require less specialized training than laboratory-developed tests or more advanced technology, like Luminex-based assays. PRNTs require a strong background in cell culture and virology, along with a laboratory of the appropriate biosafety level (BSL) for working with live virus. Molecular testing such as PCR and sequencing require deoxyribonucleic acid (DNA) amplification instrumentation and DNA visualization equipment, processing conditions to prevent contamination, and specialized training. Reference laboratories may perform vector surveillance, which requires an insectary and specialized training and equipment.

5. **Safety requirements**—Clinical samples are potentially infectious and should be processed for diagnostic testing in a biosafety cabinet (BSC) at the appropriate BSL based on the suspected agent. A higher laboratory BSL may be required for handling suspected arboviruses with higher biosafety classification and/or samples types that might contain high titers of the arbovirus, such as arthropod vectors or tissues from the amplifying host. For

ELISA, if the complete process cannot be performed in a BSC, samples should be aliquoted in the BSC and heat inactivated; if no BSC is available, the complete sample should be heat inactivated prior to processing for serological or molecular testing. ELISA plate washers or hand washing can cause aerosolization, which should be avoided unless performed in a BSC. For PRNT, because live virus is used, the complete procedure must be performed in a BSC with the laboratory BSL corresponding to the BSL classification of the virus. Specific BSL requirements for each arbovirus are listed in the earlier table.

**6. Nonhuman hosts**—Arboviruses are maintained in zoonotic transmission cycles between bird and/or small mammal vertebrate hosts and arthropod vectors. Humans become infected incidentally through a bite of an infected vector but do not develop a sustained viremia of sufficient titer to infect arthropod vectors. The exceptions are chikungunya, dengue, yellow fever, and Zika viruses, for which humans are a primary amplifying host.

**7. Sample/specimen requirements**—Serum and/or CSF are the appropriate specimen types for arbovirus serology. The ideal timing of specimens for serology is acute, 3–10 days after onset of symptoms, and convalescent, 2–3 weeks after the acute sample has been collected. Acute and convalescent specimens, if available, should be tested together. CSF is the preferable diagnostic specimen in neuroinvasive disease caused by arboviruses in the Japanese encephalitis serocomplex, the tickborne encephalitis viruses, and the equine encephalitis viruses, as IgM antibodies elicited in nonneuroinvasive flavivirus infections or following arbovirus vaccination do not enter the CSF. By testing the CSF, the effect of background IgM antibodies in the serum is eliminated. At least 0.5 mL of serum and/or 1.0 mL of CSF is required for serological testing. CSF specimens are routinely tested undiluted and therefore require larger amounts. Virus isolation and/or nucleic acid amplification testing is done on fresh frozen tissue, serum, and CSF; recently, whole blood, urine, and saliva have been shown to be appropriate specimen types for Zika RNA detection assays and may potentially be useful to test for other arboviruses. Those arboviruses for which nucleic acid detection acid assays are a sensitive method of diagnosis and the timing of sample collection are listed in the later table. For serology or nucleic acid detection testing, the specimen should be stored or transported cold or frozen. Tissue specimens should be approximately 1 $cm^3$, frozen as soon as possible at −70°C, and stored frozen or shipped on enough dry ice so that specimens remain frozen until received. Clinical samples are potentially infectious and should be processed in a biosafety cabinet or heat inactivated prior to processing. Nonclinical samples (arthropods and tissues from zoonotic hosts) should be stored at −70°C to preserve the virus viability. Because these samples may contain high concentrations of virus, they should be processed for testing in a BSC.

**8. Testing requirements**—The prioritized diagnostic tests used for some of the most commonly tested arboviruses are listed in the later table. The diagnostic testing algorithm is based on the clinical syndrome and illness phase; timing of sample collection; sample type, volume, and condition; the geographical region and season where the patient lives or traveled; the virus timeline of viremia and immune response; vaccine history; and the performance characteristics of the assay.

Nucleic acid amplification assays such as conventional or qRT-PCR are sensitive tests for samples collected in the first few days following onset of illness in which humans are the primary vertebrate host, due to high-titer, prolonged viremia but have low sensitivity for zoonotic arbovirus detection, characterized by viremia that is brief and of low titer. The qRT-PCR is highly specific and serves as a confirmatory assay, whereas conventional RT-PCR may be less specific, requiring genomic sequencing of the RT-PCR product for confirmation. A negative RT-PCR result does not rule out infection, as the timing of the specimen collection may not have been optimal for RNA detection. Detection of viral nucleic acid or antigen in brain tissue by nucleic acid amplification tests or immunohistochemistry is useful for diagnosis in fatal cases, as these patients may not have detectable IgM or immunoglobulin class G (IgG) antibodies in serum or CSF.

Detection of virus-specific IgM demonstrates recent infection, and a positive result in the MAC-ELISA, microsphere immunoassays, or other IgM detection platform is interpreted as a presumptive infection. A negative result in a specimen collected fewer than 10 days post onset of clinical symptoms does not rule out infection, as IgM may not yet have risen to detectable levels. Although it is recommended that a second sample be obtained between 1–2 weeks after the first sample to demonstrate seroconversion (negative to positive), in practice only a single acute specimen is usually obtained.

False-positive results in the MAC-ELISA are a problem in flavivirus infections due to the conserved immunogenic epitopes on flavivirus envelope proteins, which cross-react in serological assays with other flaviviral antigens. Antibodies within a flavivirus serocomplex are highly cross-reactive; those between serocomplexes are less cross-reactive but still may confound accurate diagnosis. For example, dengue and West Nile viruses, which are not in the same serocomplex, cocirculate in Africa and Asia. Dengue virus does not cause encephalitis but may have a clinical presentation of encephalopathy, and a specimen from a dengue patient submitted for West Nile testing may test positive in a West Nile Virus MAC-ELISA. The PRNT is a more specific assay and should be used to confirm or differentiate conflicting IgM ELISA results in primary flavivirus infections.

The PRNT measures virus-specific neutralizing antibodies. PRNT can also be used for differential diagnosis to discriminate between cross-reacting antibodies in primary flavivirus infections by testing samples simultaneously with multiple challenge viruses. A detectable neutralizing antibody titer to only 1 of the viruses tested corresponding to the IgM results is virus-specific and confirmatory. In patients who have been immunized against or infected with another flavivirus in the past (i.e., who have secondary flavivirus infections), neutralizing antibody titer from the primary flavivirus infection rises quickly and may be equal to or higher than that of the antibody titer from the acute flavivirus infection. Thus, serological diagnosis of secondary flavivirus infections remains problematic, as cross-reactive antibodies in IgM, IgG, and neutralization assays may make it difficult to identify which flavivirus is causing the patient's illness. In addition, IgM antibody to the second infecting virus may not rise to levels detectable by the IgM ELISA, producing a false-negative result. This is typically seen in secondary dengue virus infections. Other serological diagnostic methods are less widely used because they require appropriately timed, paired acute and convalescent specimens. These include detection of a 4-fold or greater rise in virus-specific antibody as measured by hemagglutination inhibition, IgG detection, complement fixation, or PRNT in samples collected during the acute and convalescent phase of illness, at least 14 days apart. Antigen detection assays are generally less sensitive than RT-PCR and, depending on the detection antibody used, may be less specific as well.

Validated, commercial IgM detection assays are not available for most of the arboviruses. IgM detection assays have been developed in reference laboratories for some of the most commonly tested arboviruses (see later table). For suspected arbovirus infections outside the scope and capacity of a laboratory, samples should be submitted to a reference laboratory for diagnostic testing. In-house and commercial assays that have not been validated may have low or unknown sensitivity and specificity and should not be used. Bunyavirus diagnostics are low in specificity as they are such a large, diverse group. There are not general serological assays (ELISA) or consensus primers for conventional RT-PCR.

**9. Reporting requirements**—Currently in the USA, dengue, West Nile, Chikungunya, and Zika are nationally notifiable diseases. The National Notifiable Diseases Surveillance System is a nationwide collaboration that enables all levels of public health agencies—local, state, territorial, federal, and international—to share notifiable disease-related health information (see https://wwwn.cdc.gov/nndss). Identification of an arbovirus isolate in the USA classified as a select agent (North American Eastern equine encephalitis virus and Venezuelan equine encephalitis virus subtypes IAB and IC, Rift Valley fever virus) requires registration with the Federal Select Agent Program (see https://www.selectagents.gov). Arboviral infections are also required to be reported by laboratories in a number of other countries. It is the responsibility of each laboratory to determine the disease reporting requirements within its respective country or jurisdiction.

**10. Referral network**—ArboNET (https://wwwn.cdc.gov/arbonet) is a US arboviral surveillance system managed by CDC and state health departments.

In addition to human disease, ArboNET maintains data on arboviral infections among presumptive viremic blood donors, veterinary disease cases, mosquitoes, dead birds, and sentinel animals. International referral networks include the WHO Japanese encephalitis and yellow fever within the Vaccine Preventable Diseases division and the Arbovirus Diagnosis Laboratory Network of the Americas in the WHO Pan American Health Organization.

**11. Special considerations**—None.

**Diagnostic Testing Algorithm for Most Commonly Tested Arboviruses**

| Virus | Vertebrate host | Specimen(s) to Collect | Method of Identification or Confirmation[a] |
|---|---|---|---|
| CHIKUNGUNYA, O'NYONG-NYONG, MAYARO, ROSS RIVER | Human and nonhuman primates (CHIK), unknown (ONN) zoonotic (MAY, RR) | Serum: ≤ 8 days postsymptom onset | Real-time RT-PCR or conventional RT-PCR/sequencing, virus isolation, IgM ELISA, PRNT |
| | | Serum: > 8 days postsymptom onset | IgM ELISA, PRNT |
| EASTERN EQUINE ENCEPHALITIS,[b] VENEZUELAN EQUINE ENCEPHALITIS,[b] WESTERN EQUINE ENCEPHALITIS | Zoonotic | Serum | IgM ELISA, PRNT |
| | | Cerebrospinal fluid | IgM ELISA, PRNT, real-time RT-PCR, virus isolation |
| | | Tissue specimens (e.g., brain) | Real-time RT-PCR, virus isolation |
| DENGUE (1,2,3,4), YELLOW FEVER | Human (DEN1-4, YF), nonhuman primates (YF) | Serum: ≤ 8 days postsymptom onset | Real-time RT-PCR, virus isolation, NS1 ELISA, IgM ELISA, PRNT |
| | | Serum: > 8 days postsymptom onset | IgM ELISA, PRNT, real-time RT-PCR, virus isolation |
| | | Cerebrospinal fluid | IgM ELISA, PRNT, real-time RT-PCR, virus isolation |
| | | Tissue specimens (e.g., liver, lung, lymph nodes) | Real-time RT-PCR, virus isolation |
| JAPANESE ENCEPHALITIS, MURRAY VALLEY ENCEPHALITIS, POWASSAN, ST. LOUIS ENCEPHALITIS, WEST NILE | Zoonotic | Cerebrospinal fluid | IgM ELISA, PRNT, real-time RT-PCR |
| | | Cerebrospinal fluid | IgM ELISA, PRNT, real-time RT-PCR |
| | | Tissue specimens | Real-time RT-PCR, virus isolation |
| | | Serum: < 14 days postsymptom onset | IgM ELISA, PRNT, real-time RT-PCR, virus isolation |
| | | Serum: ≥ 14 days postsymptom onset | IgM ELISA, PRNT |
| ZIKA | Human | Serum: < 14 days postsymptom onset | Real-time RT-PCR, virus isolation, IgM ELISA, PRNT |
| | | Serum: ≥ 14 days postsymptom onset | IgM ELISA, PRNT, real-time RT-PCR, virus isolation |
| | | Urine | Real-time RT-PCR |
| | | Cerebrospinal fluid | IgM ELISA, PRNT, real-time RT-PCR, virus isolation |
| | | Amniotic fluid | Real-time RT-PCR |
| | | Tissue specimens | Real-time RT-PCR, virus isolation |

*(Continued)*

**Diagnostic Testing Algorithm for Most Commonly Tested Arboviruses (Continued)**

| Virus | Vertebrate host | Specimen(s) to Collect | Method of Identification or Confirmation[a] |
|---|---|---|---|
| JAMESTOWN CANYON, LA CROSSE, SNOWSHOE HARE | Zoonotic | Serum | IgM ELISA, PRNT |
| | | Cerebrospinal fluid | IgM ELISA, PRNT, real-time RT-PCR, virus isolation |
| | | Tissue specimens (e.g., brain) | Real-time RT-PCR, virus isolation |

*Source*: Adapted from CDC (see: http://www.CDC.gov/zika or other specific arbovirus).

[a]Listed in order of priority test.
[b]North American EEEV and VEEV subtypes IAB and IC are classified as select agents in the USA. Identification of a virus isolate requires registration with the Federal Select Agent Program.

[B. W. Johnson, C. H. Goodman, B. Russell]

# ARENAVIRAL HEMORRHAGIC FEVERS, NEW WORLD

| DISEASE | ICD-10 Code |
|---|---|
| JUNIN (ARGENTINIAN) HEMORRHAGIC FEVER | ICD-10 A96.0 |
| MACHUPO (BOLIVIAN) HEMORRHAGIC FEVER | ICD-10 A96.1 |
| GUANARITO (VENEZUELAN) HEMORRHAGIC FEVER | ICD-10 A96.8 |
| SABIA (BRAZILIAN) HEMORRHAGIC FEVER | ICD-10 A96.8 |
| CHAPARE HEMORRHAGIC FEVER | NONE |

**1. Clinical features**—The clinical manifestations of the South American arenaviral hemorrhagic fevers are very similar. They are all acute febrile viral illnesses lasting 6–14 days. Onset is gradual, with malaise, headache, retro-orbital pain, conjunctival injection, and sustained but moderate fever, followed by gastrointestinal signs and symptoms. There may be petechiae and ecchymosis, accompanied by erythema flushing of the face, neck and upper thorax. An enanthem with petechiae on the soft palate is frequent. In the second week of illness, severe infections (e.g., 20%–30% in Junin infections) result in epistaxis, hematemesis, melena, hematuria and gingival hemorrhage, or neurologic manifestations: confusion, ataxia, intention tremors and convulsions and coma. Bradycardia and hypotension with clinical shock are also common findings in severe cases. Progressive leukopenia and thrombocytopenia are characteristic as well as proteinuria. Subclinical infections occur. Case-fatality rates range from 15%–30% in untreated individuals. Around 10% of the patients receiving immune plasma for Junin infection develop a late neurological syndrome with cerebellar signs and cranial nerve palsies. Due to the very limited number of cases described, the full clinical spectrum of Sabia and Chapare infections is unknown.

**2. Causative agents**—Among the 21 known New World arenaviruses (enveloped ambisense ribonucleic acid [RNA] virus in the genus *Arenavirus*, family *Arenaviridae*) belonging to the Tacaribe complex, 5 have been associated with hemorrhagic fever in humans: Junin virus in Argentina, Machupo virus in Bolivia, Guanarito virus in Venezuela, Sabia virus in Brazil, and recently Chapare virus in Bolivia. These viruses are related to the Old World arenaviruses that include lymphocytic choriomeningitis, Lassa, and Lujo viruses.

**3. Laboratory diagnosis**—Confirmation of diagnosis needs laboratory data. During the acute phase of the disease, specific diagnosis is mostly done by virus isolation, RNA detection by conventional or real-time polymerase chain reaction (PCR) or antigen detection in blood or organs (for Machupo infections). In the convalescent phase, immunoglobulin class M (IgM) capture and detection of IgG by enzyme-linked immunosorbent assay (ELISA) are very useful. Laboratory studies for virus isolation and neutralizing antibody tests require biosafety level 4 (BSL-4).

**4. Laboratory capability**—Clinical specimens from suspect patient should always be collected and handled with universal/standard precautions. Outside of endemic areas of each of the viruses, diagnostic reagents are available only at select reference laboratories. For processing clinical specimens with suspicion of viral hemorrhagic fever, trained personnel with appropriate BSL-4 facilities are mandatory. Molecular and serological techniques should be available.

**5. Safety requirements**—Junin, Machupo, Guanarito, Sabia, and Chapare viruses are BSL-4 agents. With the exception of the Junin vaccine, which is available only in Argentina, no other human vaccines are currently available. Collection and handling of infectious or suspected infectious clinical specimens should be performed by trained personnel with disposable caps, gowns, shoe covers, surgical gloves, and respirators (i.e., N99 or N100 high efficiency particulate air filters). Procedures generating aerosols (e.g., centrifugation) should be minimized. The infectivity of samples may be greatly reduced, if not totally inactivated, by the addition of 0.5% Triton X-100 and heating at 37°C for 30 minutes. Afterwards, the samples may then be safely tested by serologic or antigen capture assays in the field. RNA extraction, using the guanidinium acid-phenol method conducted in a laminar-flow safety cabinet, will inactivate the specimen. Handling of infectious diagnostic specimens should be performed by trained personnel with appropriate BSL-4 facilities. Virus isolation attempts should always be performed in a BSL-4 facility.

**6. Nonhuman hosts**—Rodents are arenavirus reservoirs. In Argentina, wild rodents of the pampas (*Calomys musculinus* and *Calomys laucha*) are the hosts for Junin virus. In Bolivia, the large vesper mouse (*Calomys callosus*) is the reservoir for Machupo virus. Cane rats (*Zygodontomys brevicauda*) have been shown to be the main reservoir of Guanarito virus. The reservoir of Sabia and Chapare viruses are not known, although a rodent host is presumed.

Arenaviruses persist in nature by chronically infecting rodents with generally a 1 virus to 1 rodent species relationship. Rodent infections result in long term virus excretion and lifelong viremia; vertical infection is also common.

**7. Sample/specimen requirements**—During the acute febrile stages of disease, virus can be detected in serum, heparinized plasma, or whole blood; serologic techniques can be performed on late acute or convalescent samples of the same type. Virus may also be detected or isolated in biopsy or autopsy specimens from various tissues. Diagnostic samples should be stored and shipped frozen, if possible on dry ice or liquid nitrogen vapor. Viral antigens from tissues can be detected by immunohistochemistry; formaldehyde-fixed tissue and paraffin-embedded blocks should be stored and shipped at room temperature.

**8. Testing requirements**—Junin, Machupo, Guanarito, Sabia, and Chapare diseases are rare, and diagnostic reagents are available only at select reference laboratories. There are no commercially available assays. As for other infectious diseases, the diagnosis should always be based on the results of a combination of clinical and laboratory data. During acute febrile stages of disease, virus can be detected by conventional or real-time PCR targeting the L gene or isolated in general cell culture (e.g., Vero cells) followed by confirmatory sequencing or antigen detection ELISA. In late acute and convalescent stages, IgM or IgG antibodies can be detected by ELISA. Virus antigens can be detected by immunohistochemistry in tissue samples collected postmortem. Direct detection of virus, viral antigens, IgM, or IgG antibodies in an individual with a clinically compatible illness or an individual with a known high-risk exposure to the virus constitutes a confirmed case of infection.

**9. Reporting requirements**—In the USA, Junin, Machupo, Guanarito, and Sabia hemorrhagic fevers are reportable as "viral hemorrhagic fevers" by guidelines of the Council of State and Territorial Epidemiologists. Suspected cases should be reported to state health authorities and if confirmed to CDC through the Nationally Notifiable Diseases Surveillance System. If any of these diseases is suspected in the USA, contact the CDC Viral Special Pathogens Branch by phone (470-312-0094, 404-639-1115) or e-mail (spather@cdc.gov).

**10. Referral network**—Even in endemic areas, testing can only be performed at select reference laboratories with BSL-4 capabilities. For shipping potentially infectious material, samples should be packaged and shipped by appropriately trained and certified staff in accordance with current recommendations (i.e., International Airline Transportation Association) and forwarded, after consultation, to one of the BSL-4 facilities with diagnostic capability for these agents. Testing could be performed at international WHO reference laboratories.

**11. Special considerations**—Occurrence of Junin, Machupo, Guanarito, Sabia, and Chapare diseases do not constitute International Health Regulations reportable events to WHO. Isolation of Junin, Machupo, Guanarito, Sabia, and Chapare viruses must be reported to the Federal Select Agent Program in the USA.

[P. E. Rollin, S. Nichol]

# ARENAVIRAL HEMORRHAGIC FEVERS, OLD WORLD

| DISEASE | ICD-10 CODE |
|---|---|
| LASSA FEVER | ICD-10 A96.2 |
| LUJO DISEASE | NONE |
| Lymphocytic choriomeningitis (see "Lymphocytic Choriomeningitis") | |

**1. Clinical features**—

1) Lassa fever patients present, after a gradual onset, with malaise, fever, headache, sore throat, cough, nausea, vomiting, diarrhea, myalgia, and chest and abdominal pain. Fever is persistent or spikes intermittently. Inflammation and exudation of the pharynx and conjunctivae are common. About 80% of human infections are mild or asymptomatic; the remaining cases have severe multisystem disease. Acute illness lasts 1–4 weeks. Aspartate aminotransferase levels above 150 and high viremia are poor prognosis indicators for the patient.

   In severe cases, hypotension or shock, pleural effusion, hemorrhage, seizures, encephalopathy, and edema of the face and neck are frequent, often with albuminuria and hemoconcentration. Early lymphopenia may be followed by late neutrophilia. Platelet counts are moderately depressed, and platelet function is abnormal. Transient alopecia and ataxia may occur during convalescence, and eighth cranial nerve deafness occurs in 25% of patients, of whom only half recover some function, after 1-3 months.

The overall case-fatality rate is about 1% but can be as high as 15% among hospitalized cases, and even higher in some epidemics. Disease is more severe in pregnancy. Fetal loss occurs in more than 80% of cases and maternal death is frequent, particularly in the third trimester of pregnancy.

Unapparent infections, diagnosed serologically, are common in endemic areas.

2) Lujo disease: the clinical description is similar to that of severe Lassa fever but is based only on observation of 5 patients, 4 of them with a fatal outcome. The incubation period varied between 7-13 days. The clinical course started by a nonspecific febrile illness, headache, and muscle pain. It then progressed rapidly, becoming more severe with a morbilliform rash on the face and trunk, face and neck swelling, pharyngitis, and diarrhea. Bleeding was not a prominent feature. In the fatal cases, a transient improvement was followed by a rapid deterioration with respiratory distress, neurological signs, and circulatory collapse. Death occurred 10-13 days after onset. Low blood platelets, low white blood cell count (at the onset, rising later on), and elevated liver function values were present in all patients.

**2. Causative agents**—Lassa and Lujo viruses are enveloped ambisense ribonucleic acid (RNA) viruses in the genus *Arenavirus*, family *Arenaviridae*. Among viruses in the *Arenavirus* genus, Lassa and Lujo viruses are considered Old World arenaviruses, which include lymphocytic choriomeningitis.

**3. Laboratory diagnosis**—Lassa fever can be confirmed by direct detection of virus in blood or tissue samples by virus isolation, conventional or real-time polymerase chain reaction (PCR), antigen-detection enzyme-linked immunosorbent assay (ELISA), immunohistochemistry (IHC) on formalin-fixed tissues, or by detection of virus-specific immunoglobulin class M (IgM) antibodies or rising IgG antibody titers. Lujo disease can be diagnosed by the same techniques, although the diagnosis experience is based on very few cases.

**4. Laboratory capability**—Clinical specimens from suspect patient should always be collected and handled with universal/standard precautions. Outside of endemic areas of West Africa, Lassa fever is rare and diagnostic reagents are available only at select reference laboratories with biosafety level 4 (BSL-4) capabilities. Laboratories capable of offering Lujo diagnostic tools are even more limited. For processing clinical specimens with suspicion of viral hemorrhagic fever, and trained personnel with appropriate BSL-4 facilities are mandatory. Molecular and serological techniques should be available.

**5. Safety requirements**—Lassa and Lujo viruses are BSL-4 agents. No human vaccines are currently available. Collection and handling of infectious or suspected infectious clinical specimens should be performed by trained personnel with disposable caps, gowns, shoe covers, surgical gloves, and respirators (e.g., N99 or N100 high efficiency particulate air filters). Procedures generating aerosols (e.g., centrifugation) should be minimized. The infectivity of samples may be greatly reduced, if not totally inactivated, by the addition of 0.5% Triton X-100 and heat treatment for 30 minutes at 65°C, and the samples may then be safely tested by serologic or antigen capture assays in the field. RNA extraction, using the guanidinium acid-phenol method conducted in a laminar-flow safety cabinet or a glove box, will inactivate the specimen. Handling of infectious diagnostic specimens should be performed by trained personnel with appropriate personal protective equipment and BSL-4 facilities. Virus isolation attempts should always be performed in a BSL-4 facility.

**6. Nonhuman hosts**—Rodents in the genus *Mastomys* are the reservoir of Lassa virus. The reservoir of Lujo virus is unknown but probably a rodent, as for other arenaviruses.

**7. Sample/specimen requirements**—During the acute febrile stages of disease, virus can be detected in serum, heparinized plasma, or whole blood, and serologic techniques can be performed on late acute or convalescent samples of the same type. Virus may also be detected or isolated in biopsy or autopsy specimens from various tissues. Diagnostic samples should be stored and shipped frozen, if possible, on dry ice or liquid nitrogen vapor. Viral antigens from tissues as well as skin can be detected by IHC; formaldehyde-fixed tissue and paraffin-embedded blocks should be stored and shipped at room temperature.

**8. Testing requirements**—Lassa and Lujo virus infections are limited in distribution, and diagnostic reagents are available only at select reference laboratories. There are no commercially available assays. As for other infectious diseases, the diagnosis should always be based on the results of a combination of clinical and laboratory data. During acute febrile stages of disease, virus can be detected by conventional PCR with primers targeting the L gene, followed by confirmatory sequencing of the amplicon; the newly proposed real-time PCR (targeting both S and L genes); virus isolation, followed by sequencing; or antigen detection ELISA. In late acute and convalescent stages, IgM or IgG antibodies can be detected by ELISA. Virus antigens can be detected by immunohistochemistry in tissue samples collected postmortem. Direct detection of virus, viral antigens, IgM or IgG antibodies in an individual with a clinically compatible illness or an individual with a known high-risk exposure to the virus constitutes a confirmed case of infection.

**9. Reporting requirements**—Lassa virus infections in the USA are reportable as "viral hemorrhagic fever" by the guidelines of the Council of State and Territorial Epidemiologists. Suspected cases should be reported to the State Health authorities, and if confirmed, to CDC through the National Notifiable Diseases Surveillance System. If Lassa or Lujo infections are suspected in the USA, contact the CDC Viral Special Pathogens Branch by phone (470-312-0094 or 404-639-1115) or e-mail (spather@cdc.gov).

**10. Referral network**—Testing can only be performed at select reference laboratories with BSL-4 capabilities. For shipping potentially infectious material, samples should be packaged and shipped by trained and competency assessed in packaging and shipping requirements personnel, in accordance with current recommendations (i.e., International Airline Transportation Association) and forwarded, after consultation, to one of the BSL-4 facilities with diagnostic capability for these agents. Testing could be performed at international WHO reference laboratories or nationally in select laboratories (e.g., European Network for Diagnostics of "Imported" Viral Diseases).

**11. Special considerations**—Occurrence of Lassa infection outside of an endemic country likely constitutes an International Health Regulations reportable event to the WHO. Isolation of Lassa or Lujo viruses must be reported to the Federal Select Agent Program in the USA.

[P. E. Rollin, S. Nichol]

# ASCARIASIS

| DISEASE | ICD-10 CODE |
|---|---|
| ASCARIASIS | ICD-10 B77 |

**1. Clinical features**—Infection with the intestinal helminth *Ascaris lumbricoides* often causes few, or no, overt clinical symptoms. The most frequent complaint of patients infected with *Ascaris* is vague abdominal pain, but some may have pulmonary manifestations (pneumonitis, Loeffler's syndrome) caused by larval migration (mainly during reinfections) and characterized by wheezing, cough, fever, and signs of eosinophilia and pulmonary infiltration. Live worms, passed in stools or occasionally from the mouth, anus, or nose, are often the first recognized signs of infection. Worm migration may be stimulated by anesthetic agents, fever, or subtherapeutic anthelmintic treatment. Heavy parasite burden may aggravate nutritional deficiency and, if chronic, may affect work and school performance. Serious complications, sometimes fatal, include bowel obstruction by a bolus of worms, particularly in children, or obstruction of bile duct, pancreatic duct, or appendix by 1 or more adult worms.

**2. Causative agents**—*A. lumbricoides* is a large intestinal roundworm and is a human parasite. However, *Ascaris suum*, a similar parasite of pigs, is probably synonymous with *A. lumbricoides*, based on morphological, biological, and molecular analyses. The degree of sharing between humans and pigs is still not clear. Ongoing studies are being conducted to elucidate under what conditions and how commonly the infection is shared between the hosts and what differences and similarities exist between their clinical signs and symptoms.

**3. Laboratory diagnosis**—*A. lumbricoides* is diagnosed primarily by the microscopic observation of eggs in concentrated stool during routine ova and parasite (O&P) examinations. Routine molecular and serologic assays are not available for ascariasis.

Fertile eggs are unembryonated when passed in feces and measure 55–75 μm long by 35–50 μm wide and have a thick shell that may have a bumpy outer layer (mammillated) or smooth surface (decorticated). Infertile eggs are 85–95 μm long by 43–47 μm wide with a thin shell and disorganized internal contents and may also be mammillated or decorticated.

Adult worms may be recovered in stool or, less frequently, expelled from the nose or mouth. Adult female worms are 20–35 cm and have 3 fleshy lips on the anterior end; males are smaller and tend to have a curved tail. Adult worms and eggs in ectopic sites are usually identified incidentally during examination of histologically prepared biopsy specimens. Third-instar larvae may be detected in respiratory washes and biopsy specimens.

**4. Laboratory capability**—Microscopy and stool concentration/centrifugation capabilities should be available. Laboratorians should be trained in the microscopic/morphologic detection of parasites and undergo regular proficiency testing.

**5. Safety requirements**—Clinical specimens should always be collected and handled with universal/standard precautions. *A. lumbricoides* is a biosafety level 2 organism. Fertile eggs are shed unembryonated in human stool and not immediately infectious; however, they may embryonate over time, even in stool preserved in 10% formalin, and may eventually become infectious. Formalin should only be used in a well-ventilated area, preferably in a chemical fume hood. Unpreserved and preserved stools should be disposed of as infectious waste.

**6. Nonhuman hosts**—Pigs can serve as a reservoir host and food, water, and fomites contaminated with infected pig feces may serve as a source of human infection.

**7. Sample/specimen requirements**—Stool should be promptly preserved in an appropriate liquid medium, such as 10% buffered formalin or sodium acetate-acetic acid-formalin. Single vial systems for O&P collection are also adequate. Adult worms should also be placed in a liquid preservative such as 10% formalin or 70% laboratory grade ethanol as soon as possible after collection to avoid desiccation and alteration of morphologic features. Specimens in the appropriate preservatives should remain intact indefinitely. To maximize O&P sensitivity, up to 3 stool specimens should be collected.

**8. Testing requirements**—Routine concentration procedures for stool (eggs) and routine examination of gross helminths (adults). A calibrated ocular micrometer should be used to measure egg size.

**9. Reporting requirements**—Ascariasis is not nationally reportable in the USA. Report to local health authority; official report not ordinarily justifiable. International reporting not required.

**10. Referral network**—None.

**11. Special considerations**—None.

[B. Mathison]

# ASPERGILLOSIS

| DISEASE | ICD-10 CODE |
|---|---|
| ASPERGILLOSIS | ICD-10 B44 |

**1. Clinical features**—Aspergillosis is an infection by the fungus *Aspergillus*. Aspergillosis describes a large number of diseases involving both infection and growth of fungus as well as allergic responses. Aspergillosis can occur in a variety of organs, both in humans and animals. All animals and many plants have highly efficient mechanisms to prevent themselves being infected by *Aspergillus* spp., and it is usually only when those mechanisms are defective in some way that *Aspergillus* spp. can grow within the body. The vast majority of people who may develop life-threatening aspergillosis are those who have had their immune system weakened by corticosteroid therapy, critical care, transplant surgery, or following treatments for cancer. Alternatively, aspergillosis can occur in an immunocompetent person (i.e., a person with no known suppression of their immune system) where previous tissue damage has occurred—for instance, heavily scarred pulmonary tissue associated with tuberculosis, chronic obstructive pulmonary disease, bronchiectasis, or some underlying lung disease.

Many different manifestations of aspergillosis are well described, including allergic aspergillosis (i.e., rhinosinusitis and bronchopulmonary; >10 million cases worldwide), chronic pulmonary and rhinosinus aspergillosis (~3 million cases worldwide), invasive aspergillosis (incidence >300,000 cases annually), and superficial disease (i.e., notably keratitis, otomycosis, and trauma or burn wound infections). These conditions are seen worldwide.

Allergic bronchopulmonary aspergillosis (ABPA) presents as poorly controlled asthma, production of mucous plugs and/or mucoid impaction, pneumonia, and serologically, in patients with asthma. Poor asthma control in severe asthma is associated with *Aspergillus* spp. sensitization. In cystic fibrosis, it presents with pulmonary infiltrates and worsening lung function. Extrinsic allergic bronchoalveolitis may be attributable to *Aspergillus* spp.

Chronic pulmonary aspergillosis (CPA) usually occurs in patients with underlying pulmonary disease and presents with persistent cough, hemoptysis, weight loss, breathlessness, and fatigue. It may lead to respiratory failure through progressive fibrosis (e.g., destroyed lung).

Invasive aspergillosis (IA) occurs in hematological malignancy after transplantation, in those with chronic obstructive pulmonary disease and in those treated with corticosteroids. IA is now reported in other immunocompromised patient populations, such as intensive care unit patients, patients given anti-tumor necrosis factor therapy, and patients with acquired immune deficiency syndrome. The early clinical features are usually silent; pyrexia is unusual, and later manifestations include chest discomfort and mild hemoptysis.

**2. Causative agents**—The genus *Aspergillus* includes over 300 species. *Aspergillus* spp. spores are commonly found in air, water, soil, plant debris, rotten vegetation, manure, sawdust litter, bagasse litter, animal feed, bark chippings on animals, and the indoor air environment.

Around 20 species have so far been reported as causative agents of opportunistic infections in humans, although many cryptic species are now implicated; therefore, the term "complex" is added to species names, unless definitive identification has been done. Among these, *Aspergillus fumigatus* is the most commonly isolated species, followed by *Aspergillus flavus* and *Aspergillus niger. Aspergillus nidulans, Aspergillus terreus, Aspergillus calidoustus,* and *Aspergillus versicolor* are among the other species less commonly isolated. If cultured at all, the fungus grows quite readily on ordinary laboratory culture media at room temperature, at 37°C, and at higher temperatures. Czapek's solution agar or Sabouraud's agar may be used.

The use of multilocus deoxyribonucleic acid (DNA) sequence analysis has led to the description of previously unknown cryptic *Aspergillus* spp., whereas classical morphology-based identification of *Aspergillus* remains limited to the section or species-complex level. The current literature highlights 2 main features concerning these cryptic *Aspergillus* spp. First, the prevalence of such species in clinical samples is relatively high compared with emergent filamentous fungal taxa such as *Mucorales*, *Scedosporium*, or *Fusarium*. Second, it is clearly important to identify these species in the clinical laboratory because of the high frequency of antifungal drug-resistant isolates of such *Aspergillus* spp. Matrix-assisted laser desorption/ionization time-of-flight mass spectrometry (MALDI-TOF MS) has recently been shown to enable the identification of filamentous fungi with an accuracy similar to that of DNA sequence-based methods. As MALDI-TOF MS is well suited to the routine clinical laboratory workflow, it facilitates the identification of these cryptic *Aspergillus* spp. in the routine mycology laboratory. The rapid establishment of enhanced filamentous fungi identification facilities will lead to a better understanding of the epidemiology and clinical importance of these previously unrecognized *Aspergillus* spp. Based on routine MALDI-TOF MS–based identification results, insights are provided into the key interpretation issues of a positive *Aspergillus* culture from a clinical sample. Which ubiquitous species frequently isolated from air samples are rarely involved in human invasive disease? Can both the species and the type of biological sample indicate *Aspergillus* carriage, colonization, or infection in a patient? Highly accurate routine filamentous fungi identification is central to enhance the understanding of these previously unknown *Aspergillus* spp., with a vital impact on further improved patient care.

**3. Laboratory diagnosis**—Diagnosis of the different forms of aspergillosis can be challenging for several reasons, especially as *Aspergillus* spp. is infrequently isolated from infected persons. Microscopy is rapid and useful for respiratory, ocular, and ear specimens.

1) Culture: the sensitivity of cultures for diagnosing invasive aspergillosis is low, varies with the patient population being tested, and may require unacceptable patient risk to obtain tissue for culture. The positive predictive value of cultures in patients receiving a hematopoietic cell transplant is at its highest 72% and the lowest in human immunodeficiency virus patients at 14%. When analyzing sputum cultures, a positive result for an *Aspergillus* spp. may reflect colonization or chronic pulmonary disease in immunocompetent patients, but in the immunocompromised host, a positive result more likely represents invasive disease. In addition to the variation in interpretation of the cultures based on at-risk populations, the slower identification of growth of *Aspergillus* spp. may delay initiation of appropriate antifungal agents and thus further compromise patient outcome. However, a positive culture does allow the laboratory to identify the species of *Aspergillus*, which may have important clinical implications. The success of culturing respiratory secretions is volume dependent. Standard sputum cultures have a low yield in the detection of *Aspergillus* spp., where a fraction of the specimen is cultured. Plating out 1–5 mL of the specimen significantly

increases the recovery rate of *Aspergillus* spp. compared with conventional culture where, typically, a small volume (1–10 μL) is inoculated. For therapeutic decisions regarding antifungal agents, the culture can be used for in vitro susceptibility testing.

2) Antibody detection: measuring *Aspergillus*-specific antibodies are key parts of the diagnostic pathway for allergic aspergillosis (e.g., the immunoglobulin class E [IgE]) and chronic aspergillosis (e.g., IgG). There are numerous techniques for quantifying antibodies. The best techniques are automated (e.g., the Siemens Immulite assay) or based on enzyme-linked immunosorbent assay (e.g., the Bio-Rad assay). Skin prick testing may be used for allergic aspergillosis. Total IgE is usually elevated, as is the eosinophil count in allergic aspergillosis.
3) Antigen detection: first successfully evaluated in hematology patients, the antigen galactomannan (GM) sensitivity in serum is low in other patient populations where the pathophysiology of the infection can be different, and the prevalence of IA is much lower. In bronchoalveolar lavage specimens, detection of *Aspergillus* antigen (usually GM) is ~80% sensitive and specific and superior to culture and microscopy for all pulmonary aspergillosis syndromes. In IA, *Aspergillus* antigen may be detected in blood especially in neutropenic patients; it is less sensitive in blood in transplant and critical care patients. In invasive aspergillosis, beta-1,3-D-glucan is often detectable in blood but is not specific to aspergillosis. A combination of beta-1,3-D-glucan and GM looks promising. Confirming the diagnosis of invasive aspergillosis is often difficult to accomplish and is usually based on a combination of clinical, radiological, microbiological, and/or histopathological findings. Certain chest computerized tomography findings are highly distinctive, notably with the halo sign in neutropenic patients.
4) Nucleic acid amplification techniques (i.e., polymerase chain reaction [PCR]): *Aspergillus* DNA detection in blood or serum (or both) has reached a certain level of acceptance thanks to consensus methods based on real-time quantitative PCR, for example, the European Aspergillus PCR Initiative. The sensitivity and specificity of PCR for detecting invasive aspergillosis vary greatly between studies. The lack of standardization of the technique between studies proves to be a recurrent factor in the variation of the test results. However, since *Aspergillus* DNA circulates as free DNA, the use of serum instead of whole blood for the detection of infection gives the advantage of reducing the processing required to extract and isolate the DNA. This allows for a reduced risk of contamination. Incorporating PCR with nonmolecular techniques, however, could be useful in creating

diagnostic strategies with high sensitivity and specificity. For example, combining PCR with a GM assay on a serum specimen in a test requiring only 1 of the 2 assays to have a positive signal for the diagnosis produces highly sensitive and specific results. PCR can also be performed using bronchoalveolar lavage (BAL) fluid with sensitivities similar to the GM assay. Sputum samples usually yield *Aspergillus* DNA by PCR in chronic and allergic aspergillosis more often than culture. A number of studies have suggested that consecutively positive results with PCR are associated with higher mortality rates in patients with suspected invasive aspergillosis. There have also been some inconclusive results regarding the utility of PCR in antifungal stewardship, suggesting that using consecutive PCR results for diagnosis may lead to a decrease in empiric antifungal agent use.

5) New diagnostic modalities (i.e., lateral flow devices and exhaled breath signatures): lateral-flow immunoassays for *Aspergillus* antigen detection potentially have the advantage of being highly accurate, easy to use, and cost efficient and can be used on serum and BAL. The simplicity and low cost of the lateral flow device for invasive aspergillosis offers a point-of-care test, both in resource-available and resource-limited clinical care centers. Electronic noses or E-noses use exhaled volatile organic compounds from patients with invasive aspergillosis as a creative and sensitive biomarker for diagnosis. In small studies, accuracy is good, and the technique is user friendly, quick, and potentially cheap once the equipment is acquired. This interesting technology will be helped by further clinical validation followed by marketing of reliable, cost-effective equipment to medical centers.

In parallel, new therapeutic strategies (mainly, azole prophylaxis in hematology) are now widely used. If the expected result is a decrease of IA prevalence, an expected bystander effect is a negative impact on the performance of biomarkers, which must be reappraised. Indeed, the prevalence of the disease directly impacts the performance of any test and GM in particular. Furthermore, this extensive use of prophylaxis, for example posaconazole, has also shed light on the occurrence of azole-resistant *A. fumigatus* isolates.

**4. Laboratory capability**—To achieve the best patient outcomes, modern clinical mycology laboratories must have both the portfolio of tests necessary for the accurate and timely diagnosis and follow-up of patients with suspected invasive fungal infections (IFIs), and the laboratory must integrate well with clinicians at the bedside. Test availability must be present in medical center and hospital laboratories who care for the seriously ill to ensure optimal patient care. Although all acute care hospitals will generally deal at times with some aspect of IFIs, it is important to emphasize that hospitals and/or medical centers vary in their number of patients at risk for IFIs, and all hospital system hospitals must be aware of their own specific fungal epidemiology.

There are a series of basic needs for the clinician by the clinical mycology laboratory today. In any hospital or medical center taking care of acute and/or immunosuppressed patients, the mycology laboratory must have or be in the process of acquiring the following skill sets:

1) Accurate fungal species identification is essential. This ability is now being switched from classical mycological descriptions and biochemistries to matrix-assisted laser desorption/ionization time-of-flight mass spectrometry and nucleic acid amplification techniques/PCR/sequencing. It has implications in treatment at the bedside and in infection control.
2) Histopathology can be insightful, and the clinical mycology laboratory needs to collaborate with the pathology department for optimization of care. Training in this area is urgently needed (see http://www.microfungi.net).
3) Rapid diagnosis is important, and therefore, mycology laboratories need to work with clinicians to understand and implement effective biomarkers tailored to the local host populations and management strategies. Biomarkers, such as beta-1,3-D-glucan can replace or reduce spiraling antifungal empiricism.
4) Culture techniques need to be carefully integrated with rapid diagnostic methods. Clinicians have validated clinical practice outcomes on viable fungi (cultures), but this must be combined with more efficient diagnostic methods. Clinicians need to embrace new technology.
5) Invasive fungal infections are deadly, but the combination of a receptive and progressive mycology laboratory and a small cadre of antifungal agents can and does save lives.
6) The clinical mycology laboratory needs to be carefully linked to clinical practices, antifungal stewardship, and infection control challenges. In general, it is a dynamic time for the clinical mycology laboratory with many tools to use and validate. What can the clinical mycology laboratory do? Used wisely, it has the ability to save the lives of our most fragile and vulnerable patients.

**5. Safety requirements**—In the USA and Canada, *Aspergillus* spp. is classified as risk group 2. This rating applies to the genus as a whole and may not apply to every species in the genus. In the UK, the Advisory Committee on Dangerous Pathogens lists *Aspergillus* spp. as hazard group 2 organisms, and containment level 2 laboratory practices are sufficient for handling the agent. Laboratory-acquired infections have not been reported. A primary hazard is inhalations of air contaminated with *Aspergillus* conidia.

**6. Nonhuman hosts**—The importance of aspergillosis in humans and various animal species has increased over the last decades. *Aspergillus* spp. are found worldwide in humans and in almost all domestic animals and birds as well as in many wild species. They cause a wide range of diseases from localized infections to fatal disseminated diseases, as well as allergic responses to inhaled conidia. Some prevalent forms of animal aspergillosis are invasive fatal infections in sea fan corals, stonebrood mummification in honey bees, pulmonary and air sac infection in birds, mycotic abortion and mammary gland infections in cattle, guttural pouch mycoses in horses, sinonasal infections in dogs and cats, and invasive pulmonary and cerebral infections in marine mammals and nonhuman primates.

**7. Sample/specimen requirements**—Upper and lower respiratory secretions (sputum, BAL, bronchial washings) are the appropriate specimens for direct microscopy, culture, GM, PCR; blood for antibody assays (specific IgG, specific IgE); blood for GM and PCR; and sinus lavage in cases of sinusitis. Under certain conditions, biopsy and postmortem tissue samples may also be appropriate.

**8. Testing requirements**—Besides direct microscopy and culture, which remain important for identification and antifungal susceptibility testing of the fungus, several biomarkers have been evaluated: GM, beta-1,3-D-glucan, and *Aspergillus* DNA. These biomarkers have been tested in blood or serum (or both) and in respiratory specimens. The main issue for the present circulating biomarkers is their poor specificity. This weak specificity is due to the analytical performance of the tests but also to the presence of the biomarkers tested in the environment, including food, inhaled air, pharmaceutical products, or blood tubes. Antibody detection has been poorly studied for IA because of the underlying immunodepression and is not considered a diagnostic criterion. Moreover, the assays are not standardized. Therefore, they will not be addressed here.

Galactomannan detection in combination with radiology is the cornerstone for the diagnosis of IA; beta-1,3-D-glucan assists in case detection, especially outside hematology units. Galactomannan is a microbiological criterion for defining IA in hematology and solid organ transplant patients, but there are difficulties related to studying its performance as an evaluation tool and as a diagnostic criterion. Galactomannan is also used as a surrogate marker to follow the efficacy of treatment. The main limitation of serum GM is the high rate of false-positive results, which fall under 2 categories: irreproducible results and detection not related to IA. The irreproducible positive results correspond to results that are not confirmed when retested and should be considered negative. Confirmed positive results are technically true positive, which corresponds to either a true IA or the presence of GM from environmental sources. There is currently no means to safely discard a GM-positive result that is not related to ongoing IA based on technical artefacts. Only the analysis of prescribed intravenous drugs or parenteral nutrition and possibly dietary products can support a false positive due to infused or ingested products. Otherwise, it is the analysis of the evolution of the disease and medical file records that allow discrimination between true-positive or false-positive results.

As highlighted earlier, the medical performance of GM is decreasing due to the increasingly widespread use of effective antimold prophylaxis. In these conditions, the screening strategy usually proposed in hematology could become inefficient and would no longer be recommended. If it is used as a confirmatory test, thresholds to define positivity could have to be reassessed for GM and also for other biomarkers. For instance, the GM positivity level of 0.5 in 2 separate serum samples is used as a screening test because the goals are to minimize the risk of IA and to limit the risk of overtreating, whereas the positivity threshold is at least 0.7–1.0 in BAL fluid sample to assess the diagnosis.

**9. Reporting requirements**—There are no regional or national reporting/notification requirements for aspergillosis. Outbreaks (≥ 2 cases in a short time frame) should be reported to the individual hospital's infection control teams. Notification to national organizations, such as Public Health England in the UK, is voluntary, but currently there is a data gathering exercise with a focus on antifungal resistance in *A. fumigatus.*

**10. Referral network**—There is a robust network of specialist mycology laboratories in some regions of the world. However, mycology reference laboratories are still needed in many areas. Within Europe, there are European Confederation of Medical Mycology Centres of Excellence, which provide expertise in diagnosing and managing aspergillosis.

**11. Special considerations—**

1) Prevention: avoidance of exposure can be achieved by restricting gardening and occupational activities. The wearing of masks is effective but rarely practicable.
2) Prophylaxis is usually used for high (>10%) and medium (3%–10%) risk patients, such as those with chronic granulomatous disease, acute myeloid leukemia, and allogeneic hematopoietic transplant recipients with graft versus host disease. The preferred agent is posaconazole, but itraconazole solution and voriconazole have been used.
3) Numerous hospital-associated outbreaks of aspergillosis have occurred. Hospital construction, indoor water damage, and improper air filtration have all been associated with these outbreaks.

[M. D. Richardson, D. W. Denning]

# BABESIOSIS

| DISEASE | ICD-10 CODE |
|---|---|
| BABESIOSIS | B60 |

**1. Clinical features**—The clinical spectrum ranges from asymptomatic to life threatening. Common manifestations include fever, other nonspecific flu-like symptoms (e.g., chills, sweats, myalgia, fatigue), and hemolytic anemia; thrombocytopenia also is common. Severe cases can be associated with hemodynamic instability, acute respiratory distress, renal failure, hepatic compromise, disseminated intravascular coagulation, altered mental status, and death. Even persons with asymptomatic infection may have low-level parasitemia for months, sometimes for longer than a year, making transmission via blood transfusion a year-round concern.

**2. Causative agents**—Intraerythrocytic protozoan parasites of the *Babesia* genus, transmitted by ticks in the genus *Ixodes*. In the USA, the identified zoonotic agents include, predominantly, *Babesia microti*; also, *Babesia duncani* (formerly, the WA1-type parasite) and related organisms, as well as *Babesia divergens*-like parasites. In Europe and China, identified agents are *Babesia divergens*, *Babesia venatorum* (formerly, the EU1 agent), and *B. microti*. In other regions of the world, poorly described *Babesia* strains have been identified causing human infections, including a *B. microti*-like agent in Taiwan and Japan and a new agent (KO1) in South Korea. Poorly characterized species of *Babesia* infecting humans have been reported from Africa, Central America, and South America. Transfusion acquired babesiosis has been documented, and blood stocks in endemic areas should be screened for the parasite.

**3. Laboratory diagnosis**—Acute cases with patent parasitemia are diagnosed by the morphological detection and identification of intraerythrocytic *Babesia* trophozoites or merozoites in patient blood. *B. microti* infections may have parasitemias as high as 85% on peripheral blood films. *Babesia* trophozoites are distinctive, small ring forms with blue cytoplasm and purple nuclei. These are often the only forms present in a blood film and may be very difficult to distinguish from ring forms of *Plasmodium falciparum*. Indicators of ring forms being *Babesia* sp. rather than *P. falciparum* are unusually small sized rings, the absence of malaria pigment granules in the cytoplasm of the ring or infected red cell, the presence of extracellular forms, the presence of abnormal or pleomorphic merozoite forms, and a patient travel history consistent with exposure to *Babesia* but not malaria. *Babesia* merozoites are mostly intracellular in the red cells, though extracellular forms may occasionally be seen. Merozoites may appear as pyriform, oval, comma shaped or other pleomorphic forms staining purple or blue in Romanowsky stains. A negatively staining internal vacuole may be present. Multiple infected red cells are common, with 4 or more parasites per red cell not being unusual. Tetrad forms, although morphologically distinctive, are rarely seen. Pyriform bodies of *B. microti* and *B. duncani* merozoites are 1.0–2.5 μm in size and morphologically indistinguishable from one another. *B. divergens* merozoites are slightly larger, between 1.0–3.0 μm.

Results based on morphology should be reported as *Babesia* spp., since morphology alone cannot distinguish between some species. Confirmation of the diagnosis and species-specific identification can be obtained by serologic or molecular assays. Several polymerase chain reaction (PCR)-based protocols are available to confirm microscopy results and provide a species-level identification; the majority of protocols amplify unique parts of the 18S ribosomal ribonucleic acid gene. Polymerase chain reaction–based detection is more sensitive than microscopy and generally highly specific. Serologic testing can be performed by indirect immunofluorescence assay (IFA) or enzyme-linked immunosorbent assay (ELISA). IFA titers of 1:64 or higher are considered indicative of current infection or past exposure to *B. microti* and *B. divergens* antigens, whereas titers of 1:256 or higher are considered positive for *B. duncani*. Gradual seroreversion after treatment is seen in most patients. *B. microti* antigen titers of 1:1024 or higher are considered indicative of infection within the past 12 months, though titers usually drop to 1:64 or less within 12 months of infection. If indicated by the epidemiologic and clinical context, the possibility of coinfection with *Borrelia burgdorferi* sensu lato (Lyme disease) or *Anaplasma phagocytophilum* (human granulocytic anaplasmosis) should be considered. If laboratory assays are inconclusive and infection is strongly suspected, inoculation into laboratory animals (e.g., hamsters and gerbils) may be required.

**4. Laboratory capability**—Regional or district level clinical diagnostic laboratory with trained blood microscopists is needed for morphological detection. Microscopists should be trained in how to distinguish *Babesia* from *Plasmodium* species. Tertiary level laboratories with PCR facilities are required for molecular techniques. Serological detection requires reference laboratory level skills. Laboratories performing diagnostic testing should participate in regular external quality assessment.

**5. Safety requirements**—Clinical specimens should always be collected and handled with universal/standard precautions. *Babesia* spp. are biosafety level 2 organisms. Blood specimens should be disposed of as infectious waste.

**6. Nonhuman hosts**—Babesiosis is a zoonotic disease that can be transmitted to humans from animals via a vector. Nonhuman animal hosts include white-footed mice (*Peromyscus leucopus*) and other small mammals for *B. microti* in the USA, as well as cattle for *B. divergens* and roe deer for

*B. venatorum* in Europe. *B. duncani* has also been identified as a parasite of dogs. The nonhuman hosts of other species of *Babesia* have not yet been definitively determined.

**7. Sample/specimen requirements**—Ethylenediaminetetraacetic acid (EDTA) anticoagulated blood specimens are required for morphologic and molecular diagnosis. Thin and thick blood smears for morphologic identification should be prepared as soon as possible and no later than 24 hours after collection. Serum or plasma are required for serology.

**8. Testing requirements**—Morphological diagnosis should be carried out on thick and thin blood smears. Smears should be stained with a Romanowsky stain (i.e., Wrights, Wright Giemsa, or Giemsa) and examined thoroughly by light microscopy. Data are not available on the sensitivity of microscopy for the detection of *Babesia* sp. in blood, though parasites may be very scarce in blood films and it is likely that molecular and serological approaches have a greater efficacy in detecting infections. A real-time PCR for the diagnosis of *B. microti* and a conventional PCR for the diagnosis of all *Babesia* spp. are available at CDC, with a reported diagnostic sensitivity and specificity of 100%. These molecular tests are performed on EDTA anticoagulated blood samples. Testing of serum or plasma for antibodies to *Babesia* spp. can diagnose recent and past infections, when the parasitemia is resolved or below the detection limits of both microscopy and PCR. IFAs for *B. microti*, *B. duncani*, and *B. divergens* are available at CDC. The diagnostic sensitivity of IFA for *B. microti* cases has been shown to be 88%–96%, while specificity has been found to be between 90%–100%, except when used to diagnose babesiosis in acquired immunodeficiency syndrome patients. Due to limited positive serum availability, sensitivity and specificity data for other species are unavailable. Enzyme-linked immunosorbent assay has been reported to have comparable diagnostic performance to IFA and may be preferred in laboratories with limited access to a fluorescent microscope or lacking the technical skills required to perform IFA. The degree of cross-reactivity between *Babesia* species is unknown but is suspected to be low for both IFA and ELISA. Diagnosis is confirmatory in specimens meeting morphologic criteria or positive in serologic or molecular testing.

**9. Reporting requirements**—Reporting requirements/criteria vary by country and local jurisdiction. In the USA, babesiosis is currently reportable in 34 states.

**10. Referral network**—Parasitic Diseases Diagnostic Reference Laboratory at CDC offers morphological, PCR, and serological diagnosis of *Babesia* infections. Laboratories testing for babesiosis outside of the USA should ascertain what referral networks are available within their respective countries or regions.

**11. Special considerations**—Cases occurring in a new geographic area deserve careful investigation to identify and characterize the *Babesia* species involved, tick vector, and reservoir hosts. Investigations of potential transfusion-associated cases require both medical and public health attention. The implicated blood donor should be investigated promptly and should refrain from future donations. In addition, recipients of cellular blood components from all potentially relevant donations from the implicated donor should be promptly evaluated for evidence of *Babesia* infection.

[Y. Qvarnstrom, H. S. Bishop, R. S. Bradbury]

# BALANTIOSIS

(balantidiasis, balantidial dysentery, balantidiosis, neobalantidiasis)

| DISEASE | ICD-10 CODE |
|---|---|
| BALANTIOSIS | ICD-10 A07 |

**1. Clinical features**—Balantiosis (formerly known as balantidiasis) is an infection of the colon characteristically producing diarrhea or dysentery, accompanied by abdominal colic, tenesmus, nausea, and vomiting. Occasionally the dysentery resembles amebiasis, with stools containing much blood and mucus but relatively little pus. Peritoneal or urogenital invasion is rare.

**2. Causative agents**—*Balantioides coli*, (formerly classified as *Balantidium coli* or *Neobalantidium coli*), the only ciliated protozoan parasite in the human host and the largest protozoan parasite of humans. Occurs worldwide.

**3. Laboratory diagnosis**—Identification of trophozoites or cysts of *B. coli* in fresh feces, or trophozoites in material obtained by sigmoidoscopy. Both cysts and trophozoites may be observed in wet mounts of concentrations or in permanently stained smears such as trichrome. Trophozoites may also be detected morphologically in colonic biopsy specimens processed for routine histology. There are no serologic nor molecular tests available for routine diagnosis.

Trophozoites of *B. coli* measure 50–200 μm long, with an average range of 50–100 μm long by 40–70 μm wide, ovoid in shape, tapering to anterior end that contains a cytostome; both a large kidney bean-shaped macronucleus and a smaller micronucleus may be visible (the latter of which may be difficult to see in unstained preparations); cilia are present and trophozoites move with a rotary, boring motion that may be rapid in fresh unpreserved specimens;

cytoplasm may contain contractile vacuoles and food particles, including yeast, protozoan cysts, and helminth eggs. Cysts are round, measuring 50–70 μm in diameter; cilia are usually visible internally through the cyst wall; both a macronucleus and micronucleus may be visible; cytoplasm may contain contractile vacuoles and food particles, especially in younger cysts.

**4. Laboratory capability**—Microscopy, stool concentration/centrifugation capabilities, and permanent staining techniques (e.g., trichrome) should be available. Laboratorians should be trained in the microscopic/morphologic detection of parasites and undergo regular proficiency testing.

**5. Safety requirements**—Clinical specimens should always be collected and handled with universal/standard precautions. *B. coli* is a biosafety level 2 organism. Formalin should only be used in a well-ventilated area, preferably in a chemical fume hood. Unpreserved and preserved stools should be disposed of as infectious waste.

**6. Nonhuman hosts**—Pigs and rats can serve as reservoir hosts. Food, water, and fomites contaminated with infected pig or rat feces may serve as a source of human infection.

**7. Sample/specimen requirements**—Stool should be promptly preserved in appropriate liquid media, such as 10% buffered formalin or sodium acetate-acetic acid-formalin (SAF) and polyvinyl alcohol (PVA). If PVA is used, zinc-based solutions are recommended over mercury-based solutions to prevent issues with disposal. Single vial systems for ova and parasite (O&P) collection are also adequate. To maximize O&P sensitivity, up to 3 stool specimens on 3 successive days should be collected.

**8. Testing requirements**—Routine concentration and staining procedures for stool. A calibrated ocular micrometer should be used to measure trophozoite and cyst size. Diagnosis is confirmatory in specimens meeting morphologic criteria.

**9. Reporting requirements**—Balantiosis is not nationally reportable in the USA. Report to local health authority; official report not ordinarily justifiable. International reporting is not required.

**10. Referral network**—None.

**11. Special considerations**—None.

Note: ICD-10 still lists the disease as balantidiasis.

[B. Mathison]

# BARTONELLA INFECTIONS

(Carrión's disease, cat scratch disease, trench fever)

| DISEASE | ICD-10 CODE |
|---|---|
| OROYA FEVER | ICD-10 A44.0 |
| VERRUGA PERUANA | ICD-10 A44.1 |
| CARRIÓN'S DISEASE (South American bartonellosis, Oroya fever, Verruga peruana) | ICD-10 A44.0 |
| ZOONOTIC BARTONELLOSIS (other forms of bartonellosis, emerging bartonellosis, rodent-borne bartonellosis, flea-borne bartonellosis) | ICD-10 A44.8 |
| CAT SCRATCH DISEASE (cat scratch fever, benign lymphoreticulosis) | ICD-10 A28.1 |
| TRENCH FEVER (quintana fever) | ICD-10 A79.0 |

**1. Clinical features**—*Bartonella* spp. can cause several diseases.

1) Carrión's disease: a bacterial infection with 2 clinical forms: a life-threatening febrile anemia (Oroya fever) and a benign dermal eruption (verruga peruana). Asymptomatic infection and a carrier state may both occur. Oroya fever is characterized by fever, headache, myalgia, arthralgia, pallor, severe hemolytic anemia (macrocytic or normocytic, usually hypochromic), and generalized nontender lymphadenopathy. Verruga peruana has a preeruptive stage characterized by shifting pains in muscles, bones, and joints; the pain, often severe, lasts minutes to several days at any one site. The dermal eruption may be miliary with widely disseminated small hemangioma-like nodules, or nodular with fewer (but larger) deep-seated lesions, most prominent on the extensor surfaces of the limbs. Individual nodules, particularly near joints, may develop into tumor-like masses with an ulcerated surface. Atypical cases of Oroya fever with milder manifestations (prolonged splenomegaly and mild anemia) may occur.

2) Cat scratch disease (CSD): a subacute, usually self-limited bacterial disease characterized by malaise, granulomatous lymphadenitis, and variable patterns of fever. Most often preceded by a cat scratch that develops into a red papular lesion(s) with subsequent development of lymphadenitis in the draining lymph nodes, usually within 2 weeks. Lymphadenitis may progress to suppuration. The papule at the inoculation site can be found in 50%–90% of cases. When the direct inoculation site is in the conjunctiva, Parinaud's oculoglandular syndrome can develop, with granulomatous conjunctivitis

and pretragal lymphadenopathy. Approximately 10% of CSD cases can be complicated by systemic disease including prolonged high fever, malaise, fatigue, myalgia, arthralgia, weight loss, neuroretinitis, or hepatosplenomegaly. Rarely neurological complications such as encephalopathy and optic neuritis can also occur. Cat scratch disease can be clinically confused with other diseases that cause regional lymphadenopathies (e.g., tularemia, brucellosis, tuberculosis, plague, pasteurellosis, and lymphoma).

In immunocompromised individuals (e.g., patients with acquired immunodeficiency syndrome [AIDS], organ transplant, or cancer), the *Bartonella* bacteria can disseminate and cause lesions distinctly different from the CSD manifestations observed in immunocompetent people: vascular cutaneous lesions (bacillary angiomatosis [BA]), hepatic vascular proliferation (bacillary peliosis hepatis), widespread lymphadenopathy, and bacteremia. In AIDS patients, BA can be clinically indistinguishable in appearance from Kaposi's sarcoma. In immunocompromised patients, *Bartonella* infection is sometimes fatal.

3) Trench fever: a typically nonfatal, febrile bacteremic disease varying in manifestations and severity, characterized by headache, malaise, shin pain, and dizziness. Onset is either sudden or gradual, and fever may be relapsing (usually with a 5-day periodicity), prolonged (typhoid-like), or limited to a single episode lasting several days. Splenomegaly, transient macular rash, and conjunctivitis may also be present. Symptoms may continue to recur many years after the primary infection; persistent bacteremia has been described. Bacteremia can be complicated by osteomyelitis, lymphadenopathy, and BA in immunocompromised patients, especially those with human immunodeficiency virus infection. Endocarditis has been associated with trench fever infections, especially among homeless or alcoholic persons.
4) Zoonotic bartonellosis acquired from wild animals: although much less common, several other *Bartonella* spp. infecting various mammalian species have been associated with human infections. Clinical presentations include vegetative endocarditis, neuroretinitis, lymphadenitis, myocarditis, fever of unknown origin, and asymptomatic bacteremia.

**2. Causative agents**—Members of the genus *Bartonella* are fastidious, hemotropic, Gram-negative bacteria of the alpha-2 subgroup of the class Proteobacteria and taxonomically closely related to *Brucella* spp. Among more than 30 reported species of *Bartonella*, 3 species account for the great majority of recognized human infections: *B. bacilliformis* (Carrión's disease),

*B. henselae* (CSD), and *B. quintana* (trench fever). However, at least a dozen other *Bartonella* spp. have been associated with various human illnesses, including *B. alsatica, B. clarridgeiae, B. doshiae, B. elizabethae, B. grahamii, B. koehlerae, B. mayotimonensis, B. rochalimae, B. schoenbuchensis, B. tamiae, B. tribocorum, B. vinsonii*, and *B. washoensis*. *B. vinsonii* subsp. *arupensis* was isolated from an American patient with acute onset of confusion, difficulty in walking, and facial numbness. Subsequently, the same subspecies was identified as an etiologic agent of blood culture-negative endocarditis and febrile illnesses in Europe and Asia. Another subspecies of *B. vinsonii* (*B. vinsonii* subsp. *berkhoffii*) has been identified as a cause of endocarditis and neurological disease. *B. washoensis* was responsible for human cases of myocarditis and meningitis in the western USA. *B. elizabethae* was originally isolated from a patient with endocarditis in Massachusetts; evidence of *B. elizabethae* infection also has been demonstrated in patients with neuroretinitis, hepatic granulomas, ulcers, endocarditis, and myocarditis. *B. alsatica* was reported as a cause of several cases of culture-negative endocarditis and lymphadenitis in France. *B. rochalimae* was diagnosed in a US traveler who presented at the hospital with fever, insomnia, myalgia, headache, and a mild cough after returning from a trip to Peru. *B. tamiae* was recognized as a new pathogen in Thailand after isolation and characterization of the strains from blood of 3 patients with fatigue, myalgia, headache, and rash. *B. schoenbuchensis, B. doshiae*, and *B. tribocorum* were identified in individuals with chronic illness, history of tick exposure, or lymphadenopathy and fever. The novel species *B. mayotimonensis* was isolated from a patient with endocarditis in the US Midwest.

**3. Laboratory diagnosis**—Methods for laboratory diagnosis include serology, culture, and polymerase chain reaction (PCR). Several techniques are available for serological diagnostics, including antibody-capture enzyme-linked immunosorbent assay and direct immunofluorescence using fluorescein-conjugated polyclonal antibodies. The indirect immunofluorescence assay (IFA) for detection of *Bartonella* antibodies is the most common and convenient serologic method, with a common cutoff value of 1:64 (sometimes 1:128 or 1:256) for most *Bartonella* spp. For most commercial laboratory IFA tests, there is substantial cross-reactivity between different *Bartonella* spp. (e.g., *B. quintana* and *B. henselae*). Titration of positive sera against several *Bartonella* antigens can greatly improve serological diagnostics and reduce a possibility of cross-reactive results, but this is rarely available in commercial laboratories. IFA immunoglobulin class G testing for *Bartonella* antibodies has been much more sensitive than IFA immunoglobulin class M testing. Isolation of the organisms is very challenging but can be accomplished by bacteriological culture of patient blood or tissue biopsies using specific agar medium enriched with mammalian blood or chocolate agar and prolonged incubation in a moist, $CO_2$-enhanced environment. Molecular techniques, particularly conventional and real-time PCR assays, increasingly have been used for detection and identification of *Bartonella* deoxyribonucleic acid (DNA) in most types of clinical materials, including tissues and body fluids. Nonspecific histological stains such as the tissue Warthin-Starry silver stain may provide presumptive evidence of infection. More specific immunohistological methods have been used for detection of *Bartonella* bacteria in cardiac valves and other tissues. Well-validated assays offered by Clinical Laboratory Improvement Amendments (CLIA)-certified reference laboratories are recommended for all clinical diagnostics.

**4. Laboratory capability**—Most commercial laboratories offer serologic testing for *B. henselae* and *B. quintana*. PCR testing is offered by several commercial laboratories and is becoming more widespread but is still not readily available in most hospital clinical laboratories. Cultures are generally available only at specialized reference laboratories.

**5. Safety requirements**—Biosafety level 2 practices, containment equipment, and facilities are recommended for all activities involving known or potentially infectious tissues, body fluids, and cultures. As with any human specimens, universal precautions should be strictly applied. Although laboratory-associated *Bartonella* infections have not been reported, the agent may be present in blood, urine, and tissues of infected animals and ectoparasites. The importance of aerosol exposure is not known but considered minimal. Vaccines are not available for use in humans or animals. None of the *Bartonella* spp. is designated as a select agent, although viable *B. quintana* shipment is regulated by the US Department of Commerce. Laboratorians working with *B. quintana* in other countries should check with their respective commerce or health officials.

**6. Nonhuman hosts**—*Bartonella* spp. persist in nature through a wide range of mammalian reservoir hosts including cats, dogs, wild carnivores, ungulates, rodents, bats, marine mammals, and nonhuman primates. They cause long-term bacteremias and can be transmitted among hosts by diverse arthropod species. Cats represent the main reservoir for *B. henselae*, *B. clarridgeiae*, and *B. koehlerae*. Dogs and wild canids are major reservoirs for *B. vinsonii* subsp. *berkhoffii*. Urban and wild rats of the genus *Rattus* constitute the main reservoir of *B. elizabethae* and other phylogenetically related species (e.g., *B. tribocorum*). In North America, rodent-borne *Bartonella* are commonly associated with a specific genus of rodent host, for example, *B. vinsonii* subsp. *arupensis* with deer mice (*Peromyscus* spp.) and *B. washoensis* with ground squirrels (*Spermophilus* spp.). In Europe, host-specific relationships between *Bartonella* spp. and rodents are less evident. *B. alsatica* has been described and isolated from the blood of wild rabbits and also detected from rabbit fleas. *B. rochalimae* has been isolated or detected from canids, raccoons, and rodents. Animal reservoirs for *B. tamiae* have not been identified, but the patients infected with this organism stated that they had previous contact with rats and *B. tamiae* DNA has been detected in chigger mites collected from rats. *B. mayotimonensis,* a recently identified etiological agent of human endocarditis, was detected in bats from Europe and North America. Recently, *B. quintana*, which was thought to be only a human pathogen, has been isolated from macaques in various Asian countries raising a possible zoonotic origin. Numerous isolates of *Bartonella* spp. have been obtained from wildlife including marsupials from Australia.

**7. Sample/specimen requirements**—Paired serum samples (the acute taken at first presentation and the convalescent taken 3-6 weeks later) should be collected for evaluation of antibodies reactive with *Bartonella* spp. The preferable specimen types for culture isolation of *Bartonella* are blood, tissues, and lymph node aspirate. The samples should be kept frozen at -20°C or below before shipping to a laboratory on dry ice. Overnight shipment of refrigerated specimens is also suitable. Blood can be collected into either ethylenediaminetetraacetic acid-anticoagulant tubes or Isolator blood lysis tubes, although blood clots can also be used for culturing and molecular detection. Check with the clinical laboratory regarding specimen submission requirement. Because of the broad susceptibility of *Bartonella* spp. to antibiotics, it is very desirable to collect blood specimens before antibiotic therapy. It was reported that growth of *B. henselae* was inhibited by concentrations of sodium polyanethol sulfonate in collection tubes. Tissue samples other than blood suitable for culture or PCR detection methods include cardiac valves from the patients suspected of having *Bartonella* endocarditis, skin biopsies, lymph nodes, liver, spleen, and osteomedullar biopsies. Tissues and fluid from affected lymph nodes can be collected by fine-needle aspiration and submitted for testing.

**8. Testing requirements**—Well-validated assays offered by CLIA-certified reference laboratories are recommended for clinical diagnostics. All isolation work should be performed in a biosafety cabinet after preparation of workplace and tools. *Bartonella* is optimally cultured at 35°C with an atmosphere containing 5% $CO_2$. However, growth of *B. bacilliformis* is optimal at a lower temperature of incubation (25°C-28°C) and in the absence of $CO_2$ enrichment. Tissue samples can be triturated in M199 medium with 20% fetal bovine serum prior to inoculation, then spread onto freshly poured agar plates. Recovery of primary isolates may require several days to several weeks. Initial identification of the bacteria is mainly based on colony and bacterium morphology with subsequent confirmation by DNA amplification and sequencing. Long term storage of the cultures is achieved by freezing at -80°C or below in a final concentration of 10% glycerol in Brain Heart Infusion. DNA extracts suitable for use as templates in PCR assays are prepared from blood samples or crushed tissues by using extraction reagents available from various manufacturers. Identification of *Bartonella* spp. needs to be carefully addressed by using 3 to 5 housekeeping loci as genetic markers. In the case of isolates, only well isolated colonies with at least 2 subcultures from single colonies are recommended for the characterization. Sensitivity and specificity of IFAs may be improved by using a variety of antigens prepared by cocultivation of *Bartonella* strains with antibiotic-free Vero cells.

**9. Reporting requirements**—*Bartonella* infection is not a nationally notifiable condition in the USA. Laboratories outside the USA should determine whether *Bartonella* infections are reportable within their respective jurisdictions.

**10. Referral network**—Testing for bartonellosis does not utilize a special tiered referral laboratory testing system. Clinical laboratories must determine if they have the requisite capability and request a confirmation of their results from CLIA-certified reference laboratories when they are available.

**11. Special considerations**—None.

[M. Kosoy, B. Chomel]

# BEJEL

(Njovera, nonvenereal endemic syphilis)

| DISEASE | ICD-10 CODE |
|---|---|
| BEJEL | ICD-10 A65 |

**1. Clinical features**—A chronic skin and tissue disease characterized by an eruption on skin and mucous membranes, usually without an evident primary sore, as seen in yaws.

During the primary stage, lesions are painless, and tiny papules or ulcers that appear on the mouth and lips often go undetected. Secondary lesions are characterized by shallow, painless mucous patches of the mouth, soon followed by moist papules in skinfolds and by drier lesions on the trunk and extremities. Other secondary skin lesions are macular or papular, often hypertrophic, and frequently circinate; lesions resemble those of venereal syphilis. Plantar and palmar hyperkeratoses occur frequently, often with painful fissuring; alopecia and patchy depigmentation/hyperpigmentation of the skin are common. Inflammatory or destructive lesions of skin, long bones, and nasopharynx are late manifestations. Unlike venereal syphilis, bejel rarely shows neurological or cardiovascular involvement. The case-fatality rate is low.

**2. Causative agents**—*Treponema pallidum* subsp. *endemicum*, a spirochete.

**3. Laboratory diagnosis**—Spirochetes are demonstrable by dark-field and direct fluorescent antibody microscopic examination of lesion exudate during early disease. Molecular methods using polymerase chain reaction (PCR) and deoxyribonucleic acid (DNA) sequencing have been developed to detect *T. pallidum* subsp. endemic-specific sequences in lesion exudate. Serological tests for syphilis usually become reactive before or during the secondary lesions, and thereafter behave as in venereal syphilis. Although not formally validated, point-of-care tests for syphilis are anticipated to also be reactive in bejel.

**4. Laboratory capability**—Serological testing can be performed in laboratories with standard equipment and minimal scientific and technical knowledge, but the high throughput tests (usually found in more sophisticated laboratories) require automation. Point-of-care serological tests can be performed by staff with minimal laboratory training and can be used at all levels of health care facilities even those without a laboratory. Specialized scientific and technical knowledge including sophisticated laboratory equipment is essential for performing PCR testing.

**5. Safety requirements**—Biosafety level 2 conditions and practices are required. Universal/standard precautions must be observed when working with blood or clinical specimens as other infectious agents may also be present.

**6. Nonhuman hosts**—No nonhuman host for bejel has been identified, although a role for fomites such as utensils has been postulated.

**7. Sample/specimen requirements**—Serum is the specimen of choice for treponemal and nontreponemal serological tests, but plasma can be used for some tests. Rapid point-of-care tests use whole blood obtained through a finger stick. Serum and plasma should be stored at 4°C if testing cannot be performed within 4 hours and at –20°C or less if testing will be done more than 5 days from collection. Serous exudate from moist lesions of primary and secondary bejel are amenable to dark-field microscopy (DF) and PCR. Specimens for DF must be tested within 20 minutes of collection. Tissue for silver staining and immunohistochemistry (IHC) should be fixed in 10% buffered formalin as soon as possible at ambient temperature and then paraffin embedded and sectioned for staining. Polymerase chain reaction can be performed on either fixed or unfixed tissue, although unfixed tissue is preferred. All samples for PCR should be stored at –70°C if testing cannot be performed immediately.

**8. Testing requirements**—Serology is the mainstay for diagnosis of bejel although serological tests maybe negative in early primary bejel. Treponemal antibody tests, such as the *Treponema pallidum* passive particle agglutination (TP-PA), *Treponema pallidum* hemagglutination assay (TPHA), and fluorescent treponemal antibody absorption (FTA-ABS), remain positive for life. Quantitative nontreponemal tests become positive following infection, and the titer then falls following successful treatment.

Traditionally samples were screened using a nontreponemal test (i.e., rapid plasma reagin [RPR] or venereal disease research laboratory [VDRL] assays) and if this test was positive, a confirmatory treponemal test was performed. Many laboratories have now adopted an alternative algorithm, the reverse syphilis screening algorithm. Using this approach, the initial test is a treponemal antibody test. When this test is positive, a quantitative nontreponemal test is then performed. If the nontreponemal test is negative, a second treponemal test can be performed. Point-of-care serological tests are now available. The majority detect only treponemal antibodies, commonly referred to as rapid syphilis tests. Point-of-care tests that detect both treponemal and nontreponemal antibodies are now available. When using a point-of-care test, it is important to ensure the kit meets appropriate quality standards. It should be noted that serological assays cannot distinguish bejel from other endemic treponematoses or syphilis. A quantitative nontreponemal test is required for assessing response to therapy. Participation in the WHO/CDC Syphilis Serology Proficiency Programme is recommended for maintaining proficiency in treponemal and nontreponemal testing. Detection of specific *T. pallidum* subsp. *endemicum* DNA targets by PCR or observation of spirochetes is definitive of bejel infection. Lesion samples should be initially screened with a pantreponemal PCR such as polA or tp47. In samples that are positive, PCR may allow differentiation of *T. pallidum* subsp. *endemicum* from other subspecies. IHC, silver stain, or PCR is used for tissue biopsies. Use of a hematoxylin counterstain with IHC allows tissue structure to be observed with localization of treponemes. With molecular testing, many clinically suspicious lesions will not have detectable treponemal DNA present.

**9. Reporting requirements**—Reactive treponemal and nontreponemal test results is consistent with current or past bejel infection but cannot distinguish from infection with an alternative treponemal infection, most importantly, syphilis. If the nontreponemal titer is lower than 1:4, this could be associated with a serofast state where nontreponemal titers neither increase nor decrease 4-fold after treatment. If the treponemal test is nonreactive, then there is no laboratory evidence of bejel infection. If the nontreponemal test is reactive but the treponemal test is nonreactive, then it is most likely a biological false-positive result. If the first treponemal test in the reverse algorithm is reactive and the nontreponemal test is nonreactive, but the second/supplemental treponemal test is reactive, then this is consistent with past or potential early infection with bejel or an alternative treponemal infection. If nonreactive, it is inconclusive for bejel infection or a false-positive result. In some endemic areas, bejel may be a reportable disease. Laboratories should determine if bejel is reportable to the public health authorities in their specific setting.

**10. Referral network**—No specific referral networks exist.

**11. Special considerations**—International measures: examine groups of children and adults who emigrate from areas of high prevalence for treponemal infections.

[M. Marks, A. Pillay]

# BLASTOMYCOSIS

(North American blastomycosis, Gilchrist's disease)

| DISEASE | ICD-10 CODE |
|---|---|
| BLASTOMYCOSIS | ICD-10 B40 |

**1. Clinical features**—A granulomatous systemic mycosis that primarily affects the lungs and is often subclinical. Hematogenous dissemination may occur, and in the majority of cases involves skin, bones, and genitourinary tract. Pulmonary blastomycosis may be acute or chronic. Acute infection, which often goes unrecognized, presents with the sudden onset of fever, cough, and a pulmonary infiltrate on chest X-ray. The acute disease usually resolves spontaneously after 1–3 weeks of illness. More commonly, there is an indolent onset of pulmonary infection that evolves into chronic disease. Some patients exhibit extrapulmonary infection during or after the resolution of pneumonia. Disseminated disease is more common in the immunocompromised. Cough and chest ache may be mild or absent, so patients may present with infection already spread to other sites, particularly the skin, and less often to bone, prostate, or epididymis. Cutaneous lesions begin as erythematous papules that become verrucous, crusted, or ulcerated and spread slowly. Most commonly, cutaneous lesions are located on the face and distal extremities. Constitutional symptoms such as weight loss, weakness, and low-grade fever are often present. Untreated disseminated or chronic pulmonary blastomycosis can eventually progress to death.

**2. Causative agents**—Thermally dimorphic fungi in the genus *Blastomyces* (*Ajellomycetacaea*). *Blastomyces dermatitidis* is mostly restricted to North America and Africa. *Blastomyces gilchristii* is found predominantly in Ontario, Wisconsin, and Minnesota. Recent taxonomic studies have identified several additional *Blastomyces* spp. and support the reclassification of some species originally placed in *Emmonsia* as *Blastomyces* spp.

**3. Laboratory diagnosis**—The clinical and radiological features of blastomycosis overlap with malignancy, tuberculosis, and infections with some other dimorphic fungal pathogens.

The organism is usually readily recovered in respiratory secretions in patients with symptomatic lung involvement. The characteristic yeast form (yeast budding on a broad base) can be seen by microscopic examination of secretions and is facilitated when optical brighteners are employed. Growth of the typical mold form of the fungus (narrow hyaline mycelium with disc-shaped aleuriocondia borne on narrow, slightly swollen stalks around the ends and sides of hyphae) on mycological media incubated at 30°C confirms the diagnosis.

The commercially available chemiluminescent deoxyribonucleic acid (DNA) probe test (Hologic AccuProbe) is the most commonly employed test to formally confirm an identification of *Blastomyces*, as it provides results within a few hours once there is sufficient growth of the organism in culture.

In disseminated blastomycosis, visualization of the yeast form in histological specimens of the affected organs is a commonly employed diagnostic approach. Congo red staining helps to distinguish the yeasts of *Blastomyces* spp. (positive) from the tissue form of *Histoplasma* spp. (negative); however, the shape and size and budding on a broad base (for *Blastomyces* spp.) are usually sufficient to allow differentiation of the 2 organisms without recourse to special stains.

A commercial assay for *Blastomyces* antigen is available and permits an alternative diagnostic approach with specimens of blood, urine, and other fluids, although cross-reactivity with other dimorphic fungal pathogens has been reported. The beta-D-glucan assay, which is a useful diagnostic adjunct in many other invasive fungal infections, appears less useful in blastomycosis, presumably because of low levels of this antigen in *Blastomyces* spp.

A variety of commercial tests for the detection of antibody to *Blastomyces* spp. are available, including complement fixation using antigens derived from the yeast phase of the organism, immunodiffusion and enzyme immunoassays. Although all tests are capable of diagnosing blastomycosis, they suffer from issues with sensitivity and/or specificity that limit their clinical value.

No standardized PCR approach exists for the diagnosis of blastomycosis. However, success has been reported using both panfungal (18S or 28S) and species-specific approaches with DNA extracted from fixed tissue and from a variety of fresh clinical specimens with apparently excellent sensitivity and specificity.

**4. Laboratory capability**—Laboratories handling clinical material that may contain *Blastomyces* spp. and confirmed cultures of the organism should be equipped with suitable biosafety level 2 (BSL-2) and BSL-3 facilities as appropriate according to local regulatory requirements. Manipulation of live cultures of *Blastomyces* spp. should be performed in a class I biosafety cabinet under BSL-3 conditions. Skilled laboratory personnel should be available for working specifically with potential dimorphic fungi, including *Blastomyces* spp.

Laboratories that are accustomed to processing tissues and fluids from usually sterile sites when fungal infection is suspected should have appropriately trained staff and expertise in the use of optical brighteners. Microscopes should be equipped with appropriate filters necessary for examining specimens treated with optical brighteners under ultraviolet light. All specimens for culture require appropriate mycological media containing selective agents to prevent bacterial growth and incubation in standard microbiological incubators maintained at 30°C and at 37°C to confirm the dimorphic nature of any fungal pathogen recovered.

**5. Safety requirements**—In the UK, the Advisory Committee on Dangerous Pathogens lists *Blastomyces* spp. as hazard group 3 organisms, and containment level 3 laboratory practices should be employed for handling cultures of the agent. In the US, BSL-2 and animal BSL-2 practices, containment equipment, and facilities should be employed when working with clinical materials, animal tissues, yeast-form cultures, and infected animals. BSL-3 practices, containment equipment, and facilities should be used for handling cultures growing the mold form of the organisms that have already been identified as *Blastomyces* spp. and environmental samples known or likely to contain infectious conidia. Laboratory-acquired infections following traumatic inoculation and following the presumptive inhalation of conidia have both been reported.

**6. Nonhuman hosts**—The natural habitat of *Blastomyces* spp. is soil, particularly in association with rotting vegetation. Interactions of *Blastomyces* spp. with soil amoebae have been suggested. Infections have been reported in a variety of other animals, including horses, dogs, cats, and marine mammals. Anecdotal reports exist of blastomycosis acquired after bites or scratches from animals. Dogs may be a sentinel species for detection of high-risk locations.

**7. Sample/specimen requirements**—Because of the high recovery of *Blastomyces* spp. from respiratory sites, the preferred specimens for the diagnosis of acute pulmonary blastomycosis are respiratory tract secretions (i.e., bronchial washings or sputum). Samples should be processed as soon as possible after collection to avoid overgrowth by other fungi that are frequently present in such samples (e.g., *Candida* spp.).

Swabs collected from ruptured pustules may be useful in cutaneous blastomycosis. For other extra-pulmonary forms of the disease, biopsy samples are useful for histological examination. In all cases, if possible, samples should be processed for both microscopic examination and for culture. Expertise is required to recognize the yeast/tissue form of the organism, which is 8–15 μm in diameter. This form has a distinctive budding pattern where the daughter cell approaches the size of the mother cell before detachment, leading to a "budding on a broad base" appearance.

Urine and serum samples may be useful for *Blastomyces* antigen detection in humans and dogs via a quantitative enzyme immunoassay, although sensitivity is higher with urine. Serum samples may also be used for serological approaches aimed at detecting circulating anti-*Blastomyces* antibodies.

Polymerase chain reaction detection of *Blastomyces* DNA from blood, serum, or tissue samples should be performed according to current best practice guidelines.

**8. Testing requirements**—Positive culture recovery rates of *Blastomyces* spp. of 86% and 100% have been reported from sputum and bronchial washings, respectively, in patients with pulmonary involvement. Although the sensitivity of microscopy is lower (50%–90%), both microscopy and culture should be performed as culture is substantially slower, and it may be 4–6 weeks before the organism is recovered.

Urinary antigen positivity by enzyme immunoassay has been reported in approximately 93% of confirmed cases of blastomycosis, but the test has poor specificity, with cross-reactivity specifically seen with *Histoplasma* spp., *Paracoccidioides* spp., and *Talaromyces marneffei*; all yield similar positivity rates. There is limited evidence that repeat testing might be useful in monitoring response to therapy in confirmed infections.

The most useful serological test for the diagnosis of blastomycosis is immunodiffusion, which is specific for the disease. However, results are negative in as many as 60% of patients with localized infections and in 10% of patients with disseminated disease (sensitivity 65%–85%). Complement fixation yields poorer results (i.e., sensitivity 57% and specificity 30%). Antibody tests may remain negative for several months after exposure and are of limited value in immunocompromised patients with suspected blastomycosis.

Limited numbers of studies have reported sensitivity and specificity of 86% and 99%, respectively, for *Blastomyces*-specific real-time PCR assays employed with a range of clinical samples, making it a potential useful adjunct for earlier diagnosis.

**9. Reporting requirements**—There are currently very few requirements for the national reporting of *Blastomyces* infections worldwide. However, in the USA, infections are reportable in 5 states (Arkansas, Louisiana, Michigan, Minnesota, and Wisconsin).

Outbreaks of blastomycosis are uncommon but do sporadically occur, usually in relation to activities that cause extensive soil disturbance. Appropriate local infection teams should be involved when unusual clusters of *Blastomyces* infections are identified in a given region so that the possibility of outbreaks can be investigated. Referral of isolates of *Blastomyces* spp. to appropriate reference centers is recommended to aid in local, national, and international epidemiological surveillance and detection of novel and emerging pathogens.

**10. Referral network**—A comprehensive network of expert mycology references laboratories exists in some countries and may be approached for help with the identification of suspected isolates of *Blastomyces* spp. *Blastomyces* antigen testing is available from at least 1 reference laboratory in the USA.

**11. Special considerations**—Importation and exportation of the agent to and from the USA may require CDC, USDA, or Department of Commerce permits. Domestic transport of confirmed cultures of *Blastomyces* spp. requires special arrangements in many countries.

[A. M. Borman]

# BOTULISM

| DISEASE | ICD-10 CODE |
|---|---|
| BOTULISM | ICD-10 A05.1 |

**1. Clinical features**—Botulism is a severe neuroparalytic illness resulting from irreversible blockade of acetylcholine release from presynaptic nerve endings by botulinum toxin. Beyond infancy (i.e., > 1 year), it manifests as bilateral cranial nerve palsies followed by bilateral descending flaccid paralysis. Signs and symptoms typically include some or all of the following: ptosis, diplopia, blurred vision, dysphagia, dysarthria, and ophthalmoplegia. Autonomic symptoms such as constipation commonly occur. Patients maintain their baseline mental status. Gastrointestinal symptoms, including nausea, vomiting, and diarrhea, can occur in foodborne botulism. Illness may include respiratory failure and death if mechanical ventilation and supportive care are not provided. Most patients recover if diagnosed and treated promptly, but recovery may take months, and some have residual weakness.

Symptoms in infants younger than 1 year typically start with constipation and may include poor suck, altered cry, weakness, and loss of head control. Infant botulism ranges from a mild illness with gradual onset to severe paralysis and respiratory failure. Mortality from infant botulism is rare, about 0.1% during 2000–2009 in the USA, where 85% of all reported infant botulism cases occur.

**2. Causative agents**—Botulinum toxin is a potent neurotoxin that is one of the most lethal substances known. Botulinum toxin is produced by *Clostridium botulinum* but is also produced by some strains of *Clostridium butyricum*, *Clostridium baratii*, and *Clostridium argentinense*. These Gram-positive spore formers are present in the environment. They only grow and produce toxin under specific conditions in food products, in contaminated wounds, and in the intestinal tract of infants and adults with structurally or functionally compromised intestinal tracts (e.g., intestinal surgery, antibiotic use). Of the 7 recognized serotypes of botulinum toxin (types A–G), the most common serotypes associated with naturally occurring human illness are A, B, E, and F.

**3. Laboratory diagnosis**—Botulism is clinically diagnosed and laboratory confirmed. Other neurological disorders resembling botulism in noninfants include myasthenia gravis and Guillain-Barré syndrome, and in infants, sepsis and electrolyte imbalances. Illnesses confused with botulism can be hard to differentiate in the early workup. Botulism should be considered, and antitoxin administered, early in the workup as more common diseases are evaluated. Routine hospital laboratory studies are not helpful in diagnosing botulism but may help rule out other illnesses. Electromyography can support the clinical diagnosis of botulism.

1) Foodborne: confirmed by detecting botulinum toxin in serum, stool, or gastric aspirate, or through culture of botulinum toxin producing clostridia from gastric aspirate or stool in a clinically compatible case. Laboratory confirmation of a foodborne case can also be achieved by detecting botulinum toxin in a food source known to have been consumed by the patient. Botulism is considered confirmed in persons with a consistent clinical syndrome who consumed a food item implicated in a laboratory-confirmed case.
2) Infant intestinal: confirmed by detecting botulinum toxin in clinical specimens (serum or stool) or by isolating botulinum toxin producing clostridia from stool specimens from an infant younger than 1 year.
3) Wound: confirmed by culture of botulinum toxin producing clostridia from a wound or detection of botulinum toxin in serum in a patient with a history of a contaminated wound or injection drug use within 2 weeks of onset of symptoms.
4) Other: a designation as "other" botulism occurs when a clinically compatible case is laboratory confirmed in a patient aged 1 year or older who has no history of ingestion of suspect food and has no wounds. Some of these cases are suspected to be adult intestinal colonization cases due to complicating medical factors and/or prolonged excretion of botulinum toxin producing clostridia in stool.

**4. Laboratory capability**—There are no point-of-care or commercially available methods to confirm botulism; therefore, botulism testing is generally performed in regional public health laboratories where the expertise exists. The primary laboratory test used to confirm botulism requires the use of laboratory animals (i.e., mouse bioassay). Laboratories must comply with applicable animal care and use regulations. In the USA, the Animal Welfare Act regulates the care and use of animals in research, which requires institutions to have an Institutional Animal Care and Use Committee review protocols and research projects that involve animals. Additionally, the laboratory must be in compliance with applicable national regulations for testing human clinical specimens using assays of high complexity for which national compliance organizations have not reviewed performance characteristics. The Centers for Medicare & Medicaid Services regulates all laboratory testing (except research) performed on humans in the USA through the Clinical Laboratory Improvement Amendments (CLIA). Laboratories must meet specific personnel and quality assurance requirements as defined by CLIA.

**5. Safety requirements**—Biosafety level 2 practices, containment equipment, and facilities are recommended for activities that involve the organism or the toxin, including the handling of potentially contaminated food. Latex gloves (or latex alternatives) should be worn when handling material known or suspected to contain botulinum toxin to prevent introduction of botulinum toxin into broken skin. Additional primary containment, such as use of a class II biosafety cabinet (BSC), and personnel precautions, such as use of respiratory protection, should be considered for activities with a high potential for aerosol or droplet production. Currently there is no vaccine available for immunization of laboratory personnel who handle botulinum toxin. A heptavalent (A, B, C, D, E, F, and G) botulism antitoxin product (BAT) is available for specific treatment of botulism in the USA. This product is not approved as a postexposure prophylactic; however, CDC may consider the release of this product for administration to individuals exposed to botulinum toxin and who are at high risk of developing botulism symptoms (e.g., accidental injection or ingestion of a highly concentrated toxin material). Other antitoxin products are available in Europe. It is the responsibility of the laboratory director to ensure that all safety procedures and practices are adequate to prevent exposure of laboratory personnel. Additionally, laboratory directors should consider developing emergency response guidelines for staff conducting tests for botulism. These guidelines should include information on the process for access to treatment including antitoxin, if available.

1) The primary risks to laboratory personnel in conducting these tests are injection while handling needles during testing for toxicity by mouse bioassay. Needles must not be recapped. Syringes and needles must be discarded in a puncture-resistant sharps container.
2) Ingestion during processing food and clinical specimens or during transfer or other manipulations of highly toxic cultures. Mechanical devices must be used to pipette material. Eye, nose, and mouth protection such as goggles and a respirator or a BSC for manipulation of toxin contaminated samples or cultures must be used.

3) Inhalation during processing samples, including unloading samples from centrifuge. Eye protection must be used when operating a centrifuge, and the use of sealed rotors or safety cups is required. Rotors or cups must only be opened within a BSC. Respiratory protection must be worn in the event of a centrifuge failure.
4) Ocular mucous membrane exposure (not yet proven a laboratory risk) during procedures which generate droplets or aerosols. Eye protection or a BSC is required when manipulating liquid materials containing botulinum toxin.

**6. Nonhuman hosts**—Botulism occurs in cattle, horses, water fowl, and other animals in addition to humans; however, botulism is not a zoonotic disease.

**7. Sample/specimen requirements**—

1) Suitable specimens include the following:

- Foodborne botulism: suitable specimens for examination are serum, feces, vomitus, gastric contents, and suspected foods.
- Wound botulism: suitable specimens for examination are serum and debrided tissue or swab samples from wounds. Feces can also be submitted for testing if foodborne botulism is also suspected.
- Infant intestinal: suitable specimens for examination are feces. It is not necessary to collect serum samples from infant botulism cases as circulating toxin levels are usually too low to detect.

2) Clinical specimens: these should be collected prior to patient treatment of any kind and are most useful if collected within 7 days of exposure. Plasmapheresis, used for other diagnosis, reduces the circulatory level of botulinum toxin. Early administration of botulinum antitoxin assists in toxin clearance from circulation thereby limiting the number of neuronal cells effected; however, antitoxin treatment prior to serum collection will prohibit the detection of toxin. Administration of some drugs may cause unexpected symptoms in mice and prevent the confirmatory identification of botulinum toxin, so any drugs provided to the patient prior to specimen collection should be reported to the testing laboratory. Clinical specimens should be submitted to a testing laboratory within 2–4 days of collection.

- Serum: collect enough blood (i.e., ~50 mL) without anticoagulant to provide at least 20 mL of serum for toxin neutralization tests. Allow blood to clot in the refrigerator; centrifuge, and transfer serum to a sterile vial or test tube with a leak-proof cap prior to submission to the testing facility. Alternatively, commercially available serum separator tubes may be used to collect and separate red blood cells from serum. Refrigerate at 4°C. Serum must be collected prior to administration of antitoxin treatment as this treatment will prevent the detection of botulinum toxin in the specimen. Examination of postantitoxin treatment (within 8–24 hours) serum may also be helpful in some cases to determine if additional antitoxin treatment is necessary. Botulinum toxin is considered stable in serum held at 4°C for at least 1 week. Stability of the toxin in serum held at temperatures greater than 4°C is not known.

- Feces: collect 25 g of the patient's feces in a sterile, unbreakable, leak-proof container; smaller quantities may be submitted for testing. Preferably, use a screw-cap wide-mouth plastic bottle. Seal caps with waterproof tape. Cardboard containers are not acceptable. Refrigerate specimens at 4°C until examined. If a passed stool is not available, a request may be submitted to collect an enema with sterile water only. Botulinum toxin and *C. botulinum* are considered stable in stool held at 4°C for at least 1 week. Stability of the toxin in stool held at temperatures greater than 4°C is not known. Recovery of *C. botulinum* from stool held in a nonanaerobic environment for more than 1 week at any temperature is not known.
- Miscellaneous clinical specimens: vomitus or gastric aspirate should be collected within 24 hours of the exposure to botulinum toxin. Tissue samples from contaminated wounds may be collected for suspect wound botulism cases. All specimens should be collected in sterile leak-proof containers and refrigerated at 4°C.
- Culture: cultures isolated in hospital laboratories with a preliminary identification of *C. botulinum* may be submitted for confirmatory testing. These cultures may be stored and transported at ambient temperature or 4°C with or without an anaerobic transport medium.

3) Nonclinical samples: foods suspected to be associated with botulism should be collected as soon as possible. Any food remnants known to be consumed by the patient within 36 hours (typical incubation period for foodborne botulism ranges from 18–36 hours) of symptom onset should be collected from the home. Any commercial food suspected to be the cause of botulism should be reported to the appropriate food regulatory authority (e.g., FDA or USDA in the USA). Whenever possible, food samples should be kept in their original container. However, if the sample cannot be

transported without spilling, then the food should be transferred to a sterile, closable container. The secondary container should be clearly marked as to the contents, including the original container information. The original container should be placed in a plastic, closable bag (double bag is preferred) and transported with the food sample. If laboratory testing later identifies botulinum toxin in the remnants of a food, then similar unopened products (e.g., home or commercially canned food) should be retrieved from the home for possible additional testing. Unopened commercial food products should only be tested by a food regulatory authority approved testing facility. *C. botulinum* may be stable indefinitely in food products, even if unrefrigerated. Stability of botulinum toxin depends on several factors, including type of food and storage conditions.

**8. Testing requirements**—The mouse bioassay is the only universally accepted method for identification of botulinum toxin in clinical specimens, food samples, and cultures. This assay is unique in that it incorporates all aspects of toxin function and identifies the presence of botulinum toxin in samples by demonstration of signs of botulism in the injected animals. Use of specific antisera to neutralize the effects of the toxin identifies the botulinum toxin serotype involved. Detection of botulinum toxin in serum or stool is diagnostic of botulism. The minimum detectable limit in serum and stool is 5–10 $mLD_{50}$ per mL and 10–20 $mLD_{50}$ per mL, respectively. Still, less than 50% of serum from patients clinically diagnosed with botulism are positive and less than 40% of stool samples are positive. Approximately 70% of stool cultures are positive. While a positive result confirms the clinical diagnosis of botulism, a negative result cannot be used to rule out botulism in a patient with compatible signs/symptoms. Standard methods for conducting the mouse bioassay are available in *Compendium of Methods for Microbiological Examination of Foods* (https://ajph.aphapublications.org/series/books) and *Bacteriological Analytical Manual.*[1,2]

If foodborne botulism is suspected, laboratories should test serum, stool, and suspect food for the presence of botulinum toxin. Culture of stool specimens increases the chance of laboratory confirmation of botulism. Culture of food which is known to contain botulinum toxin is also helpful for an outbreak investigation as molecular subtyping (pulsed field gel electrophoresis or whole genome sequencing) can help establish a link between clinical and food isolates. Culture of food which does not contain botulinum toxin is not useful since spores are ubiquitous in food and the environment.

Because of the need to reduce animal testing, a number of alternative assays have been developed as either screening assays prior to mouse bioassay or as full replacement. Alternative or ancillary methods include the following: (1) polymerase chain reaction (PCR)-based methods for detecting the toxin gene in culture, (2) enzyme-linked immunosorbent assay (ELISA)-based methods for detection of toxin, (3) protein A bead based capture systems (ALISSA), (4) detection of toxin based on mass spectrometry identification of peptide cleavage products (Endopep-mass spectrometry), and (5) cell-based assays using primary neurons or human-induced stem cell production of neurons. However, these methods have not been reviewed or cleared by regulatory agencies responsible for diagnostic testing. Some have been validated for food and food culture testing. In order to use these alternative methods for clinical specimen testing, an individual laboratory must perform internal validation studies which meet their specific regulatory requirements. Any alternative assay being considered should meet the minimal detectable limits of the mouse bioassay and not produce false-positive results. Methods based on the detection of the toxin gene (i.e., real-time PCR) should not be used in the absence of a toxin detection method since (1) bacteria may contain more than 1 toxin gene but only produce 1 toxin and (2) identification of a toxin gene does not always correlate with the presence of toxin in the sample.

**9. Reporting requirements**—Identification of a case of botulism is reportable in the USA and in the EU member states and in 3 European Economic Area/European Free Trade Association countries (Iceland, Liechtenstein, and Norway) according to case definitions established in the USA or EU. Botulism is also reportable in other countries (e.g., Argentina, Canada). Laboratory directors should ensure that all reporting requirements are met including notification of potentially contaminated commercially produced and distributed food products. Since botulinum toxin and botulinum neurotoxin producing-*Clostridia* are considered tier 1 select agents in the USA, any laboratory identifying these agents in clinical or food samples must immediately report to the Federal Select Agent Program. Transport restrictions also apply to samples identified to contain these agents. It is the laboratory director's responsibility to be aware of any national notification or transport restrictions as a result of laboratory identification of these biological agents.

**10. Referral network**—There are no specific restrictions on who is authorized to test for botulinum toxin; however, the use of the mouse bioassay in the USA is limited to reference laboratories at the state or national level primarily due to the high costs of maintaining animal testing facilities. Laboratories must adhere to the botulism testing referral process within their respective countries or regions.

**11. Special considerations**—Botulism is covered by the International Health Regulations (IHR). Events must be reported if a contaminated food product has or could be imported to other countries and determined by WHO as meeting the IHR criteria. Additionally, in the EU, the Rapid Alert System for Food and Feed and Early Warning and Response System are used for rapid notification of potential risky food products that are exported. In the USA, either the FDA or USDA initiate product recalls and notifications. In the event of intentional contamination of food, national security agencies become involved in investigations.

## References

1. Maslanka SE, Solomon HM, Sharma S, Johnson EA. *Clostridium botulinum* and its toxins. In: Salfinger Y, Tortorello ML, eds. *Compendium of Methods for the Microbiological Examination of Foods*. 5th ed. Washington, DC: American Public Health Association; 2012:391-400.
2. Solomon HM, Lilly T Jr. Clostridium botulinum. In: *Bacteriological Analytical Manual*. US Food and Drug Administration. 2001. Available at: http://www.fda.gov/Food/FoodScienceResearch/LaboratoryMethods/ucm070879.htm. Accessed June 20, 2018.

[S. E. Maslanka, C. Lúquez, J. Dykes]

# BRUCELLOSIS

(undulant fever, Malta fever, Mediterranean fever)

| DISEASE | ICD-10 CODE |
|---|---|
| BRUCELLOSIS | ICD-10 A23 |

**1. Clinical features**—A systemic bacterial disease that has an acute or insidious onset, with continued, intermittent, or irregular fever of variable duration, headache, weakness, profuse sweating, arthralgia, myalgia, fatigue, anorexia, and weight loss. Localized suppurative infections of organs, including liver and spleen, may occur, as well as chronic localised infections; subclinical infection has been reported. The disease may last days, months, or occasionally a year or more if not adequately treated. Osteoarticular complications occur in 20%–60% of cases; sacroiliitis is the most frequent joint manifestation. Genitourinary involvement is seen in 2%–20% of cases, with orchitis and epididymitis as common manifestations. Recovery is usual, but disability is often pronounced. Neurobrucellosis is a less common but more severe manifestation, which occurs in 3%–7% of cases. The case-fatality rate of untreated brucellosis is 2% or less and usually results from endocarditis caused by *Brucella melitensis* (most virulent) infection. Part of, or the entire original syndrome, may reappear as relapses.

**2. Causative agents**—*Brucella abortus, B. melitensis, Brucella suis, Brucella canis, Brucella ceti*, and *Brucella pinnepedialis* (nov. sp.).

**3. Laboratory diagnosis**—Microbial isolation of *Brucella* spp. from blood, bone marrow, or other tissues or discharges is considered the gold standard for patient diagnosis. Several polymerase chain reaction (PCR) assays are currently available for isolates to identify *Brucella* at the species level.

A 4-fold rise in titer on an agglutination assay is the serologic method of choice in diagnosing acute, noncomplicated cases of brucellosis caused by *B. abortus*, *B. melitensis*, or *B. suis*. For chronic, complicated or neurobrucellosis cases, serologic assays other than agglutination, such as enzyme-linked immunosorbent assay (ELISA), are recommended. Serologic tests to detect *B. canis* antibodies are not performed routinely in diagnostic laboratories.

**4. Laboratory capability**—Pathology and microbiology laboratories equipped with biosafety level 3 (BSL-3) facilities are required for diagnosis of brucellosis. Personnel trained to work in BSL-3 facilities and trained to handle dangerous organisms are required.

**5. Safety requirements**—*Brucella* spp. are extremely infectious, and brucellosis is the most common bacterial infection acquired in a laboratory. If brucellosis is suspected, samples should be handled in a BSL-3 laboratory by trained personnel. If a culture that is handled on the open bench is subsequently suspected of containing *Brucella* spp., the culture should be placed immediately in a BSL-3 laboratory, and all personnel who handled the culture on the open bench should be monitored for symptoms.

**6. Nonhuman hosts**—Brucellosis is a zoonotic infection acquired from contact with infected domesticated or wild animals. Human brucellosis is strongly associated with the management of domesticated animals and ingestion of their products. Certain *Brucella* spp. are associated with different animal species as follows: *B. abortus, B. melitensis, B. ovis* (goats, cattle, sheep, and hippos); *B. suis* biotypes 1–4 (pigs, boar, and reindeer); *B. suis* biotype 5 (rodents); *B. canis* (dogs); and *B. ceti* and *B. pinnepedialis* (marine mammals).

**7. Sample/specimen requirements**—*Brucella* spp. are most commonly isolated from blood and blood cultures. *Brucella* spp. can also be isolated from other clinical matrices such as bone marrow, cerebrospinal fluid, wounds, purulent discharge, and joint fluid. Serological tests are common for the diagnosis of brucellosis and paired (i.e., acute and convalescent) serum samples are required. When sending specimens of suspected brucellosis to the laboratory for testing, the laboratory must be made aware of the suspected diagnosis due to the risk for laboratory workers of handling samples containing *Brucella* spp. Samples with suspected *Brucella* for diagnostics should be shipped as UN category B.

**8. Testing requirements**—Diagnosis of brucellosis is mainly by serological testing, although culture can be used to isolate the organism from clinical samples. PCR is becoming increasingly common and is considered to be sensitive. PCR can be used in acute cases on blood samples but works best in later stages of disease on samples from affected body parts (see earlier sample details).

1) Culture: *Brucella* spp. can be cultured from blood and bone marrow tissue in the acute phase of illness, with the likelihood of

obtaining positive blood cultures in this phase of 70%-90%. In subacute or chronic infections, culture may be successful from other tissues depending on the clinical symptoms, or serological tests may be required to establish the diagnosis. *Brucella* spp. are slow growing and may require prolonged incubation up to 6 weeks to grow, although when using automated blood culture methods, the cultures may be positive after 7 days. The recommended culture method is Castaneda biphasic medium. Gram stain of positive cultures yields clumps of Gram-negative cocco-bacilli, which may be difficult to see. Biochemical tests, particularly for urease, can distinguish *Brucella* spp. from other look-alike bacteria such as *Salmonella* spp.

2) Serological tests: serological tests are the tests of choice for brucellosis, but many available serological tests will not detect *B. canis*. *B. canis* has a rough O-polysaccharide layer in its outer cell membrane as opposed to the smooth O-polysaccharide layer present in the outer cell membrane of other *Brucella* spp., which is the major immunodominant epitope. Serology procedures are divided into 2 categories: conventional tests and primary binding assays. Conventional tests include agglutination tests, rapid agglutination tests, precipitation tests, and complement fixation tests. Agglutination tests such as standard tube agglutination (STA) with and without addition of reducing agents such as 2-mercaptoethanol or ethylenediaminetetraacetic acid, STA with addition of antiglobulin to enhance agglutination, and the milk ring test using a mixture of bacterial antigens incubated with the test serum. The tests are performed at a nearly neutral pH and are sensitive at detecting immunoglobulin class M (IgM) antibodies, but less sensitive for IgG antibodies, particularly IgG1 antibodies, resulting in low assay specificity. It is generally recommended that the tests be used in combination with other tests. Rapid agglutination test methods include acidified antigen modifications of agglutination tests, where the test pH is reduced to an acid test environment to enhance the agglutination of IgG antibodies, particularly IgG1 antibodies. These assays typically use antigens from *B. abortus*, since *B. abortus, B. melitensis,* and *B. suis* all contain smooth O-polysaccharide, and therefore, cross-react in these tests. Examples of rapid agglutination tests include the rose bengal test (RBT), modified RBT test, buffered antigen plate agglutination test (BPAT), and card test. RBT and BPAT tests are the most widely used of these tests. Precipitation tests, agar gel immunodiffusion, and radial immunodiffusion can distinguish between serum from antibodies resulting from vaccination and antibodies resulting from infection and are

thus better for veterinary diagnostics than clinical diagnostics. The methods are labor-intensive and not widely used. Complement fixation tests are technically challenging but are widely used as a confirmation test for brucellosis. The test specificity is high, as only IgG1 antibody isotypes fixes complement efficiently. Primary binding assays include radioimmunoassays, fluorescence immunoassays, particle counting fluorescent immunoassays, indirect ELISA, competitive ELISA, and fluorescence polarizing immunoassays. The 2 most commonly used of these are the indirect and competitive ELISA. Indirect ELISA assays are available commercially and are considered to be very sensitive, but with lower specificity, and can cross-react with the immune response from other infections. Competitive ELISA assays were developed to overcome the lower specificity and cross-reactivity of the indirect ELISA. The resulting assays are highly specific but have lower sensitivity. The assay is generally used as a confirmatory assay, and these assays are available from various commercial sources.

3) Molecular methods: PCR is currently the most efficient way of finding organisms in appropriate clinical samples. A number of single plex and multiplex PCR assays are described for the diagnosis of brucellosis, and several commercial PCR assays are available. For single plex assays, sensitivity and specificity varies widely depending on different primer sets used. For clinical diagnosis, primers targeting the bcsp31 gene are commonly used. Combined PCR assays targeting the bcsp31 and selected outer membrane proteins (omp2a, omp31) have been used to differentiate the 4 different *Brucella* spp. causing human infection. A number of multiplex PCR assays have been described in the literature, including the Bruce-ladder PCR, which can distinguish between all *Brucella* spp. at genus level. More recently, real-time PCR assays have been developed, and a number of real-time PCR assays are commercially available. Real-time PCR assays are rapid and sensitive, being able to detect bacteria in the femtogram range. A distinct advantage of PCR over serology is the ability to detect *B. canis*, as there are no current serological tests available for *B. canis*.

The gold standard test for brucellosis remains isolation of the organism from the host by culture, but this is time consuming and potentially dangerous because of the risk of laboratory acquired infection. Not all laboratories are equipped with the high-security laboratories required to handle *Brucella* spp. Serological tests are widely available and widely used. Each individual test has its disadvantages, and therefore, most laboratories use a combination of agglutination and primary antigen test methods to increase sensitivity and specificity. PCR assays, particularly real-time PCR assays, are becoming increasingly more common, and published papers have reported high sensitivity and specificity with these assays. Commercial serological and real-time PCR assays are widely available.

**9. Reporting requirements**—Brucellosis in domestic animals (cattle, sheep, pigs, dogs) must be reported under World Organisation for Animal Health regulations. Human brucellosis is a notifiable disease in some countries, such as the USA and the UK. Confirmed cases should be reported according to national or local regulations for notifiable diseases. Cases of suspected or laboratory confirmed brucellosis should be reported as required by local health regulations. Isolates for confirmatory testing should be sent on solid media in tightly sealed containers (e.g., slants).

**10. Referral network**—The WHO/FAO Collaborating Centre for Reference and Research on Brucellosis is the Animal and Plant Health Agency located in Weybridge, UK. Each country may have national or regional referral networks.

**11. Special considerations**—*B. melitenis, B. suis,* and *B. abortus* are considered to be potential biothreat agents and are listed in the Select Agents and Toxins, 7 CFR Part 331, 9 CFR Part 121, and 42 CFR Part 73 (http://www.selectagents.gov). In the USA, confirmed isolates of select agents identified in a clinical or diagnostic laboratory must be reported. Each country may have specific registration requirements for laboratories working with *Brucella* for human or animal pathogen regulations, and these should be checked. For example in the UK, *Brucella* sp. are regulated as animal pathogens by the Department for Environment, Food & Rural Affairs.

[J. Duggan]

# BURULI ULCER

| DISEASE | ICD-10 CODE |
|---|---|
| BURULI ULCER | ICD-10 A31.1 |

**1. Clinical features**—Classically presents as a chronic painless skin ulcer, with undermined edges, and a necrotic white or yellow base (cotton wool appearance). Secondary bacterial infection may occur, causing the ulcer to become painful. Most lesions are located on the extremities and tend to be seen more frequently on lower extremities rather than upper. It often starts as a painless nodule or a papule, which eventually ulcerates. Other presentations may be seen, such as indurated plaques or edematous lesions; the latter represents a rapidly disseminated form that does not pass through a nodular stage. Bones and joints may be affected by direct spread from an overlying cutaneous lesion or through the bloodstream. Long-neglected or poorly managed patients usually present with scars that are sometimes hypertrophic or keloid, with partially healed areas or disabling contractures, especially for lesions that cross joints. Marjolin ulcers (squamous cell carcinoma) may develop in unstable or chronic non-pigmented scars.

The differential diagnosis includes the following, by dermatologic manifestation:

1) Minor infections: insect bites and a variety of dermatological conditions.
2) Nodules: cysts, lipomas, boils, onchocercomas, lymphadenitis, mycoses.
3) Plaques: leprosy, cellulites, mycoses, psoriasis.
4) Edematous forms: cellulites, elephantiasis, actinomycosis.
5) Ulcers: tropical phagedenic ulcer, diabetic ulcer, leishmaniasis, neurogenic ulcer, yaws, squamous cell carcinoma, pyoderma gangrenosum, noma.

**2. Causative agents**—*Mycobacterium ulcerans* is a slow growing environmental mycobacterium that requires temperatures of 29°C–33°C for growth and produces mycolactone, a polyketide derived macrolid toxin. Mycolactone is cytotoxic, immunosuppressive, and induces analgesia by targeting the angiotensin pathway. Human strains from Africa predominantly produce the structural variant A/B (the most cytotoxic congener), and the Australian and Asian strains produce the C and D variants, respectively. Temperature requirements and mycolactone production account for the characteristics of infection (i.e., development of painless lesions in skin and subcutaneous tissue as well as tissue destruction through apoptosis, necrosis, and suppression of local host immune responses). *M. ulcerans* is closely related to the *Mycobacterium marinum* complex that contains non-mycolactone producing *M. marinum* as well as mycolactone producing mycobacterial species (i.e., *Mycobacterium liflandii,* structural variant E, some unusual clades of *M. marinum,* and *Mycobacterium pseudoshotsii*, structural variant F), which are pathogenic for aquatic vertebrates. Based on complete genomic sequencing, the causative agent of Buruli ulcer in Japan has been defined as *M. ulcerans* subsp. *shinshuense*. Like other mycolactone producing mycobacteria, *M. ulcerans* acquired the insertion sequences IS*2404* (present in >200 copies in its genome), IS*2606*, and the plasmid pMUM that confers the ability to synthesize mycolactone.

**3. Laboratory diagnosis**—The clinical diagnosis of Buruli ulcer is usually straightforward if symptomatic patients present with typical painless ulcers with undermined edges and either originate from endemic areas or have an appropriate travel history. However, due to the various clinical manifestations, a range of differential diagnoses must be borne in mind, and in areas where health professionals do not regularly see cases of Buruli ulcer the accuracy of clinical diagnosis may be challenging. Before initiation of antimycobacterial treatment, microbiological confirmation is essential to confirm that the disease is Buruli ulcer. Currently laboratory diagnosis of Buruli ulcer includes 4 standard laboratory tests: (1) direct smear examination for acid fast bacilli (AFB), (2) in vitro culture, (3) IS*2404* polymerase chain reaction (PCR), and (4) histopathology. About 20% of patients present with paradoxical reactions (i.e., an inflammatory response caused by treatment-induced recovery of the immune system, which leads to worsening of existing lesions or development of secondary lesions during or after treatment). Laboratory assessment (i.e., culture or alternative viability assays and histopathology) is required to distinguish these paradoxical reactions (characterized by the absence of viable bacilli and characteristic histopathologic features such as granulomas and massive immune cell infiltrates) from treatment failures, recurrences, or reinfection (the latter characterized by the presence of viable organisms).[1]

**4. Laboratory capability**—Direct smear examination can be done in any clinical laboratory routinely performing AFB microscopy. Cultivation of *M. ulcerans* requires a laboratory with experience in mycobacterial culture techniques, preferably including isolation of nontuberculous mycobacteria. Due to the growth requirements of *M. ulcerans*, capacity for incubation at 29°C–33°C must be available, and access to PCR facilities is necessary as identification of colonies is done by IS*2404* PCR. Regarding the PCR laboratory, the 3-room principle (i.e., deoxyribonucleic acid [DNA] extraction, PCR reaction mix, and PCR amplification) should be strictly observed to avoid false-positive results. Preparation and staining of tissue samples for histopathological analysis requires a fully equipped histopathological laboratory, and examination must be done by a pathologist.

**5. Safety requirements**—In the USA, *M. ulcerans* is classified as a biosafety level 2 (BSL-2) pathogen. As with other *Mycobacterium* spp., excluding *M. tuberculosis* complex and *Mycobacterium leprae*, BSL-2 practices, including appropriate containment practices and facilities, are recommended for activities with clinical material and cultures of *M. ulcerans*. Person-to-person transmission has not been observed; however, the mode of transmission has not yet been fully elucidated. Mechanical transmission caused by inoculating events such as insect bites or trauma is considered likely; therefore, the use of sharps should be strictly avoided. Potentially aerosolizing procedures such as opening of sample containers, grinding of tissue, or decontaminating samples for culture should be conducted exclusively in a biosafety cabinet (BSC). Polymerase chain reaction samples should be subjected to heat inactivation at 95°C for 15 minutes (e.g., in a thermomixer) before further processing outside a BSC.

6. **Nonhuman hosts**—*M. ulcerans* DNA has been found in various mosquitoes (e.g., *Aedes, Coquilletidae, and Culex* spp. from Australia) and in aquatic insects from West Africa (e.g., creeping and giant water bugs, water beetles, water striders) with successful cultivation from a water strider from Benin. Furthermore, various mollusks, fish, and shellfish (among those a freshwater crayfish found in a water channel in the backyard of a Japanese family with 3 cases of Buruli ulcer) have tested positive. Natural infections of domestic and wildlife mammals (e.g., horses, dogs, cat, alpaca) and marsupials (e.g., koalas, long-footed potoroo, ringtailed and brushtailed possums) have occurred in Australia.

7. **Sample/specimen requirements**—Clinical samples for laboratory confirmation should be collected before starting antimycobacterial therapy. Appropriate sample types for routine confirmation of Buruli ulcer are swabs (ulcerative lesions) and fine needle aspirates (nonulcerative lesions and late stage ulcers with scarred edges). Punch biopsies (3 mm or 4 mm in diameter) are not the first choice for diagnostic samples but may be required for histopathological analyses, with the aim of establishing the differential diagnosis or the monitoring of treatment response. Swabs are collected by circling the entire undermined edge of an ulcer. Fine needle aspirates and punch biopsies are taken from the center of nonulcerative lesions or from the edge of ulcers, preferably from the end of the undermined edge. In cases requiring surgical intervention, surgical biopsies may be taken from the same locations during surgical excision. All tissue samples must contain necrotic tissue! Laboratory confirmation of osteomyelitis is possible by assessment of bone biopsy samples, curetted bone, or pus from fistulas. Conditions for transport and storage of clinical samples depend on time to processing and subsequent diagnostic tests. Acid-fast bacilli smears for microscopic analysis can be prepared directly after collection and transported to the laboratory. Punch biopsies for histopathological analysis should be stored in 10% neutral or buffered (pH 7.4) formaldehyde immediately after collection. As a rule, when microbiological analysis can be performed within 24 hours, clinical specimens should be kept at 4°C. Otherwise, transport media should be used. It is to be noted that some transport media are suitable for culture and PCR analysis (e.g., Liquid Middlebrook 7H9 or BBL mycobacteria growth indicator tube [MGIT; Becton Dickinson, Sparks, MD] supplemented with OADC enrichment [oleic acid, albumin, dextrose, catalase; Becton Dickinson] and PANTA [polymyxin B, nalidixic acid, trimethoprim, azlocillin; Becton Dickinson], Dubos broth base [Becton Dickinson] supplemented with

Dubos medium albumin [Becton Dickinson] and PANTA or supplemented with OADC and PANTA). Some transport media, however, are appropriate for PCR only (e.g., phosphate buffered saline, Tris-ethylenediaminetetraacetic acid-buffer, Gentra Puregene cell lysis solution [CLS; QIAGEN, Hilden, Germany], and alcohol), but not all media and subsequent extraction procedures are mutually compatible (e.g., Gentra Puregene procedures require compatible cell lysis solutions). Stability of samples for PCR analysis is greatest if alcohol or CLS is used as transport medium.[2]

**8. Testing requirements**—Currently 4 standard diagnostic tests are applied for laboratory confirmation of Buruli ulcer. The positivity rates or sensitivities of different tests depend on the quality of samples and may vary according to the type of sample and the clinical form of the disease.

1) Direct smear examination for AFB: the method is rapid and easy and can be performed on swab samples, fine needle aspirates, and tissue samples (i.e., ground tissue or material subjected to decontamination procedures for culture). The sensitivity however is less than 60%. Microscopic examination cannot distinguish *M. ulcerans* from other mycobacteria possibly involved in the etiology of skin lesions, nor can it be used to ascertain bacterial viability. AFB smears are stained with the staining technique locally used for laboratory diagnosis of tuberculosis (TB) such as the Ziehl-Neelsen hot staining method, and Kinyoun, or auramine-rhodamine stain. Likewise, quantitation of AFB smears should be in accordance with the method locally used for the diagnosis of TB, and laboratories should participate in external quality assurance programs for AFB microscopy according to local standards.[2]
2) In vitro culture: cultures can be performed on swab samples, fine needle aspirates, and tissue samples. The maximum sensitivity is 70%. *M. ulcerans* grows on several culture media (i.e., Loewenstein-Jensen, Ogawa, Brown and Buckle, Middlebrook 7H10 or 7H11). Recommended decontamination procedures are the oxalic acid method, the modified Petroff method, or the N-acetyl-cysteine-sodium hydroxide technique. Cultures are usually positive after 9–12 weeks, but incubation times of up to 9 months or more may be required. Species identification is done by IS*2404* PCR. Due to the long generation time of *M. ulcerans*, cultures are inappropriate for rapid laboratory confirmation but constitute the reference method for the assessment of bacterial viability in patients with paradoxical reactions or suspected treatment failures, recurrences, or reinfection. Furthermore, cultures are required for conventional susceptibility testing and other downstream applications.[2]

3) PCR: due to its high sensitivity and specificity (>90%) and the availability of diagnostic results within a few days, PCR targeting the insertion sequence IS*2404* is considered the method of choice for laboratory confirmation of Buruli ulcer. However, PCR cannot distinguish between viable and dead bacilli and is not suitable for treatment monitoring as *M. ulcerans* DNA may persist for months. PCR can be performed on all types of clinical samples as well as on culture material. Several IS*2404* PCR protocols have been described. Most commonly used are conventional single-step gel-based PCR and real-time qPCR. Compared with gel-based PCR, the advantages of real-time qPCR are increased sensitivity due to a considerable (up to 100 times) lower limit of detection, increased specificity, decreased risk of cross-contamination due to the closed-tube format, as well as shorter turnaround times. DNA extraction is a crucial step of the PCR process, and various in-house and commercial extraction procedures employing physical and/or chemical lysis followed by precipitation and purification procedures are available. According to current expertise, the Maxwell method and the Gentra Puregene procedure are most suitable for use with IS*2404* PCR.[2]

   Diagnostic PCR procedures generally require stringent quality control measures. Laboratories performing PCR diagnosis of Buruli ulcer have the possibility to participate in an external quality assurance program organized by the Institute of Tropical Medicine, Mycobacteriology Unit, Antwerp, Belgium (WHO Collaborating Centre for the Diagnosis and Surveillance of *Mycobacterium Ulcerans* Infection).

4) Histopathological examination: Histopathological analysis is conducted on tissue specimens (3 mm or 4 mm punch biopsies, surgical biopsies) in 10% neutral or buffered (pH7.4) formalin stained with hematoxylin and eosin, Ziehl-Neelsen, or other stains suitable for the detection of pathogens other than *M. ulcerans*. As punch biopsies are not considered first-line diagnostic samples, and in most cases diagnostic confirmation can be achieved by less invasive methods, histopathology normally is reserved for issues beyond initial diagnosis. Distinctive histopathological features of Buruli ulcer comprise hyperplasia of the epidermis, inflammation and vasculitis, contiguous coagulation necrosis of lower dermis, subcutaneous tissue and fascia, characteristic fat cell ghosts, and the presence of extracellular AFB, often in clusters, in necrotic subcutaneous tissue. Whereas progressing active disease shows a poor inflammatory response, granulomatous responses occur in healing stages and paradoxical reactions. With a sensitivity of approximately 90%,

histopathology provides reliable results and can identify late/healing stages in which bacilli are scarce or absent, and direct detection methods are not effective. Histopathology can establish differential diagnoses and is useful in monitoring treatment progress; however, it may not always provide unambiguous identification.[2]

5) New test methods include the following:

- For the detection of *M. ulcerans* DNA from all types of clinical samples, LAMP assays targeting IS*2404*, including a dry-reagent based LAMP format, are available. LAMP is highly specific, and its sensitivity is comparable to that of PCR. The robust, fast, and unsophisticated technology can be run on a portable fluorimeter in decentralized laboratories, thus providing the possibility for Point-of-Care-Testing.
- Molecular viability assay: in view of the drawbacks of culture and the inability of PCR to differentiate viable and dead bacilli, ribonucleic acid (RNA) assays provide an alternative to determine bacterial viability. To monitor treatment responses in Buruli ulcer patients and to distinguish paradoxical reactions from treatment failures, recurrences, and reinfection, a 16S rRNA RT qPCR is available. In combination with IS*2404* real-time qPCR, the assay is 100% *M. ulcerans* specific and highly sensitive. Fine needle aspirates or swab samples stored in RNA protecting transport media (e.g., RNA*later*; Qiagen) are suitable sample types.[3,4]

**9. Reporting requirements**—For Buruli ulcer control programs, WHO provides standardized recording and reporting forms that include information on diagnostic samples and test results.[5] Outside endemic regions, in any event, the type and origin of diagnostic samples and corresponding laboratory results should be recorded and provided to relevant health authorities.

**10. Referral network**—For all suspected cases of Buruli ulcer occurring in the USA, CDC constitute the main reference laboratory, and clinical samples should be sent to CDC for final confirmation. Current WHO recommendations require that at least 70% of all reported cases globally are PCR confirmed and that a network of laboratories specialized in the PCR diagnosis of Buruli ulcer has been established. The network currently comprises 14 laboratories in Africa, Asia, Australia, Europe, and South America, including 2 WHO collaborating centers in Belgium and Australia. These laboratories can be contacted with any further questions related to the laboratory diagnosis of Buruli ulcer.[6]

**11. Special considerations**—Although neither notifiable nor contagious from person to person, it is recommended that cases be reported to local health authorities to track down the provenance of infection and generate further epidemiological information on imported Buruli ulcer in the USA.

## References

1. World Health Organization. Treatment of *Mycobacterium ulcerans* disease (Buruli ulcer). Guidance for health workers. 2012. Available at: http://apps.who.int/iris/bitstream/10665/77771/1/9789241503402_eng.pdf?ua=1. Accessed June 21, 2018.
2. Portaels F, ed. Laboratory diagnosis of Buruli ulcer: a manual for health care providers. World Health Organization. 2014. Available at: http://apps.who.int/iris/bitstream/10665/111738/1/9789241505703_eng.pdf?u.http:a=1. Accessed June 21, 2018.
3. Beissner M, Symank D, Phillips RO, et al. Detection of viable *Mycobacterium ulcerans* in clinical samples by a novel combined 16S rRNA reverse transcriptase/IS*2404* real-time qPCR assay. *PLoS Negl Trop Dis*. 2012;6(8):e1756.
4. Sarpong-Duah M, Frimpong M, Beissner M, et al. Clearance of viable *Mycobacterium ulcerans* from Buruli ulcer lesions during antibiotic treatment as determined by combined 16S rRNA reverse transcriptase/IS*2404* qPCR assay. *PLoS Negl Trop Dis*. 2017;3;11(7):e0005695.
5. World Health Organization. New recording and reporting forms. Available at: http://www.who.int/buruli/control/forms_2/en. Accessed June 21, 2018.
6. World Health Organization. Global Network of laboratories for confirming *Mycobacterium ulcerans* disease (Buruli ulcer). Table 2. 2014. Available at: http://www.who.int/buruli/Global_network_laboratories_PCR_2014.pdf?ua=1. Accessed June 21, 2018.

[M. Beissner, G. Bretzel]

# CAMPYLOBACTER ENTERITIS

| DISEASE | ICD-10 CODE |
|---|---|
| CAMPYLOBACTER ENTERITIS | ICD-10 A04.5 |

**1. Clinical features**—The disease is characterized by diarrhea that may be bloody, abdominal pain, fever, malaise, and nausea, sometimes with vomiting. A prodromal period of fever and malaise may precede diarrhea by a day or more. Severe abdominal pain may be mistaken for acute appendicitis or inflammatory bowel disease. Symptoms usually persist for several days to 2 weeks. Gross or occult blood with mucus and white blood cells is often present in liquid stools. Extraintestinal infection is rare, usually occurring in immunocompromised patients. Rare postinfectious complications include reactive arthritis (~1% of cases) and Guillain-Barré syndrome (~0.1% of cases). Postinfectious irritable bowel syndrome has also been linked to *Campylobacter* infection. The number of campylobacteriosis cases is comparable to or higher than the number of cases of nontyphoidal salmonellosis in most developed countries. Many infections are asymptomatic, and most are self-limited. Case-fatality rates have been estimated from 0.01% to 1%.

**2. Causative agents**—*Campylobacter jejuni* and, less commonly, *Campylobacter coli* are the usual causes of campylobacter diarrhea. Other *Campylobacter* spp., including *Campylobacter lari*, *Campylobacter fetus*, and *Campylobacter upsaliensis*, have been associated with illness in both normal and immunocompromised hosts.

**3. Laboratory diagnosis**—Definitive diagnosis is based on isolation of the organism from clinical specimens using selective media, microaerobic growth conditions, incubation at 42°C (107.6°F), phenotypic identification using oxidase and catalase tests, and Gram staining. Standard culture methods may not detect all strains of *C. fetus* and *C. upsaliensis*. Visualization of motile and curved, spiral, or S-shaped rods similar to those of *Vibrio cholerae* in stool by phase contrast or dark-field microscopy can provide rapid presumptive evidence for *Campylobacter* enteritis. Culture-independent nucleic acid and antigen-based methods for detection of *C. jejuni* and, in some cases, *C. coli* in stool specimens have also been developed for early diagnosis. The relatively low specificity described to date for antigen-based diagnostic methods suggests that high false-positive rates may limit the usefulness of these tests. Diagnosis through whole genome sequencing is likely to be available at central hospital level in many countries in the near future.

**4. Laboratory capability**—A contained, purpose-built, microbiological facility with the capacity to autoclave microbiological waste is required to handle this pathogen. Staff should be trained and competent to handle potentially hazardous biological material and should be able to carry out basic phenotypic techniques. *Campylobacter* spp. are fastidious organisms having specific atmospheric and temperature growth requirements and, therefore, can be difficult to isolate, grow, and identify. The use of rapid diagnostic methods such as polymerase chain reaction (PCR) and enzyme immunoassays (EIAs) for campylobacteriosis may be restricted to more specialized laboratories, although PCR testing for gastrointestinal pathogens is becoming widely available in general pathology laboratories.

*Campylobacter* is predominantly a foodborne pathogen, and specialized staff and facilities are required for its recovery and isolation from food. Since *Campylobacter* is a serious public health concern, the detection of this bacterium in food is a routine capability in many food and water microbiology testing laboratories both in the public and private sectors.

**5. Safety requirements**—Employers have a responsibility to protect their workers from the risks related to exposure to hazardous biological agents.[1] *Campylobacter* spp. are hazard group 2 organisms and require biosafety containment level 2 (BSL-2) laboratories. The infectious dose for *Campylobacter* is low (< 500 organisms can cause disease), and there have been several reports of laboratory-acquired infection. Dependent upon the risk assessment for the procedure being undertaken, appropriate personal protective equipment, including a laboratory coat and safety glasses, should be worn at all times. Safe working practices, including good hand washing techniques to minimize the risk of exposure, should be adopted by laboratory workers.

**6. Nonhuman hosts**—Campylobacteriosis is a zoonotic illness. The 2 species most frequently associated with human disease, *C. jejuni* and *C. coli*, are commonly found in the gastrointestinal tract of many warm-blooded animals, particularly poultry, cattle, sheep, pigs, wild birds, and domestic animals such as cats and dogs. They often exist in animals as commensals and are shed in feces, with food animals and especially poultry becoming contaminated at slaughter. Other *Campylobacter* spp. (e.g., *C. fetus*) are associated with reproductive disease in cattle and can cause gastroenteritis and septicemia in humans. The main route of infection for acute gastroenteritis in humans is through ingestion of contaminated, undercooked poultry or other ready-to-eat foods that have been cross-contaminated via raw poultry and the consumption of raw, unpasteurized dairy products.

**7. Sample/specimen requirements**—A stool specimen is required for diagnosis of *Campylobacter* gastroenteritis and should be collected during the acute phase of the diarrheal illness. Specimens should be processed within 2 hours of collection, as the organisms are fastidious, and a delay in processing may affect recovery. When processing cannot be performed within 2 hours, the sample should be added to a suitable transport medium (e.g., Cary-Blair) and stored at 4°C before being sent to the testing laboratory. *Campylobacter* spp. can also be isolated from blood in patients with bacteremia and from cerebrospinal fluid in cases of meningitis.

For investigating food or water borne outbreaks of *Campylobacter* enteritis, the suspected food and water samples should be collected, refrigerated, and transported to a food microbiology testing laboratory for processing.

**8. Testing requirements**—All testing facilities must adhere to the quality standards set out by their accreditation body, and diagnostic laboratories must follow the manufacturer's instructions for any assay being performed. There are a variety of methods for diagnostic detection of *Campylobacter*, which have differing levels of specificity and sensitivity, including culture, antigen testing, and PCR.

Culture methods are most widely used enabling species identification, antibiotic susceptibility testing, and typing for public health purposes. However, identification to species level is challenging, and many diagnostic clinical microbiology laboratories identify to genus level only using basic phenotypic methods. The 2 most common *Campylobacter* spp. associated with acute gastroenteritis, *C. jejuni,* and *C. coli*, can be isolated by direct plating of fecal specimens onto selective media and incubating at 42°C for 48–72 hours under microaerobic atmosphere (85% $N_2$, 10% $CO_2$, and 5% $O_2$). A variety of selective blood-based or charcoal-based media with antibiotics is available, such as cefoperazone-vancomycin-amphotericin B agar, Skirrow agar, or modified charcoal cefoperazone deoxycholate agar. However, it should be remembered that because these media favor isolation of *C. jejuni* and *C. coli*, the incidence of gastroenteritis caused by other species may be underestimated. There is currently no single method to isolate all *Campylobacter* spp., and additional methods such as microfiltration of stool specimens and subsequent microaerobic incubation at 37°C on nonselective media should be considered for isolation of species other than *C. jejuni* and *C. coli*. Once cultured, *Campylobacter* cells can be rapidly identified by Gram staining, oxidase, and catalase testing. Characteristically, by Gram stain, *Campylobacter* appear as slender, spiral or curved Gram-negative rods that look S- or gull-shaped when 2 or more cells group together. Most *Campylobacter* are both catalase and oxidase positive.

Nonculture methods for detection of *Campylobacter* include several commercially available EIAs for the detection of *Campylobacter* specific antigens in fecal samples. The antigen detected is common to *C. jejuni* and *C. coli*, and thus EIA detects both species; however, EIA does not distinguish between the species and does not detect all *Campylobacter* spp. While these assays are rapid, there are reports of cross reactivity and false positives. Therefore, they are not currently recommended for use as stand-alone methods for diagnostic purposes.

There are a number of commercially available multiplex nucleic acid amplification tests for the detection of gastrointestinal pathogens that include *Campylobacter* as one of the target organisms. Several of these have FDA approval and their increasing use is providing evidence that they offer a rapid, sensitive alternative to culture for *Campylobacter* as well as other gastrointestinal pathogens. However, the current deoxyribose nucleic acid-based detection assays may not detect all *Campylobacter* spp. associated with human disease.

Alternative identification methods such as multiplex PCR and matrix-assisted laser desorption/ionization time-of-flight mass spectrometry have increasingly been shown to provide rapid alternatives for identification of *Campylobacter* sp. Nevertheless, isolation of *Campylobacter* from positive stool specimens is still required for antibiotic sensitivity testing and for typing for epidemiological investigations.

Specialized methods are required for the isolation of *Campylobacter* from foods, and these are available in many food and water microbiology testing laboratories. Similar to those described for pathology laboratories, the methods here utilize microaerobic incubation at 42°C with selective and enrichment culture techniques. There is no single isolation method for all food sample types.

**9. Reporting requirements**—Notification of *Campylobacter* infections is via active laboratory reporting of confirmed cases, and national surveillance data is available in the USA and the UK. While the majority of *Campylobacter* gastrointestinal infections are sporadic, outbreaks do occur. When suspected, isolates from clinical cases and foods should be referred for further characterization and typing to assist epidemiological investigations in identifying the source and prevent further transmission.

**10. Referral network**—Isolates may be sent to specialized reference laboratories for species identification, for antimicrobial sensitivity testing, and for typing in outbreak situations. Molecular typing methods have superseded phenotypic typing methods with pulsed-field gel electrophoresis being commonly used for short-term epidemiological investigations, although discriminatory limitations make it less useful for surveillance purposes. Multilocus sequence typing, which enables source attribution of *Campylobacter* causing human disease to poultry, other food, and wild animals, has been shown to be valuable for long-term surveillance, although not always sufficiently discriminatory for short-term outbreak investigations. The use of whole genome sequencing, which provides rapid high-powered strain resolution together with phylogenetic information, offers the ultimate typing tool for the epidemiological surveillance of *Campylobacter*.

**11. Special considerations**—There is a risk of common source outbreaks occurring when mass feeding and poor sanitation coexist. Clusters of cases and outbreaks should be reported to the local health authority and investigated to identify the source, vehicle, and transmission route.

## References

1. EUR-Lex. Directive 2000/54/EC of the European Parliament and of the Council of 18 September 2000. Available at: https://eur-lex.europa.eu/legal-content/EN/ALL/?uri=CELEX%3A32000L0054. Accessed February 15, 2019.

[K. A. Grant, C. Swift]

# CANDIDIASIS

(moniliasis, thrush, candidosis)

| DISEASE | ICD-10 CODE |
|---|---|
| CANDIDIASIS | ICD-10 B37 |

**1. Clinical features**—A mycosis usually confined to the superficial layers of skin or mucous membranes, presenting clinically as oral thrush, intertrigo, vulvovaginitis, paronychia, or onychomycosis. Ulcers or pseudomembranes may form in the esophagus, stomach, or intestine. Invasive candidiasis, including candidemia, usually occurs in patients with specific risk factors for infection, such as central venous catheters, immunosuppression, antibiotic therapy, abdominal surgery, or critical illness. Repeated clinical skin or mucosal eruptions are common. Candidemia may be uncomplicated or may disseminate and cause deep-seated infection in many organs, including the eyes, kidneys, liver, spleen, heart, and central nervous system.

**2. Causative agents**—Most commonly *Candida albicans, Candida glabrata, Candida parapsilosis, Candida tropicalis,* and *Candida krusei*. However, more than 100 less common *Candida* spp. have been implicated in human disease, including *Candida dubliniensis*. Most recently, a novel *Candida* spp., *Candida auris*, has been described as a significant emerging pathogen on several continents (see Special Considerations section in this chapter).

**3. Laboratory diagnosis**—For superficial candidiasis affecting mucosal surfaces, diagnosis requires both clinical and laboratory evidence of infection. Swabs or smears taken from the affected areas should contain the relevant morphological forms of the yeast and should yield the organism after culture. However, as *Candida* spp. can be normal commensals of the oral cavity and vagina, isolation alone is not diagnostic of infection. Severe or recurrent oropharyngeal candidiasis in an adult with no other underlying immunosuppressive condition should suggest the possibility of human immunodeficiency virus infection. The diagnosis of *Candida* intertrigo, paronychia, nail infections, and lesions in chronic mucocutaneous candidiasis is best achieved by microscopic examination of scrapings from lesions. Culture of *Candida* spp. from swabs of affected areas is less useful, as the organism is frequently present as a colonizing component of the normal flora. For deep-seated candidiasis, the single most useful laboratory test is microscopic demonstration of pseudohyphae or budding yeast cells in infected tissue or normally sterile body fluids. Culture confirmation is important, as it will permit antifungal susceptibility testing, which is recommended in all such cases. In candidemic patients, blood cultures are frequently positive (50%–75%). High resolution imaging is useful for detecting deep-seated foci of infection in the liver and spleen; transthoracic echocardiograms should be employed with suspected *Candida* endocarditis; patients with candidemia should undergo ophthalmological examination to exclude *Candida* endophthalmitis. *Candida*-specific polymerase chain reaction (PCR) may play a role in early detection of candidemia or in those patients who have blood cultures that are negative for *Candida*. Specific biomarkers (beta-D-glucan and *Candida* mannan antigen) may be useful for starting empirical therapy in some classes of high-risk, critically ill patients, although false-positive results are not uncommon with beta-D-glucan testing. High titers of anti-mannan antibodies are detectable in patients with *Candida* endocarditis.

The employment of chromogenic agar is recommended for organisms isolated from deep, usually sterile sites and from blood cultures to aid detection of mixed infections caused by more than 1 *Candida* spp.

**4. Laboratory capability**—Laboratories that are accustomed to processing dermatology specimens should have staff sufficiently trained to examine swabs and scrapings collected from suspected cases of superficial candidiasis and to examine tissues and fluids from usually sterile sites when deep-seated candidiasis is suspected. Microscopes should be equipped with appropriate filters necessary for examining specimens treated with optical brighteners under ultraviolet light. Most clinical microbiology laboratories will be equipped with blood culture systems suitable for the isolation of *Candida* spp. All specimens for culture require appropriate mycological media containing selective agents to prevent bacterial growth and incubation in standard microbiological incubators maintained at 30°C. Chromogenic agars should be considered with samples from sites likely to contain more than 1 *Candida* spp.

**5. Safety requirements**—In the UK, the Advisory Committee on Dangerous Pathogens lists *Candida* spp. as hazard group 2 (biosafety level 2) organisms, and containment level 2 laboratory practices are sufficient for handling the agent. Equivalent recommendations (risk group 2) have been issued in the following publications: CDC's *Biosafety in Microbiology and Biomedical Laboratories* and the European Economic Community Directives (2000/50/EC and 90/679/EEC).[1,2]

**6. Nonhuman hosts**—*Candida* spp. have worldwide occurrence. They have been isolated from water, plants, and insects in anthropic marine and terrestrial environments and all animals sympatric with humans, including wild and pet birds.

**7. Sample/specimen requirements**—Swabs of affected mucosal surfaces are adequate for the microscopic and cultural diagnosis of superficial candidiasis (i.e., oral thrush, vulvovaginitis). Swabs in viral transport medium should be avoided due to the presence of antifungal agents in the medium. Skin or nail scrapings/clippings collected from suspected cases of *Candida* intertrigo and paronychia and lesions from patients with chronic mucocutaneous candidiasis should be transported dry using approved receptacles. In the laboratory, a representative proportion of the sample should be digested with potassium hydroxide to soften keratinized material prior to microscopic examination with optical brighteners, with the rest of the sample processed for mycological culture. Since isolation of *Candida* spp. from blood or other normally sterile body site is indicative of deep infection, samples from such sites should be processed as soon as possible after collection to avoid proliferation of other organisms that may have contaminated samples during collection. Blood cultures should be pursued in all cases of suspected candidemia and repeated regularly if initially negative. Positive cultures from blood collected by peripheral venipuncture are indicative of candidemia. Positive cultures from intravascular devices might represent contamination or colonization of devices, especially if peripheral blood cultures are negative. Recovery of *Candida* spp. from cerebrospinal fluid provides a reliable diagnosis of *Candida* meningitis. Serum samples for beta-D-glucan and mannan antigen detection should preferably be transported on ice and processed immediately upon receipt (i.e., < 48 hours after collection). PCR detection of *Candida* deoxyribonucleic acid (DNA) from blood or serum samples should be performed according to current best practice guidelines.

**8. Testing requirements**—To confirm clinical diagnosis, the collection and investigation of samples from suspected cases of superficial candidiasis is recommended in all symptomatic cases. For oropharyngeal, vulvovaginal, and chronic mucocutaneous candidiasis, the identification of organisms recovered to species level is recommended, accompanied by antifungal susceptibility testing in recurrent and/or complicated cases and in cases where patients have had prior exposure to antifungals, in particular the triazoles. Daily blood cultures are recommended when candidemia is suspected and should be incubated for at least 5 days. Sensitivity of blood culture depends upon the culture system used and the *Candida* spp. involved. When optimal conditions are employed, sensitivity has been reported to be 50%–75%; thus, blood culture is not necessarily an early diagnostic approach. In addition, not all yeasts recovered in blood culture are *Candida* spp. Emerging and rare non-*Candida* yeasts and the yeast form of dimorphic fungal pathogens account for up to 5% of positive blood cultures. The combined detection of mannan and anti-mannan antibodies specifically detects *Candida* spp. in serum, with sensitivity and specificity rates of approximately 80% and 85%, respectively, and a high negative predictive value (> 85%) when serial testing is performed. Similar sensitivity and specificity rates and negative predictive values have been reported for beta-D-glucan testing (> 65%, > 80%, and > 85%, respectively), although the beta-D-glucan antigen is not specific to *Candida* spp. Twice weekly determinations are recommended. Both mannan and beta-D-glucan detection assays can be positive several days before blood cultures. Although similar sensitivity and specificity (> 85%) have been reported for PCR-based techniques to detect *Candida* DNA, lack of standardization of techniques hinders a thorough evaluation of the clinical utility of these approaches. Microscopic examination of tissue samples and fluids from sterile sites is useful in diagnosing deep-seated candidiasis if samples are collected aseptically and processed promptly, although sensitivity is limited by sample quality. Tissue biopsies should be pursued in chronic disseminated candidiasis, as blood cultures are rarely positive. Swabs from affected lesions in oropharyngeal candidiasis should be examined microscopically and by culture on selective media to avoid bacterial overgrowth.

In all cases, microscopic detection of *Candida* spp. is facilitated by the use of fluorescent enhancers/optical brighteners and requires expertise for interpretation. Species identification and antifungal susceptibility should be performed in all cases of suspected disseminated and deep-seated candidiasis and in cases of recurrent or complicated superficial infections. Accurate identification of less common *Candida* spp. can be achieved using either molecular approaches (ribosomal DNA [rDNA] sequencing) or matrix-assisted laser desorption/ionization time-of-flight (MALDI-TOF).

Regular updated guidelines for the diagnosis and management of both superficial and systemic *Candida* infections are provided by the Infectious Disease Society of America and the European Society of Clinical Microbiology and Infectious Diseases.

**9. Reporting requirements**—There are currently no requirements for the national reporting of *Candida* infections diagnosed by local or regional microbiology laboratories. Appropriate local infection control teams should be involved when unusual clusters of deep *Candida* infections are identified in a given health care setting, so that the possibility of nosocomial transmission/outbreaks can be investigated. Referral of isolates of rare *Candida* spp. to appropriate reference centers is recommended to aid in local, national, and international epidemiological surveillance and detection of novel and emerging pathogens. (See Special Considerations section in this chapter).

**10. Referral network**—A comprehensive network of expert mycology reference laboratories exists both nationally and globally. They may be approached for help with the identification and antifungal susceptibility testing of unusual *Candida* spp. and for assistance with suspected outbreaks of deep *Candida* infections in high risk populations.

**11. Special considerations**—*C. auris* was first described as a novel species in 2009 and appears to be unlike other pathogenic yeast species in its propensity for transmission between hospital patients. It has since been associated with a wide range of clinical manifestations ranging from colonization to candidemia and disseminated candidiasis. Large nosocomial outbreaks have to date been described in high-risk settings in India, South Africa, South America, the UK, and Spain, with sporadic cases and smaller clusters reported in several additional Western European countries and the USA. Significantly, it is commonly resistant to fluconazole and can rapidly develop resistance to other classes of antifungal agents.

*C. auris* is a germ tube test-negative, budding yeast that is microscopically indistinguishable from many other *Candida* spp. Current commercially available biochemical-based tests (e.g., API AUX 20C and VITEK-2 YST) frequently misidentify *C. auris* as *Candida haemulonii, Saccharomyces cerevisiae*, *Candida famata*, *Candida sake,* or *Rhodotorula glutinis.* Therefore, it is recommended that *Candida* isolates from invasive infections, from superficial sites in patients in high intensity settings, and from patients transferred from an affected hospital should be identified to species level. If *C. haemulonii, C. famata*, *C. sake,* or *S. cerevisiae* are identified, further work should be undertaken to exclude *C. auris*. This would involve either molecular sequencing of rDNA genes or MALDI-TOF analysis using a platform that contains *C. auris* reference spectra. Antifungal susceptibility testing is recommended for all confirmed *C. auris* isolates.

Culture and identification of all *Candida* spp. recovered from surveillance swabs (e.g., nose, axilla, groin) taken from patients who are contacts with known *C. auris*-positive patients is important to control or reduce nosocomial spread. Specific guidelines concerning *C. auris* screening, identification, and management have been issued by CDC, Public Health England, and the European Centre for Disease Prevention and Control.

## References

1. US Department of Health and Human Services, Centers for Disease Control and Prevention; National Institutes of Health. *Biosafety in Microbiological and Biomedical Laboratories*. 5th ed. 2009. Available at: https://www.cdc.gov/labs/pdf/CDC-BiosafetyMicrobiologicalBiomedicalLaboratories-2009-P.PDF. Accessed March 7, 2019.
2. EUR-Lex. EUR-Lex homepage. Available at: https://eur-lex.europa.eu/homepage.html?locale=en. Accessed March 19, 2019.

[A. M. Borman]

# CAPILLARIASIS

| DISEASE | ICD-10 CODE |
|---|---|
| INTESTINAL CAPILLARIASIS | ICD-10 B81.1 |
| HEPATIC CAPILLARIASIS | ICD-10 B83.8 |
| PULMONARY CAPILLARIASIS | ICD-10 B83.8 |

**1. Clinical features**—Capillariasis is a zoonotic parasitic disease caused by infection with 1 of 3 *Capillaria* spp. Clinical features depend on the location in the human body where the worm resides—intestines, liver, and respiratory tract.

1) Intestinal capillariasis is an enteropathy with fever, eosinophilia, massive protein loss due to diarrhea, and a malabsorption syndrome, leading to progressive weight loss and emaciation. Fatal cases are characterized by the presence of great numbers of parasites in the small intestine together with ascites, pleural transudate, and abnormalities in electrolytes. Case-fatality rates of 10% have been reported. Subclinical cases also occur but usually become symptomatic over time.
2) Hepatic capillariasis is an uncommon and occasionally fatal infection of the liver. The picture is that of an acute, or subacute, hepatitis, with hepatomegaly and marked eosinophilia resembling that of visceral larva migrans; the organism can disseminate to the lungs and other viscera.
3) Pulmonary capillariasis is associated with fever, cough, shortness of breath, and other symptoms of lower respiratory tract infection. Eggs may appear in the sputum in 4 weeks; symptoms may appear earlier or later. Pneumonitis may be severe; heavy infections may be fatal.

**2. Causative agents**—Intestinal capillariasis is caused by infection with *Capillaria philippinensis*, hepatic capillariasis by *Capillaria hepatica* (*Hepaticola hepatica*), and pulmonary capillariasis by *Capillaria aerophila* (*Thominx aerophila*). *C. hepatica* and *C. aerophila* occur worldwide; *C. philippinensis* occurs in Southeast Asia, the Middle East, and parts of South America, including Colombia and Peru.

**3. Laboratory diagnosis**—Diagnosis of intestinal capillariasis is based on clinical findings plus the identification of eggs, larvae, or adult parasites in the stool. Jejunal biopsy may show worms in the mucosa. Eggs measure 36–45 μm long by 21 μm wide, have a thick, striated shell, and possess polar prominences at each end. Eggs are usually unembryonated or in a 2-cell state of division when passed in feces. Eggs need to be distinguished from those of the related species, *Trichuris trichiura*. Adult worms are 2.2–4.3 mm in length and have typical trichuroid features, including stichocytes around the esophagus and modified lateral chords forming bacillary bands.

Hepatic capillariasis is diagnosed by demonstrating eggs or the parasite in a liver biopsy or at necropsy. Eggs are not passed in feces as part of the natural life cycle, and eggs resembling those of *C. hepatica* in stool represent spurious passage after eating infected liver or food and water contaminated with eggs. Subsequent specimens should be collected and analyzed. Eggs of *C. hepatica* are 51-67 μm long by 30-35 μm wide and have a distinctly striated shell and bipolar prominences. Eggs may be in various stages of embryonation when spuriously passed in feces.

Pulmonary capillariasis is diagnosed by demonstrating eggs in the sputum or through eggs seen on bronchial biopsy. Eggs of *C. aerophila* are 60 μm long by 30 μm wide and have a granular shell and bipolar plugs.

There are no serologic or molecular tests available for routine clinical diagnosis of any of the 3 species.

**4. Laboratory capability**—Microscopy and stool concentration capabilities are required. Laboratorians should be trained in the microscopic detection of parasites and undergo regular proficiency testing.

**5. Safety requirements**—Clinical specimens should always be collected and handled with universal/standard precautions. *Capillaria* spp. are biosafety level 2 organisms. Formalin should only be used in a well-ventilated area, preferably in a chemical fume hood. Unpreserved and preserved stools, respiratory specimens, and biopsy specimens should be disposed of as infectious waste.

**6. Nonhuman hosts**—For *C. philippinensis*, fish-eating birds are the primary natural definitive hosts in nature, while fish serve as paratenic hosts; humans are usually infected when consuming raw or undercooked fish harboring infective larvae.

For *C. hepatica*, rodents are the natural definitive hosts. The entire life cycle takes place within the liver, and carnivores that eat infected rodents may spuriously pass eggs into the environment via their feces. Humans become infected when ingesting embryonated eggs in food or fomites contaminated soil containing infective eggs.

The natural hosts for *C. aerophila* are cats, dogs, and other carnivores. Humans become infected when ingesting embryonated eggs in food or fomites contaminated with soil containing infective eggs.

**7. Sample/specimen requirements**—Stool should be promptly preserved in an appropriate liquid medium, such as 10% buffered formalin or sodium acetate-acidic acid-formalin (SAF). Single vial systems for ova and parasite (O&P) collection are also adequate. Specimens in the appropriate preservatives should remain intact indefinitely. To maximize O&P sensitivity, up to 3 stool specimens should be collected on 3 successive days.

Biopsy specimens should be collected and prepared per standard histological procedures.

**8. Testing requirements**—Routine concentration procedures for stool (eggs) and routine examination of gross helminths (adults). A calibrated ocular micrometer should be used to measure egg size. Diagnosis is confirmatory in specimens meeting morphologic criteria.

**9. Reporting requirements**—Eggs of *C. hepatica* in stool may be reported to the requesting authority, although it should be understood their presence in that specimen type represents spurious passage. Capillariasis is not nationally reportable in the USA. Report to local health authority; official report not ordinarily justifiable. International reporting is not required.

**10. Referral network**—None.

**11. Special considerations**—None.

[B. Mathison]

# CHANCROID
(ulcus molle, soft chancre)

| DISEASE | ICD-10 CODE |
|---|---|
| CHANCROID | ICD-10 A57 |

**1. Clinical features**—An acute, sexually transmitted bacterial infection usually localized in the genital area and characterized clinically by a single, or multiple, painful, necrotic ulcers that bleed on contact. Chancroid ulcers are more frequently found in uncircumcised men on the foreskin or in the coronal sulcus and may cause a phimosis. These lesions are frequently accompanied by painful, swollen, and suppurating regional lymph nodes. In women, asymptomatic carriage is rare, but minimally symptomatic or painless lesions may occur on the vaginal wall or cervix. Extragenital lesions have been reported. Chancroid ulcers, like other genital ulcers, are associated with an increased risk of human immunodeficiency virus infection.

**2. Causative agents**—*Haemophilus ducreyi*, a Gram negative coccobacillus.

**3. Laboratory diagnosis**—The clinical diagnosis of chancroid lesions is difficult, as the lesions are similar in size to the primary chancre of syphilis. There is some distinction in that the edges of chancroid lesions are ragged, undermined, and pliable, whereas syphilis lesions are firm, round, and painless. Direct microscopic examination from the lesion is not ideal owing to the low number of *H. ducreyi* organisms present in the exudate and the confounding presence of nonpathogenic genitourinary and perirectal flora. Under ideal circumstances, a direct Gram stain of *H. ducreyi* will reveal Gram-negative slender rods or coccobacilli, often seen in clustered groups in arrangements described as thumb prints, school of fish, or railroad tracks. Definitive diagnosis requires cultivation of the organism or detection by a polymerase chain reaction (PCR)-based assay.

**4. Laboratory capability**—Only laboratories that meet certain conditions of experience and capability should attempt to isolate *H. ducreyi* or detect *H. ducreyi* using PCR techniques. The cultivation of *H. ducreyi* should not be attempted unless the specimen can be transported at 2°C–8°C in suitable transport medium and the special media and proper atmospheric conditions required are available in the laboratory. Due to the fastidious nature of *H. ducreyi*, molecular detection is the preferred method of identification. Currently there are no FDA-cleared *H. ducreyi* PCR tests available in the USA. As a consequence, the molecular testing for this organism is only available in laboratories that have validated their own laboratory developed test.

**5. Safety requirements**—Biosafety level 2. The following precautions should be implemented when working with this organism: appropriate personal protective equipment, including gloves and coat, as well as eye protection as needed. Any procedure that may produce aerosols or splashes should be performed within a biological safety cabinet.

**6. Nonhuman hosts**—Humans are the primary host of *H. ducreyi*. That said, flies have been implicated in the transmission of *H. ducreyi* in pediatric cases of cutaneous ulcers in Papua, New Guinea.[1]

**7. Sample/specimen requirements**—Optimally, samples should be collected from the base and undermined margins of the ulcer using a swab moistened with either saline or transport medium. The specimen should be collected by vigorously swabbing the base of the lesion. Suboptimal specimens for culture include ulcer material, lymph node aspirates, pus, and aspirates from buboes. The specimen should be transported on ice and submitted to the laboratory within 4 hours of collection. Suitable transport media include Amies transport medium and specially formulated thioglycolate/hemin—based media.[2] If extended transport is required, then the specimen should be directly inoculated to selective agar plates (see Testing Requirements section in this chapter).

**8. Testing requirements**—

1) Gram stain: a direct Gram stain from the sample is not recommended owing to the poor sensitivity and specificity of the smear. Gram stains from culture show Gram-negative pleomorphic coccobacilli. Culture: the cultivation of *H. ducreyi* requires specialized media. For the

best recovery of this organism the following media formulations are recommended:

- GC agar base with 1% IsoVitaleX (BD Diagnostic Systems, Sparks, MD), 5% fetal bovine serum, 1%–2% hemoglobin, and 3 μg of vancomycin per mL
- Mueller-Hinton agar with 5% lysed horse blood, 1% IsoVitaleX, and 3 μg of vancomycin per mL
- Columbia agar base with 1% hemoglobin, activated charcoal, 5% fetal calf serum (optional), 1% IsoVitaleX (BD Diagnostic Systems), and 3 μg of vancomycin per mL
- GC agar base with 5% Fildes enrichment, 5% horse blood, and 3 μg of vancomycin per mL
- 5% fresh rabbit blood agar with 3 μg of vancomycin per mL

Growth on these media is strain dependent, so it is recommended that at least 2 different selective media be utilized. In addition, the use of nonselective media is advisable as some strains of *H. ducreyi* can be inhibited by vancomycin.

*H. ducreyi* cultures should be incubated at 33°C in 5% $CO_2$ (exceeding an incubation temperature of 35°C may inhibit growth) and examined for growth after at least 48 hours. Plates with no growth should be held for 5 days. The colonies of *H. ducreyi* are gray, yellow, or tan in color, and the shape of the colony are typically round, entire, and convex. Colonies will slide across the plate when pushed and are difficult to pick up. Note that *H. ducreyi* grown in broth forms tight small clumps, in contrast to other *Haemophilus* spp., which form a homogenous layer in the broth. The addition of 0.002% Tween 80 may aid in dispersion of the *H. ducreyi*. Definitive identification is based on the Gram stain and appropriate biochemical reactions (i.e., catalase, oxidase, indole, 6-aminolaevulinic acid, growth on MacConkey agar, and sodium polyanetholesulfonate). The laboratory identification of *H. ducreyi* can also be made using manual identification systems such as the RapID NH (Remel, Lenexa, KS) and the RapID ANA (Remel).

2) Molecular detection: the fastidious nature of *H. ducreyi* makes it an ideal candidate for detection using nucleic acid amplification, although at this time there are no FDA-cleared molecular assays available. Investigational PCR assays for *H. ducreyi* have shown sensitivities at around 95%.

**9. Reporting requirements**—A chancroid case is typically a health care reportable disease in most countries. Case classification is usually defined as either confirmed or probable. A case is considered "confirmed" if proven by laboratory testing. A case is "probable" if the individual has 1 or more painful genital ulcers, laboratory testing excludes *Treponema pallidum* infection by darkfield examination of ulcer exudate or by serologic test for syphilis performed at least 7 days after onset of ulcers, and either the clinical presentation of ulcer(s) is not typical disease caused by herpes simplex virus (HSV) or HSV culture is negative.

Empiric treatment of high-risk groups, including sex workers, contacts to sex workers, and patients with genital ulcers, may be required to control outbreaks. Periodic presumptive treatment of sex workers and their clients has resulted in reduced incidence in some settings.

**10. Referral network**—None.

**11. Special Considerations**—None.

## References

1. Houinei W, Godornes C, Kapa A, et al. *Haemophilus ducreyi* DNA is detectable on the skin of asymptomatic children, flies and fomites in villages of Papua New Guinea. *PLoS Negl Trop Dis*. 2017;11(5):e0004958.
2. Dangor Y, Radebe F, Ballard RC. Transport media for *Haemophilus ducreyi*. *Sex Transm Dis*. 1993;20(1):5–9.

[A. B. Mochon]

# CHLAMYDIAL INFECTIONS

| DISEASE | ICD-10 CODE |
|---|---|
| CHLAMYDIAL DISEASE, SEXUALLY TRANSMITTED | ICD-10 A56 |
| NONSPECIFIC URETHRITIS | ICD-10 N34.1 |
| Conjunctivitis (see "Conjunctivitis/Keratitis") | |
| Lymphogranuloma venereum (see "Lymphogranuloma Venereum") | |
| Pneumonia due to *Chlamydia pneumonia* (see "Pneumonia") | |
| Pneumonia due to *Chlamydia trachomatis* (see "Pneumonia") | |
| Psittacosis (see "Psittacosis") | |

**1. Clinical features**—Most chlamydial infections are asymptomatic. Symptomatic infections are difficult to distinguish clinically from gonorrhea and manifest in males primarily as urethritis (moderate or scanty mucopurulent discharge, dysuria, urethral itching), and in females as cervicitis (mucopurulent endocervical discharge, cervical friability). Rectal infections (asymptomatic or with symptoms of proctitis) can be acquired through receptive anal intercourse, or possibly via contiguous spread from the vagina. Less common manifestations of chlamydial infections include epididymitis in males; urethral syndrome (dysuria and pyuria), periphepatitis (Fitz-Hugh-Curtis syndrome), and bartholinitis in females; and conjunctivitis (acquired through contact with infected genital secretions) in either sex.

In women, untreated infection can ascend from the cervix to the uterus, fallopian tubes, and ovaries, causing pelvic inflammatory disease (PID), which may be asymptomatic (i.e., subclinical) or acute, with abdominal and pelvic pain, and adenexal, uterine, and cervical motion tenderness. Both subclinical and acute PID can lead to long-term sequelae of chronic pelvic pain, ectopic pregnancy, and infertility. Infection during pregnancy has been associated with preterm delivery and can result in conjunctival and pneumonic infection of the newborn.

Chlamydial infection has been associated with an increased risk of human immunodeficiency virus acquisition. Reactive arthritis occurs as a sequel in a minority of chlamydial infections.

**2. Causative agents**—*Chlamydia trachomatis* serovars B and D through K are responsible for sexually acquired genital infections in the adult and perinatally transmitted infections of the neonate and infant. While *C. trachomatis* is the most frequently isolated causal agent of nongonococcal urethritis (NGU) in men (isolated 15%–40% of cases), other agents have been implicated. These include *Mycoplasma genitalium* (15%–25% of nongonococcal urethritis cases in the USA), *Trichomonas vaginalis*, herpes simplex virus, adenovirus, *Ureaplasma urealyticum*, and enteric bacteria.

**3. Laboratory diagnosis**—Culture is technically difficult and not as sensitive as molecular assays. Antigen detection using enzyme immunoassay (EIA) has been shown not to be as sensitive as the molecular assays. Nucleic acid amplification tests (NAATs) offer excellent sensitivity (usually well > 90%) and high specificity. Nucleic acid amplification tests can be used with a variety of specimen types including vaginal (patient and provider-collected), endocervical, urethral, rectal and oropharyngeal swabs, and urine specimens.

**4. Laboratory capability**—Culture isolation and identification requires a microbiology laboratory with an epifluorescent microscope and personnel trained in cell culture and aseptic technique. More stringent environments involving unidirectional workflow from specimen processing to testing and highly skilled technical staff are required for laboratories using open NAATs. By contrast, enclosed NAATs may be performed by personnel with minimal training and in basic environments. Commercially available EIAs can be performed in most laboratory environments, but direct immunofluorescence assays require an epifluorescent microscope. Serological testing can be performed in laboratories proficient in serological analysis but are often limited to research settings due to the lack of commercially available reagents.

No standard procedures exist to assess in vitro susceptibility of *C. trachomatis* to antibiotics.

**5. Safety requirements**—Biosafety level 2 facilities are required for *C. trachomatis* testing. All specimens, microbial cultures, and inoculated products should be considered infectious and handled appropriately. Aseptic technique and universal/standard precautions for handling the bacterial group studied should be observed throughout testing.

**6. Nonhuman hosts**—Humans are the only known reservoir for *C. trachomatis*. Primate animal models have been used to investigate pathogenesis but are limited by the inability to establish chronic infections similar to those observed in humans. Contrived animal models ranging from murine to ovine species investigate naturally occurring chlamydial infections with non-*C. trachomatis* spp. have been useful in describing the pathogenesis of human chlamydial infections.

**7. Sample/specimen requirements**—Specimen collection swabs for *C. trachomatis* culture must have a plastic or wire shaft and either rayon, dacron, or cytobrush tip. Other materials might inhibit isolation. Specimen collection for *C. trachomatis* culture is invasive, requiring insertion of a swab 2–3 cm into the male urethral or 1–2 cm into the endocervical canal followed by 2 or 3 rotations to collect sufficient columnar or cuboidal epithelial cells. Following the collection, culture samples should be stored in an appropriate transport media such as sucrose phosphate glutamate buffer or M4 media and transported at ≤4°C to the laboratory within 24 hours of collection to maximize recovery of viable organisms. If transport is delayed more than 24 hours, the transport media containing the specimen should be stored at -70°C.

Swab and urine specimens can be used to test for *C. trachomatis* by NAATs. Vaginal swabs can be collected by either the patient or heath care provider. More invasive cervical and urethral swabs must be collected by a health care provider. These specimens can be stored frozen or at temperatures up to 25°C for several months prior to testing according to product inserts.

Cervical and urethral swabs can be tested by EIAs. The direct fluorescent antibody (DFA) is the only test currently cleared by the FDA for testing ocular swabs. Specimen material for the DFA is obtained with a swab or endocervical brush, which is then rolled over the specimen well of a slide. After the slide has dried and the fixative applied, the slide can be stored or shipped at ambient temperature. The laboratory should process the slide within 7 days after the specimen has been obtained.

**8. Testing requirements**—NAATs are recommended by CDC for the detection of urogenital, rectal, and oropharyngeal infections caused by *C. trachomatis* infections in women and men with and without symptoms. However, FDA has not cleared NAATs for the detection of *C. trachomatis* infections in the rectum and oropharynx. Laboratories that use NAATs for rectal and oropharyngeal specimens of *C. trachomatis* will need to establish the performance of the assay in accordance to the Clinical Laboratory Improvement Amendments. The sensitivity of NAATs range from 90% to 100% and the specificity exceeds 97% across all specimens and tests. Because NAATs are so sensitive, efforts are warranted to prevent contamination of specimens in the clinic or spread of environmental amplicon in the laboratory. Laboratories should follow standard molecular method techniques, clean workspaces and equipment frequently, include multiple negative controls in each run, and monitor the rate of indeterminate and positive results, as a change in monthly trends might indicate a need to investigate the accuracy of the results. Environmental monitoring might be required as recommended by the manufacturer. If environmental amplicons are found, robust cleaning of the laboratory is needed until negative results are obtained. Steps to prevent cross-contamination include proper testing of laboratory workflow design and strict adherence to testing and quality assurance protocols.

Cell culture specimens should be inoculated by centrifugation onto a confluent monolayer of McCoy, HeLa 229, or Buffalo Green Monkey Kidney cells that support growth of *C. trachomatis*. Once the specimen has been inoculated, 2 μg/mL of cycloheximide should be added to the growth medium to suppress protein synthesis by the host eukaryotic cell. Cultivated cell lines are harvested after 48–72 hours of growth; infected cells develop characteristic intracytoplasmic inclusions that contain substantial numbers of *C. trachomatis* elementary and reticulate bodies. The cell monolayers are reacted with either genus specific or species-specific fluorescein-conjugated monoclonal antibodies to allow specific visualization of the chlamydial inclusions with an epifluorescent microscope. Cell culture detection of *C. trachomatis* is highly specific if a *C. trachomatis* major outer membrane protein (MOMP)-specific stain is used. Monoclonal antibodies directed against the family specific lipopolysaccharide (LPS) of *Chlamydiaceae* cost less but might stain bacteria that share LPS antigens. Lipopolysaccharide stains might be suitable for routine use, but a species-specific (i.e., MOMP) stain is recommended in situations requiring increased specificity. Less specific inclusion-detection methods using iodine or Giemsa are not recommended. *C. trachomatis* EIA tests detect chlamydial LPS, and there is the potential for false-positive results caused by cross-reaction with LPS of other microorganisms. The sensitivity and specificity of EIAs is approximately 60%–70%. Depending on the commercial product used, the antigen that is detected by the antibody in the *C. trachomatis* DFA procedure is either the MOMP or LPS molecule. Staining consists of flooding the smear with fluorescein-labeled monoclonal antibody that binds to *C. trachomatis* elementary bodies. Stained elementary bodies are then identified by fluorescence microscopy. Only *C. trachomatis* organisms will stain with the anti-MOMP antibodies used in commercial kits. The anti-LPS monoclonal antibodies will react with family specific epitopes found within the LPS of *Chlamydiaceae* and might cross-react with LPS of other bacteria. The procedure requires an experience microscopist and is labor-intensive and time-consuming.

**9. Reporting requirements**—Results should be reported based on bacterial identification or NAATs. Chlamydial infections are required to be reported to the public health authorities in many states/provinces and countries. Laboratories must determine their obligation to report.

**10. Referral network**—No specific referral networks exist.

**11. Special considerations**—NAATs have not been cleared by the FDA for the detection of rectal and oropharyngeal infections caused by *C. trachomatis*. Laboratories must establish performance specifications to meet federal, state, and local regulatory requirements prior to reporting results for patient management.

[J. R. Papp]

# CHOLERA AND OTHER VIBRIOSES

| DISEASE | CAUSATIVE AGENT | ICD-10 CODE |
|---|---|---|
| CHOLERA | Toxigenic *Vibrio cholerae* serogroups O1 and O139 | ICD-10 A00 |
| *VIBRIO PARAHAEMOLYTICUS* INFECTION | *Vibrio parahaemolyticus* | ICD-10 A05.3 |
| *VIBRIO VULNIFICUS* INFECTION | *Vibrio vulnificus* | ICD-10 A05.3 |
| OTHER *VIBRIO* INFECTIONS | Other non-01 and -0139 serogroups of *Vibrio cholerae*, *Vibrio mimicus*, *Vibrio alginolyticus*, and others | ICD-10 A05.81 |

Of the more than 200 recognized *Vibrio cholerae* serogroups, only cholera toxin-producing O1 and O139 serogroups have caused large epidemics and are defined as causing cholera.

Infection with other *Vibrio* spp. has been associated with sporadic diarrhea and rare outbreaks, as well as with wound and septicemic infections. These include *Vibrio parahaemolyticus*, *Vibrio vulnificus*, and other vibrios such as *V. cholerae* of serogroups other than O1 and O139 (*Vibrio mimicus, Vibrio alginolyticus, Vibrio fluvialis, Vibrio furnissii*) and *Grimontia hollisae*. The main *Vibrio* diseases are profiled later.

# I. CHOLERA

**1. Clinical features**—An acute bacterial enteric disease characterized in its severe form by sudden-onset, profuse, painless watery stools. Massive loss of fluids is caused by release of an enterotoxin that affects the small intestine. Nausea and profuse vomiting occur early in the course of illness. In most cases, infection is asymptomatic or causes mild diarrhea, especially with organisms of the El Tor biotype; asymptomatically infected persons can transmit the infection.

In untreated severe disease, rapid dehydration, acidosis, circulatory collapse, hypoglycemia in children, and renal failure can lead rapidly to death. In severely dehydrated cases (cholera gravis), death may occur within a few hours, and the case-fatality rate may reach 50%. With proper and timely rehydration, case-fatality rates should be less than 1%.

**2. Causative agents**—Toxigenic *V. cholerae* serogroups O1 and O139. Serogroup O1 occurs as 2 biotypes—classical and El Tor—each of which occurs as 3 serotypes (Inaba, Ogawa, and, rarely, Hikojima). The clinical illnesses caused by *V. cholerae* O1 and O139 are alike because these 2 serogroups produce similar enterotoxins; however, infections caused by serogroup O1 of the classical biotype are associated with more severe disease, although these strains are not currently circulating. In recent years, an El Tor variant that has characteristics of both the classical and El Tor biotypes and may be more virulent than older El Tor strains has emerged in Asia and spread to Africa and the Caribbean.

In any single epidemic, one particular serogroup and biotype tends to be dominant, but serotype switching (e.g., from Inaba to Ogawa or Ogawa to Inaba) is commonly seen in cholera epidemics worldwide and is thought to be driven primarily by the development of population immunity to the circulating serotype.

**3. Laboratory diagnosis**—The etiology is confirmed by isolation of *V. cholerae* serogroups O1 or O139 from a stool specimen. Ideally, serogroup O139 isolates and all *V. cholerae* isolates from sporadic illness should be tested for cholera toxin production or cholera toxin gene sequences (*ctxA*). Strains of *V. cholerae* O1 or O139 that do not possess the cholera toxin gene can cause acute watery diarrhea but do not cause cholera or epidemic disease. In nonendemic areas, organisms isolated from initial suspected cases should be confirmed in a reference laboratory.

For clinical purposes, a quick presumptive diagnosis can be made by dark-field or phase microscopic visualization of vibrios in stool moving like "shooting stars," inhibited by preservative-free, serotype-specific antiserum. When acute and convalescent serum specimens are collected, a presumptive diagnosis can be based on the demonstration of a significant rise in titer of anticholera toxin or vibriocidal antibodies. One-step dipstick tests for rapid antigen detection of *V. cholerae* O1 and O139 are available and have shown promise in initial field evaluations; however, these tests do not yield isolates for subtyping or antimicrobial resistance testing that may be useful for some epidemiologic and treatment decisions and are not recommended for individual patient diagnosis.

In epidemics, once laboratory confirmation and antibiotic susceptibility have been established, it is unnecessary to confirm all subsequent cases. A shift should then be made to primary use of proposed WHO clinical case definitions for cholera surveillance as follows:

1) Disease unknown in area: severe dehydration or death from acute watery diarrhea in a patient aged 5 years or older.
2) Endemic cholera: acute watery diarrhea with or without vomiting in a patient aged 5 years or older.
3) Epidemic cholera: acute watery diarrhea with or without vomiting in any patient.

Prolonged outbreaks should include periodic laboratory confirmation and antimicrobial susceptibility testing of a small proportion of cases to monitor for antimicrobial resistance.

**4. Laboratory capability**—A contained, purpose-built, microbiological facility is required to handle this pathogen with the capacity to autoclave microbiological waste. Staff should be trained and shown to be competent to handle potentially hazardous biological agents and should be able to carry out molecular and basic phenotypic techniques.

**5. Safety requirements**—Employers have a responsibility to protect their workers from the risks related to exposure to hazardous biological agents.[1] *V. cholerae* is a hazard group 2 bacterium and should be handled within a biosafety level 2 laboratory. *V. cholerae* transmission is via the fecal-oral route but can also enter the body via wounds. Therefore, gloves should be worn when handling fecal samples, and the importance of good hand washing techniques must be emphasized to laboratory staff. In addition to gloves, other personal protective equipment should be worn, including a laboratory coat and laboratory safety glasses. Finally, it is recommended to use a class I or class II microbiological safety cabinet when handling this pathogen, particularly where there is a risk of aerosol production.

**6. Nonhuman hosts**—Transmission is through the fecal-oral route and a person can get cholera by drinking water or eating food contaminated with *V. cholerae* bacterium. There are no known animal hosts for *V. cholera*, and brackish and marine waters are the natural environment. The disease is occasionally spread through eating raw or undercooked shellfish that are naturally contaminated, but large epidemics are often related to fecal contamination of water supplies or street vended foods.

**7. Sample/specimen requirements—**A stool sample is the sample of choice, and ideally a diarrheal stool sample should be collected within the first few days of a patient becoming symptomatic. In resourced limited countries with few testing facilities and poor transport and storage facilities, rectal swabs can be used and ideally tested within a few days of becoming symptomatic. Bacterial recovery will be improved if samples are taken before any antibiotic treatment is given. Stool/swab samples should be placed into appropriate sterile containers labeled with patient details (to ensure sample integrity). UN regulations stipulate that samples should be kept in appropriate stool containers to prevent leaking and transported according to the UN Transport of Infectious Substances Regulations.[2]

**8. Testing requirements—***V. cholerae* infections in the field are currently diagnosed by rapid diagnostic tests such as dipstick in feces. The rapid diagnostic test Crystal VC (Span Diagnostics, Surat, India) is widely used during outbreaks and detects lipopolysaccharide antigens of *V. cholerae* O1 and O139.[3] Laboratory diagnosis involves culturing *V. cholerae* from fecal specimens and confirming epidemic strains with biochemistry and serology.[4] Alternatively, polymerase chain reaction (PCR) of deoxyribonucleic acid (DNA) from fecal samples and/or culture targeting the toxin (*ctxA, ctxB*), transcriptional factors that regulate expression of virulence factors (*toxR*), El Tor biotype (*tcpA* El Tor), and classical biotype (*tcpA* classical) or serogroup specific O1 (*wbe*/O1*rfb*) and O139 (*wbe*/O139*rfb*) genes can be used but have not been widely up taken in the frontline laboratories.

Testing facilities must adhere to the quality standards set by their accreditation body, and diagnostic laboratories must follow the manufacturer's instructions for any assay being performed. Once a sample has arrived at the testing facility, patient identifiers on the request form and the sample should be checked. Ideally, samples will be tested on arrival. If this is not possible, fecal/swab samples can be stored at refrigerated temperatures (between 4°C–8°C) to prevent overgrowing of other organisms. Whichever method is used, full characterization of *V. cholerae* is essential to ensure robust public health surveillance and typing is carried out. There are basic cholera tests available that can be carried out in countries with limited resources.[4] The stages of testing are as follows:

1) Screening and diagnostic: testing should be carried out using rapid diagnostic test kits or PCR of toxigenic *V. cholerae* genes in fecal DNA extracts.
2) Presumptive: cases can be identified by the detection of *V. cholerae* genes in fecal DNA extracts.
3) Confirmation: isolation of *V. cholerae* by culture using selective agar plates such as thiosulfate citrate bile-salt sucrose (TCBS) agar and confirmation of identification (serotype and biotype) with biochemistry, serology, and/or PCR of *V. cholerae* genes.

**9. Reporting requirements**—*V. cholerae* is a notifiable organism and reporting varies from country to country as does the likelihood of testing. Some countries will test all diarrheal stool samples from the community setting, whereas other countries will only test stool samples from patients during cholera outbreaks. This disparity in international testing practices therefore affects the level of cholera reporting. Significant outbreaks of cholera should be reported on international platforms, such as the Epidemic Intelligence Information System–Food and Waterborne Diseases and Zoonoses (EPIS-FWD) platform to assess whether current and emerging public health threats have a potential impact in the EU, in registered countries such as the USA, and on organizations such as CDC and WHO.

**10. Referral network**—The increased interest in the use of rapid diagnostic test kits in resourced limited countries has markedly improved the diagnosis of cholera particularly in outbreak settings. These nonculture methods are useful for diagnosing but currently should not fully replace culture-based methods as a pure isolate is still needed for *V. cholerae* characterization allowing surveillance and public health management of outbreaks. Isolates are referred to reference laboratories to confirm O1 or O139 strains associated with toxin production and epidemic strains. There are limited subtyping methods available and restricted to mainly serotyping and biotyping. There are now multilocus sequence typing (MLST) schemes available and whole genome sequencing where facilities are available.

**11. Special considerations**—Due to the potential severity of the disease, local public health services should be notified rapidly of all cholera cases to allow identification of sources and to apply appropriate preventative measures to control the spread of this infection. Case reporting of *V. cholerae* infection is obligatory in many countries. Hygiene advice should be given to infected individuals, family members, and any institutions involved with patients to prevent person-to-person spread, with a particular emphasis on frequent hand washing (particularly post-defecation) with soap and water, disposal of diapers, human waste, and prevention of contamination of food and drink. During acute illness, enteric precautions must be enforced, and symptomatic cholera cases should be excluded from work until they are symptom free for 48 hours. Education of the community during outbreaks should be encouraged, and eating raw fruits, vegetables, street raw or undercooked seafood, food from street vendors, and drinking water from contaminated areas should be highlighted as potential risk factors. General preventative and control measures include the following:

1) Provision of safe water, proper sanitation, and food safety, all critical for preventing occurrence of cholera.
2) Health education aimed at communities adopting preventive behavior for averting contamination.
3) Proper and timely case management in cholera treatment centers.

4) Specific training for proper case management, including avoidance of nosocomial infections.
5) Vaccination.

## II. *VIBRIO PARAHAEMOLYTICUS* INFECTION

**1. Clinical features**—An intestinal disorder characterized by watery diarrhea and abdominal cramps in most cases, often with nausea, vomiting, and headache. About one-quarter of patients experience a dysentery-like illness with bloody or mucoid stools. Wound infections can also occur. Typically, it is a disease of moderate severity lasting 1–7 days; systemic infection and death rarely occur.

**2. Causative agents**—*V. parahaemolyticus* is a natural inhabitant of estuarine and marine environments. Isolates may be subtyped into O and K serotypes. Over 30 different O:K serotypes are found in the USA, but O3:K6, O4:K12, and O6:K18 have been identified from recent outbreaks. Clinical isolates from humans are generally (but not always) capable of producing a characteristic hemolytic reaction (Kanagawa phenomenon) and carriage of 2 hemolysin genes correlate with diarrheal disease. Over 90% of isolates from ill persons carry one or both of these genes compared with less than 1% of isolates from food or environmental sources.

**3. Laboratory diagnosis**—By isolation of *V. parahaemolyticus* from stool, blood, or other clinical specimen. No serodiagnostic or rapid tests have been developed.

**4. Laboratory capability**—A contained, purpose-built, microbiological facility is required to handle this pathogen with the capacity to autoclave microbiological waste. Staff should be trained and shown to be competent to handle potentially hazardous biological agents and should be able to carry out molecular and basic phenotypic techniques.

**5. Safety requirements**—Employers have a responsibility to protect their workers from the risks related to exposure to hazardous biological agents.[1] *V. parahaemolyticus* is a hazard group 2 bacterium and should be handled within a biosafety level 2 laboratory. *V. parahaemolyticus* transmission is via the fecal-oral route but can also enter the body via wounds, and therefore gloves should be worn when handling fecal samples, and the importance of good hand washing techniques must be emphasized to laboratory staff. In addition to gloves, other personal protective equipment should be worn, including a laboratory coat and laboratory safety glasses. Finally, it is recommended to use a class I or class II microbiological safety cabinet when handling this pathogen, particularly where there is a risk of aerosol production.

**6. Nonhuman hosts**—*V. parahaemolyticus* naturally occurs in warm coastal areas and can also be found in fish and shellfish. During the summer months, the bacteria can be found free floating in coastal waters (and therefore can infect open wounds). During the cooler months, the organism is commonly found in silt or mud on the bottom of marine environments.

**7. Sample/specimen requirements**—A stool sample is the sample of choice, and ideally a diarrheal stool sample should be collected within the first few days of a patient becoming symptomatic. In resourced limited countries with few testing facilities, poor transport, and lack of storage facilities, rectal swabs can be used and ideally tested within a few days of becoming symptomatic. Bacterial recovery will be improved if samples are taken before any antibiotic treatment is given. Stool/swab samples should be placed into appropriate sterile containers labeled with patient details (to ensure sample integrity). UN regulations stipulate that samples should be kept in appropriate stool containers to prevent leaking and transported according to the UN Transport of Infectious Substances Regulations.[2]

**8. Testing requirements**—Testing facilities must adhere to the quality standards set by their accreditation body, and diagnostic laboratories must follow the manufacturer's instructions for any assay being performed. Once a sample has arrived at the testing facility, patient identifiers on the request form and the sample should be checked. Ideally samples will be tested on arrival. If this is not possible, fecal/swab samples can be stored at refrigerated temperatures (between 4°C–8°C) to prevent overgrowing of other organisms. Whichever method is used, accurate identification of *V. parahaemolyticus* is essential to ensure robust public health surveillance and typing is carried out. Only culture-based methods are commonly used, and therefore screening, diagnostic, and confirmation testing involves the isolation of *V. parahaemolyticus* by culture using selective agar plates such as TCBS and confirmation of identification with biochemistry tests.

**9. Reporting requirements**—*V. parahaemolyticus* is a notifiable disease, and reporting varies from country to country, as does the likelihood of testing. Some countries will test all diarrheal stool samples from the community setting, whereas other countries will only test stool samples from patients during outbreaks. This disparity in international testing practices therefore affects the level of *V. parahaemolyticus* reporting. Significant outbreaks of *V. parahaemolyticus* should be reported on international platforms, such as the EPIS-FWD platform, to assess whether current and emerging public health threats have a potential impact in the EU, in registered countries such as the USA, and on organizations such as CDC and WHO.

**10. Referral network**—Isolates are referred to reference laboratories to confirm identification. There are limited subtyping methods available including MLST schemes and whole genome sequencing where facilities are available.

**11. Special considerations**—Case reporting to local health authorities is recommended. Effective prevention measures include refrigerating raw seafood within 8 hours of marine acquisition, hand washing with soap and water after handling raw shellfish, and thoroughly cooking seafood before consumption. Avoiding open-wound (burns, fresh piercings, fresh tattoos, and cuts) contact with warm saltwater is also recommended.

## III. INFECTION WITH *VIBRIO VULNIFICUS*

**1. Clinical features**—Typically produces septicemia in persons with chronic liver disease, chronic alcoholism, hemochromatosis, or immunocompromising conditions. Intestinal infection rarely occurs. Fever, chills, hypotension, and distinctive bullous skin lesions that progress to necrotic ulcers are common. About 50% of patients with septicemia die. *Vibrio vulnificus* can also cause wound infection when preexisting or new skin lesions are exposed to sea or brackish water or to sea life; these infections range from mild, self-limited lesions to rapidly progressive cellulitis, myositis, and septicemia. Others can be infected and can develop gastroenteritis but do not usually present with septicemia.

**2. Causative agents**—*V. vulnificus* is halophilic and is commonly found in marine environments. Three biogroups have been identified. Biogroup 1 is an opportunistic human pathogen usually associated with the consumption of raw oysters, although wound infections can occur after trauma and exposure to a contaminated marine environment. Biogroup 2 strains are rarely found outside of Europe and are isolated predominantly from diseased eels, but they are occasionally isolated from human septicemia and wound infections acquired from handling eels. Biogroup 3 has been isolated only from Israeli patients with wound infections and bacteremia. These cases are associated with exposure to live fish (tilapia and carp) grown in aquaculture environments.

**3. Laboratory diagnosis**—*V. vulnificus* infection is usually diagnosed by isolation of the organism from blood or a wound usually on blood agar. No serodiagnostic or rapid tests have been developed.

**4. Laboratory capability**—A contained, purpose-built, microbiological facility is required to handle this pathogen with the capacity to autoclave microbiological waste. Staff should be trained and shown to be competent to handle potentially hazardous biological agents and should be able to carry out molecular and basic phenotypic techniques.

**5. Safety requirements**—Employers have a responsibility to protect their workers from the risks related to exposure to hazardous biological agents.[1] *V. vulnificus* is a hazard group 2 bacterium and should be handled within a biosafety level 2 laboratory. *V. vulnificus* transmission is via the fecal-oral route but can also enter the body via wounds, and therefore gloves should be worn when handling fecal samples, and the importance of good hand washing techniques must be emphasized to laboratory staff. In addition to gloves, other personal protective equipment should be worn, including a laboratory coat and laboratory safety glasses. Finally, it is recommended to use a class I or class II microbiological safety cabinet when handling this pathogen, particularly where there is a risk of aerosol production.

**6. Nonhuman hosts**—*V. vulnificus* inhabits brackish and salt water and naturally occurs in warm coastal areas and can also be found in fish and shellfish. During the summer months, the bacteria can be found free floating in coastal waters (and therefore can infect open wounds).

**7. Sample/specimen requirements**—A stool sample is the sample of choice and ideally a diarrheal stool sample should be collected within the first few days of a patient becoming symptomatic. In resourced limited countries with few testing facilities, poor transport, and lack of storage facilities, rectal swabs can be used and ideally tested within a few days of becoming symptomatic. Bacterial recovery will be improved if samples are taken before any antibiotic treatment is given. Stool/swab samples should be placed into appropriate sterile containers labeled with patient details (to ensure sample integrity). UN regulations stipulate that samples should be kept in appropriate stool containers to prevent leaking and transported according to the UN Transport of Infectious Substances Regulations.[2]

**8. Testing requirements**—Testing facilities must adhere to the quality standards set by their accreditation body, and diagnostic laboratories must follow the manufacturer's instructions for any assay being performed. Once a sample has arrived at the testing facility, patient identifiers on the request form and the sample should be checked. Ideally samples will be tested on arrival; however, if this is not possible, fecal/swab samples can be stored at refrigerated temperatures (between 4°C–8°C) to prevent overgrowing of other organisms. Whichever method is accurate, identification of *V. vulnificus* is essential to ensure robust public health surveillance and typing is carried out. Isolation of *V. vulnificus* is by culture using selective agar plates such as TCBS and confirmation of identification with biochemistry tests. Though biotyping and genotyping methods are available,[5] these are not routinely used in testing laboratories for surveillance.

**9. Reporting requirements**—*V. vulnificus* is a notifiable disease and reporting varies from country to country as does the likelihood of testing. Some countries will test all diarrheal stool samples from the community setting, whereas other countries will only test stool samples from patients during outbreaks. This disparity in international testing practices therefore affects the level of *V. vulnificus* reporting. Significant outbreaks of *V. vulnificus* should be reported on international platforms, such as the EPIS-FWD platform, to assess whether current and emerging public health threats have a potential impact in the EU, in registered countries such as the USA, and on organizations such as CDC and WHO.

**10. Referral network**—Isolates are referred to reference laboratories to confirm identification. There are limited sub-typing methods available including MLST schemes and whole genome sequencing where facilities are available.

**11. Special considerations**—Case reporting to local health authorities is recommended. Effective prevention measures include refrigerating raw seafood within 8 hours of marine acquisition, washing hands with soap and water after handling raw shellfish, and thoroughly cooking seafood before consumption. Avoiding open-wound (burns, fresh piercing, fresh tattoos, and cuts) contact with warm saltwater is also recommended.

## IV. INFECTION DUE TO OTHER *VIBRIOS*

**1. Clinical features**—Infection with vibrios other than those discussed earlier causes a range of clinical syndromes. *V. cholerae* of serogroups other than O1 and O139, as well as *V. mimicus*, nontoxigenic *V. cholerae* O1, and others, cause gastroenteritis that ranges from mild to severe, but they have not caused large epidemics. *V. alginolyticus* causes otitis externa, otitis media, and cellulitis. Other less commonly identified vibrios cause wound and septicemic illnesses.

**2. Causative agents**—Isolates of *V. cholerae* O1 and O139 that do not produce cholera toxin are known to occur, but, as is the case with non-toxigenic non-O1/non-O139 strains, these strains do not cause large cholera epidemics but are usually associated with sporadic diarrheal disease. Isolates of non-O1/non-O139 *V. cholerae* can cause illness because they can possess a variety of virulence factors, sometimes including production of cholera toxin. However, cholera toxin–producing strains of non-O1 *V. cholerae* are rarely encountered. In the USA, toxigenic strains of *V. cholerae* serogroups O75 and O141 are associated with sporadic cholera like illness that is usually attributed to consumption of undercooked seafood; on average fewer than 10 cases a year are detected. Some *V. cholerae* strains that do not agglutinate in O1 or O139 antiserum and produce a heat-stable enterotoxin (ST) are referred to as nonagglutinable-ST strains. Certain other species in the family *Vibrionaceae* can cause human illness, including diarrhea, septicemia, and other extraintestinal infections. These include *V. mimicus, G. hollisae* (formerly *Vibrio hollisae*), *V. furnissii, V. fluvialis, V. alginolyticus*, and *Photobacterium damselae* (formerly *Vibrio damsela*). Some strains of *V. mimicus* produce cholera toxin and have been associated with outbreaks of severe watery diarrhea. Most septicemic infections occur in immunocompromised individuals or persons with underlying liver disease.

**3. Laboratory diagnosis**—Diagnosis is by isolation of the organism from clinical specimens. No serodiagnostic or rapid tests have been developed.

**4. Laboratory capability**—A contained, purpose-built, microbiological facility is required to handle this pathogen with the capacity to autoclave microbiological waste. Staff should be trained and shown to be competent to handle potentially hazardous biological agents and should be able to carry out molecular and basic phenotypic techniques.

**5. Safety requirements**—Employers have a responsibility to protect their workers from the risks related to exposure to hazardous biological agents.[1] *Vibrio* spp. are hazard group 2 bacteria and should be handled within a biosafety level 2 laboratory. *Vibrio* spp. transmission is via the fecal-oral route but can also enter the body via wounds, and therefore gloves should be worn when handling fecal samples, and the importance of good hand washing techniques must be emphasized to laboratory staff. In addition to gloves, other personal protective equipment should be worn, including a laboratory coat and laboratory safety glasses. Finally, it is recommended to use a class I or class II microbiological safety cabinet when handling this pathogen, particularly where there is a risk of aerosol production.

**6. Nonhuman hosts**—*Vibrio* spp. inhabit brackish and salt water and naturally occur in warm coastal areas. They can also be found in fish and shellfish as well as chitinous zooplankton.

**7. Sample/specimen requirements**—A stool sample is the sample of choice and ideally a diarrheal stool sample should be collected within the first few days of a patient becoming symptomatic. In resourced limited countries with few testing facilities and poor transport and storage facilities, rectal swabs can be used and ideally tested within a few days of becoming symptomatic. Bacterial recovery will be improved if samples are taken before any antibiotic treatment is given. Stool/swab samples should be placed into appropriate sterile containers labeled with patient details (to ensure sample integrity). UN regulations stipulate that samples should be kept in appropriate stool containers to prevent leaking and transported according to the UN Transport of Infectious Substances Regulations.[2]

**8. Testing requirements**—Testing facilities must adhere to the quality standards set by their accreditation body, and diagnostic laboratories must follow the manufacturer's instructions for any assay being performed. Once a sample has arrived at the testing facility, patient identifiers on the request form and the sample should be checked. Ideally samples will be tested on arrival; however, if this is not possible, fecal/swab samples can be stored at refrigerated temperatures (between 4°C–8°C) to prevent overgrowing of other organisms. Whichever method is used, accurate identification of *Vibrio* spp. is essential to ensure robust public health surveillance and typing is carried out. Isolation of *Vibrio* spp. is by culture using selective agar plates such as TCBS and confirmation of identification with biochemistry tests.

**9. Reporting requirements**—Vibriosis is a notifiable disease and reporting varies from country to country as does the likelihood of testing. Note that non-O1 or non-O139 *V. cholerae* strains should not be reported as cholera but as vibriosis. Some countries will test all diarrheal stool samples from the community setting, whereas other countries will only test stool samples from patients during outbreaks. This disparity in international testing practices therefore affects the level of vibriosis reporting. Significant outbreaks of vibriosis should be reported on international platforms. These include the EPIS-FWD platform, to assess whether current and emerging public health threats have a potential impact in the EU, in registered countries such as the USA, and on organizations such as CDC and WHO.

**10. Referral network**—Isolates are referred to reference laboratories to confirm identification. There are limited subtyping methods available including MLST schemes and whole genome sequencing where facilities are available.

**11. Special considerations**—Case reporting to local health authorities is recommended. Effective prevention measures include refrigerating raw seafood within 8 hours of marine acquisition, washing hands with soap and water after handling raw shellfish, and thoroughly cooking seafood before consumption. Avoiding open-wound (burns, fresh piercings, fresh tattoos, and cuts) contact with warm saltwater is also recommended.

## References

1. EUR-Lex. Directive 2000/54/EC of the European Parliament and of the Council of 18 September 2000. Available at: https://eur-lex.europa.eu/legal-content/EN/ALL/?uri=CELEX%3A32000L0054. Accessed February 15, 2019.
2. United Nations Economic Commission for Europe. UN Recommendations on the Transport of Dangerous Goods. Available at: http://www.unece.org/trans/danger/publi/unrec/rev18/18files_e.htm. Accessed March 19, 2019.
3. Martinez-Pino I, Luquero FJ, Sakoba K, et al. Use of a cholera rapid diagnostic test during a mass vaccination campaign in response to an epidemic in Guinea, 2012. *PLoS Negl Trop Dis*. 2013;7(8):e2366.
4. Chattaway MA, Kamara A, Rhodes F, et al. Establishing an enteric bacteria reference laboratory in Sierra Leone. *J Infect Dev Ctries*. 2014;8(7):933-941.
5. Jones MK, Oliver JD. Vibrio vulnificus: disease and pathogenesis. *Infect Immun.* 2009;77(5):1723-1733.

[M. A. Chattaway]

# CHROMOMYCOSIS
(dermatitis verrucosa)

| DISEASE | ICD-10 CODE |
|---|---|
| CHROMOMYCOSIS | ICD-10 B43 |

**1. Clinical features**—A chronic spreading mycosis of the skin and subcutaneous tissues, usually of the lower extremities, although other areas can be involved. The initial lesion appears as a papule or a nodule. Progression to the contiguous tissues is slow, over a period of years, with eventual large, nodular, verrucous, or even cauliflower-like masses. Invasion to muscle or bone can occur, although disseminated disease is rare. Rarely is a cause of death.

**2. Causative agents**—Dematiaceous fungi, including *Fonsecaea (Phialophora) pedrosoi, Phialophora verrucosa, Cladophialophora carrionii, Rhinocladiella aquaspersa, Botryomyces caespitatus, Exophiala spinifera*, and *Exophiala jeanselmei*.

**3. Laboratory diagnosis**—Microscopic examination of the scrapings or biopsies from lesions shows characteristic muriform cells, large, brown, thick-walled rounded cells that divide by fission into 2 planes. Confirmation of diagnosis should be made by biopsy and attempted cultures of the fungus.

**4. Laboratory capability**—Laboratories with mycology testing capability are the most appropriate for receipt and testing of specimens. Laboratories that do not have mycology testing capability should refer all specimens and testing requests to their respective reference laboratory.

**5. Safety requirements**—These agents should be handled in a class II biological safety cabinet under at least biosafety level 2 conditions.

**6. Nonhuman hosts**—The fungus is found in soils and plant materials in the tropical and subtropical regions of the world.

**7. Sample/specimen requirements**—Most commonly specimens come from proliferation of skin layers at infected wound sites. The limbs are areas of particular interest due to the high likelihood of lesion development and because they often show presence of secondary infections. Brain, sinus/nasal cavity, skin, and tissue are all possible sources for specimen submission. Specimens should be collected in sterile, leak-proof containers and transported to the testing laboratory as soon as possible.

**8. Testing requirements**—*F. pedrosoi*, *P. verrucosa*, and *C. carrionii* account for the majority of chromomycosis cases. There are several stains which may assist in visualizing the morphologic characteristics of the organisms, such as calcofluor white, Giemsa, Wright, Gram, periodic acid-Schiff, or hematoxylin and eosin. A hallmark found in wet preparation is the presence of muriform cells as indicated by thick-walled cells which can develop a septum. Cultures may be proliferated on potato dextrose agar or cornmeal dextrose agar to detect enhanced conidiation. Under microscopic examination, *F. pedrosoi* conidiophores are septate and sympodial. Elongated conidiophores may form into an asterisk-like shape. No budding cells are routinely found on the routine media utilized. The cultures are slow growing at 14 days maturation with a downy brownish-black surface and brownish-black reverse. *P. verrucosa* phialides are vase-like with collarettes with little or no conidiation (i.e., appears as a vase of flowers). The culture is slow growing with 14 days to maturation with dark green-brownish with a reverse black color. Some strains may be heaped and granular while others are flat. *C. carrionii* is a slow grower with a maturation of 21 days with a velvety brownish-black surface and brownish-black reverse. The conidiophores are brown, fragile chains that have a black scar present at the points of attachment.

**9. Reporting requirements**—Diagnosis is difficult since the etiological agents of chromomycosis are not well known to most clinicians or laboratorians. The recovery of an etiological agent, especially those repeatedly recovered from multiple specimens or recovered from a normally sterile site, should be considered significant. A correlation between culture and histopathology may be important for diagnosis. Public health authorities may require notification of potential or confirmed cases; check with state/provincial authorities for requirements.

**10. Referral network**—When assistance with testing is required, reference laboratories may be contacted. If shipping of specimens is required, then all applicable International Air Transport Association dangerous goods regulations should be followed.

**11. Special considerations**—When assessing clinical features, it should be noted that lesions generally appear on the arms, legs, feet, and upper trunk of patients, which may lead to secondary infections of these areas. In some texts chromomycosis is also referred to as chromoblastomycosis.

[M. Soehnlen]

# COCCIDIOIDOMYCOSIS

(valley fever, San Joaquin fever, desert fever, desert rheumatism, coccidioidal granuloma)

| DISEASE | ICD-10 CODE |
|---|---|
| COCCIDIOIDOMYCOSIS | ICD-10 B38 |

**1. Clinical features**—The primary infection may be entirely asymptomatic or may resemble an acute influenza-like illness with fever, chills, cough, rash, and (rarely) pleuritic pain. About 1 in 5 clinically recognized cases (an estimated 5% of all primary infections) develop erythema nodosum. Primary infection may heal completely without detectable sequelae; may leave fibrosis, a pulmonary nodule that may or may not have calcified areas;

may leave a persistent thin-walled cavity; or, most rarely, may progress to the disseminated form of the disease.

Less than 1% of symptomatic coccidioidomycosis becomes disseminated. Disseminated coccidioidomycosis is a progressive, severe granulomatous disease characterized by lesions in nearly any part of the body, especially in subcutaneous tissues, skin, bone, and meninges. Coccidioidal meningitis can resemble tuberculous meningitis but runs a more chronic course. Disseminated infection is uniformly fatal without treatment.

**2. Causative agents**—*Coccidioides immitis* and *Coccidioides posadasii*. The dimorphic fungus *Coccidioides* contains 2 species, *C. immitis* and *C. posadasii*, delisted from the select agent category in 2012. Although both species are endemic to the new world (i.e., the Southwest USA, as well as portions of Mexico and South America), *C. immitis* seems limited to the West Coast of the USA (i.e., Southern California and recently an area in inland Washington State). *C. posadasii* is found in the other endemic regions, including Arizona. In its saprophytic phase in soil, *Coccidioides* spp. produce septate hyphae with thick-walled arthroconidia (2 × 4 μm) formed along the length of the hyphae and separated by empty, thin-walled cells called disjunctors. These disjunctors allow for the easy release and dissemination of the arthroconidia due to soil disturbance and wind. Upon entry into alveoli or tissue, the arthroconidia transform into multinucleated, spherical structures called spherules, which increase in size (60 > 100 μm in diameter) and form thick outer walls. As they grow, the spherules divide internally through endosporulation, producing numerous (600–1,000) uninucleated endospores of 2–5 μm in size. Upon release from the spherule, the endospore matures into new spherules in the adjacent tissue or, if not contained locally after migration via the lymphatics, matures in other areas of the body.

**3. Laboratory diagnosis**—Diagnosis of coccidioidomycosis is most beneficial in sicker patients who may maximally benefit from therapy. However, other benefits of diagnosis may include avoidance of use of antimicrobial agents, avoidance of corticosteroid use, avoidance of use of added expensive diagnostics, and reducing patient anxiety.

1) Serology: coccidioidomycosis induces 2 main immunological responses in human infections. The first is a cell-mediated immune response that usually provides lasting immunity against further infection and can be measured by Spherusol, a commercially available skin test (Nielsen BioSciences, San Diego, CA). The skin test antigen has been FDA-approved for use in individuals 18–64 years of age. The second is a humoral antibody response that increases if immunity is not initially established and the infection continues to grow. Measurement of antibodies is useful for the diagnosis and prognosis of coccidioidomycosis. The humoral serologic response includes production of (a) early immunoglobulin class M (IgM), or

tube precipitin, antibody, which becomes measurable earlier in the acute phase of infection, usually between the first (50% of cases) and third (90% of cases) weeks of onset; and (b) late IgG or complement fixation (CF) antibody, which becomes measurable between the second and twenty-eighth week post onset. The IgG antibody may remain for several months and is usually related to the level of fungal activity during infection and not to any form of protection. Serologic studies are less sensitive than previously thought (especially in self-limited clinical cases or the immunocompromised patient). Although positive serologies may be helpful in the diagnosis of coccidioidomycosis, negative serologies cannot be used to rule out the disease (especially early in the acute phase).

Three major techniques are now available for measurement of the antibody serologic response to coccidioidomycosis in the clinical laboratory:

- Enzyme immunoassays (EIA) detect both IgM and IgG antibodies separately and are the most sensitive of the methods. Negative results by EIA do not normally have to be confirmed by any of the other methods. However, positive EIA results, especially those for the IgM class of antibody, may be less specific (2%–4% false-positive results). These may be confirmed by the immunodiffusion test. At this time, the EIA test does not provide quantitative data.
- Immunodiffusion (IMDF) detects both IgM and IgG but requires longer incubation periods ($\leq 4$ days) to rule out negatives. Although these test systems are not considered quantitative, they can be modified to quantify titers if a tube or microtiter well CF for IgG is not available.
- Complement fixation (CF) studies for IgG class of antibody may be useful in the diagnosis of more severe forms of coccidioidomycosis but should normally be limited to the evaluation of fungal activity and the prognosis of the disease in severe cases. Increasing CF titers in sequentially collected serum specimens suggest dissemination of the infection; decreasing titers indicate the amelioration of the infection. Variability in commercially available reagents used in CF tests can result in very different results from different laboratories, and test results from different laboratories should not be compared. The CF test is not as sensitive as the EIA or IMDF tests. It should not be used alone for the diagnosis of milder forms of the disease or in its early acute stages. At this time, the CF test is a primary serologic test for the diagnosis of meningeal coccidioidomycosis. However, recent data on the *Coccidioides* antigen test (MiraVista Diagnostics,

Indianapolis, IN) indicate it may be a far more sensitive and efficacious test than the CF test.

There are significant discrepancies between EIA, IMDF, and CF study results, especially between IgM results using either EIA or IMDF methods. There is a paucity of comparative data showing how quickly the various classes of antibody convert to positive by the differing methods of testing currently available and how long they remain detectable. It has, however, been documented that both CF and IMDF titers decrease as clinical disease abates. For serologic diagnosis, blood in the appropriate tubes for serum separation should be collected. It has been reported that serum concentration can help decrease time to IgM and IgG detection but is not practiced routinely.

2) Culture and direct microscopic detection: laboratory diagnosis of more severe or disseminated diseases may include direct visualization of spherules, endospores, and possible mycelia (in association with cavitary lesions) in specimens using histopathologic stains such as hematoxylin and eosin (least sensitive), Grocott's methenamine silver (GMS; more sensitive) and calcofluor white fluorescent fungal stains. Culture of sputum, bronchoalveolar lavage (BAL), tissue biopsies, or other appropriate specimens may also be indicated in more severe cases. The best specimens for diagnosis depend on the clinical presentation and the affected organ system or tissue. Blood for culture is not normally indicated, as fungemia may be fleeting. When the respiratory tract is involved, sputum, BAL, or lung tissue biopsies are the best specimens to submit as necessary. When the skin or other organs are involved, biopsies of the effected sites are most efficacious. In cases of meningitis, cerebrospinal fluid for serologic diagnosis (CF testing) has been the standard approach to diagnosis as culture has poor recovery of the organism even when large volumes are submitted. Recently, a *Coccidioides* antigen EIA test was introduced that may be far more sensitive than the CF test for diagnosis of meningitis. Unfortunately, it is not yet commercially available, or FDA-approved in a kit form, but is available through a commercial reference laboratory (MiraVista Diagnostics, Indianapolis, IN).

There is no phenotypic test that can conclusively separate the 2 *Coccidioides* spp. Although molecular methods are required to conclusively identify an isolate to species, such effort is not needed for routine laboratory diagnosis as differences in the severity of infection for the 2 species have not been reported. Research polymerase chain reaction (PCR) assays and whole genome sequencing have been reported that can provide a correct species identification, but these are not widely used in the clinical or public health laboratories. One of the most widely used methods for identification is the AccuProbe *Coccidioides* ribonucleic acid (RNA) hybridization method (Hologic, San Diego, CA), but this method also does not differentiate between the 2 species. In vitro susceptibility testing with the primary therapeutic agents such as fluconazole and amphotericin B is rarely indicated, and in vitro antifungal results do not correlate with clinical outcomes. Specialized specimen collection, processing, or transportation methods are not necessary, and methods used for usual diagnosis of other bacterial and fungal infections may be used.

**4. Laboratory capability**—Clinical, private reference, and public health laboratories staffed by personnel trained in mycologic techniques can culture and identify *Coccidioides* spp. and perform serologic assays. Specialized molecular techniques including PCR and sequencing are required to determine species but are not necessary for routine clinical diagnosis. Positive RNA hybridization testing of culture isolates can be reported as *Coccidioides* spp. Presence of spherules with endospores in histopathologic preparations is presumptive evidence for coccidioidomycosis and further identification is not routinely necessary.

**5. Safety requirements**—Use of biosafety level 2 (BSL-2) or BSL-3 facilities is needed for culture of *Coccidioides* using a class II biological safety cabinet for manipulation of cultures. Plates should be sealed if held for any length of time, and all recommendations of the Clinical and Laboratory Standards Institute's document on fungal cultures should be followed. (See: *M54-A: Principles and Procedures for Detection of Fungi in Clinical Specimens—Direct Examination and Culture; Approved Guideline*.)

**6. Nonhuman hosts**—A wide variety of domesticated and wild animal species may be infected by *Coccidioides* spp., including dogs, cats, cattle, sheep, swine, llamas, coyotes, monkeys, sea otters, and other rodents. Although, coccidioidomycosis is not classified as a zoonotic disease, because animals do not normally transmit to humans, its presence in the environment may be perpetuated by infection of endemic rodents such as the cactus mouse and kangaroo rat.

**7. Sample/specimen requirements**—For serologic studies, whole blood or serum separator tube collections for serum are to be stored at refrigerator temperate for no longer than one week and then frozen at −20°C or lower if further retention is required. For histopathologic evaluation and culture, sputum, BALs, and specimens, such as tissues and normally sterile fluids (including cerebrospinal fluid) from other involved sites as clinically indicated, should be held at refrigerator temperature and processed promptly. Culture can only be attempted on unpreserved tissue specimens.

**8. Testing requirements**—Serum specimens collected in the acute phase can be tested for IgM and IgG antibodies by IMDF, EIA, and CF methods. It must be remembered that serologic response may be absent or diminished in early disease presentation or in immunocompromised patients. Serial CF titers should be used to evaluate the prognosis and status of the disease; they should not be used alone for primary diagnosis of coccidioidomycosis. A negative serology should not be immediately interpreted as negative for coccidioidomycosis. Tissue specimens may be submitted for histopathologic exams and culture. Fungal structures including characteristic endospore-containing spherules may be visualized by potassium hydroxide (KOH) wet mounts, which lack sensitivity but require just an ordinary light microscope, or the calcofluor white fluorescent stain that is more sensitive ( 40% overall) than the KOH but requires a fluorescent microscope and specialized filters. Reading the slides requires well-trained personnel and strict attention to morphologic detail. Inflammation in coccidioidomycosis is characterized by early infiltration of polymorphonuclear cells, which is replaced predominantly by a granulomatous reaction, as granulomas are formed with multinucleated giant cells at the site. For staining of fungal elements, the GMS stain is considered most sensitive. Other commonly used histological stains, including the periodic acid-Schiff and the hematoxylin eosin, are not considered as sensitive as GMS. At times, the Giemsa, Papanicolaou, and mucicarmine stains may be useful. The Gram stain does not adequately stain *Coccidioides* spp. and should not be used as the sole staining method. A diagnosis of coccidioidomycosis may be made by the presence of endospore-containing spherules in the specimen. Mycelial forms may also be observed. However, when specimens are collected from peripheries of cavitary lesions or other lesions abutting open spaces, spherules must be observed to provide a conclusive diagnosis of coccidioidomycosis.

**9. Reporting requirements**—Coccidioidomycosis is a laboratory and physician reportable finding in many states. As of 2017, 21 US states required reporting of *Coccidioides* infection findings by laboratories. In addition, it is on the list of reportable agents under the CDC National Notifiable Diseases Surveillance System. Laboratories testing for *Coccidioides* should determine if voluntary or required reporting of results are in place at the state, provincial, or national level. National reference laboratories should comply with the reporting requirements under the WHO International Health Regulations.

**10. Referral network**—There are several different referral options for the laboratory testing of *Coccidioides*. They include the following:

1) University of California, Davis: performs *Coccidioides* serology by both IMDF and CF testing.
2) MiraVista Diagnostics, Indianapolis, IN: performs *Coccidioides* antigen and antibody detection tests, both qualitative and quantitative.
3) Fungus Testing Laboratory, University of Texas Health Science Center at San Antonio: performs *Coccidioides* spp. identification and referral antimicrobial susceptibility testing.

Note: specimen submission should follow the individual referral laboratory's instructions.

**11. Special considerations**—None.

## Bibliography

Galgiani JN, Ampel NM, Blair JE, et al. 2016 Infectious Diseases Society of America (IDSA) clinical practice guideline for the treatment of Coccidioidomycosis. *Clin Infect Dis*. 2016;15;63(6):e112-146.

*M54-A: Principles and Procedures for Detection of Fungi in Clinical Specimens—Direct Examination and Culture; Approved Guideline*. 1st ed. Wayne, PA: Clinical and Laboratory Standards Institute; 2012.

Saubolle MA. Laboratory aspects in the diagnosis of coccidioidomycosis. *Ann N Y Acad Sci*. 2007;1111:301-314.

Saubolle MA, McKellar PP, Sussland D. Epidemiologic, clinical, and diagnostic aspects of coccidioidomycosis. *J Clin Microbio*. 2007;45(1):26–30.

[J. L. Beebe, M. A. Saubolle]

# COMMON COLD AND OTHER ACUTE VIRAL RESPIRATORY DISEASES

| DISEASE | ICD-10 CODE |
|---|---|
| COMMON COLD | ICD-10 J00 |
| OTHER ACUTE FEBRILE RESPIRATORY ILLNESSES | ICD-10 J01–J06, J12 |
| Influenza (see "Influenza") | |
| SARS (see "MERS, SARS, and Other Human Coronavirus Infections") | |
| Streptococcal pharyngitis (see "Streptococcal Diseases") | |

Numerous acute respiratory illnesses of known and presumed viral infection etiology are grouped here. Clinically, infections of the upper respiratory tract (above the epiglottis) can be designated as acute viral rhinitis or acute viral pharyngitis (common cold), and infections involving the lower respiratory tract (below the epiglottis) can be designated as croup (laryngotracheitis), acute viral tracheobronchitis, bronchitis, bronchiolitis, or acute viral pneumonia. These respiratory syndromes are associated with a large number of viruses. As a group, acute respiratory diseases are one of the leading causes of death from any infectious disease.

The illnesses, caused by known agents, have important common epidemiological attributes, such as reservoir and mode of transmission (respiratory droplet/aerosol). Many of the viruses involved can invade any part of the respiratory tract; others show a predilection for certain anatomical sites. Some predispose to bacterial complications. Morbidity and mortality from acute respiratory diseases are especially significant in children. In adults, relatively high incidence and resulting disability, with consequent economic loss, make acute respiratory diseases a major health problem worldwide.

Several infections of the respiratory tract are presented as separate chapters because they are sufficiently distinctive in their manifestations and occur in regular association with a single infectious agent. Examples include influenza, psittacosis, hantavirus pulmonary syndrome, chlamydial pneumonia, vesicular pharyngitis (herpangina), epidemic myalgia (pleurodynia), and severe acute respiratory syndrome (SARS). Symptoms of upper respiratory tract infection, mainly pharyngotonsillitis, can be produced by bacterial agents, among which group A streptococcus is the most common and for which specific antimicrobial measures are available, whereas most acute viral respiratory infections have no specific treatments.

**1. Clinical features—**

1) Common cold (acute viral rhinitis, rhinitis, coryza [acute]): an acute catarrhal infection of the upper respiratory tract characterized by coryza, sneezing, lacrimation, irritation of the nasopharynx, chills, and malaise lasting 2–7 days. Fever is uncommon in children older than 3 years and rare in adults. White blood cell counts are usually normal. Illness may be accompanied by laryngitis, tracheitis, or bronchitis and may predispose to more serious complications, such as sinusitis and otitis media. Fatalities are not associated with common colds, although severe illness may progress through a catarrhal phase, such as in debilitated persons or with secondary infections. Disability due to common colds is important because it affects work performance and industrial and school absenteeism.
2) Other acute febrile respiratory illnesses: viral diseases of the respiratory tract may be characterized by fever, cough, increased respiratory rate, chills, headache, general aches, malaise, anorexia, and, occasionally, gastrointestinal symptoms. Localizing signs also occur at various sites in the respiratory tract, either alone or in combination, such as rhinitis, pharyngitis or tonsillitis, laryngitis, laryngotracheitis, bronchitis, bronchiolitis, pneumonitis, or pneumonia. There may be associated conjunctivitis. Upper respiratory tract infection symptoms and signs usually subside in 2–5 days without complications. Lower respiratory tract infections may be severe or complicated by bacterial infections.

**2. Causative agents—**Acute viral respiratory syndromes are associated with a large number of viruses including influenza (A, B, C), respiratory syncytial virus (RSV), human metapneumovirus (hMPV), parainfluenza virus 1–4, enteroviruses, rhinoviruses, coronaviruses, and adenovirus. The morphology and replication strategies of these viruses are very diverse, involving mostly viruses with enveloped or nonenveloped ribonucleic acid (RNA) genomes but also some deoxyribonucleic acid viruses. Many of these viruses show a predilection for certain anatomical sites (e.g., parainfluenza viruses and the glottis, RSV and the bronchiolar epithelia; others such as adenoviruses have the capability of infecting upper and lower respiratory tract). Some predispose to bacterial complications.

A spectrum of clinical illness involving a wide range of symptoms such as febrile illness, cough, and sneezing is usually present with a rapid onset within days. It is usually very difficult distinguish the infectious cause through clinical examination. Symptoms and signs overlap and do not allow differentiation on clinical grounds, and illness spectrum and severity may differ between adults and children. A clinical distinction of lower respiratory tract infection is made based on presence of bronchiolitis or pneumonia. Viral pneumonia may cause radiographic changes on chest X-ray. In very young infants, the presence of bronchiolitis and wheezing in conjunction with upper respiratory infection is strongly suggestive of RSV or hMPV.

A clinician may have some help in determining which is the most likely etiology if there is knowledge of which viruses are circulating viruses through the use of local or national surveillance data. Viruses such as influenza and RSV, rhinoviruses, and parainfluenza have distinct seasonal patterns in temperate climates. Laboratory diagnostic testing is required to determine causality of acute viral respiratory disease with accuracy.

**3. Laboratory diagnosis**—Laboratory investigations are unusual mainly because illness is recognized as acute and self-limiting. Diagnostic tests are expensive and may be hard to access for the wide range of organisms involved. Less than 0.1% of community respiratory infections have sampling for diagnosis undertaken, and clinical management is usually directed toward empirical symptom relief. The question of whether to treat presumed viral respiratory tract infection with antibiotics remains a clinical challenge, balancing concerns about unnecessary antibiotic treatment against host susceptibility, predisposing to secondary bacterial infections.

The foundation of laboratory diagnosis is the detection of viral material in respiratory secretions taken early during illness. Serology plays little part in diagnosis. If undertaken, it requires the use of paired acute illness and convalescent samples around 21 days apart. In recent years, there has been a shift toward the use of nucleic acid amplification testing (NAAT) and away from traditional methods of viral detection such as immunofluorescence (IF) or virus isolation. The diversity of possible agents requires that if laboratory testing is undertaken, it will be for a wide range of agents, both bacterial and viral, and may be because illness is prolonged or severe.

Making a specific laboratory diagnosis for the individual common viruses associated with these syndromes (influenza A and B, RSV, rhinoviruses, parainfluenza 1-4, hMPV, coronaviruses, enteroviruses, adenoviruses) requires the ability to undertake NAAT testing as this is the method of choice for detection of a wide range of respiratory viruses, the majority of which are RNA viruses. Although very accurate, cost considerations require that samples are usually batched, giving rise to a turnaround time of approximately 24-48 hours, with results available too late to influence clinical management decisions.

Typically, once influenza and RSV are excluded, the most common pathogens found in common cold syndromes are rhinoviruses, with others in varying frequency combinations according to age and seasonality.

There is increasing interest in the use of rapid point-of-care tests (PoCT) for influenza and RSV, which can be applied in emergency room and other acute care settings and may be used as a simple single test, close to the patient, to exclude these viruses as a common cause of acute respiratory illness. The format and costs of the tests vary but usually involve a closed cassette and small-footprint, shoebox-sized instrumentation that does not require specialized skill to operate to provide detection of a range of 4-10 organisms within 15-20 minutes (typically influenza A, influenza B, RSV, rhinovirus, and parainfluenza viruses).

4. **Laboratory capability**—Laboratory facilities required to undertake viral diagnostics tests for this group of viruses are dependent on the types of testing undertaken. Traditional methods of virus isolation require specialized virology laboratories, with stringent attention to laboratory safety associated with virus propagation and the ability to work with mammalian cell cultures. Together these capabilities are found in very few hospital facilities and require highly trained and experienced staff with specialist knowledge. Such facilities are gradually disappearing from mainstream health care settings.

By contrast, although capability for NAAT testing does require specialist facilities that have thermocycler equipment, freezers and centrifuges, and a complex infrastructure staffed by individuals skilled in molecular techniques, NAAT testing for respiratory samples is increasingly available on commercial platforms that run in a fully automated manner. Capabilities are widely available in tertiary referral hospitals with large pathology departments where there may be combined microbiology and virology service provision, allowing implementation of multiplex testing algorithms to detect a long list of individual organisms, both bacterial and viral. The staff skills required for both bacteriology and virology are generic, involving the use of automation and nucleic acid manipulation and allowing for more interoperability of equipment and staffing

An alternative to the use of NAAT testing in resource limited settings is the use of IF or enzyme-linked immunosorbent assay techniques for detection of viral proteins in clinical respiratory material, which also requires the availability of specialist equipment and facilities, although the laboratory infrastructure and staff training requirements may be much simpler. These approaches are limited by sensitivity, and even in these settings there is a trend toward the use of NAAT technologies in their simplest format.

**5. Safety requirements**—The widespread use of NAAT testing in clinical virology laboratories worldwide, even in resource-poor settings, means that there has been a shift away from traditional methods of virus diagnosis involving viral propagation, where some of the greatest operator hazards lie. The majority of safety issues relating to work with clinical samples containing the respiratory viruses (excluding SARS, Middle East respiratory syndrome, and influenza) are generic. Clinical sample handling should be done within a class I biological safety cabinet (BSC) to prevent aerosol spread in an open laboratory or inadvertent infection of operator prior to nucleic acid extraction from clinical material. Downstream processing of nucleic acid can be undertaken in a wide range of facilities, including clean rooms that are not designated as specialist microbiology laboratories. Safety requirements therefore relate to the following:

1) Use of specialist facilities with BSC
2) Engineering controls for BSC
3) Use of personal protective equipment (gloves, eyewear, and laboratory coats)
4) Staff training in procedures and safe use of BSC
5) Safety training for equipment associated with workflow process (e.g., thermocyclers, centrifuges)
6) Risk assessment of clinical samples

**6. Nonhuman hosts**—Respiratory viruses involved in human disease described in this chapter are generally restricted to the human host. This excludes influenza viruses and viruses such as SARS and Middle East respiratory syndrome (MERS), which cause common respiratory illness following from a zoonotic transmission event.

**7. Sample/specimen requirements**—Respiratory samples need to be taken at a time close to illness onset, as respiratory viral shedding with the range of viruses under consideration tends to be maximum within 1–5 days of illness onset and gradually wanes for up to 10–14 days postillness onset. Specimens for diagnosis of respiratory viruses can be taken from upper or lower respiratory tract and should contain a mixture of respiratory epithelial cells and secretions. Typically, this would involve nasopharyngeal aspirates in very young children or individual nose or nasopharyngeal swabs in older children or adults taken into viral transport medium or saline prior to processing. Lower respiratory tract samples such as sputum, endotracheal aspirates, or bronchoalveolar lavage are excellent samples for diagnosis using NAAT testing, but sputum is not desirable for IF detection of viral-infected cells or propagation of viruses. When considering RSV and hMPV as a likely diagnosis, it is very important to ensure that the biological sample taken has sufficient quantity of epithelial cells, as these viruses are highly cell-associated.

**8. Testing requirements**—This involves the ability to detect viral genomic material using NAAT techniques on samples taken in the early phase of illness or, alternatively, viral antigen detection through IF or ELISA testing. Targets for NAAT testing tend to be conserved regions of viral genomes. NAAT testing typically has high sensitivity and high specificity (>95%) for samples taken early in infection, whereas the sensitivity and specificity of ELISA techniques and IF decrease significantly to about 60% on optimum samples. NAAT testing extends the duration of viral detection through illness as well as sensitivity. However, each individual NAAT test will only target a single agent, and it is necessary to undertake a multiplex or parallel processing approach to ensure that a wide range of organisms are covered. Confirmatory strategies for each target virus that has been identified through NAAT testing could involve sequencing of polymerase chain reaction products, detecting second nucleic acid targets in the same samples, or alternatively testing different samples.

Rapid molecular PoCT platforms for respiratory viruses have been developed with broadly equivalent diagnostic accuracy to laboratory PCR and are starting to be deployed in emergency room settings, using nasopharyngeal swab samples.

Quality assurance for the accuracy of diagnostic tests arises from the application of internal and external quality assurance programs and regular proficiency testing of the laboratory staff. Testing may be undertaken as part of a screening protocol when there are outbreaks in closed communities where early diagnosis would be beneficial for infection control measures or for severely immunocompromised individuals who may not be very symptomatic in the early stages of illness.

**9. Reporting requirements**—There are no requirements for any laboratory to report testing for the range of viruses considered in this chapter to notify detection, although some infections and illnesses (e.g., SARS, MERS, influenza) are much more closely monitored through clinical and laboratory-based reporting. In the UK, the outputs of all hospital laboratory tests is collected through data capture systems into a national surveillance system that collects all positive detections (numerator). These are reported in a weekly aggregated report.

Monitoring trends in detection of all respiratory viral targets through centralized report analysis improves understanding of circulating respiratory pathogens and the ability to provide a snapshot of what is circulating seasonally. There are no International Health Regulations or statutory reporting requirements for any of the respiratory viruses described in this chapter; however, for SARS, MERS, and influenza, see "MERS, SARS, and Other Human Coronavirus Infections" and "Influenza." Specific enhanced surveillance schemes are likely to be introduced in preparation for major public health campaigns, such as RSV vaccination when available, which will require specific sampling from particular case definitions.

**10. Referral network**—The respiratory viral pathogens do not have specific laboratory referral network pathways as there are very few public health or clinical interventions designed for them and therefore little need for specific reference laboratory activities. However, nearly all of the infections can be associated with significant nosocomial outbreaks-particularly in immunocompromised individuals-where tracing the pathway of person-to-person transmission may be important in understanding spread. This may require specialized and detailed molecular epidemiology to determine what is present. If there is licensure of an RSV-specific vaccine, it is likely that monitoring arrangements for detection of RSV will be enhanced.

**11. Special considerations**—The viruses described have diverse replication strategies and multiple different subtypes. It is unlikely that any single intervention could be designed. Typically the illnesses are mild and self-resolving; thus, none of these agents are of specific public health interest for population control measures unless there are outbreaks in hospitals, other care facilities, or institutional settings such as schools.

Symptomatic relief is the cornerstone for treatment in the community, for which no specific microbiological diagnosis is usually possible, and avoidance of contact, hand washing hygiene, and surface hygiene are important in infection control practice in secondary care facilities where infections due to any of these agents can be devastating in cohorts of immunosuppressed individuals. In this situation, stringent infection control and respiratory droplet precautions, cohorting of individuals, and restricting access is usually the way in which outbreaks are brought under control.

Differences in viral morphology may impact on the environmental stability and therefore infection control strategies (e.g., nonenveloped viruses such as adenoviruses are more stable in the environment than enveloped viruses such as RSV and may require more stringent decontamination measures).

The prolonged detection of a virus postillness onset, through the use of NAAT testing, may pose some difficulties in regard to understanding true infectious period for infection control purposes, as detection by NAAT testing may not equate to the detection of infectious virus. Prolonged detection of viral genomes in asymptomatic patients is particularly noted for rhinoviruses.

With age and the development of the immune system, respiratory viral infection typically becomes less severe until in older age waning immune function blunts the adaptive immune response in ways that are not well understood, and there is again a rise in severity of illness associated with these infections.

Respiratory viruses are detectable in around 40%–50% of hospitalized adults with acute respiratory illness, and it is likely that they account for a similar or higher proportion of acute respiratory episodes seen in primary care.

## Bibliography

Clark TW, Medina MJ, Batham S, Curran MD, Parmar S, Nicholson KG. Adults hospitalised with acute respiratory illness rarely have detectable bacteria in the absence of COPD or pneumonia; viral infection predominates in a large prospective UK sample. *J Infect.* 2014;69:507–515.

Falsey AR, Becker KL, Swinburne AJ, et al. Bacterial complications of respiratory tract viral illness: a comprehensive evaluation. *J Infect Dis.* 2013;208:432–441.

Self WH, Williams DJ, Zhu Y, et al. Respiratory viral detection in children and adults: comparing asymptomatic controls and patients with community-acquired pneumonia. *J Infect Dis.* 2015;213:584–591.

[M. C. Zambon]

# CONJUNCTIVITIS/KERATITIS

| DISEASE | ICD-10 CODE |
|---|---|
| CONJUNCTIVITIS, BACTERIAL | ICD-10 A48.4 |
| KERATOCONJUNCTIVITIS, ADENOVIRAL | ICD-10 B30.0 |
| KERATOCONJUNCTIVITIS, MICROSPORIDIAL | ICD-10 B60 |
| HEMORRHAGIC CONJUNCTIVITIS, ADENOVIRAL AND ENTEROVIRAL | ICD-10 B30.1 (adenoviral) ICD-10 B30.3 (enteroviral) |
| CHLAMYDIAL CONJUNCTIVITIS | ICD-10 A74.0 |
| Gonococcal conjunctivitis (see "Gonococcal Infections") | |
| Trachoma (see "Trachoma") | |

## I. CONJUNCTIVITIS, BACTERIAL (pinkeye, sticky eye, Brazilian purpuric fever)

**1. Clinical features**—A clinical syndrome beginning with lacrimation, irritation, and hyperemia of the palpebral and bulbar conjunctivae of one or both eyes, followed by edema of eyelids and mucopurulent discharge. In severe cases, ecchymoses of the bulbar conjunctiva and marginal infiltration of the cornea with mild photophobia may occur. Nonfatal (except as noted later), the disease may last from 2 days to 2–3 weeks; many patients have no more than hyperemia of the conjunctivae and slight exudate for a few days.

**2. Causative agents**—*Haemophilus influenzae*, *Streptococcus pneumoniae*, *Moraxella catarrhalis*, and *Staphylococcus aureus* are common etiologic agents of bacterial conjunctivitis; others include *Haemophilus aegyptius*, *Neisseria meningitidis*, and *Corynebacterium diphtheriae*. *H. influenzae*, *Neisseria gonorrhoeae* (see "Gonococcal Infections"), *S. pneumoniae*, viridans group streptococci, various Gram-negative enteric bacilli and, rarely, *Pseudomonas aeruginosa* may produce the disease in newborn infants.

**3. Laboratory diagnosis**—Diagnosis is often made clinically, and bacterial cultures are not routinely necessary. Bacterial cultures could be considered for neonatal infections, recurrent infections, conjunctivitis that has not responded to therapy, severe purulent discharge, and suspected cases of gonococcal infection.

**4. Laboratory capability**—Most bacteria that cause conjunctivitis can be recovered in standard clinical microbiology laboratories using routine media, such as blood agar, chocolate agar, and/or enriched media containing X and V factors.

**5. Safety requirements**—Bacteria that cause conjunctivitis can be safely recovered and identified using biosafety level 2 (BSL-2) precautions, including the use of protective laboratory coats and gloves.

**6. Nonhuman hosts**—Bacterial conjunctivitis is generally not due to zoonosis; however, other animals may suffer from a similar infection caused by the same organisms.

**7. Sample/specimen requirements**—Conjunctival scrapings are the most common type of specimen. These can be obtained using a soft-tipped applicator containing artificial fiber (cotton may be bacteriostatic) that has been moistened with sterile media such as saline or broth, a commercially available sterile applicator used for bacterial culture, or a sterile spatula or other blunt metallic device. The collection device is applied across the affected areas. Specimens from both eyes may be collected even if only one eye is symptomatic. Topical anesthetic may be used prior to sample collection but is not required. For optimal results, specimens should be sent to the laboratory as soon as possible, and refrigeration should be considered if delays are expected.

**8. Testing requirements**—The diagnostic laboratory test for bacterial conjunctivitis is microscopic examination of a stained smear and bacterial culture. Isolation of the causative agent also allows for antimicrobial susceptibility testing, if warranted. Standard quality assurance practices used for routine bacterial culture and antimicrobial susceptibility testing should be followed.

**9. Reporting requirements**—Bacterial conjunctivitis is generally caused by common pathogens and does not need to be reported. However, recovery of certain organisms (*N. gonorrhoeae* or *C. diphtheria*) or particularly severe infections (invasive *H. influenzae* or invasive *S. pneumoniae*) may require reporting to local, state, and/or federal authorities.

**10. Referral network**—Public health laboratories may provide assistance in isolating and identifying less common agents of bacterial conjunctivitis, like *C. diphtheriae*, if needed. Additionally, such laboratories may request submission of isolates for further testing, such as antimicrobial susceptibility testing for *N. gonorrhoeae*. Requirements for reporting and isolate submission should be determined in conjunction with the relevant authorities.

**11. Special considerations**—None.

## II. KERATOCONJUNCTIVITIS, ADENOVIRAL (epidemic keratoconjunctivitis, shipyard conjunctivitis, shipyard eye)

**1. Clinical features**—An acute viral disease of the eye, with unilateral or bilateral inflammation of conjunctivae and edema of the lids and periorbital tissue. Onset is sudden with pain, photophobia, blurred vision, and, occasionally, low-grade fever, headache, malaise, and tender preauricular lymphadenopathy. Approximately 7 days after onset in about half the cases, the cornea exhibits several small, round subepithelial infiltrates; these may eventually form punctate erosions that stain with fluorescein. Duration of acute conjunctivitis is about 2 weeks; it may continue to evolve, leaving discrete subepithelial opacities that may interfere with vision for a few weeks. In severe cases, permanent scarring may result.

**2. Causative agents**—Typically, adenovirus types 8, 19, and 37 are responsible, though other adenovirus types have been involved. Most severe disease has been found in infections caused by types 8, 5, and 19.

**3. Laboratory diagnosis**—Confirmed by the recovery of virus from appropriate cell cultures inoculated with eye swabs or conjunctival scrapings; virus may be visualized through fluorescent antibody (FA) staining of scrapings or through immune electron microscopy; viral antigen may be detected by enzyme-linked immunosorbent assay (ELISA) testing. Serum neutralization or hemagglutination inhibition tests may identify type-specific titer rises. Laboratory developed nucleic acid amplification assays (NAATs) are increasing in use due to superiority in detecting virus.

**4. Laboratory capability**—The detection of adenovirus from ocular specimens tends to be limited to larger microbiology and reference laboratories due to low testing volumes, the laborious nature of cell culture, the need for experienced technologists to microscopically identify the viral cytopathic effect, and the nature of laboratory developed NAAT testing.

**5. Safety requirements**—A class II biosafety cabinet should be used in handling patient specimens or adenovirus-infected cell cultures to prevent infection of laboratory personnel or contamination of specimens via aerosols, splashes to mucous membranes, and hand-to-face actions.

**6. Nonhuman hosts**—Adenoviruses have a broad range of vertebrate hosts including bats, dogs, horses, cattle, and birds.

**7. Sample/specimen requirements**—Use a cotton, Dacron, or rayon swab with a metal or plastic shaft that is premoistened with saline to obtain epithelial cells from the conjunctival surface. Other swab types, such as calcium alginate or wooden-shafted swabs, may be toxic to the organism and inhibit isolation. For direct detection techniques (immunofluorescence [IF]), immediately transfer the swab contents by rolling back and forth onto a glass slide. For culture and NAATs, place the swab in viral transport medium (VTM), and for culture, transport to the laboratory as quickly as possible under refrigerated conditions, ideally within 4 hours of collection. If cultures cannot be set up within 48 hours, the specimen should be frozen at -70°C to maintain viability of the organisms.

**8. Testing requirements**—While no FDA-cleared NAAT exists on any commercial platform for detection of adenovirus from ocular specimens, laboratories have validated such tests and show acceptable performance characteristics across molecular platforms. Advantages include the specimen no longer requiring viable virus, easing stringent transportation requirements, not needing an experienced technologist to detect cytopathic effect, and superior sensitivity/specificity compared with direct detection or culture techniques. Isolation of adenovirus in cell culture can be done using A549, Hep2, and HeLa 229 cell lines. After 1–5 days of incubation at 37°C, the monolayer can be stained with antibodies with a fluorescent tag and viewed under a fluorescent microscope. Cell culture is falling out of favor due to difficulties in preserving viability via transport, prolonged turnaround times, high costs, and relatively low sensitivity. Antigen detection can be used for rapid detection of adenoviruses in ocular specimens, although the sensitivity is poor as compared with that of molecular methods. Immunofluorescence, enzyme immunoassays (EIAs), and lateral-flow immunochromatography are the most common test formats for antigen detection.

**9. Reporting requirements**—Obligatory reporting to local health authorities of epidemics is required in some countries; normally individual case reporting is not required. CDC recommends health care providers report unusual clusters of conjunctivitis to state or local health departments.

**10. Referral network**—Larger reference laboratories are more likely to have the resources to validate a NAAT.

**11. Special considerations**—None.

# III. HEMORRHAGIC CONJUNCTIVITIS, ADENOVIRAL (pharyngoconjunctival fever), ENTEROVIRAL (Apollo 11 disease, acute hemorrhagic conjunctivitis)

**1. Clinical features**—In adenoviral hemorrhagic conjunctivitis, lymphoid follicles usually develop, the conjunctivitis lasts 7–15 days, and there are frequently small subconjunctival hemorrhages. In one adenoviral syndrome, pharyngoconjunctival fever (PCF), there is upper respiratory disease and fever with minor corneal epithelial inflammation (epithelial keratitis). In enteroviral acute hemorrhagic conjunctivitis (AHC), onset is sudden, with redness, swelling, and pain often in both eyes; the course of inflammatory disease is 4–6 days, during which subconjunctival hemorrhages appear on the bulbar conjunctiva as petechiae that enlarge to form confluent subconjunctival hemorrhages. Large hemorrhages gradually resolve over 7–12 days. In major outbreaks of enteroviral origin, there has been a low incidence of a polio-like paralysis, including cranial nerve palsies, lumbosacral radiculomyelitis, and lower motor neuron paralysis.

Neurological complications start a few days to a month after conjunctivitis and often leave residual weakness.

**2. Causative agents**—Adenoviruses and picornaviruses. Most adenoviruses can cause PCF, but types 3, 4, and 7 are the most common causes. The most prevalent picornavirus type is enterovirus 70; this and a variant of coxsackievirus A24 have caused large outbreaks of AHC.

**3. Laboratory diagnosis**—Laboratory confirmation of adenovirus infections requires isolation of the virus from conjunctival swabs in cell culture, rising antibody titers, detection of viral antigens through IF, or identification of viral nucleic acid with a deoxyribonucleic acid (DNA) probe or NAAT. Enterovirus infection is diagnosed by isolation of the agent in cell culture, IF, demonstration of a rising antibody titer, or NAAT.

**4. Laboratory capability**—The detection of adenovirus or enterovirus from ocular specimens tends to be limited to larger microbiology and reference laboratories due to low testing volumes, the laborious nature of cell culture, the need for experienced technologists to microscopically identify the viral cytopathic effect, and the nature of laboratory developed NAAT testing.

**5. Safety requirements**—A class II biosafety cabinet should be used in handling patient specimens or adenovirus-infected cell cultures to prevent infection of laboratory personnel or contamination of specimens via aerosols, splashes to mucous membranes, and hand-to-face actions.

**6. Nonhuman hosts**—Adenoviruses have a broad range of vertebrate hosts including bats, dogs, horses, cattle, and birds. Enteroviruses have been isolated from nonhuman primates.

**7. Sample/specimen requirements**—Use a cotton, Dacron, or rayon swab with a metal or plastic shaft that is premoistened with saline to obtain epithelial cells from the conjunctival surface. Other swab types, such as calcium alginate or wooden-shafted swabs, may be toxic to the viruses and inhibit isolation. For direct detection techniques (IF), immediately transfer the swab contents by rolling back and forth onto a glass slide. For culture and NAATs, place the swab in VTM, and, for culture, transport to the laboratory as quickly as possible under refrigerated conditions, ideally within 4 hours of collection. If cultures cannot be set up within 48 hours, the specimen should be frozen at -70°C to maintain viability of the virus.

**8. Testing requirements**—While no FDA-cleared NAAT exists on any commercial platform for detection of adenovirus or enterovirus from ocular specimens, laboratories have validated such tests and show acceptable performance characteristics across molecular platforms. Advantages include the fact that the specimen no longer requires viable virus, easing stringent transportation requirements, and an experienced technologist is not needed to detect cytopathic effect. Sensitivity and specificity are superior to direct detection or culture techniques. Isolation of adenovirus in cell culture can be done using A549, Hep2, and HeLa 229 cell lines. After 1-5 days of incubation at 37°C, the monolayer can be stained with antibodies with a fluorescent tag and viewed under a fluorescent microscope. A combination of cell lines is used for enterovirus isolation including human derived and primate cell lines. Isolation of enterovirus typically takes 4-8 days but may be shorter from sites with higher viral titers. Cell culture is falling out of favor due to difficulties in preserving viability via transport, prolonged turnaround times, high costs, and relatively low sensitivity. Antigen detection can be used for rapid detection of adenoviruses in ocular specimens, although the sensitivity is poor as compared with that of molecular methods. Immunofluorescence, EIAs, and lateral-flow immunochromatography are the most common test formats for antigen detection.

**9. Reporting requirements**—Obligatory reporting to local health authorities of epidemics is required in some countries; normally individual case reporting is not required. CDC recommends health care providers report unusual clusters of conjunctivitis to state or local health departments.

**10. Referral network**—Larger reference laboratories are more likely to have the resources to validate a NAAT.

**11. Special considerations**—None.

## IV. CHLAMYDIAL CONJUNCTIVITIS (inclusion conjunctivitis, paratrachoma, neonatal inclusion blennorrhea, sticky eye)

**1. Clinical features**—In the newborn, an acute conjunctivitis with purulent discharge, usually recognized within 5–12 days after birth. The acute stage usually subsides spontaneously in a few weeks; inflammation of the eye may persist for more than a year if untreated, with mild scarring of the conjunctivae and infiltration of the cornea (micropannus). Chlamydial pneumonia (see "Pneumonia" and "Chlamydial Infections") occurs in some infants with concurrent nasopharyngeal infection. Gonococcal infection must be ruled out.

In children and adults, an acute follicular conjunctivitis is seen typically with preauricular lymphadenopathy on the involved side, hyperemia, infiltration, and a slight mucopurulent discharge, often with superficial corneal involvement. In adults, there may be a chronic phase with scant discharge and symptoms that sometimes persist for more than a year if untreated. The agent may cause symptomatic infection of the urethral epithelium and the cervix, with or without associated conjunctivitis.

**2. Causative agents**—*Chlamydia trachomatis* of serovars D through K. Feline strains of *Chlamydia psittaci* have also caused acute follicular keratoconjunctivitis in humans.

**3. Laboratory diagnosis**—Laboratory methods to assist diagnosis include isolation in cell culture, antigen detection using IF staining of direct smears, EIA methods, and DNA probe. Laboratory developed NAATs for *C. trachomatis* are increasing in use due to superiority in detection of organisms.

**4. Laboratory capability**—The detection of *C. trachomatis* from ocular specimens tends to be limited to larger microbiology and reference laboratories due to low testing volumes, the laborious nature of cell culture, the need for experienced technologists to microscopically identify the chlamydial inclusions, and the nature of laboratory developed NAAT testing.

**5. Safety requirements**—A class II biosafety cabinet should be used in handling patient specimens or *C. trachomatis*-infected cell cultures to prevent infection of laboratory personnel or contamination of specimens via aerosols, splashes to mucous membranes, and hand-to-face actions. *C. psittaci* is a BSL-3 organism.

**6. Nonhuman hosts**—Sexually transmitted *C. trachomatis* only causes infection in humans. *C. felis*, a species endemic to domestic cats, has been documented as causing zoonotic infections in humans, including acute follicular keratoconjunctivitis.

**7. Sample/specimen requirements**—Use a cotton, Dacron or rayon swab with a metal or plastic shaft that is premoistened with saline to obtain epithelial cells from the conjunctival surface. Purulent exudate alone is not sufficient. Other swab types, such as calcium alginate or wooden-shafted swabs, may be toxic to the organism and inhibit isolation. For direct detection techniques (i.e., IF), immediately transfer the swab contents by rolling back and forth onto a glass slide. For culture and NAATs, place the swab in chlamydial transport medium or manufacturer approved collection media, and for culture, transport to the laboratory as quickly as possible under refrigerated conditions, ideally within 4 hours of collection. If cultures cannot be set up within 48 hours, the specimen should be frozen at -70°C to maintain viability of the organisms.

**8. Testing requirements**—While no FDA-cleared NAAT exists on any commercial platform for detection of *C. trachomatis* from extragenital specimens, numerous laboratories have validated such tests for the diagnosis of chlamydial conjunctivitis and shown acceptable performance characteristics across molecular platforms. Advantages include that the specimen no longer has to contain viable organisms, easing stringent transportation requirements, an experienced technologist is not needed to detect inclusions, and sensitivity/specificity is superior to direct detection or culture techniques. Isolation of *C. trachomatis* and *C. psittaci* in cell culture can be done using HeLa 229 and McCoy cell lines. After 48–72 hours of incubation at 37°C, the monolayer can be stained with antibodies with a fluorescent tag and viewed under a fluorescent microscope for the characteristic intracytoplasmic elementary and reticulate bodies. Cell culture is falling out of favor due to difficulties in preserving viability via transport, prolonged turnaround times, high costs, and relatively low sensitivity. While antigen detection from direct smears is FDA-cleared for ocular *C. trachomatis* infections, is less laborious, and relatively rapid to perform, the need for a fluorescent microscope, an experienced laboratory technologist, and poor sensitivity limits its clinical utility. DNA probe tests are no longer widely available. EIA tests have shown cross reactivity with the lipopolysaccharide of other microorganisms, and the use of both DNA probe and EIA testing is not recommended.

**9. Reporting requirements**—As of 2010, reporting of *C. trachomatis* infections is a nationally notifiable disease, and as such, laboratories should follow individual state's reporting requirements.

**10. Referral network**—Depending on the area, the reporting of positive results may authorize health departments to notify and screen sexual partners of the index case.

**11. Special considerations**—Laboratory criteria for diagnosis of a confirmed case: isolation of *C. trachomatis* by culture or demonstration of *C. trachomatis* in a clinical specimen by detection of antigen or nucleic acid.

## V. MICROSPORIDIA KERATOCONJUNCTIVITIS

**1. Clinical features**—Clinical symptoms include foreign body sensations, moderate to intense pain, redness, light sensitivity, excessive tearing, swelling of eyelid, itchiness, and impaired eyesight. Ocular manifestations include superficial punctate keratoconjunctivitis and corneal stromal keratitis. Duration of symptoms lasts between 4 days and 18 months. Disease commonly causes symptoms in immunocompromised patients but also has been documented in immunocompetent persons.

**2. Causative agents**—Microsporidia; obligate, intracellular, spore-forming, parasitic fungi belonging to the phylum *Microsporidia*. Keratoconjunctivitis is caused by genus *Encephalitozoon*, and stromal keratitis is caused by genus *Nosema* and *Microsporidium*. *Vittaforma corneae* (formerly *Nosema corneum*) cause keratoconjunctivitis and urinary tract infections in humans.

**3. Laboratory diagnosis**—Laboratory confirmation is performed by examining corneal scrapings or a conjunctival smear for microsporidia. Culture is used to exclude other causative agents. Laboratory methods to assist diagnosis include light microscopy using various stains including Gram stains (microsporidia spores are Gram-positive, stain dark violet, and become readily visible under the microscope), modified trichrome stains (e.g., trichrome blue), Warthin-Starry silver stains, Giemsa, and chemofluorescent agents like Calcofluor.

*V. corneae* and *Nosema* spp. measure 1.5–4 μm under the microscope. Immunofluorescence assays (IFAs) and molecular techniques are emerging methods for diagnosis. Transmission electron microscopy is the gold standard for identifying specific species.

**4. Laboratory capability**—Various staining procedures, IFAs and polymerase chain reaction (PCR) techniques tend to be limited to larger microbiology and reference laboratories due to low testing volumes, the need for experienced technologists to identify the organisms microscopically, and the nature of laboratory developed testing. Transmission electron microscopy is limited to facilities that possess these capabilities and experienced staff to identify species level characteristics of microsporidia. CDC offers PCR assays and species specific sequencing identification on a case by case basis.

**5. Safety requirements**—If drying is prevented, the spores of microsporidia remain infectious for prolonged periods of time. As such, BSL-2 practices, containment equipment, and facilities are recommended, including working in a biological safety cabinet and donning personal protection (e.g., gown, gloves, face shield).

**6. Nonhuman hosts**—Microsporidia are capable of causing infection in almost all animal groups including insects, birds, fish and mammals. While direct zoonotic transmission has not been confirmed, there is potential as there are common microsporidial species that infect both humans and animals.

**7. Sample/specimen requirements**—The spores of microsporidia can be detected from a corneal scraping, conjunctival smear, ocular fluid or vitreous fluid. The specimen should be collected in a sterile container or with a swab. If fluid is collected, at least 0.5 mL is recommended. Specimens should be refrigerated and ideally processed within 3 days for staining-based techniques.

**8. Testing requirements**—Commonly performed diagnostic microscopic tests include various staining procedures, including chromotrope-based and chemofluorescent agents, and IFAs. These tests require an experienced technologist, specific microsporidial quality control material with each run, and only allow for the identification of microsporidial spores as the spores of various genera and species are indistinguishable. In general, these tests suffer from lower sensitivity. Chemofluorescent agents tend to be more sensitive, with the risk of false-positive results, while the chromotrope based stains are highly specific for the presence of spores. The use of PCR, transmission electron microscopy, and sequencing can confirm the diagnosis and allow for genus and species level identification. Due to the small sample size, transmission microscopy can be relatively insensitive. Molecular based methodologies for the diagnosis of microsporidia are considered to be sensitive and specific.

**9. Reporting requirements**—It is not required that laboratories routinely report the identification of microsporidia to public health authorities.

**10. Referral network**—No formal laboratory referral networks exist for microsporidia.

**11. Special considerations**—None.

[C. Wojewoda, L. Stempak, D. Chen]

# CRYPTOCOCCOSIS
(torula)

| DISEASE | ICD-10 CODE |
|---|---|
| CRYPTOCOCCOSIS | ICD-10 B45 |

**1. Clinical features**—In immunocompetent persons, primary pulmonary infection commonly presents with fever and dry cough. In immunocompromised persons, signs and symptoms often develop after hematogenous spread to the meninges, with subacute or chronic meningitis, and include headache, visual disturbance, and confusion. Other sites of disseminated infection include the kidneys, prostate, bone, and skin (pustules, papules, plaques, ulcers, or subcutaneous masses). Untreated meningitis leads to death within weeks to months.

**2. Causative agents**—*Cryptococcus neoformans* var. *neoformans* and *C. neoformans* var. *grubii*, and *Cryptococcus gattii*. Seven lineages within *C. neoformans* and *C. gattii* have been described as distinct species.[1] However, the legitimacy and diagnostic value of some of these designations are controversial. Current recommendations are to recognize and report the *C. neoformans* and *C. gattii* spp. complexes.[2]

**3. Laboratory diagnosis**—Cryptococcal meningitis diagnosis is aided by the evidence of the characteristic capsular halo or budding forms on microscopic examination of cerebrospinal fluid (CSF) mixed with India ink. Tests for antigen in serum and CSF are highly sensitive and specific. Diagnosis is confirmed through histopathology or culture; media containing cycloheximide inhibit the agent and should not be used. *Cryptococcus* can be stained using Gomori-methenamine silver or periodic acid-Schiff staining; mucicarmine helps to differentiate it from other yeasts, especially *Blastomyces* and *Histoplasma*.

**4. Laboratory capability**—Specimens and cultures from suspected cryptococcosis cases must be handled within a biosafety level 2 (BSL-2)/physical containment 2 (PC-2) facility. Specimens should be processed in a class II biosafety cabinet. However, it is recognized that despite international efforts, such facilities and training may not always be possible in developing countries, which often have the highest burden of cryptococcal infection. Laboratory staff must be trained to recognize and differentiate cryptococci from other yeasts, including what might otherwise be dismissed as oral flora.

**5. Safety requirements**—*C. neoformans* and *C. gattii* are classified as risk group 2 organisms, and specimens and cultures should be handled and stored in a BSL-2/PC-2 facility using BSL-2 precautions. Manipulations attempting to induce mating/sporulation (sexual state) should be performed with BSL-3 precautions. Inhalation of aerosolized yeast cells or basidiospores must be avoided.

**6. Nonhuman hosts**—Cryptococcal disease has been identified in a wide range of companion, livestock, and wild animals including land mammals, marine mammals, birds, reptiles, and some invertebrates. Infections are common in domestic cats and dogs, ferrets, birds, horses, and koalas. Cryptococcosis is not known for zoonotic spread. However, the incidence and prevalence of animal infection serves as a good sentinel for human cryptococcosis.

**7. Sample/specimen requirements**—Aseptically collected blood and CSF should be submitted for cryptococcal antigen testing, microscopy (India ink), and culture as soon as cryptococcal infection is suspected; it should be noted that the CSF profile may be unremarkable. If the latex agglutination (LA) method is to be used for antigen detection, CSF (1 mL; minimum 0.5 mL) should be centrifuged at 1,000 × *g* for 15 minutes to obtain the supernatant; this is not necessary for the lateral flow assay (LFA). Blood (4 mL; minimum 1.4 mL) should be collected without anticoagulants, clotted, and centrifuged to obtain the serum component for antigen testing. Automated blood culture systems may be used for culture. Centrifuged CSF sediment should be used for culture. While testing should be performed as soon as possible upon arrival in the laboratory, if this is not possible, specimens may be stored at 2°C–8°C for up to 72 hours. Serum and CSF may be stored for longer periods at or below −20°C, but repeated freeze-thawing must be avoided. Sputum, bronchial fluids, and urine are also useful for cryptococcal culture; care should be taken to adequately communicate to the laboratory that cryptococcal infection is suspected. Where appropriate, cutaneous lesions should be biopsied and submitted for fungal stains and cultures.

**8. Testing requirements**—Antigen detection, microscopy and culture, and histopathological staining are part of the recommended practice. Antigen detection to detect capsular proteins by LA, enzyme immunoassay (EIA), or LFA is associated with high sensitivity and specificity. Overall the sensitivity in cryptococcal meningitis (CM) is 94% for CSF and 93.5% for serum.[3] Positive results assist in establishing preliminary/presumptive diagnosis. However, false-positive results have been reported, and these are not a reliable diagnostic test for non-*neoformans/gattii* spp. The somewhat superior performance of LFA compared with LA and EIA, along with its low cost, point-of-care potential, and minimal training and equipment requirements recently led to the designation of LFA as a WHO-preferred method for rapid presumptive diagnosis of cryptococcal disease.[4] India ink stain for direct examination of CSF, urine, and other body fluids allows visualization of the polysaccharide capsule. Sensitivity in CSF specimens is 60%–80% in the setting of human immunodeficiency virus (HIV)-related CM.[5] False-positive results may be due to confusion of encapsulated yeast cells with fat droplets or lymphocytes. Within tissue sections, mucicarmine or alcian blue stains the cryptococcal capsule to distinguish it from yeasts with similar morphologies. Immunohistochemical staining permits reliable identification and discrimination of *C. neoformans* from *C. gattii* in formalin-fixed tissues.[6]

Positive antigen and/or microscopy results should be confirmed with culture, although this may take 1–3 weeks or longer. Nonsterile site specimens should be cultured on media containing antibiotics, but not cycloheximide. In HIV related CM, the sensitivity of CSF and blood cultures is 80%–90% and 47%–70%, respectively. Cerebrospinal fluid culture sensitivity is dependent on inoculum volume.[7,8] *C. neoformans/gattii* may be identified using commercial carbohydrate assimilation tests. *C. gattii* can be differentiated from *C. neoformans* by its growth and blue color reaction on canavanine-glycine-bromothymol blue (CGB) agar. While generally reliable for distinguishing *C. gattii* from *C. neoformans*, other yeasts may return a positive

CGB result, including *Cryptococcus* spp., *Candida parapsilosis*, and *Trichosporon* spp.[9] Creatinine dextrose bromothymol blue thymine agar may be used for differentiation of *C. neoformans* var. *neoformans* and *C. neoformans* var. *grubii*. Matrix-assisted laser desorption/ionization time-of-flight mass spectrometry can provide reliable species and subspecies level identification of *Cryptococcus* spp., depending on database quality.[10] Sequencing of the ribosomal deoxyribose nucleic acid internal transcribed spacer regions and/or the large subunit D1/D2 domains may also assist in molecular subspecies typing and identification of non-*neoformans/gattii* spp.

**9. Reporting requirements**—Positive cryptococcal antigen, India ink, or culture results should be actively communicated to clinicians within 2 hours. When known, reporting to *C. neoformans* or *C. gattii* spp. complex level is recommended.[2] *C. gattii* infections confirmed by definitive culture identification, nucleic acid detection from clinical specimen, or demonstration of *C. gattii* in clinical specimen by immunohistochemistry are notifiable to state health authorities of Washington and Oregon within 24 hours; culture submission is required within 2 business days. Additionally, animal cases in Washington and Oregon are notifiable within 7 days. While not listed as notifiable diseases in other US states, it is highly desirable that confirmed human *C. gattii* cases and cultures be submitted to CDC.

Culture-confirmed cases are also reportable to the British Columbia Centre for Disease Control for residents of British Columbia with accompanying culture.

**10. Referral network**—None.

**11. Special considerations**—None.

## References

1. Hagen F, Khayhan K, Theelen B, et al. Recognition of seven species in the *Cryptococcus gattii/Cryptococcus neoformans* species complex. *Fungal Genet Biol.* 2015;78:16–48.
2. Kwon-Chung KJ, Bennett JE, Wickes BL, et al. The case for adopting the "species complex" nomenclature for the etiologic agents of cryptococcosis. *mSphere.* 2017;2(1):e00357-416.
3. Antinori S, Radice A, Galimberti L, et al. The role of cryptococcal antigen assay in diagnosis and monitoring of cryptococcal meningitis. *J Clin Microbiol.* 2005;43(11):5828–5829.
4. World Health Organization. Rapid advice: Diagnosis, prevention and management of cryptococcal disease in HIV-infected adults, adolescents and children. 2011. Available at: http://apps.who.int/iris/bitstream/10665/44786/1/9789241502979_eng.pdf. Accessed June 22, 2018.
5. AIDS*info*. Guidelines for the prevention and treatment of opportunistic infections in HIV-infected adults and adolescents. Available at: https://aidsinfo.nih.gov/contentfiles/lvguidelines/adult_oi.pdf. Accessed February 26, 2019.
6. Krockenberger MB, Canfield PJ, Kozel TR, et al. An immunohistochemical method that differentiates *Cryptococcus neoformans* varieties and serotypes in formalin-fixed paraffin-embedded tissues. *Med Mycol.* 2001;39(6):523–533.

7. Antinori S. New insights into HIV/AIDS-associated cryptococcosis. *ISRN AIDS*. 2013:471363.
8. Boulware DR, Rolfes MA, Rajasingham R, et al. Multisite validation of cryptococcal antigen lateral flow assay and quantification by laser thermal contrast. *Emerg Infect Dis*. 2014;20(1):45–53.
9. Klein KR, Hall L, Deml SM, et al. Identification of *Cryptococcus gattii* by use of L-canavanine glycine bromothymol blue medium and DNA sequencing. *J Clin Microbiol*. 2009;47(11):3669–3672.
10. Posteraro B, Vella A, Cogliati M, et al. Matrix-assisted laser desorption ionization-time of flight mass spectrometry-based method for discrimination between molecular types of *Cryptococcus neoformans* and *Cryptococcus gattii*. *J Clin Microbiol*. 2012;50(7):2472–2476.

[S. E. Kidd]

# CRYPTOSPORIDIOSIS

| DISEASE | ICD-10 CODE |
|---|---|
| CRYPTOSPORIDIOSIS | ICD-10 A07.2 |

**1. Clinical features**—This parasitic infection primarily affects epithelial cells of the gastrointestinal (GI), biliary, and respiratory tracts. The major symptom is diarrhea, which may be profuse and watery and is associated with cramping abdominal pain. The diarrhea is preceded by anorexia and vomiting in children, but general malaise, fever, anorexia, nausea, and vomiting occur less often in adults. Symptoms often wax and wane but remit in less than 30 days in most immunologically healthy people. Immunocompetent people may have asymptomatic or self-limited symptomatic infections; it is not clear whether reinfection and latent infection with reactivation can occur. Immunodeficient individuals generally clear their infections when factors contributing to immunosuppression (including malnutrition or intercurrent viral infections such as measles) are ameliorated or controlled. In those with human immunodeficiency virus infection, the clinical course may vary, and asymptomatic periods may occur, but the infection usually persists throughout the illness unless highly active antiretroviral therapy is successful. Symptoms of cholecystitis may occur in biliary tract infections; the relationship between respiratory tract infections and clinical symptoms is unclear.

**2. Causative agents**—*Cryptosporidium* spp. (*Cryptosporidium hominis* and *Cryptosporidium parvum* are the 2 most common species infecting humans), an apicomplexan protozoan parasite related to coccidian protozoa. Cryptosporidia are cosmopolitan and occur worldwide. While human-to-human transmission is common, depending on the local conditions, zoonotic transmission may be more frequent.

**3. Laboratory diagnosis**—Generally, through identification of oocysts in fecal specimens or of life cycle stages of the parasites in intestinal biopsy sections. Oocysts are small (4–6 μm), round-to-oval, and contain 4 naked sporozoites (not contained within a sporocyst). The oocysts may be confused with yeast unless appropriately stained or labeled. *Cryptosporidium* may not be detected by standard ova and parasite examinations, and testing requires a specific request. Most commonly used stains include the modified acid-fast stain (e.g., Kinyoun's modified acid fast), hot safranin-methylene blue, and auramine O (acid-fast fluorescent stain). Parasite antigen detection assays include commercially available antibody-based enzyme-immunoassays (EIA/ELISA) as well as immunochromatographic assays (widely known as rapid diagnostic tests or point-of-care tests). Direct or indirect immunofluorescent detection of oocysts using a fluorescent dye-tagged monoclonal antibody is considered the most sensitive microscopical assay and is useful for detecting oocysts in stool and in environmental samples. Unlike *Cyclospora* oocysts, cryptosporidial oocysts do not autofluoresce under ultraviolet light. Infection with this organism is not easily detected unless looked for specifically.

Nucleic acid-based tests, such as polymerase chain reaction (PCR), are increasingly being used and are incorporated in commercial multipathogen panels (e.g., FilmArray Gastrointestinal Panel, BioFire Diagnostics, Salt Lake City, UT). Performance of nucleic acid-based methods show high sensitivity (comparable to or better than immunofluorescence assays) and high specificity. While not required for clinical care guidance, molecular methods can identify species and provide genotyping data valuable in epidemiologic investigations. There are no serologic assays (i.e., antibody detection) for routine clinical diagnosis of cryptosporidiosis. Noncommercial, research laboratory serological assays are available to support epidemiological studies.

**4. Laboratory capability**—Microscopy, stool concentration/centrifugation, and permanent staining capabilities should be available. Laboratorians should be trained in the microscopic/morphologic detection of parasites and undergo regular proficiency testing. Laboratories that perform fluorescent acid-fast staining (e.g., auramine O) or immunofluorescence assays typically use common filter sets for visualizing targets labeled with fluorescent dyes (e.g., fluorescein [green], rhodamine [red], or similar). Commercial assays may require specialized equipment including microplate readers (ELISA), fluorescent microscopes, PCR systems, or custom hardware platforms that will require routine maintenance.

Laboratorians trained in performing nucleic acid-based diagnostic assays are needed for molecular detection of cryptosporidiosis. Specific equipment required will depend on the type of assay selected (e.g., standard thermocycler, real-time PCR thermocycler, or multiplex molecular platform). Deoxyribonucleic acid extraction processes should include a step for mechanical disruption (e.g., bead beating) of the tough oocysts to ensure release of nucleic acids. A unidirectional workflow should be implemented to reduce risk of false-positive results because of amplicon contamination.

**5. Safety requirements**—Clinical specimens should always be collected and handled with standard precautions. *Cryptosporidium* spp. is a biosafety level 2 organism. Oocysts are immediately infective when shed in stool. Cryptosporidial oocysts are very resistant to chemical inactivation by routine disinfectants (e.g., bleach, quaternary ammonium, alcohols) and can remain infectious for 6 or more months in moist, cool environments. Formalin, as a stool fixative, should only be used in a well-ventilated area, preferably in a chemical fume hood. Scant data are available for the persistence of oocyst infectivity in standard stool fixative/preservatives, consequently unpreserved and preserved stools should be disposed of as infectious waste.

**6. Nonhuman hosts**—*Cryptosporidium* spp. infect more than 45 vertebrate hosts, including birds, fish, reptiles, and mammals. However, the majority of human infections are caused by *C. hominis* (essentially restricted to humans) and *C. parvum* (a zoonotic species especially common in livestock). Infections transmitted from pets or companion animals, including dogs and cats, have been reported rarely but most often occur in immunocompromised patients.

**7. Sample/specimen requirements**—Stool should be promptly preserved in a liquid medium appropriate for microscopical examination or for antigen detection (e.g., EIA/ELISA or immunochromatographic assays). Formalin-based fixatives are suitable for microscopical assays. Single vial alcohol-based systems for ova and parasite collection are also appropriate (e.g., EcoFix [Meridian Bioscience, Cincinnati, OH] and TotalFix [Medical Chemical Corporation], Torrance, CA). If nucleic acid-based assays are to be utilized, stool may be left unpreserved or placed in a medium that is acceptable for molecular detection (i.e., lacking formalin or mercury). To maximize microscopy sensitivity, up to 3 separate stool specimens should be collected on different days.

**8. Testing requirements**—Diagnostic assays are based on identification of the parasite (whole organism, antigen, or nucleic acids) in stool as no culture methods for diagnosis are available. Microscopical assays typically include routine concentration procedures (e.g., formalin ethyl acetate sedimentation) and permanent staining of stool. A calibrated ocular micrometer should be used to measure oocyst size. Diagnosis is confirmatory in specimens meeting morphologic criteria in laboratories with appropriate training; however, antigen or nucleic acid-based assays are more suitable for confirmation of diagnosis.

Molecular diagnosis can be useful for clarification of suspicious microscopy findings and for providing a more sensitive detection compared with brightfield microscopy. For in-house assays, cutoff values for what should be considered a positive result should be established based on a laboratory-specific validation using known positives and negatives.

Assay sensitivity and specificity follows this general pattern: if immunofluorescence microscopy is used as a reference (gold standard), brightfield microscopy is approximately 70%–75% sensitive, fluorescent acid-fast microscopy is approximately 90%–95% sensitive, antigen detection assays (e.g., EIA, immunochromatographic) are approximately 70%–100% sensitive, and nucleic acid-based assays (e.g., PCR) are essentially 100% sensitive. Specificity can vary considerably for nonspecific staining methods, depending on microscopist skills, but antigen and nucleic acid-based assays show high specificity, approaching 100%, especially when used as confirmation of positive results.

Serology is not available for routine clinical diagnosis.

**9. Reporting requirements**—Reporting requirements/criteria vary by country and local jurisdiction. In the USA, cryptosporidiosis (confirmed and probable) is included in the National Notifiable Diseases Surveillance System (https://wwwn.cdc.gov/nndss). Positive cases in humans may be reported as *Cryptosporidium* spp. It is not necessary to report the species name (if determined) since clinical care and therapy is the same for symptomatic cryptosporidiosis, regardless of infecting species. For epidemiologic or genotyping studies, if the species is identified in molecular assays, this additional data can be provided. In jurisdictions where formal reporting mechanisms are not yet established, clinicians and laboratory workers who identify cases of cryptosporidiosis are encouraged to inform the appropriate health departments.

**10. Referral network**—CryptoNet, a multidisciplinary, molecular-based surveillance system, facilitates the systematic collection and molecular characterization of *Cryptosporidium* isolates to further understand cryptosporidiosis epidemiology (see: https://www.cdc.gov/parasites/crypto/cryptonet.html).

**11. Special considerations**—Health care providers should consider the diagnosis of *Cryptosporidium* infection in persons with prolonged diarrheal illness and should request stool specimens so that specific tests for this parasite can be made. Conduct an epidemiological investigation of clustered cases in an area or institution to determine source of infection and mode of transmission. A common vehicle should be sought, such as recreational water, drinking water, raw milk, or other potentially contaminated food or drink, or association with a day care center. Institute applicable prevention or control measures. Control of person-to-person or animal-to-person transmission requires special emphasis on personal cleanliness and sanitary disposal of feces.

[M. J. Arrowood, B. Mathison]

# CYCLOSPORIASIS

| DISEASE | ICD-10 CODE |
|---|---|
| CYCLOSPORIASIS | ICD-10 A07.8 |

**1. Clinical features**—An infection of the upper small bowel with a clinical syndrome that consists of watery diarrhea, nausea, anorexia, abdominal cramps, fatigue, myalgia, and weight loss; fever is rare. Persistence of symptoms, with remittance and relapse episodes, is typical: if untreated, diarrhea in the immunocompetent usually lasts for 10–24 days but is self-limited; in the immunocompromised, who appear more susceptible to infection, diarrhea can last for months in some patients. *Cyclospora* infection occurring in individuals who are not treated or not treated promptly is also associated with chronic complications including Guillain-Barré syndrome and Reiter's syndrome. Health care providers should consider the diagnosis of *Cyclospora* infection in persons with prolonged diarrheal illness and should request stool specimens so that specific tests for this parasite can be made.

**2. Causative agents**—*Cyclospora cayetanensis*, a coccidian protozoan.

**3. Laboratory diagnosis**—*C. cayetanensis* is primarily diagnosed by finding oocysts during the microscopic examination of stool. Nucleic acid-based assays, such as real-time polymerase chain reaction (PCR), are available for cyclosporiasis, and there are commercial molecular platforms that include *Cyclospora* in their intestinal panels (e.g., FilmArray Gastrointestinal Panel, BioFire Diagnostics, Salt Lake City, UT).

Oocysts of *C. cayetanensis* are spherical and measure 8–10 µm in diameter. They are unsporulated (immature, noninfectious) when passed in human stool and usually contain refractile globular cytoplasm. *C. cayetanensis* does not stain consistently with conventional stains for routine ova and parasite examinations, such as trichrome stain. Specialty stains such as the modified hot safranin, Kinyoun's modified acid-fast (MAF), and auramine O fluorescent stain can be used to enhance detection. Oocysts stain variably with Kinyoun's MAF, and many oocysts may not take up the stain and appear colorless (ghost forms). The hot safranin method yields more consistently stained oocysts but is sometimes accompanied by higher background issues. Oocysts on permanent stained smears will often have a wrinkled or ground-glass appearance to the oocyst wall. Oocysts in wet mounts may be easily overlooked due to their small size and having few defined morphologic features. *Cyclospora* oocysts autofluoresce under ultraviolet (UV) light illumination in wet mount preparations and detection is enhanced by using a fluorescence microscope with a UV filter set (340–380 nm excitation filter, 420 nm barrier filter, typically used with the nuclear stain

4',6-diamidino-2-phenylindole[DAPI]). This autofluorescence phenomenon occurs in many other protozoan cysts and some helminth eggs, and may be employed for rapid screening of intestinal parasites after brightfield scan of ova and parasite (O&P) wet mount slide preparations.

There are no serologic assays (i.e., antibody detection) for routine clinical diagnosis of cyclosporiasis.

**4. Laboratory capability**—Microscopy, stool concentration/centrifugation, and permanent staining capabilities should be available. Laboratorians should be trained in the microscopic/morphologic detection of parasites and undergo regular proficiency testing. Laboratories that perform immunofluorescence assays typically use common filter sets for visualizing targets labeled with fluorescent dyes (e.g., fluorescein [green], rhodamine [red], or similar). The UV or DAPI filter set is less commonly installed in fluorescence microscopes but can be added as a one-time purchase at modest cost.

Laboratorians trained in performing nucleic acid-based diagnostic assays are needed for molecular detection of cyclosporiasis. Specific equipment required will depend on the type of assay selected (e.g., standard thermocycler, real-time PCR thermocycler or multiplex molecular platform). Deoxyribonucleic acid (DNA) extraction processes should include a step for mechanical disruption (e.g., bead beating) of the tough oocysts to ensure release of the DNA. A unidirectional workflow should be implemented to reduce risk of false-positive results because of amplicon contamination.

**5. Safety requirements**—Clinical specimens should always be collected and handled with universal/standard precautions. *C. cayetanensis* is a biosafety level 2 organism. Oocysts are not immediately infective when shed in stool but may sporulate over time. The factors affecting sporulation and infectivity are not well understood, and precautions should be taken when handling specimens that may contain sporulated oocysts. Formalin should only be used in a well-ventilated area, preferably in a chemical fume hood. Scant data are available for the persistence of oocyst viability and infectivity in standard stool fixative/preservatives, consequently unpreserved and preserved stools should be disposed of as infectious waste.

**6. Nonhuman hosts**—Unknown. Several other *Cyclospora* spp. are known to infect primates; whether this is the case for *C. cayetanensis* is still unclear. No compelling evidence of zoonotic transmission has been reported.

**7. Sample/specimen requirements**—Stool should be promptly preserved in a liquid medium appropriate for microscopical examination. Single vial alcohol-based systems for O&P collection are also appropriate (e.g., EcoFix, Meridian Bioscience, Cincinnati, OH; TotalFix, Medical Chemical Corporation, Torrance, CA). If nucleic acid-based assays are to be utilized, stool may be left unpreserved or placed in a medium that is acceptable for molecular detection (i.e., lacking formalin or mercury). To maximize microscopy sensitivity, up to 3 separate stool specimens should be collected on different days.

**8. Testing requirements**—Diagnostic assays are based on identification of the parasite (whole organism or nucleic acids) in stool as no culture methods for diagnosis are available. Microscopical assays typically include routine concentration procedures (e.g., formalin ethyl acetate sedimentation) and permanent staining of stool or immediate examination of wet mounts under UV illumination. A calibrated ocular micrometer should be used to measure oocyst size. Diagnosis is confirmatory in specimens meeting morphologic criteria in laboratories with appropriate training; however, nucleic acid-based assays are more suitable for confirmation of diagnosis.

Molecular diagnosis can be useful for clarification of suspicious microscopy findings and for providing a more sensitive detection, especially compared with brightfield microscopy. For in-house assays, cutoff values for what should be considered a positive result should be established based on a laboratory-specific validation using known positives and negatives.

**9. Reporting requirements**—Reporting requirements/criteria vary by country and local jurisdiction. In jurisdictions where formal reporting mechanisms are not yet established, clinicians and laboratory workers who identify cases of cyclosporiasis are encouraged to inform the appropriate health departments. In the USA, cyclosporiasis (confirmed and probable) is included in the National Notifiable Diseases Surveillance System. Positive cases from humans may be reported as *C. cayetanensis*.

**10. Referral network**—None.

**11. Special considerations**—Institute an epidemiological investigation of clustered cases in an area or institution to determine source of infection and mode of transmission. A common vehicle, such as water or food should be sought; institute applicable preventive or control measures. While direct person-to-person transmission is unusual with cyclosporiasis, the sanitary disposal of feces is nevertheless important as a control measure.

[M. J. Arrowood, Y. Qvarnstrom, D. Mathison]

# DENGUE

(dengue fever, dengue hemorrhagic fever/dengue shock syndrome, severe dengue)

| DISEASE | ICD-10 CODE |
|---|---|
| DENGUE FEVER | ICD-10 A90 |
| DENGUE HEMORRHAGIC FEVER | ICD-10 A91 |

**1. Clinical features**—Dengue is a mild to moderately severe acute febrile illness that usually follows 3 phases: febrile, critical, and convalescent. Patients with dengue often have sudden onset of fever, which lasts for 2–7 days and may be biphasic. Other signs and symptoms include intense headache, myalgia, arthralgia, bone pain, retro-orbital pain, anorexia, vomiting, macular or maculopapular rash, and minor hemorrhagic manifestations, including petechiae, ecchymosis, purpura, epistaxis, bleeding gums, hematuria, or a positive tourniquet test. Some patients have injected oropharynx and facial erythema in the first 24–48 hours after onset. Warning signs of progression to severe dengue occur in the late febrile phase, around the time of defervescence, and include persistent vomiting, severe abdominal pain, mucosal bleeding, difficulty breathing, signs of hypovolemic shock, and rapid decline in platelet count with an increase in hematocrit (hemoconcentration).

The critical phase of dengue begins at defervescence and typically lasts 24–48 hours. Most patients clinically improve during this phase, but those with significant plasma leakage develop severe dengue as a result of a marked increase in vascular permeability. Initially, physiologic compensatory mechanisms maintain adequate circulation, which narrows pulse pressure as diastolic blood pressure increases. Patients may appear to be well despite early signs of shock. However, once hypotension develops, systolic blood pressure rapidly declines, and irreversible shock and death may ensue despite resuscitation. Patients with severe plasma leakage have pleural effusions or ascites, hypoproteinemia, and hemoconcentration. Patients can also develop hemorrhagic manifestations, including severe frank hemorrhage, hematemesis, hematochezia, melena, or menorrhagia, especially if they have prolonged shock. Patients with severe dengue may also present clinically as hepatitis, myocarditis, pancreatitis, and encephalitis.

The convalescent phase begins when plasma leakage subsides, and extravasated fluids (pleural, abdominal) reabsorb, hemodynamic status stabilizes, and diuresis ensues. The hematocrit stabilizes or may fall because of the dilutional effect of the reabsorbed fluid, and the white cell count usually starts to rise, followed by a slow recovery of platelet count. Patients may develop a generalized erythematous rash with circular areas of nonerythematous skin. This convalescent-phase rash may desquamate and be pruritic.

Laboratory findings commonly include leucopenia, thrombocytopenia, hyponatremia, elevated aspartate aminotransferase and alanine aminotransferase, and a normal erythrocyte sedimentation rate. Some patients may have an elevated partial thromboplastin time and a decreased fibrinogen level (with a normal prothrombin time).

Differential diagnosis includes chikungunya and other epidemiologically relevant diseases listed under "Arboviral Fevers"; influenza; measles; rubella; malaria; leptospirosis; melioidosis, typhoid; scrub typhus; and other systemic febrile illnesses, especially those accompanied by rash.

Dengue hemorrhagic fever and dengue shock syndrome are now classified as subsets of severe dengue according to the 2009 WHO Guidelines. Timely identification of dengue patients with warning signs is critical to ensure proper anticipatory guidance and initiation of supportive treatment. Severe dengue can occur in both children and adults.

**2. Causative agents**—Dengue viruses (DENV) are flaviviruses and include 4 types (serotypes; DENV-1, -2, -3, -4). All 4 DENV serotypes can cause dengue and have been associated with severe dengue, including dengue hemorrhagic fever/dengue shock syndrome with a fatal outcome. It is important to note, however, that the majority (~75%) of DENV infections are asymptomatic in both children and adults. Long-term, serotype-specific protective immunity is produced by infection with each serotype, but there is no long-term, cross-protective immunity following infection. An increased risk of severe dengue is associated with the presence of heterotypic antibody and with viral strains that have greater virulence and/or epidemic potential. DENV serotypes can be further defined into genotypes based on differences in the envelope gene sequence; molecular epidemiologic studies may assist in tracking disease transmission patterns.

**3. Laboratory diagnosis**—Laboratory confirmation of the clinical diagnosis of dengue can be made using a single serum specimen obtained during the febrile phase of the illness (days 0–7 after onset of fever) with diagnostic testing to detect DENV and immunoglobulin class M (IgM) anti-DENV. DENV viremia occurs for 5–6 days before and after fever onset. Molecular diagnostics by nucleic acid amplification, such as by reverse transcription polymerase chain reaction (RT-PCR), can detect DENV ribonucleic acid (RNA) with a higher sensitivity than virus isolation by cell culture, and multiplex RT-PCR provides serotype-specific results. Molecular diagnostics are now available in many dengue endemic areas. DENV can also be detected by an immunoassay for the nonstructural protein 1 (NS1) antigen; a soluble antigen present during the viremic period. While somewhat less sensitive than DENV detection by RT-PCR, NS1 antigen detection tests have become commercially available in many dengue endemic areas. Detection of IgM anti-DENV in the febrile phase may indicate a current or recent DENV infection, or in some settings, infection with another flavivirus because of antibody cross-reactivity. Immunoglobulin class M anti-DENV becomes detectable in about 30% of dengue patients on the third day after fever onset and in almost all patients 6–7 days after fever onset. Immunoglobulin class M capture anti-DENV enzyme-linked immunosorbent assay (ELISA) testing is widely available, and evaluation studies have identified commercially available microplate tests with high sensitivity and specificity and low cross-reactivity with other flaviviruses.

Testing for IgG anti-DENV is not useful for dengue diagnosis since a high proportion of persons in endemic areas have preexisting, cross-reactive IgG antibody from previous DENV infections (secondary DENV infection).

**4. Laboratory capability**—Diagnostic tests for dengue require differing laboratory capabilities. NS1 antigen immunochromatography tests can be used as bedside point-of-care tests. They contain a sample flow control to help ensure that the test strip has been used correctly and can be used by unskilled staff outside laboratory settings. However, such rapid diagnostic tests tend to have lower sensitivity and specificity characteristics than assays that can only be performed in a laboratory.

Enzyme-linked immunosorbent assays for dengue antibodies, or NS1 antigen and real-time RT-PCR assays for dengue RNA, require a functioning laboratory with trained staff and robust quality assurance processes. In most countries, real-time RT-PCR is only performed in specialist centers with access to a functional molecular laboratory. A variety of molecular methods including RT-PCR and sequencing can be used to establish dengue serotype, but, as this is only necessary for epidemiological and research purposes, typing is rarely performed outside national reference laboratories. However, it is essential to maintain this capability in endemic areas to enable rapid detection of outbreaks caused by new dengue serotypes.

**5. Safety requirements**—In the USA and Canada, dengue is categorised as a risk group 2 organism based on its ability to cause human disease, mitigated by the fact that it is unlikely to pose a serious risk to laboratory workers or the wider community. Dengue should be handled in a biosafety level 2 (BSL-2) laboratory by staff trained in handling infectious pathogenic agents. Procedures which generate aerosol or splash should be performed in a biosafety cabinet. Viral culture of dengue should be conducted in a BSL-3 facility because of the possibility of generating high concentrations of virus.

Note that European guidelines classify dengue as a risk/hazard group 3 organism on the basis of it being able to cause severe disease, and therefore, potentially posing a serious hazard to employees. However, local risk assessment may allow for initial diagnostic work on primary samples that potentially contain dengue virus being performed in a BSL-2 laboratory.

**6. Nonhuman hosts**—No animal hosts have been identified.

**7. Sample/specimen requirements**—A fresh serum sample is the most appropriate specimen on which to perform dengue serology. Either serum or plasma is suitable for molecular diagnostics. Other specimen types may occasionally be tested using molecular assays, for instance, post-mortem tissue samples, provided the assay used has been validated for the relevant sample type.

The timing of samples is important. The form that accompanies the specimen should contain pertinent details including date of symptom onset and specimen collection together with clinical symptoms and salient travel history with dates. This allows accurate interpretation of results.

Diagnostic samples for dengue virus testing can be transported as category B infectious substances. The primary receptacle should be surrounded by absorbent material inside a secondary leak-proof receptacle, which should be contained in the appropriately labeled outer packaging. Staff need to be trained and certified in national packaging and shipping requirements. If virus culture is to be attempted, it is important to keep blood samples refrigerated or frozen to −20°C in order to preserve the viability of the virus throughout transport from the patient to the laboratory. However, for routine diagnostic testing, samples can usually be transported to the laboratory at ambient temperature.

**8. Testing requirements**—For hospitalized patients, a correct diagnosis of dengue is essential to optimize clinical care and, in areas where the mosquito vector is present, to support disease control activities. Other viral infections such as chikungunya and Zika may present with a similar clinical syndrome, and, as the global distribution of these viruses overlap in many areas, it is prudent to test for all 3 diseases in patients with an appropriate geographical exposure.

The virus can be directly detected by RT-PCR or by detection of viral antigen, both of which confirm a diagnosis of acute dengue but cannot differentiate between primary and secondary episodes of dengue. Real-time RT-PCR is extremely sensitive in the first 4 to 5 days of illness with diagnostic sensitivity and specificity values usually over 98%. The limit of detection in these assays is typically around $10^3$ plaque forming units/mL.[1] It is therefore the optimal method of early diagnosis, and results can be obtained within 6 hours. In areas in which other arboviruses such as Zika virus and chikungunya are endemic, multiplex assays that distinguish between these infections are very valuable. RT-PCR methods can also be used to distinguish between the various serotypes, which is useful for epidemiological investigations. However, RT-PCR is expensive, requires a fully functional molecular laboratory with quality assurance controls, and requires laboratory staff with considerable expertise.

The most commonly used viral antigen tests detect NS1 antigen, which is detectable for the first 5–6 days of clinical illness. NS1 ELISA sensitivity ranges from 45%–57% with a specificity of 93%–100%.[2] Rapid immunochromatography tests are easier to perform and yield results in less than 1 hour but are likely to be less sensitive and specific.

The most widely used serological tests are IgG/IgM ELISAs, although commercial rapid immunochromatography tests are also available. In primary dengue infection (i.e., in an individual who has not previously been infected with or immunized against a flavivirus infection), IgM becomes positive around day 4 of clinical illness and remains positive for up to 90 days. Dengue IgG becomes positive around day 7 of clinical illness and remains positive for many months and probably for life; however, in an individual with a second dengue infection, dengue IgM may fail to become detectable, while dengue IgG rises to high titer very rapidly. As with all flaviviruses, there is considerable serological cross-reactivity; therefore, positive dengue antibody tests alone will usually only confirm a diagnosis of recent dengue infection if recent exposure to other flavivirus antigens (including yellow fever vaccine and Zika virus infection) can be excluded serologically. Enzyme-linked immunosorbent assays are cheap, relatively easy to perform, and highly amenable to automation for high throughput.

Neutralizing assays such as the plaque reduction and neutralisation test can be used when a serotype-specific serological diagnosis is required. However, these assays are difficult to standardize and require considerable technical infrastructure and expertise. Therefore, they are not amenable for routine diagnostic use.

Virus isolation in cell culture usually takes several days and similarly can only be performed in laboratories with the necessary infrastructure and technical expertise. Therefore, this technique too is used predominantly for research rather than for diagnosis.

External quality assurance schemes are available for RT-PCR, antigen detection, and serology.

RT-PCR or NS1 antigen testing is particularly recommended within the first 5 days of illness. In patients presenting after day 5 of illness, serological tests should be performed, preferably with a convalescent sample 14 days after symptoms begin. Dengue diagnostics are often only available at regional or national reference laboratories. Local laboratories should have standard operating procedures and protocols for referral of samples to these laboratories.

**9. Reporting requirements**—Dengue is a nationally notifiable disease in the USA. Clinical cases should be reported to CDC in accordance with Council of State and Territorial Epidemiologist's case definitions. State health departments should report laboratory confirmed cases to the National Surveillance System for Arboviral Disease.

WHO collects data from member states including the number of suspected and confirmed dengue cases, number of deaths from dengue, and the serotype in circulation. Changes in dengue activity, such as a case of locally acquired dengue in an area previously free of dengue, should be reported by the responsible national agency to WHO.

**10. Referral network**—Dengue diagnostics are often only available at regional or national reference laboratories. Local laboratories should have standard operating procedures and protocols in place for referral of samples to these laboratories and should have means of accessing dengue diagnostics urgently.

**11. Special considerations**—Case definitions are available on the CDC website: https://wwwn.cdc.gov/nndss/conditions/dengue-virus-infections/case-definition/2015.

Extensive additional laboratory guidance is available on the CDC website: https://www.cdc.gov/dengue/clinicallab/laboratory.html.

In the absence of a highly effective vaccine to protect against dengue, people residing or travelling to endemic areas should avoid exposure to *Aedes (Stegomyia) aegypti* by using an effective mosquito repellent such as N,N-Diethyl-meta-toluamide and reducing the amount of skin exposed during daytime hours. Public authorities in endemic areas can reduce infection by controlling *A. aegypti* populations through reducing breeding sites, larval control, and use of insecticide.

## References

1. Centers for Disease Control and Prevention. CDC DENV-1-4 real-time RT-PCR assay. Available at: http://www.cdc.gov/dengue/resources/rt_pcr/CDCPackageInsert.pdf. Accessed June 22, 2018.
2. Blacksell SD, Jarman RG, Gibbons RV, et al. Comparison of seven commercial antigen and antibody enzyme-linked immunosorbent assays for detection of acute dengue infection. *Clin Vaccine Immunol*. 2012;19(5):804–810.

[L. E. B. Nabarro, E. J. Aarons]

# DIPHTHERIA

| DISEASE | ICD-10 CODE |
|---|---|
| DIPHTHERIA | ICD-10 A36 |

**1. Clinical features**—An acute bacterial disease primarily involving the mucous membrane of the upper respiratory tract (nose, tonsils, pharynx, larynx), skin, or rarely other mucous membranes (e.g., conjunctivae, vagina or ear). Inapparent infections (colonization) outnumber clinical cases. The characteristic lesion, caused by reaction to a potent exotoxin, is an asymmetrical adherent greyish white membrane with surrounding inflammation. In moderate to severe cases of respiratory diphtheria, the throat may be moderately to severely sore with enlarged and tender cervical lymph nodes and, together with marked swelling of the neck, can give rise to a bull neck appearance. Pharyngeal membranes may extend into the trachea or progress to cause airway obstruction. Nasal diphtheria can be mild and chronic with one-sided serosanguinous nasal discharge and excoriations. The lesions of cutaneous diphtheria are variable and may be indistinguishable from impetigo. Absorption of diphtheria toxin can lead to myocarditis with heart block and progressive congestive failure beginning about 1 week after onset. Neurologic complications may occur about 2 weeks after onset of illness and include polyneuropathies that can mimic Guillain-Barré syndrome. The case-fatality rate is 5%–10% for respiratory diphtheria even with treatment and has changed little in the past 50 years.

Respiratory diphtheria should be suspected in the differential diagnosis of membranous pharyngitis that includes streptococcal pharyngitis, Vincent angina, infectious mononucleosis, oral syphilis, oral candidiasis, and adenoviruses.

**2. Causative agents**—Toxin-producing strains of the human pathogen *Corynebacterium diphtheriae* and also the zoonotic pathogens, *Corynebacterium ulcerans* and *Corynebacterium pseudotuberculosis*. There are 4 biovars of *C. diphtheriae*: gravis, mitis, intermedius, and belfanti. Toxin production results when bacteria are infected by corynebacteriophage containing the diphtheria toxin gene *tox*. Nontoxigenic strains may cause sore throat but rarely produce membranous lesions; however, they are increasingly associated with infective endocarditis.

**3. Laboratory diagnosis**—Presumptive diagnosis is based on observation of an asymmetrical, adherent grayish membrane associated with tonsillitis, pharyngitis, or a serosanguinous nasal discharge. The diagnosis is confirmed by bacteriological examination of lesions. If respiratory diphtheria is strongly suspected, specific treatment with antitoxin and antibiotics should be initiated without awaiting laboratory confirmation by culture and continues even if the laboratory report is negative. Delay in starting treatment is associated with increased risk for complications and death.

**4. Laboratory capability**—The main aim of the laboratory is to provide rapid, specific, and reliable methods to confirm a clinical diagnosis of diphtheria. In advanced stages of the disease, a clinical diagnosis normally precedes the microbiologic diagnosis. The laboratory will also aid the clinician by eliminating suspected cases or contacts of diphtheria from further investigation, thus avoiding unnecessary treatment or control measures such as isolation. Guidelines for the laboratory diagnosis have been published and are being revised to include novel and up-to-date methods.[1] Personnel should have received specialized training in diphtheria diagnostics ideally through the various workshops that are held via the WHO Collaborating Centre for Reference and Research on Diphtheria or under the auspices of the various networks such as the European Diphtheria Surveillance Network (EDSN) and the WHO/European Laboratory Working Group on Diphtheria (ELWGD) or equivalent training. Training is key in maintaining awareness and microbiologic expertise particularly in countries where the disease is perceived to be rare. It is crucial to maintain laboratory capability in this specialized area via training workshops and external quality assurance (EQA) programs for microbiologic diagnosis and seroprevalence.

Ideally a laboratory skilled in testing for diphtheria should have adequate space to safely perform all activities and is usually within a state or government center or institute or is recognized as qualified to test for diphtheria by the country's ministry of health or equivalent. There should be sufficient infrastructure and management to allow enough space to separate infectious from noninfectious work (e.g., the culture of *Corynebacterium* vs. serology). Testing for diphtheria toxin requires special reference laboratory capabilities and expertise.

**5. Safety requirements**—The potentially toxigenic corynebacteria, notably *C. diphtheriae, C. ulcerans*, and *C. pseudotuberculosis*, are designated as hazard group 2 pathogens requiring containment biosafety level 2 facilities, equipment, and operational practices for work involving infected or potentially infected materials, animals, or cultures. Each laboratory should have available their own safety manual which should describe the essential biosafety, chemical, fire, and electrical safety requirements to protect staff, the community, and the environment. All staff should be familiar with the manual and should proceed accordingly. All new staff should be made aware of the risks involved in working in a diphtheria laboratory before starting work and are required to have read the manual, the standard operating protocols, safety protocols, and risk assessments. It is advisable that all laboratory staff handling potentially toxigenic corynebacteria have immunity levels greater than 0.1 IU/mL, and that these levels must be monitored and checked by the gold standard serology vero cell assay every 3 years.

All laboratory procedures that may produce aerosols or involve high concentrations or large volumes should be conducted in a biological safety cabinet. The use of needles, syringes, and other sharp objects should be strictly limited. Additional precautions should be considered with work involving animals or large-scale activities.

For transportation, human samples and cultures of potentially toxigenic corynebacteria are classified as category B (UN3373) biological substances.

**6. Nonhuman hosts**—The 2 zoonotic species that can produce diphtheria toxin are *C. ulcerans* and *C. pseudotuberculosis. C. ulcerans* was originally associated with unpasteurized dairy products or rural farm contact with animals, such as cattle. It has been identified as an infrequent cause of bovine mastitis, and raw milk has been recognized as a source of human infection. In the last few years, *C. ulcerans* has also been recovered from clinically affected and healthy wild and domesticated animal species including cats (chronic rhinitis), dogs (chronic labial ulceration, sneezing and rhinorrhea), horses, goats, pigs, and many others. Diphtheria in humans caused by *C. ulcerans* has been documented by several countries where diphtheria incidence is low, in addition to reports of transmission between humans and companion pets. *C. pseudotuberculosis* causes caseous lymphadenitis in sheep and goats, ulcerative lymphadenitis in cattle and horses, and also external and internal abscesses in horses. However, it is a rare cause of human disease and usually produces a localized suppurative granulomatous lymphadenitis with a long and recurrent course. It is usually an occupational disease of shepherds, abattoir workers, and butchers with infection believed to occur through cuts. Consumption of unpasteurized milk can also be a risk for human infection.

7. **Sample/specimen requirements**—The successful isolation of *C. diphtheriae* and other potentially toxigenic strains is dependent upon the collection of specimens and their transfer to the laboratory. As diphtheria is most commonly an upper respiratory tract infection, throat, ear, nasopharyngeal, and/or nasal swabs should be taken. If present, membranous material should also be examined. In cases of cutaneous infection, swabs should be taken from any wounds or skin lesions. Postmortem specimens from the upper respiratory tract and vital organs may be examined in extreme cases where autopsy is required to confirm the cause of death as diphtheria. After collection, the swabs, ideally cotton tipped, must be sent to the laboratory immediately, as rapid inoculation of special culture media is important. At the same time, the clinician should inform the laboratory of any presumptive diagnosis of diphtheria. Animals with pyogenic skin and visceral lesions should be investigated for evidence of infection with *C. ulcerans* and *C. pseudotuberculosis*. Nasal and/or oropharyngeal swabs, and swabs from skin lesions should be collected depending upon the clinical signs displayed. Where there is evidence of clinical or subclinical (i.e., elevated milk somatic cell counts) mastitis, individual or pooled quarter milk samples are aseptically taken from the affected animals. *C. pseudotuberculosis* may be confirmed by culture of lymph node, lung, or swab from the outer portion of the abscess. Culture of aspirated abscess contents may also be attempted in the live animal using a sterile needle through shaved, disinfected skin, thus avoiding contamination of the environment. If specimens cannot be transported to the laboratory immediately, the use of a transport medium such as Amies should be considered; it is commercially available. If transit times are to exceed 24 hours, the use of a silica gel transport medium should be considered.[2] Silica gel packs are very useful and will work at room temperature;

therefore, there is no requirement for dry ice, and they are less expensive to transport.

**8. Testing requirements**—The potentially toxigenic corynebacteria can be difficult to diagnose as they are not easily identified on primary culture. Clinical specimens are usually cultured onto blood and tellurite agars, followed by screening tests such as cystinase (i.e., Tinsdale medium) and pyrazinamidase.[1] See the figure later in this chapter. Species identification and biovars of *C. diphtheriae* (gravis, mitis, intermedius, belfanti) are biochemically identified using commercial kits and in more developed countries using new technologies such as the matrix-assisted laser desorption/ionization time-of-flight mass spectrometry. This is based upon the protein composition of microbial cells, and the method allows rapid and reliable identification of clinically relevant and potentially toxigenic corynebacteria provided that a quality-controlled database of reference spectra is available.[3] However, bio vars cannot be differentiated, and toxigenicity of the organism is not detected. Therefore, full identification and toxigenicity testing is still required and performed in the National Diphtheria Reference or specialist laboratory within each country or referred to the WHO Collaborating Centre for Reference and Research on Diphtheria (see Referral Network section in this chapter).

The key test for laboratory diagnosis of diphtheria is the detection of the lethal diphtheria toxin, undertaken only by specialized laboratories. The Elek immunoprecipitation test is the standard reference test for toxin detection that is the expression of a biologically active protein. The conventional Elek test was first described in 1949, and a modified version was introduced in the late 1990s. Polymerase chain reaction (PCR) technologies have considerably contributed towards the timeliness of diphtheria diagnostics with the rapid detection of the toxin gene. More recently, the development of real-time PCR assays has allowed an even faster turnaround time; however, occasionally *C. diphtheriae* strains are detected that possess the *tox* gene but do not express the active protein. Therefore, PCR alone cannot provide definitive results for clinical purposes and should only be used in combination with the Elek test. However, a positive PCR result is a good indicator to initiate control and public health measures.

Quality assurance is essential for all laboratory procedures but in particular for specialized areas such as diphtheria diagnostics. Diphtheria diagnostic schemes, in particular EQA, provide significant benefit to the majority of laboratories. All tests require careful validation with the use of appropriate controls. External quality assurance programs for diphtheria diagnostics have been in place since 2001, coordinated by the International/European global network. Similar diphtheria EQA programs should be in place in other settings where diphtheria testing is performed. The results have clearly demonstrated the importance of regular training along with EQA programs to all countries globally to maintain laboratory capacities and awareness.

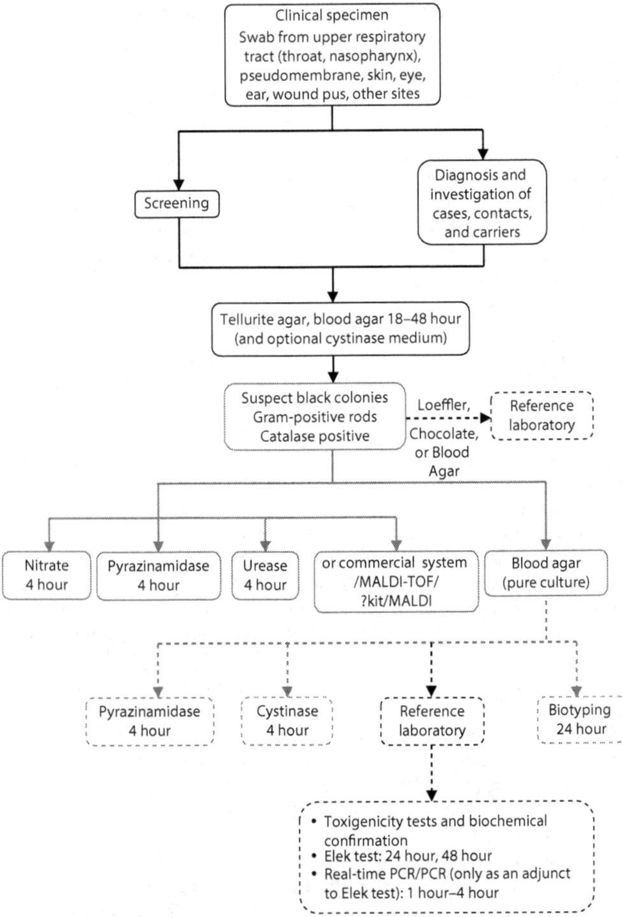


*Note:* MALDI-TOF = matrix-assisted laser desorption/ionization time-of-flight.

**Algorithm for the Laboratory Diagnosis of Diphtheria**

As the morbidity of diphtheria is almost entirely due to diphtheria toxin, protection against disease is dependent on antibodies against the toxin. Accurate determination of diphtheria antibodies is essential to obtain reliable information on the immune status of a given population and allows for the identification of susceptible individuals to facilitate the provision of recommendations for vaccination policies and schedules. It is therefore of critical importance to have serologic methods that are accurate, reproducible, specific, and sensitive. The vero cell Toxin Neutralization assay (TNT) is the recommended in vitro method. This is undertaken by only a few laboratories globally as it is time consuming and requires cell culture facilities. Diagnostic laboratories prefer to use simple format indirect enzyme-linked immunosorbent assays (ELISA), which offer significant advantages in terms of cost, speed, ease of use, and automation. However, they are not as accurate as the TNT and vary according to manufacturer, so the use of ELISA kits needs to be carefully considered as there are intrinsic problems related to the nature of these assays.[4]

**9. Reporting requirements**—Upon isolation of a toxigenic strain of *C. diphtheriae*, *C. ulcerans*, or *C. pseudotuberculosis* from a human, the following personnel must be informed immediately:

1) The clinician responsible for the case.
2) The local public health physician.
3) The local consultant for the control of communicable diseases.
4) The national communicable disease surveillance unit.

Veterinary or reference laboratories isolating the zoonotic species from animal sources should also consider the public health risks from zoonotic transmission and inform the veterinary practitioner as early as possible.

**10. Referral network**—The European Laboratory Working Group on Diphtheria (ELWGD) was established at the request of the WHO Regional Office for Europe in 1993 in response to the devastating epidemics of diphtheria in the former Soviet Union. ELWGD comprised selected representatives from different diphtheria reference centers in France, Finland, Germany, Russia, Romania, Ukraine, the UK, and the USA. The aims of ELWGD were to assess laboratory capabilities, develop laboratory guidelines, and outline future study needs. The group now encompasses more than 40 countries globally. In 2003, a European dedicated surveillance network of microbiologists and key epidemiologists responsible for diphtheria within their country was established as the Diphtheria Surveillance Network (DIPNET) and continued until 2010, when the network transferred to the European Centre for Disease Control and Prevention (ECDC) as the EDSN. In 1998, the WHO Collaborating Centre for Reference and Research on Diphtheria and Streptococcal Infections was designated by WHO and continues to be the main and only WHO reference center for these pathogens globally. The Centre is hosted within Public Health England. Full contact and terms of reference can be found at: http://apps.who.int/whocc/Detail.aspx?cc_ref=UNK-194&cc_code=unk. The WHO Reference Centre, along with some of the specialized laboratories within the network, can also provide molecular subtyping methods that will allow the identification of clonal groups and epidemiologically related strains, thus providing information on their geographic origin. Various typing methods have been evaluated, and new methods have been developed over the years for the potentially toxigenic corynebacteria. During the 1998-mid-2002 period, ribotyping was deemed as the gold standard for molecular characterization. The method was standardized globally, and an international database exists and is hosted by Public Health England (http://www.dipnet.org). More recently multilocus sequence typing is being increasingly used for these pathogens, and a database exists encompassing a large collection of strains (http://www.pubmlst.org/cdiphtheriae).

**11. Special considerations**—If a contact is positive for toxigenic *C. diphtheriae*, the person will require full treatment and follow-up cultures as per symptomatic cases. Infection control measures should be implemented (i.e., isolation with standard, contact, and droplet precautions) until 2 cultures (taken at least 24 hours apart) from both nose and throat taken more than 24 hours after completing antibiotic therapy are negative for *C. diphtheriae.* Disinfection of toys, pacifiers, and other fomites that the patient used or touched should also be done. However, it is imperative to refer cultures of the organism as rapidly as possible to the relevant laboratory for toxigenicity testing. Veterinary practitioners attending the animals should discuss possible zoonotic hazards with the animal owners so that they may take appropriate measures to minimize the risk. The 2005 International Health Regulations state the requirements for international reporting of diphtheria cases according to the official case definition to WHO and also to ECDC (for European member states only). The disease is notifiable in all countries, and once a case has been identified, the following procedures should be actioned: (a) conduct a detailed case investigation, (b) identify contacts, conduct laboratory investigation of close contacts and eligible at-risk contacts, and (c) administer chemoprophylaxis to close contacts and at-risk contacts. Cases are classified as possible, probable, or confirmed according to the EU case definition; the WHO case definition classifies cases as suspected, probable, and confirmed. In all instances, a confirmed case would be the isolation of toxigenic *C. diphtheriae* from respiratory diphtheria (WHO) or the isolation of toxigenic *C. diphtheriae*, *C. ulcerans,* or *C. pseudotuberculosis* (EU) from all forms of diphtheria (e.g., respiratory, cutaneous). The infectious dose of toxin for susceptible humans and animals is 0.1 μg/kg bodyweight.

Biological risk assessments to assess exposure and deliberate release should be undertaken by each laboratory. In such circumstances, the measures to be taken are to thoroughly disinfect the exposed area using a spill kit with fresh 10,000 ppm hypochlorite solution or presept granules (disinfectant granules that are effervescent containing the active ingredient sodium dichloroisocyanurate; they react with water in blood spillages to produce a rapid acting, broad spectrum disinfectant effective against vegetative bacteria, fungi, viruses, and bacterial spores) for all biological spillages and disinfection of blood and body fluids and 70% ethyl alcohol to wipe benches and cabinet surfaces. Provide antibiotic therapy for postexposure prophylaxis and/or if infection occurs, in addition to considering antitoxin therapy. The person must be reviewed by occupational health and an infectious disease specialist.

## References

1. Efstratiou A, Maple PAC; World Health Organization. Laboratory diagnosis of diphtheria. 1994. Available at: http://apps.who.int/iris/handle/10665/108108. Accessed June 23, 2018.
2. Facklam RR, Lawrence DN, Sottnek FO. Modified culture technique for *Corynebacterium diphtheriae* isolation from desiccated swabs. *J Clin Microbiol.* 1978; 7(2):137-138.
3. Konrad R, Berger A, Huber I, et al. Matrix-assisted laser desorption/ionisation time-of-flight (MALDI-TOF) mass spectrometry as a tool for rapid diagnosis of potentially toxigenic *Corynebacterium* species in the laboratory management of diphtheria-associated bacteria. *Euro Surveill.* 2010;15(43):pii:19699.
4. Di Giovine P, Pinto A, Olander RM, et al. External quality assessment for the determination of diphtheria antitoxin in human serum. *Clin Vaccine Immunol.* 2010;17(8):1282-1290.

[A. Efstratiou]

# DRACUNCULIASIS

| DISEASE | ICD-10 CODE |
|---|---|
| DRACUNCULIASIS | ICD-10 B72 |

**1. Clinical features**—An infection of the subcutaneous and deeper tissues by a large nematode. A blister appears, often on a lower extremity (especially the foot) when the gravid, adult (60-100 cm long) female worm is ready to discharge its larvae. Burning and itching of the skin in the area of the lesion and, frequently, fever, nausea, vomiting, diarrhea, dizziness, generalized urticaria, and eosinophilia may accompany or precede vesicle formation. After the vesicle ruptures, the worm discharges larvae whenever the affected part is immersed in fresh water. The prognosis is good unless bacterial infection of the lesion occurs; such secondary infections may produce arthritis, synovitis, ankylosis, and contractures of the involved limb. Tetanus infections may occur via the site of the lesion. Infection may be life threatening as a result of complications from secondary infections.

**2. Causative agents**—*Dracunculus medinensis*, a nematode.

**3. Laboratory diagnosis**—Diagnosis is generally by visual inspection of the adult worm recovered from a skin lesion by a qualified reference laboratory. *Onchocerca volvulus* has been reported as presenting in similar manner to *D. medinensis* and thus correct morphologic identification of worms protruding from skin in endemic areas is indicated. *Dracunculus* can also be identified by microscopic identification of larvae within a worm specimen. Definitive species identification may be achieved by a published polymerase chain reaction (PCR) targeting the *D. medinensis* 18s rRNA gene, though this method is considered as being for research use only. Crude antigen from adult *D. medinensis* has been used to prepare an immunofluorescence assay serology test. This test showed a sensitivity of 97% and a specificity of 92% for the detection of patent infection (worms emerging from the skin); cross-reaction occurred with some *O. volvulus* infected persons.

**4. Laboratory capability**—Due to the significance of any identified infection in the context of attempts for global eradication, tertiary level reference facilities should be consulted for any diagnosis of human dracunculiasis.

**5. Safety requirements**—Physical containment 2 or biosafety level 2 for cultures of larval stage 3 (L3) larva-infected copepods. L1 larva directly released from adults are not infective.

**6. Nonhuman hosts**—Natural definitive hosts are humans and dogs. There are reports of natural infection in cats and baboons. Experimental infections in dogs, monkeys, and cats have been successful. Intermediate hosts are fresh water copepods (various genera including *Thermocyclops*, *Mesocyclops*, and others). Frogs and some primitive fish may act as natural paratenic hosts.

**7. Sample/specimen requirements**—For morphological identification, adult worm preserved in 70% ethanol or other fixative, not formalin as PCR, should be performed to definitively identify species. For serology, serum or plasma.

**8. Testing requirements**—Morphological identification of adults should be performed by highly experienced reference laboratories. Due to the significance of infection in the context of the global eradication campaign, it is recommended that any specimen should be confirmed by PCR.

**9. Reporting requirements**—Report exact species based only upon adult worm morphology and molecular identification. Due to the significance of infection in the context of the global eradication campaign, report confirmed cases in the USA to CDC. Outside the USA report to the national public health authorities as well as WHO.

**10. Referral network**—Networks vary among countries. Highly skilled reference laboratories may perform molecular analysis or morphological species identification of adult worms. CDC DPDx service in the USA will identify adult worms to species level both morphologically and by PCR.

**11. Special considerations**—The identification of any *D. medinensis* infection is highly significant in the context of the global elimination campaign. Any suspect case in the USA should be reported to CDC for further investigation. Any suspect case outside the USA should be reported to WHO.

[R. S. Bradbury]

# EBOLA-MARBURG VIRAL DISEASES

(African hemorrhagic fever, Ebola virus hemorrhagic fever, Marburg virus hemorrhagic fever)

| DISEASE | ICD-10 CODE |
|---|---|
| EBOLA HEMORRHAGIC FEVER | ICD-10 A98.4 |
| MARBURG HEMORRHAGIC FEVER | ICD-10 A98.3 |

**1. Clinical features**—Severe acute viral illnesses, usually with sudden onset of fever, malaise, myalgia and headache, followed in most cases by pharyngitis, vomiting, diarrhea and maculopapular rash. In severe and fatal forms, a hemorrhagic diathesis is often accompanied by hepatic damage, renal failure, central nervous system involvement and terminal shock with multi-organ dysfunction. Laboratory findings usually show lymphopenia, severe thrombocytopenia and transaminase elevation (aspartate aminotransferase [AST] > alanine transferase [ALT]), sometimes with hyperamylasemia, elevated creatinine and blood urea nitrogen levels during the final renal failure phase. Case-fatality rates for Ebola infections in well-studied outbreaks in Africa have ranged from 32% to nearly 88%. In Marburg outbreaks, case-fatality rates have ranged from 22%–90%.

**2. Causative agents**—Ebola and Marburg viruses are negative-stranded ribonucleic acid (RNA) viruses in the family *Filoviridae*. Virions are pleomorphic virions with branched, circular, or coiled shapes; are frequent on electron microscopy preparation; and may reach micrometers in length. Five Ebola virus species have been identified, and viruses in 4 of these (*Zaire ebolavirus*, *Sudan ebolavirus*, *Taï Forest ebolavirus*, and *Bundibugyo ebolavirus*) have been shown to cause disease in humans. Virus from the fifth Ebola species, *Reston ebolavirus*, which originated in the Philippines, causes fatal hemorrhagic disease in nonhuman primates. A single Marburg virus species, *Marburg marburgvirus*, has been identified.

**3. Laboratory diagnosis**—Ebola or Marburg infection can be confirmed in blood or tissue samples by virus isolation, conventional or real-time polymerase chain reaction (PCR), antigen-detection enzyme-linked immunosorbent assay (ELISA), immunohistochemistry on formalin-fixed tissues, or by detection of virus-specific immunoglobulin class M (IgM) antibodies or rising IgG antibody titers. Rapid antigen detection assays are in development. In fatal cases, when blood or tissues are not available, conventional or real-time PCR could be done from oral swabs specimens. The laboratory diagnosis should always be considered in combination with the clinical evaluation and epidemiological investigation.

**4. Laboratory capability**—Clinical specimens from unknown patients suspected of having Ebola or Marburg fever should always be collected and handled with universal/standard precautions, including the use of personal protective equipment. For processing clinical specimens with suspicion of viral hemorrhagic fever, trained personnel with appropriate protocols and containment facilities are mandatory. Molecular and serological techniques should be available. Biohazardous waste management protocols and procedures should be in place.

**5. Safety requirements**—Ebola and Marburg viruses are biosafety level 4 (BSL-4) agents. No human vaccines are currently available. Collection and handling of infectious or suspected infectious clinical specimens should be performed by trained personnel with disposable caps, gowns, shoe covers, surgical gloves, and face masks (N99 or N100 high-efficiency particulate air filters). Procedures generating aerosols (e.g., centrifugation) should be minimized. RNA extraction, using the guanidinium acid-phenol method, which also inactivate the specimen, must be conducted in a laminar-flow safety cabinet or a class III biosafety cabinet. The infectivity of samples may be greatly reduced, if not totally inactivated, by the addition of Triton X-100 and heating, and the samples may be safely tested by serologic or antigen capture assays in the field. Handling of infectious diagnostic specimens should be performed by trained personnel with appropriate BSL-4 facilities. Virus isolation attempt should always be performed in a BSL-4 laboratory.

**6. Nonhuman hosts**—Forest-dwelling fruit bats are believed to be the reservoir of Ebola viruses, and viral RNA has been detected in 3 bat species in central Africa (*Hypsignathus monstrosus*, *Epomops franqueti*, and *Myonycteris torquata*). Cave-dwelling fruit bats are believed to be the reservoir of Marburg virus, and numerous virus isolates have been acquired from a particular species, *Rousettus aegyptiacus*. Ebola and Marburg viruses have been identified in multiple species of nonhuman primates, although these are likely incidental hosts and not reservoirs of these viruses. Swine, responsible for the Ebola Reston virus epidemic in 2008 in the Philippines, are considered to be intermediary hosts.

**7. Sample/specimen requirements**—During acute febrile stages of disease, virus or viral RNA can be detected in serum, heparinized plasma, or whole blood, and serologic techniques can be performed on late acute or convalescent samples of the same type. Virus and viral RNA may also be isolated or detected in biopsy or autopsy specimens from various tissues, including oral swabs collected after death. Diagnostic samples should be stored and shipped frozen, if possible, on dry ice or liquid nitrogen vapor. Viral antigens from tissues, including skin biopsies, can be detected by immunohistochemistry. Formaldehyde-fixed tissue and paraffin-embedded blocks should be stored and shipped at room temperature.

**8. Testing requirements**—Ebola and Marburg virus infections rarely occur. Diagnostic reagents are only available at select reference laboratories. Molecular assays for Ebola virus (*Zaire ebolavirus*) have been made available during the recent West African outbreak, but there are no commercially available assays for the other filoviruses. As for other infectious diseases, the diagnosis should always be based on the results of a combination of clinical and laboratory data. During acute febrile stages of disease, virus can be detected by conventional or real-time PCR (detection of 2 genes targets is considered optimal) or virus isolation followed by sequencing. In late acute and convalescent stages, IgM or IgG antibodies can be detected by ELISA. Antibodies are cross-reactive between the different Ebola species, but no cross-reaction has been seen between Ebola and Marburg antibodies. Virus antigens can be detected by immunohistochemistry in tissue samples collected post-mortem. Direct detection of virus, viral antigens, IgM or IgG antibodies in an individual with a clinically compatible illness or an individual with a known high-risk exposure to the virus constitutes a confirmed case.

**9. Reporting requirements**—Ebola and Marburg virus infections in the USA are reportable as "viral hemorrhagic fever" by guidelines of the Council of State and Territorial Epidemiologists. Suspected cases should be reported to the local and state health authorities and CDC through the National Notifiable Diseases Surveillance System. If Ebola or Marburg hemorrhagic fever is suspected, contact the CDC Viral Special Pathogens Branch by phone (470-312-0094 or 404-639-1115; after hours, 770-488-7100) or e-mail (spather@cdc.gov). Isolation of Ebola or Marburg viruses (tier 1 select agents) must be reported to the Federal Select Agent Program in the USA. Laboratorians in countries other than the USA should confirm what laboratory-based reporting requirements exist for viral hemorrhagic fevers, including Ebola and Marburg. Occurrence of Ebola or Marburg infection likely constitutes an International Health Regulations reportable event to WHO.

**10. Referral network**—For shipping potentially infectious material, samples should be packaged in accordance with current recommendations (International Airline Transportation Association) and forwarded, after consultation, to one of the BSL-4 facilities with diagnostic capability for these agents. Testing should be performed at international WHO reference laboratories or nationally in select laboratories (e.g., European Network for Diagnostics of "Imported" Viral Diseases laboratory network in Europe; Laboratory Response Network located throughout the USA [Ebola virus only]).

**11. Special considerations**—None.

[P. E. Rollin, S. Nichol]

# ECHINOCOCCOSIS

| DISEASE | ICD-10 CODE |
|---|---|
| CYSTIC ECHINOCOCCOSIS | ICD-10 B67.0–B67.4 |
| ALVEOLAR ECHINOCOCCOSIS | ICD-10 B67.5–B67.7 |
| POLYCYSTIC ECHINOCOCCOSIS | ICD-10 B67.9 |

**1. Clinical features**—The larval stages (hydatid cyst or solid/multivesiculated lesions) of *Echinococcus* spp. tapeworm produce disease in humans and animals; disease characteristics depend upon the infecting species. Cysts/lesions usually develop in the liver or the lungs but also develop in other viscera, nervous tissue, or bone. They can be cystic, alveolar, and/or polycystic.

1) Cystic: larval stages of the tapeworm *Echinococcus granulosus*, the most common *Echinococcus* spp., cause cystic echinococcosis or hydatid disease. Hydatid cysts enlarge slowly and require several years for development. Developed cysts range from 1–15 cm in diameter but may be larger. Infections may be asymptomatic until cysts cause noticeable mass effect; signs and symptoms vary according to location, cyst size, cyst type, and numbers. Ruptured or leaking cysts can cause severe anaphylactoid reactions and may release protoscolices that can produce secondary echinococcosis. One or several cysts, typically spherical, thick-walled, and consisting of a single cavity (unilocular), are most frequently found in the liver and lungs, although they may occur in other organs. Differential diagnoses include benign tumor, malignancies, amebic abscesses, and congenital cysts.
2) Alveolar: a highly invasive, destructive disease. Lesions are usually found in the liver; because a thick laminated cyst wall does not

restrict their growth, they expand at the periphery to produce solid, tumor-like masses. Metastases can result in secondary cysts and larval growth in other organs. Clinical manifestations depend on the size and location of cysts but are often confused with hepatic carcinoma and cirrhosis.

3) Polycystic: this disease occurs in the liver, lungs, and other viscera. Symptoms vary depending on cyst size and location. The polycystic lesion is unique in that the germinal membrane proliferates externally to form new cysts and internally to form septae that divide the cavity into numerous microcysts. Brood capsules containing many protoscolices develop in the microcysts.

**2. Causative agents—**

1) Cystic: *Echinococcus granulosus* (dog tapeworm), is found worldwide, except for Southeast Asia and the Pacific region, where it is only reported as present on the mainland of Australia. It also has not been reported from Greenland. *E. granulosus* is uncommon in Central America and in South America north of Peru and Brazil. It is rarely documented in the USA, with the exception of Alaska, where it is common.
2) Alveolar: *Echinococcus multilocularis* (fox tapeworm) is found in northern regions throughout the Northern Hemisphere, including the Arctic Circle. This parasite is also present in Central Western Europe, Central Asia, northern Japan, Russia, China, Canada, Alaska, and the north-central USA.
3) Polycystic: *Echinococcus vogeli* and *Echinococcus oligarthrus* infection in humans is rare. Distribution is limited to South America and Central America.

**3. Laboratory diagnosis**—The diagnosis of echinococcosis relies mainly on findings by ultrasonography and/or other imaging techniques supported by positive serologic tests. In seronegative patients with hepatic image findings compatible with echinococcosis, ultrasound-guided fine needle aspiration/biopsy may be useful for confirmation of the diagnosis by demonstration of protoscolices or *Echinococcus* deoxyribonucleic acid (DNA). See Special Considerations section in this chapter regarding precautionary measures for such procedures. Protoscolices can sometimes be demonstrated in sputum or bronchial washings; identification of hooklets is facilitated by acid-fast stains.

Immunodiagnostic tests can be very helpful in the diagnosis of echinococcal disease and should be used before invasive methods. False-positive reactions may occur in persons with other helminthic infections, cancer, or chronic immune disorders. Negative test results do not rule out echinococcosis because some cyst carriers do not have detectable antibodies.

Whether the patient has detectable antibodies depends in part on the physical location, integrity, and viability of the larval cyst(s). Hepatic cysts are more likely than pulmonary cysts to elicit an antibody response. Regardless of where the cysts are located, antibody detection tests are the least sensitive in patients who have intact hyaline cysts. Cysts in the lungs, brain, and spleen are associated with lower serodiagnostic reactivity than seen in liver cysts, whereas those in bone appear to more regularly stimulate production of detectable antibody. Fissuration, or rupture of a cyst, is followed by an abrupt stimulation of antibody production. A patient with senescent, calcified, or dead cysts is generally found to be seronegative.

1) Cystic echinococcal disease (*E. granulosus*): indirect fluorescent antibody tests, indirect hemagglutination (IHA) tests, and enzyme immunoassays (EIAs) are sensitive tests for detecting antibodies in serum of patients with cystic disease; sensitivity rates vary from 60%–90%, depending on the characteristics of the cases. Crude hydatid cyst fluid is generally employed as antigen. CDC has an immunoblot assay that uses camel hydatid cyst fluid. The presurgery sensitivities of the assay for liver and lung cysts are 91% and 33%, respectively, with a combined assay sensitivity of 86%. This assay also cross-reacts in 39% of *E. multilocularis* and 100% of *E. vogeli*. The immunoblot is 98% specific, with rare cross-reactions in patients with cysticercosis or paragonimiasis. Antibody responses have also been monitored as a way of evaluating the response to treatment, but with mixed results. Following successful radical surgery, antibody titers decline and sometimes disappear; titers rise again if secondary cysts develop. Chemotherapy has not been followed by consistent declines in antibody titers. Consequently, the usefulness of serology to monitor the course of infection is limited; imaging techniques provide a more accurate assessment of the patient's status.
2) Alveolar echinococcal disease (*E. multilocularis*): most patients with alveolar disease have detectable antibodies in serologic tests using heterologous *E. granulosus* or homologous *E. multilocularis* antigens. With crude *Echinococcus* antigens, nonspecific reactions create the same difficulties described earlier; however, immunoaffinity-purified *E. multilocularis* antigens (Em2) used in EIA allow the detection of antibody reactions in more than 95% of alveolar cases. Comparing serologic reactivity to Em2 antigen with that to antigens containing components of both *E. multilocularis* and *E. granulosus* permits discrimination of patients with alveolar from those with cystic disease. Combining 2 purified *E. multilocularis* antigens (Em2 and recombinant antigen II/3-10) in a single

immunoassay optimized sensitivity and specificity. These antigens are sold in a commercial EIA kit in Europe, but not in the USA. As in cystic echinococcosis, Em2 tests are more useful for postoperative follow-up than for monitoring the effectiveness of chemotherapy.

Few data are available regarding serological reactions for *E. vogeli* and *E. oligarthrus* infections. Antibodies to these organisms appear to cross-react with *E. granulosus* antigens, but there are no data available on the sensitivity or specificity. An antigen for the serological detection of *E. vogeli* infections, Ev2, has been used in a research setting but has not been validated for diagnostic use. This antigen differentiates between *E. vogeli* and *E. granulosus* but not between *E. vogeli* and *E. multilocularis* (although the geographic ranges of these 2 species do not overlap).

Observation of the distinctive *Echinococcus* hooklets by microscopy or detection of *Echinococcus* DNA within cyst fluid obtained via percutaneous aspiration is very useful for helping to confirm the diagnosis of echinococcal infection for patients with negative serologic results. Ultrasound may allow determination of the clinical type of echinococcosis. Histopathology results may allow determination of the causative agent in cases where the brood capsule can be identified and examined morphologically.

4. **Laboratory capability**—Ultrasonography-based detection could be conducted in regional or district-level clinics. Laboratories should be equipped to perform serologic assays including indirect fluorescent antibody tests, IHA tests, and EIAs.

5. **Safety requirements**—Clinical specimens should always be collected and handled with standard precautions. *Echinococcus* spp. are biosafety level 2 organisms. Formalin should only be used in a well-ventilated area, preferably in a chemical fume hood. Unpreserved and preserved tissue specimens, blood, and sera should be disposed of as infectious waste.

6. **Nonhuman hosts**—*E. granulosus* definitive hosts are canines; intermediate hosts include sheep, goat, swine, cattle, horses, and camels. *E. multilocularis* definitive hosts are foxes and, to a lesser extent, dogs, cats, coyotes, and wolves; intermediate hosts are small rodents. Definitive hosts for *E. vogeli* are bush dogs and, rarely, domestic dogs; intermediate hosts are pacas and agoutis (wild rodents). Definitive hosts for *E. oligarthrus* are wild felids; intermediate hosts are pacas, spiny rats, and agoutis.

7. **Sample/specimen requirements**—Blood without anticoagulant should be collected and the serum separated for serological testing. Molecular analysis: fresh or frozen aspirated cyst fluid. Microscopic analysis: tissue or aspirated cyst fluid preserved in 10% neutral buffered formalin.

8. **Testing requirements**—Morphological or molecular identification of protoscolices in cyst fluid is both diagnostic and confirmatory. *E. granulosus*

serology by Western blot is 86% sensitive and 98% specific. Currently, CDC does not have a Clinical Laboratory Improvement Amendments-approved immunodiagnostic test for *E. multilocularis*.

**9. Reporting requirements**—Report as *Echinococcus* spp. Species may not be easily determined by standard diagnostic serology and microscopy techniques. Species may be reported where confirmed by histological examination of the brood capsule. Sequencing of selected mitochondrial genes may allow definitive species identification.

Report to local health authority in selected endemic areas; not a reportable disease in many states or countries.

**10. Referral network**—The available networks vary among countries. Enzyme immunoassay testing, histopathological analysis, and microscopy for hooklets is available in many laboratories worldwide. Reference laboratories conduct molecular diagnostic testing. *E. granulosus* serological testing, confirmation of histopathological findings, and mitochondrial DNA amplification and sequencing is available through CDC's Parasitic Diseases Reference Diagnostic Laboratory.

**11. Special considerations**—In seronegative patients with hepatic image findings compatible with echinococcosis, ultrasound-guided fine needle aspiration/biopsy may be useful for confirmation of the diagnosis. However, because of the risk for leakage of hydatid fluid/protoscolices during invasive procedures, precautionary measures include giving anthelmintic coverage and being prepared to treat an allergic (anaphylactoid) reaction.

[B. Mathison, R. S. Bradbury, I. T. McAuliffe, B. Herwaldt, S. Handali]

# *E. COLI* DIARRHEAL DISEASES

(diarrheal diseases caused by various strains of the bacterium, *Escherichia coli*)

| DISEASE | ICD-10 CODE |
|---|---|
| ENTEROPATHOGENIC *E. COLI* (EPEC) | ICD-10 A04.0 |
| ENTEROTOXIGENIC *E. COLI* (ETEC) | ICD-10 A04.1 |
| ENTEROINVASIVE *E. COLI* (EIEC) | ICD-10 A04.2 |
| SHIGA TOXIN-PRODUCING *E. COLI* (STEC) | ICD-10 A04.3 |
| INTESTINAL E. COLI INFECTION, OTHER | ICD-10 A04.4 |

# I. ENTEROPATHOGENIC *E. COLI* (EPEC)

**1. Clinical features**—Infection is mainly among children younger than 2 years, in whom it causes watery diarrhea with mucus, fever, and dehydration. It can be severe and prolonged or persistent, and in developing countries may be associated with high case-fatality rates.

**2. Causative agents**—Enteropathogenic *Escherichia coli* (EPEC) strains have traditionally been defined as certain *E. coli* serotypes epidemiologically associated with severe diarrhea in infants but that do not produce Shiga toxin (Stx) or enterotoxin and are not invasive. Traditional EPEC strains that have caused outbreaks fall into these serogroups: O55, O111, O114, O119, O125, O127, O128, O142, and O157 (non-Stx-producing O157:H45). These strains demonstrate a distinct pattern of localized adherence to HeLa and Hep-2 cells and have the chromosomal locus of enterocyte effacement, which mediates the attaching-and-effacing phenotype and for which the intimin gene (*eae*) serves as a marker. Located on the EPEC adherence factor plasmid, the bundle-forming pilus subunit (*bfpA*) gene encodes a fimbrial adhesion that mediates the localized Hep-2 adherence pattern. The term "typical EPEC" has been suggested for those organisms harboring both the EPEC adherence factor plasmid and the locus of enterocyte effacement pathogenicity island and therefore having both *eae* and *bfpA* markers (usually detected by polymerase chain reaction [PCR]). More recently, atypical EPEC have been implicated as enteric pathogens; these strains possess *eae* but not *bfpA*. Many Stx-producing *E. coli* (STEC) and *Escherichia albertii* also have the *eae* gene and express intimin.

**3. Laboratory diagnosis**—EPEC infections are currently diagnosed either by real-time PCR of deoxyribonucleic acid (DNA) extracts from fecal samples or by culturing *E. coli* from fecal specimens and testing individual isolated colonies for the presence of EPEC-specific genes. The most common target is the *eae* gene, which can be found in EPEC and STEC; it is therefore important to rule out STEC infection if the *eae* gene has been detected.

**4. Laboratory capability**—A contained, purpose-built, microbiological facility is required to handle this pathogen with the capacity to autoclave microbiological waste. Staff should be trained and shown to be competent to handle potentially hazardous biological agents and should be able to carry out molecular and basic phenotypic techniques.

**5. Safety requirements**—Employers have a responsibility to protect their workers from the risks related to exposure to hazardous biological agents.[1] In the USA, laboratories must comply with all applicable Occupational Safety and Health Administration (OSHA) regulations available at: https://www.osha.gov/laws-regs/regulations/standardnumber/1910/1910.1030#1910.1030(b). EPEC is a hazard group 2 (HG2) bacterium and should be handled within a biosafety level 2 laboratory (BSL-2). EPEC transmission is via the fecal-oral route.

Gloves should be worn when handling fecal samples, and the importance of good hand washing techniques must be emphasized to laboratory staff. In addition to gloves, other personal protective equipment (PPE) should be worn including laboratory coat and laboratory safety glasses. Finally, it is recommended to use a class I or class II microbiological safety cabinet when handling this pathogen, particularly where there is a risk of aerosol production.

**6. Nonhuman hosts**—Transmission is fecal-oral, and the reservoir for EPEC can vary from a human source for typical EPEC to both humans and animals (e.g., cats, dogs, cattle) for atypical EPEC.

**7. Sample/specimen requirements**—A stool sample is the sample of choice, and ideally a diarrheal stool sample should be collected within the first few days of a patient becoming symptomatic. Bacterial recovery will be improved if samples are taken before any antibiotic treatment is given. Stool samples should be placed into appropriate sterile containers labeled with patient details (to ensure sample integrity). UN regulations stipulate that verotoxigenic samples should be kept in appropriate stool containers to prevent leaking and transported according to the UN Transport of Infectious Substances Regulations.[2]

**8. Testing requirements**—Testing facilities must adhere to the quality standards set by their respective accreditation body, and diagnostic laboratories must follow the manufacturer's instructions for any assay being performed. Once a stool sample has arrived at the testing facility, patient identifiers on the request form and sample container should be checked. Ideally samples will be tested on arrival; if this is not possible, fecal samples can be stored at refrigerated temperatures (between 4°C–8°C) to prevent overgrowing of other organisms.

Screening and diagnostic testing should be carried out using real-time PCR for *eae* genes from DNA extracted from stool samples. Presumptive cases can be identified by the detection of EPEC genes in fecal DNA extracts. Confirmation of EPEC requires isolation of single *E. coli* colonies followed by specific PCR for the *eae* gene. Full characterization of EPEC for public health surveillance and typing can be carried out using serotyping or a whole genome sequencing-based methodology.

**9. Reporting requirements**—There are currently no formal programs in place either for primary testing or for the surveillance of EPEC. Owing to the pathogenic nature of this gastrointestinal bacterium, it is important to consider the presence of this pathogen in symptomatic patients, particularly those with a history of travel or residence in high-incidence countries. EPEC is not a notifiable disease, though significant outbreaks of EPEC should be considered for reporting on international platforms. These include the Epidemic Intelligence Information System, Food and Waterborne

Diseases and Zoonoses (EPIS-FWD) platform to assess whether current and emerging public health threats have a potential impact in the EU, in registered countries such as the USA, and on organizations such as CDC and WHO.

**10. Referral network**—It is recommended to send pure isolates to the appropriate reference laboratories for typing and characterization. Some laboratories will offer PCR testing on fecal DNA extracts and primary isolation of EPEC from stool samples. This would usually be carried out when other tests have ruled out the presence of another pathogen and an enterovirulent *E. coli* infection is suspected as the etiological agent.

**11. Special considerations**—Outbreaks (particularly those in hospitals, nurseries, and other institutions) should be investigated by local health-protection teams; enteric precautions should be followed for known or suspected cases. Good hand hygiene needs to be maintained. Where necessary, institutions should be closed to discharge and admissions. To determine how transmission is occurring, epidemiological investigations should be carried out with a focus on the number and type of cases, the geographical distribution of cases, the time period involved, and common exposures.

## II. ENTEROTOXIGENIC *E. COLI* (ETEC)

**1. Clinical features**—Enterotoxigenic *E. coli* (ETEC) strains are an important cause of diarrhea in developing countries, particularly among young children. ETEC are a frequent cause of travelers' diarrhea. The severity of illness can range from mild watery diarrhea to severe cholera-like purging as the enterotoxigenic strains may behave like *Vibrio cholerae* in producing a profuse watery diarrhea without blood or mucus. Abdominal cramping, vomiting, acidosis, prostration, and dehydration can occur; low-grade fever may or may not be present; and symptoms usually last less than 5 days but may last longer in previously unexposed travelers. ETEC are responsible for significant rates of morbidity and mortality among children in developing countries, where mortality rates may be as high as 16%–32% in children aged 4 years old or younger.

**2. Causative agent**—ETEC are a heterogeneous group of noninvasive *E. coli* that colonize the small intestine and produce a heat-labile enterotoxin (LT), a heat-stable enterotoxin (ST), or both toxins (LT/ST). Serotypes O6:H16 and O169:H41 have been implicated in most North American ETEC outbreaks, but more than 20 O antigens and more than 30 H antigens have been identified. *E. coli* enterotoxins have been purified and sequenced and are on plasmids. Strains that produce ST only or ST in combination with LT have caused most North American ETEC outbreaks.

**3. Laboratory diagnosis**—ETEC infections are currently diagnosed either by real-time PCR of DNA extracts from fecal samples or by culturing *E. coli* from fecal specimens and testing individual isolated colonies for the presence of ETEC-specific genes. The common targets are the LT and ST (human and porcine) genes, which are all used for detection because ETEC can have a combination of these genes. Immunoassays for the identification of ST or LT from culture supernatants are available from commercial sources; however, testing for ETEC typically is available only through reference or public health laboratories.

ETEC strains have been reported to be found in controls in cohort studies, and so other gastrointestinal pathogens should be ruled out first and clinical features assessed before diagnosing an ETEC infection.

**4. Laboratory capability**—A contained microbiological facility is required to handle this pathogen with the capacity to autoclave microbiological waste. Staff should be trained to handle biological agents and undertake molecular and basic phenotypic techniques.

**5. Safety requirements**—Employers have a responsibility to protect their workers from the risks related to exposure to hazardous biological agents.[1,3] ETEC is an HG2 organism and should be handled in a BSL-2 laboratory. ETEC transmission is via the fecal-oral route, and therefore gloves should be worn when handling fecal samples. The importance of good hand washing techniques must be emphasized to laboratory staff. In addition to gloves, other PPE should be worn including laboratory coat and laboratory safety glasses. Finally, it is recommended to use a class I or class II microbiological safety cabinet when handling this pathogen, particularly where there is a risk of aerosol production.

**6. Nonhuman hosts**—Humans are the major reservoir for ETEC as transmission is by the fecal-oral route; exposure to ETEC usually occurs from contaminated foods and water. ETEC has been shown to survive in freshwater for up to 3 months.

**7. Sample/specimen requirements**—A clinical stool sample is required for testing. For optimal chance of isolation, ideally a sample should be taken within a few days of the start of symptoms, though ETEC can be detected after this period. Samples must be taken before any antibiotic treatments are undertaken. Samples should be kept in appropriate stool containers to prevent leaking and transported according to the UN Transport of Infectious Substances Regulations.[2]

Stool samples should be tested as soon as possible to obtain viable culture. Feces can be stored at refrigerated temperatures (between 4°C–8°C) to prevent overgrowth of other microorganisms, but testing feces after a week postcollection and/or storing at inappropriate temperatures will reduce the likelihood of successfully detecting and/or isolating this pathogen.

**8. Testing requirements**—Testing facilities must adhere to the quality standards set by their respective accreditation body, and diagnostic laboratories must follow the manufacturer's instructions for any assay being performed. Once a stool sample has arrived at the testing facility, patient identifiers on the request form and sample container should be checked. Ideally samples will be tested on arrival; if this is not possible, fecal samples can be stored at refrigerated temperatures (between 4°C–8°C) to prevent overgrowing of other organisms.

Screening and diagnostic testing should be carried out using real-time PCR for ST and LT genes from DNA extracted from stool samples or commercial immunoassay. Presumptive cases can be identified by the detection of ETEC genes in fecal DNA extracts. Confirmation of ETEC requires isolation of single *E. coli* colonies followed by specific PCR for the ST and LT genes. Full characterization of ETEC for public health surveillance and typing can be carried out using serotyping or a whole genome sequencing-based methodology.

**9. Reporting requirements**—There are currently no surveillance programs for ETEC nor is it a notifiable disease. It is an important pathogen with travelers and can cause similar symptoms to other notifiable gastrointestinal pathogens. It is recommended that pure isolates be sent to the reference laboratory for typing (where this option is available in each country or region). This will enable a greater understanding of ETEC infection and detection of atypical outbreaks. Significant outbreaks of ETEC should be considered for reporting on international platforms. These include the EPIS-FWD platform, to assess whether current and emerging public health threats have a potential impact in the EU, in registered countries such as the USA, and on organizations such as CDC and WHO.

**10. Referral network**—ETEC will only be detected by facilities that test samples or isolates via PCR for ETEC genes. If local facilities do not offer PCR-based methods, the sample may be referred to the local regional or reference laboratory for testing to detect all enterovirulent *E. coli*. This is usually carried out when other major gastrointestinal pathogens have been ruled out and enterovirulent *E. coli* is suspected as the etiological agent.

**11. Special considerations**—Outbreaks (particularly those in hospitals, nurseries, and other institutions) should be investigated by the local health protection teams, and enteric precautions should be followed for known or suspected cases. Good hand hygiene needs to be maintained, and where necessary institutions should be closed to discharge and admissions. To determine how transmission is occurring, epidemiological investigations should be carried out with a focus on the number and type of cases, the geographical distribution of cases, the time period involved and common exposures.

## III. ENTEROINVASIVE *E. COLI* (EIEC)

**1. Clinical features**—This inflammatory disease of the gut mucosa and submucosa closely resembles that produced by *Shigella*. The organisms possess the same plasmid-dependent ability to invade and multiply within epithelial cells. Enteroinvasive *E. coli* (EIEC) is much more likely to cause watery diarrhea than dysentery (90% vs. 10% of patients). The O antigens of EIEC may cross-react with *Shigella* O antigens. Illness begins with severe abdominal cramps, malaise, watery stools, tenesmus, and fever.

**2. Causative agent**—EIEC strains invade cells of the colon by a pathogenic mechanism similar to that of *Shigella* but do not produce enterotoxins or demonstrate adherence in cell culture. They are associated with a few characteristic serogroups including O124, O143, and O164.

Enteroinvasive *E. coli* (EIEC) are facultative intracellular pathogens, shares biochemical, genetic and pathogenic properties with *Shigella*, and both can be the etiological agents of bacillary dysentery. This highly invasive pathogen has multiple virulence determinants that are encoded by both chromosomal and plasmid loci and include a type 3 secretion system (Mxi-Spa proteins), chaperones (Ipg subunits and Spa15), transcriptional regulators (VirF, VirB, and MxiE), and translocators (ipAB, IpaC, and IpaD).

EIEC are recognized as containing the *Ipa* invasive effector genes and other genetic elements present on a large invasive mosaic plasmid. The detection of the *ipa*H gene is used by the UK reference laboratories for characterization of this pathotype. These virulence factors facilitate EIEC to invade the colonic epithelial cell, lyse the phagosome, and move through the cell by nucleating actin microfilaments.

**3. Laboratory diagnosis**—EIEC infections are currently diagnosed either by real-time PCR of DNA extracts from fecal samples or by culturing *E. coli* from fecal specimens and testing individual isolated colonies for the presence of EIEC specific genes. The common target is the *ipaH* gene also found in *Shigella* spp., and therefore *Shigella* must also be ruled out as the etiological agent when this gene is detected. Testing for EIEC typically is available only through reference or public health laboratories. Reporting of EIEC isolations provides a retrospective diagnosis.

**4. Laboratory capability**—A contained microbiological facility with the capacity to autoclave microbiological waste is required to handle this pathogen. Staff should be trained to handle biological agents and undertake molecular and basic phenotypic techniques.

**5. Safety requirements**—Employers have a responsibility to protect their workers from the risks related to exposure to hazardous biological agents.[1,3] EIEC is an HG2 organism and should be handled in a BSL-2 facility. EIEC transmission is via the fecal-oral route, and therefore gloves should be worn when handling fecal samples, and the importance of good hand washing techniques must be emphasized to laboratory staff. In addition to gloves, other PPE should be worn including laboratory coat and laboratory safety glasses. Finally, it is recommended to use a class I or class II microbiological safety cabinet when handling this pathogen, particularly where there is a risk of aerosol production.

**6. Nonhuman hosts**—Transmission is fecal-oral, and exposure to EIEC is via contamination of food. As with *Shigella*, it is likely that EIEC is host restricted as no reservoir outside of the human host has been described.

**7. Sample/specimen requirements**—A clinical stool sample is required for testing. For optimal recovery of viable isolates, ideally a diarrheal stool should be collected within a few days of the start of symptoms, though EIEC can be detected after this period. Samples must be taken before any antibiotic treatments are undertaken. Samples should be kept in appropriate stool containers to prevent leaking and transported according to the UN Transport of Infectious Substances Regulations.[2]

Stool samples should be tested as soon as possible to obtain viable culture; feces can be stored at 4°C–8°C to prevent overgrowth of other microorganisms. Testing feces after a week postcollection or storing at inappropriate temperatures will reduce the chance of successfully detecting and/or isolating the pathogen.

**8. Testing requirements**—Testing facilities must adhere to the quality standards set out to them by their respective accreditation body, and diagnostic laboratories must follow the manufacturer's instructions for any assay being performed. Once a stool sample has arrived at the testing facility, patient identifiers on the request form and sample container should be checked. Ideally samples will be tested on arrival; if this is not possible, fecal samples can be stored at refrigerated temperatures (between 4°C–8°C) to prevent overgrowing of other organisms.

Screening and diagnostic testing should be carried out using real-time PCR for *ipaH* gene from DNA extracted from stool samples. Presumptive cases can be identified by the detection of EIEC genes in fecal DNA extracts, but *Shigella* should also be considered at this stage. Confirmation of EIEC requires isolation of single *E. coli* colonies followed by specific PCR for the *ipa*H gene where *Shigella* has been ruled out. Full characterization of EIEC for public health surveillance and typing can be carried out using serotyping or a whole genome sequencing-based methodology.

Sensitivity and specificity of PCR methods vary among different laboratories and the primers and probes and assays used need to be validated in each facility. Due to EIEC colony morphology being identical to other *E. coli* commensals, it is essential that single colonies are tested by PCR to ensure accurate confirmation.

**9. Reporting requirements**—There are currently no surveillance programs for EIEC nor is it a notifiable disease. It is an important pathogen that causes severe disease and can cause similar symptoms to other notifiable gastrointestinal pathogens. EIEC has started to recently emerge in outbreaks causing severe disease. It is recommended that pure isolates be sent to the reference laboratory for typing (where this option is available in each country or region). This will enable a greater understanding of EIEC infection and detection of atypical outbreaks. Significant outbreaks of EIEC should be considered for reporting on international platforms. These include the EPIS-FWD platform to assess whether current and emerging public health threats have a potential impact in the EU, in registered countries such as the USA, and on organizations such as CDC and WHO.

**10. Referral network**—EIEC will only be detected by facilities that test samples or isolates via PCR for EIEC genes. If local facilities do not offer PCR-based methods, then the sample may be referred to the local regional or reference laboratory for testing to detect all enterovirulent *E. coli.* This is usually carried out when other main gastrointestinal pathogens have been ruled out and enterovirulent *E. coli* is suspected as the etiological agent.

**11. Special considerations**—The epidemiology of EIEC is not well known because the focus in the diagnostic laboratory is to detect *Shigella*, which tends to have more severe clinical manifestations. EIEC has not been found in surveillance studies in the UK over the past 15 years and is not thought to play a major role in diarrheal disease. Outbreaks (particularly those in hospitals, nurseries, and other institutions) should be investigated by the local health protection teams, and enteric precautions should be followed for known or suspected cases. Good hand hygiene needs to be maintained, and, where necessary, institutions should be closed to discharge and admissions. To determine how transmission is occurring, epidemiological investigations should be carried out with a focus on the number and type of cases, the geographical distribution of cases, the time period involved, and common exposures.

## IV. SHIGA TOXIN–PRODUCING *E. COLI* (STEC) (verotoxin-producing *E. coli*, *E. coli* O157:H7, enterohemorrhagic *E. coli*)

**1. Clinical features**—The diarrhea may range from mild and nonbloody to stools that are virtually all blood; abdominal cramps are often severe. The most severe manifestation of shiga toxin–producing *E. coli* (STEC) infection is hemolytic uremic syndrome (HUS), a thrombotic microangiopathy occurring in both children and adults that is characterized by hemolytic anemia, thrombocytopenia, and acute renal dysfunction. The term D+HUS is used to describe HUS that follows a diarrheal illness, and it may be associated with neurologic abnormalities. STEC is the primary cause of D+HUS. Adults with D+HUS are often misdiagnosed as having thrombotic thrombocytopenic purpura, a different thrombotic microangiopathy unrelated to STEC infection. Most D+HUS patients with an identified etiology show evidence of infection with STEC that produce Stx2. Stx2 is produced by virtually all STEC O157 strains causing human illness. STEC O157 causes the most D+HUS cases worldwide. About 15% of young children and a much smaller proportion of adults with STEC O157 diarrhea develop D+HUS. However, in an outbreak in Germany of a rare enteroaggregative STEC O104:H4 infection, principally among adults, the reported percentage who developed D+HUS was 22%. About 55% of patients with STEC O157 D+HUS require dialysis and 5% die; rates vary for other serotypes.

**2. Causative agents**—STEC is a heterogeneous group of bacteria that express potent cytotoxins called Stx1 and Stx2 (Stx1 and Stx2 are also called verocytotoxins or verotoxins). Stx1 is essentially identical to the toxin produced by *Shigella dysenteriae* 1; D+HUS is also a complication of *S. dysenteriae* 1 infection. STEC that produce certain Stx2 subtypes (e.g., Stx2a and Stx2d) tend to be more virulent. In North America, approximately 70% of D+HUS cases have laboratory evidence of antecedent STEC infection; approximately 95% of these are STEC O157. The percentage of D+HUS attributable to STEC O157 in industrialized countries is generally 50% or greater, but ranges from nearly 100% in the UK to approximately 20%–80% in other European countries and less than 20% in Australia. Over 70 STEC serogroups have been isolated from ill persons. After O157, the most common serogroups isolated from persons with diarrheal illness in North America are O26, O111, O103, O45, O145, and O121. STEC strains vary considerably in their virulence, from strains of no apparent human virulence detected primarily in animals to others causing severe human disease and outbreaks. The pathogenesis of STEC is complex and involves several virulence factors. In addition to Stx, STEC must also express intestinal adherence factors to cause disease. A common adherence factor among STEC is intimin (encoded by *eae*; see Enteropathogenic *E. Coli* [EPEC] section in this chapter).

**3. Laboratory diagnosis**—Rapid diagnosis of STEC infections (particularly *E. coli* O157:H7) is essential for patient management and infection control. STEC infections are currently diagnosed by (a) PCR-based methods targeting Stx1 and Stx2 present in fecal DNA extracts; (b) enzyme immunoassay (EIA); (c) culturing fecal specimens for *E. coli* (e.g., use of a specialized selective isolation medium such as cefixime-tellurite sorbitol MacConkey Agar or CHROMAgar O157), followed by detection of the somatic antigen (O157); or (d) by culturing *E. coli* from fecal specimens and testing individual isolated colonies for the presence of Stx1- and Stx2-specific genes.

Specimens should be collected as close to the onset of symptoms as possible to avoid loss of the phages that carry the Stx genes. Positive findings should be reported promptly for patient management and to public health authorities for the detection and control of outbreaks

**4. Laboratory capability**—A contained, purpose built, microbiological facility is required to handle this pathogen with the capacity to autoclave microbiological waste. Staff should be trained and shown to be competent to handle potentially containment level 3 hazardous biological agents and should be able to carry out molecular and phenotypic techniques.

**5. Safety requirements**—Employers have a responsibility to protect their workers from the risks related to exposure to hazardous biological agents.[1,3] STEC is a hazard group 3 bacterium and ideally should be handled within a BSL-3 laboratory. As STEC transmission is via the fecal-oral route, gloves should be worn by laboratory staff when handling fecal samples, and the importance of good hand washing techniques must be emphasized. In addition to gloves, other PPE should be worn including laboratory coat and laboratory safety glasses. Finally, it is recommended to use a class I or class II microbiological safety cabinet when handling this pathogen, particularly once it has been grown from the original diagnostic specimen and is at a high bacterial load.

**6. Nonhuman hosts**—STEC transmission is via the fecal-oral route, with ruminant animals, particularly cattle and sheep, being the major natural reservoir for this pathogen. Therefore, exposure to animals or their feces in the farming environment (including petting farms) is a risk factor.[4] Although considered less important, other wild and domestic animals can also carry STEC in their intestinal tract, including birds, horses, dogs, and cats.

**7. Sample/specimen requirements**—A stool sample is the sample of choice, and ideally a diarrheal stool sample should be collected within the first few days of a patient becoming symptomatic. Bacterial recovery will be improved if samples are taken before any antibiotic treatment is given. Stool samples should be placed into appropriate sterile containers labeled with patient details (to ensure sample integrity). UN regulations stipulate that a STEC culture is a category A (UN 2814) infectious substance in a form capable of causing permanent disability or life-threatening or fatal disease in otherwise healthy humans or animals when exposure to the substance occurs.[2] The International Air Transportation Association and US Department of Transportation recommend shipping of STEC as a category A infectious substance (see "Transport of Infectious Specimens"). Staff who package, ship, or transport category A infectious substances should have formal, documented training every 2 years.

STEC infections have been associated with a wide range of food products, including undercooked beef, unpasteurized milk and cheese, and uncooked salad and fruit products; therefore the collection and processing of food and environmental samples can be useful in outbreak investigations.

**8. Testing requirements**—Testing facilities must adhere to the quality standards set out by their respective accreditation body, and diagnostic laboratories must follow the manufacturer's instructions for any commercial assays being performed. Once a stool sample has arrived at the testing facility, patient identifiers on the request form and sample containers should be checked. Ideally samples will be tested on arrival. If this is not possible, fecal samples can be stored at refrigerated temperatures (between 4°C–8°C) to prevent overgrowing of other organisms.

Detection of STEC and in particular *E. coli* O157:H7 is of particular importance due to the prevalence and severity of the disease caused by this pathogen. However, many clinical laboratories do not routinely culture stool specimens for O157 STEC, and this test may only be carried out in patients with HUS or severe disease. Therefore, it is recommended that any stool sample submitted for microbiology testing from a patient with acute community-acquired diarrhea should also be cultured for O157 STEC on selective and differential agar.

Screening and diagnostic testing should be carried out using the following:

1) Culturing fecal specimens for *E. coli* followed by detection of the somatic antigen (O157). Most *E. coli* strains (including other STEC isolates) ferment sorbitol; however, *E. coli* O157:H7 is a nonsorbitol fermenter (in 24 hours). This phenotypic feature allows a sorbitol containing growth medium (most commonly sorbitol MacConkey or SMAC) to be used as a rapid screening method. Once nonsorbitol fermenting colonies have been isolated, there are several commercial kits that can be used to detect the somatic O antigens, thus allowing identification of nonsorbitol fermenting *E. coli* as a presumptive O157. One limitation of relying on sorbitol fermentation is the existence of sorbitol fermenting O157 strains; therefore, there are alternative chromogenic media that can be used in addition to the SMAC medium.
2) Real-time PCR for Stx1 and Stx2 genes in fecal and food DNA extracts is a popular method for the detection of STEC. Other gene targets that can be used in addition to the Stx genes include the gene coding for hemolysin (*hly*A), the attaching and effacing (*eae*) gene and the specific O antigen genes (*rfb*) for common STEC. A syndromic approach for the diagnosis of gastrointestinal pathogens has led to the development of multiplex-PCR methods. These methods can simultaneously detect the presence of STEC plus other gastrointestinal microbial pathogens in fecal samples from patients with diarrhea.
3) Enzyme immunoassay (EIA) method allows detection of Stx directly from stool samples or on an enrichment broth culture incubated overnight (16–24 hours at 37°C); however, for samples in which O157 STEC bacteria have not been detected by EIA, it is recommended to use one of the alternative methods to rule out a STEC infection.

Confirmation of STEC requires isolation of single *E. coli* colonies that have been confirmed by specific PCR for the Stx1, Stx2, *hly*A, *rfb*, and *eae* genes followed by serotyping either by direct traditional agglutination with antisera or via deriving the serotype from whole genome sequencing. Whichever method is used, full characterization of STEC is essential to ensure robust public health surveillance and typing is carried out.

**9. Reporting requirements**—Reporting varies from country to country as does the likelihood of testing. Some countries will test all diarrheal stool samples from the community setting, whereas other countries will only test stool samples from patients presenting with HUS. This disparity in international testing practices therefore affects the level of STEC reporting. Significant outbreaks of STEC should be reported on international platforms. These include the EPIS-FWD platform to assess whether current and emerging public health threats have a potential impact in the EU, in registered countries such as the USA, and on organizations such as CDC and WHO.

**10. Referral network**—The increased interest in the use of PCR to detect the Stx genes (Stx1 and Stx2) has markedly improved the diagnosis of STEC O157 and non-O157 infections. These nonculture methods are useful for diagnosing but currently should not fully replace culture-based methods, as a pure isolate is still needed for STEC characterization allowing surveillance and public health management of outbreaks. A variety of subtyping methods are in use including traditional phenotypic phage-typing, MLVA, and PFGE for STEC O157. More recently the use of whole genome sequencing has been implemented into routine service in some countries, allowing the serotype to be derived, virulence gene to be detected and subtyped and isolates to be characterized down to single nucleotide polymorphisms for all STEC strains.

**11. Special considerations**—Due to the potential severity of the disease, local public health services should be notified rapidly of all STEC cases, to allow identification of sources, and to apply appropriate preventative measures to control the spread of this infection. Case reporting of STEC infection is obligatory in many countries. Hygiene advice should be given to infected individuals, family members, and any intuitions involved, to prevent person-to-person spread, with a particular emphasis on frequent hand washing (particularly postdefecation) with soap and water, disposal of nappies (diapers) and human waste, and prevention of contamination of food and drink. During acute illness, enteric precautions must be enforced and symptomatic STEC cases should be excluded from work until they are symptom free for 48 hours. High-risk groups should not be allowed to return to work until they are clear of STEC carriage (e.g., if their job includes handling unwrapped food or they are employed in clinical, social care, or nursery environments).

To determine how transmission is occurring, epidemiological investigations should be carried out with a focus on the number and type of cases, the geographical distribution of cases, the time period involved, and common exposures. The results of the microbiological and epidemiological investigations should be used to guide specific control measures. General preventative and control measures include (a) managing slaughterhouses/abattoirs to reduce the likelihood of meat being contaminated by animal intestinal content; (b) discouraging the consumption of raw milk and dairy products; (c) washing fruit and vegetables if to be eaten raw; (d) hand washing thoroughly with soap and water after contact with farm animals or a farming environment (including petting farms); (e) cooking meat (especially ground or minced beef products) adequately; (f) provision of clean, chlorinated public water supplies; (g) removal of suspected food products from supply chains; (h) closure of affected institutions or business to further admission; and (i) communication of hand washing to the general public.

For helpful advice pertaining to the control of infection during mass catering, see: http://whqlibdoc.who.int/hq/1994/WHO_FNU_FOS_94.5.pdf.[5]

## V. INTESTINAL *E. COLI* INFECTION, OTHER (enteroaggregative *E. coli* [EAEC], diarrhea caused by diffuse-adherent *E. coli* [DAEC])

**1. Clinical features**—Enteroaggregative *E. coli* (EAEC) is a cause of epidemic and sporadic diarrhea, yet its role as an enteric pathogen is not fully understood. EAEC is associated with persistent infant diarrhea (continuing unabated for 14 days). EAEC has also been associated with acute diarrhea. Diarrhea is watery with mucous. Bloody diarrhea has been reported in 3%–31%.

The pathogenicity of diffuse-adherent *E. coli* (DAEC) is uncertain. They have been implicated as a cause of diarrhea in some studies but not in others. The ability to cause epithelial cells to secrete a high amount of chemokine IL-8 seems to be linked to disease for certain strains. In a retrospective case-control study the majority of infected children had watery diarrhea without blood or fecal leukocytes.

**2. Causative agent**—EAEC strains are a heterogeneous group of bacteria defined by their ability to adhere to Hep-2 cells in a pattern resembling stacked bricks. EAEC strains vary considerably in their virulence with subsets of pathogenic strains identified through studies and outbreak investigations. The pathogenesis of EAEC is complex and involves the production of various adhesins and accessory proteins that mediate adherence throughout the entire intestinal tract; the elaboration of 1 or more enterotoxins, cytotoxins, and proteases that mediate cytopathic effects on the epithelium; and the induction of cellular factors that may lead to mucosal inflammation. The adherence of EAEC to the intestinal epithelium results in increased mucus secretion, which forms a biofilm that entraps the bacteria onto the small intestinal epithelium. The adhesins for many EAEC have not been identified.

DAEC strains comprise a heterogeneous group of organisms that exhibit a diffuse pattern of adherence to Hep-2 cells in culture. A recent study showed that DAEC was significantly associated with diarrheal disease in children older than 12 months of age but not in children younger than

12 months of age. This finding is consistent with the fact that the cellular receptor (decay accelerating factor or CD55) for the adhesion produced by most DAEC (F1845 adhesin) is not expressed until about 1 year of age. Binding of the bacteria to this receptor induces a cytopathic effect and is accompanied by activation of signal transduction cascades. Independently of this binding, DAEC may cause diarrhea by impairing the activities and reducing the abundance of brush border-associated enzymes (sucrase-isomaltase and dipeptidylpeptidase intravenous ). A role has been proposed for DAEC in inflammatory bowel disease by promoting proinflammatory responses through the interaction of their adhesions with host membrane-bound receptors.

**3. Laboratory diagnosis**—EAEC infections are currently diagnosed either by real-time PCR of DNA extracts from fecal samples or by culturing *E. coli* from fecal specimens and testing individual isolated colonies for the presence of EAEC-specific genes. The most common target is the *aggR* gene (responsible for regulating many of the EAEC genes) to detect typical EAEC. Other common EAEC genes used for detection include *aat* (antiaggregative transporter gene responsible for transporting a protein called dispersin across the membrane) or the *aaiC* gene (chromosomal gene in a genomic island encoding a type VI secretion system). For suspected hybrid EAEC/STEC strains, detection of the Stx gene would also be required.

Due to the heterogeneity of EAEC, the key set of characterizing EAEC genes has yet to be agreed upon by experts in the field. To date there is no single gene or combination of genes that are EAEC specific and found in all EAEC strains.

Not all strains of EAEC are pathogenic, and the presence of EAEC in the stool does not confirm the etiological agent. Around 40% of EAEC found in the stool are associated with coinfections with other pathogens. Other gastrointestinal pathogens should be ruled out first and clinical features assessed before diagnosing an EAEC infection.

DAEC infections are currently diagnosed either by real-time PCR of DNA extracts from fecal samples or by culturing *E. coli* from fecal specimens and testing individual isolated colonies for the presence of DAEC-specific genes. The most common target is the *Afa* genes though this does not confirm DAEC infection and may be associated with carriage.

Not all strains of DAEC are pathogenic and presence of DAEC in the stool does not confirm the etiological agent. Detection methods are still being developed for diarrheagenic strains of DAEC, and there is no current universal method; thus the epidemiology of diarrheagenic DAEC remains unclear.

Other gastrointestinal pathogens should be ruled out first and clinical features assessed before diagnosing a DAEC infection.

**4. Laboratory capability**—A contained microbiological facility with the capacity to autoclave microbiological waste is required to handle this pathogen. Staff should be trained to handle biological agents and undertake molecular and basic phenotypic techniques.

**5. Safety requirements**—Employers have a responsibility to protect their workers from the risks related to exposure to hazardous biological agents.[1,3] EAEC is an HG2 organism and should be handled in a BSL-2. It should also be noted that hybrid EAEC/STEC strains are an HG3 pathogen and should be handled in a BSL-3. EAEC transmission is via the fecal-oral route, and therefore gloves should be worn when handling fecal samples. The importance of good hand washing techniques must be emphasized to laboratory staff. In addition to gloves, other PPE should be worn including laboratory coat and laboratory safety glasses. Finally, it is recommended to use a class I or class II microbiological safety cabinet when handling this pathogen, particularly where there is a risk of aerosol production.

**6. Nonhuman hosts**—For EAEC, transmission is fecal-oral, and though atypical EAEC (strains lacking *aggR* gene) have been found in animals such as cattle and EAEC strains have been associated with sprouts and vegetables, the reservoir of clinically relevant EAEC is generally thought to be human.

For DAEC, transmission is fecal-oral, but it is unknown whether there are any nonhuman reservoirs for DAEC.

**7. Sample/specimen requirements**—A clinical stool sample is required for testing; for optimal chance of isolation, ideally a sample should be taken within a few days of the start of symptoms though EAEC can be detected after this period. Samples must be taken before any antibiotic treatments are undertaken. Samples should be kept in stool containers to prevent leaking and transported according to the UN Transport of Infectious Substances Regulations.[2] It should also be noted that hybrid EAEC/STEC strains are an HG3 pathogen and therefore classified as a category A agent. (See Shiga Toxin-Producing *E. Coli* [STEC] section in this chapter.)

Stool samples should be tested as soon as possible to obtain viable culture. Feces can be stored at refrigeration temperatures (4°C–8°C) to prevent overgrowing of other organisms, but testing feces after a week postcollection and/or storing at inappropriate temperatures will reduce the chance of successfully detecting and/or isolating the pathogen.

**8. Testing requirements**—Testing facilities must adhere to the quality standards set out to them by their respective accreditation body, and diagnostic laboratories must follow the manufacturer's instructions for any assay being performed. Once a stool sample has arrived at the testing facility, patient identifiers on the request form and sample containers should be checked. Ideally samples will be tested on arrival. If this is not possible, fecal samples can be stored at refrigerated temperatures (between 4°C–8°C) to prevent overgrowing of other organisms.

Screening and diagnostic testing should be carried out using real-time PCR for EAEC or DAEC gene targets from DNA extracted from stool samples. Presumptive cases can be identified by the detection of EAEC or DAEC genes in fecal DNA. Confirmation of EAEC or DAEC requires isolation of single *E. coli* colonies followed by specific PCR. Full characterization of EAEC or DAEC for public health surveillance and typing can be carried out using serotyping or a whole genome sequencing-based methodology.

Sensitivity and specificity of PCR methods vary among different laboratories and the primers and probes and assays used need to be validated in each facility. Due to EIEC colony morphology being identical to other *E. coli* commensals, it is essential that single colonies are tested by PCR to ensure accurate confirmation.

**9. Reporting requirements**—There is currently no surveillance programme for EAEC, nor is it a notifiable disease. Due to EAEC adaptability to cause severe disease and extraintestinal infections, it is recommended to isolate and send the pure isolate to the reference laboratory for typing (where this option is available). This will enable a greater understanding of EAEC infection and detection of atypical outbreaks. Significant outbreaks of EAEC should be considered for reporting on international platforms. These include the EPIS-FWD platform to assess whether current and emerging public health threats have a potential impact in the EU, in registered countries such as the USA, and on organizations such as CDC and WHO.

**10. Referral network**—EAEC will only be detected by facilities that test samples or isolates via PCR for EAEC genes. If local facilities do not offer PCR-based methods, then the sample should be referred to the local regional or reference laboratory for testing to detect all enterovirulent *E. coli*. This is usually carried out when other main gastrointestinal pathogens have been ruled out and enterovirulent *E. coli* is suspected as the etiological agent.

**11. Special considerations**—There are several toxins that EAEC can produce including a plasmid encoded toxin, which has enterotoxic activity and can lead to changes in the epithelial-cell and cytoskeletal protein spectrin; an enteroaggregative *E. coli* heat-stable toxin, which could contribute to watery diarrhea; and a *Shigella* enterotoxin 1 thought to contribute to secretory diarrhea. However, not all EAEC strains produce all, if any, of these toxins, and the encoding genes for numerous adhesions and proteins associated with virulence are highly variable among strains. Even the site of infection is not uniform; some strains infect the small bowel while others infect the small bowel and colon.

There have been rare incidences of a hybrid form of EAEC containing the phage-encoding Stx genes associated with STEC and causing more severe disease (see Shiga Toxin-Producing *E. Coli* [STEC] section in this chapter). EAEC has also been found to cause extraintestinal infections such as urinary tract infections and septicemia. Though EAEC pathogenicity factors are heterogeneous in nature, a general 3-part model of EAEC pathogenesis has emerged: (a) adherence to the intestinal mucosa, (b) production of enterotoxins and cytotoxins, and (c) mucosal inflammation.

Outbreaks (particularly those in hospitals, nurseries, and other institutions) should be investigated by the local health protection teams, and enteric precautions should be followed for known or suspected cases. Good hand hygiene needs to be maintained and where necessary institutions should be closed to discharge and admissions. To determine how transmission is occurring, epidemiological investigations should be carried out with a focus on the number and type of cases, the geographical distribution of cases, the time period involved, and common exposures.

## References

1. EUR-Lex. Directive 2000/54/EC of the European Parliament and of the Council of 18 September 2000. Available at: https://eur-lex.europa.eu/legal-content/EN/ALL/?uri=CELEX%3A32000L0054. Accessed February 15, 2019.
2. United Nations Economic Commission for Europe. UN Model Regulations: UN Recommendations on the Transport of Dangerous Goods.Available at: http://www.unece.org/trans/danger/publi/unrec/rev18/18files_e.html. Accessed March 20, 2019.
3. US Occupational Safety and Health Administration. Bloodborne pathogens. Available at: https://www.osha.gov/laws-regs/regulations/standardnumber/1910/1910.1030#1910.1030(b). Accessed March 20, 2019.
4. Chase-Topping ME, McKendrick IJ, Pearce MC, et al. Risk factors for the presence of high-level shedders of Escherichia coli O157 on Scottish farms. *J Clin Microbiol.* 2007;45(5):1594–603.
5. World Health Organization. Hygiene in food-service and mass catering establishments. Available at: http://whqlibdoc.who.int/hq/1994/WHO_FNU_FOS_94.5.pdf. Accessed February 27, 2019.

[M. A. Chattaway, D. Ready]

# EHRLICHIOSIS/ANAPLASMOSIS

| DISEASE | ICD-10 CODE |
|---|---|
| EHRLICHIOSIS | ICD-10 A77.40 |
| EHRLICHIA CHAFFEENSIS | ICD-10 A77.41 |
| RICKETTSIOSIS DUE TO EHRLICHIA SENNETSU | ICD-10 A79.81 |
| ANAPLASMOSIS | ICD-10 A77.49 |
| OTHER SPECIFIED RICKETTSIOSIS | ICD-10 A79.89 |

| DISEASE IN HUMANS | CAUSATIVE AGENTS | RESERVOIRS | GEOGRAPHIC DISTRIBUTION OF HUMAN ILLNESS |
|---|---|---|---|
| EHRLICHIOSIS | *Ehrlichia chaffeensis* and *Ehrlichia ewingii* | White-tailed deer, dogs, rodents | North America |
| | *Ehrlichia muris eauclairensis* | Rodents | Minnesota and Wisconsin, USA |
| | *Ehrlichia muris muris* | Rodents | Asia |
| | *Ehrlichia canis* | Dogs | Venezuela and Costa Rica |
| ANAPLASMOSIS | *Anaplasma phagocytophilum* | Ruminants, deer, rodents, dogs | North America, Asia, Europe |
| | *Anaplasma platys* | Dogs | Venezuela and USA |
| | *Anaplasma ovis* | Sheep | Cyprus and Iran |
| | *"Anaplasma capra"*[a] | Goats | China |
| SENNETSU FEVER | *Neorickettsia sennetsu* | Trematodes that live in aquatic hosts such as snails, insects, and fish | Western Japan and Malaysia |
| NEOEHRLICHIOSIS | *"Candidatus Neoehrlichia mikurensis"*[a] | Rodents, dogs | Northern Europe and Asia |

[a]Denotes a taxon designation that has not been named according to formal bacteriological rules.

**1. Clinical features**—Acute, febrile illnesses caused by a group of small, pleomorphic, obligate intracellular, Gram-negative bacteria (family *Anaplasmataceae*) that survive and reproduce in the phagosomes of mononuclear or polymorphonuclear leukocytes of the infected host. The clinical spectrum of ehrlichiosis infections ranges from mild illness to severe, life-threatening, or fatal disease. Ehrlichiosis caused by *E. chaffeensis* presents with nonspecific symptoms, including fever, headache, malaise, and myalgia. It may be confused clinically with Rocky Mountain spotted fever (due to *Rickettsia rickettsii*), although rash is less commonly reported with ehrlichiosis. Laboratory findings include leukopenia, thrombocytopenia, and elevation of hepatocellular enzymes. Encephalitis or meningitis may occur. Infection with *E. chaffeensis* can be severe, and a 1.9% case-fatality rate is reported. There is no current evidence for persistent infection in humans. Signs and symptoms of *E. ewingii*, *Ehrlichia muris muris, and E. muris eauclairensis* infections are usually nonspecific and commonly include fever, headache, anorexia, nausea, myalgia, and vomiting. To date, *E. ewingii* or *E. muris* infections have not been reported to be associated with fatalities.

Anaplasmosis, caused by *Anaplasma phagocytophilum*, is characterized clinically by acute and usually self-limited fever, headache, malaise, and myalgia. Common laboratory findings may include thrombocytopenia, leukopenia, and increased hepatic transaminases. Meningoencephalitis is rare. Illness ranges from mild to severe, with a 0.6% case-fatality rate. Coinfections with *Borrelia burgdorferi*, *Borrelia myiamotoi*, *Babesia* spp., and tick-borne encephalitis viruses may occur because *Ixodes* spp. of ticks transmit all these organisms. There is no current evidence for persistent infection in humans.

Sennetsu fever, caused by *Neorickettsia sennetsu* is characterized by the sudden onset of fever, chills, malaise, headache, muscle and joint pain, sore throat, and sleeplessness. Generalized lymphadenopathy with tenderness of the enlarged nodes is common. Atypical lymphocytosis with postauricular and posterior cervical lymphadenopathy is similar to that seen in infectious mononucleosis. The course is usually benign; fatal cases have not been reported.

Infection with the proposed species "*Neoehrlichia mikurensis*" has recently been described in Europe and Asia. General clinical features have included recurrent fever, erysipelas-like rashes, arthralgias, sepsis, and thromboembolism. Most severe illnesses have occurred in immunocompromised people.

The veterinary pathogens *Ehrlichia canis* and *Anaplasma platys* have been reported to infect a few humans in Venezuela and Costa Rica. Recently, a new species, "*Anaplasma capra*" (proposed name, not yet formally adopted) was found infecting humans and goats in China. Clinically, the *E. canis* patients were asymptomatic or showed signs compatible with ehrlichiosis, while *A. platys* and *"A. capra"* infected humans had nonspecific febrile illnesses similar to *A. phagocytophilum* infections. These etiologies have not been reported from other areas.

Differential diagnosis for all these infections includes various viral syndromes, Rocky Mountain spotted fever, sepsis, toxic shock syndrome, gastroenteritis, meningoencephalitis, tularemia, Colorado tick fever, tick-borne encephalitis, Powassan virus disease, babesiosis, Lyme borreliosis, leptospirosis, viral hepatitis, typhoid fever, acute Q fever, murine typhus, and blood malignancies. Blood transfusions donated during the early, pre-symptomatic phase of infections with both *A. phagocytophilum* and *E. ewingii* have caused infections in blood recipients, and solid organ transplants pose a risk. There is no evidence of other person-to-person transmission with these agents

**2. Causative agents**—See the earlier table for causative agents. These organisms are members of the family Anaplasmataceae, order Rickettsiales.

**3. Laboratory diagnosis**—While the diagnosis may be based on clinical and epidemiologic features, supportive laboratory findings will contribute to the diagnosis. Due to the life-threatening nature of these infections, treatment should not be delayed while awaiting laboratory test results. Confirmatory laboratory findings include a 4-fold change in immunoglobulin class G (IgG) antibody titers detected between acute and convalescent serum samples (2–4 weeks apart). Serology may be conducted by using organism-specific antigens for *A. phagocytophilum* or *E. chaffeensis* or by using *E. chaffeensis* as surrogate antigen for *E. ewingii* and *E. muris*. Commonly observed laboratory findings in patients with anaplasmosis and ehrlichiosis include leukopenia, lymphopenia, thrombocytopenia, and elevated hepatic enzymes. Bacterial clusters (called morulae) of *A. phagocytophilum*, *E. chaffeensis*, and *E. ewingii* may be seen on stained peripheral blood smears or buffy coat examination during the acute stage of illness and may be highly specific when identified by a skilled and experienced microscopist, but this is not recommended as the most sensitive method of detection. *Ehrlichia chaffeensis* infects primarily mononuclear phagocytes, while *Ehrlichia ewingii* and *Anaplasma phagocytophilum* affect the neutrophils. *Neorickettsia sennetsu* infects mononuclear cells, while the target cells for *Neoehrlichia mikurensis* and *Ehrlichia muris* have not yet been determined (suspected of being the endothelial cells or macrophages, respectively).

Other, highly sensitive diagnostic techniques, especially during the acute febrile phase of illness, include deoxyribonucleic acid (DNA) amplification by polymerase chain reaction (PCR) assays. Culture and immunohistochemistry (IHC) of blood marrow or necropsy tissues can be used for diagnosis in fatal cases. The later table provides information on available laboratory testing options for the diagnosis of ehrlichiosis.

**4. Laboratory capability**—Most clinical laboratory procedures including serologic testing, DNA extraction/amplification, and culture should be conducted in a facility with biosafety level-2 (BSL-2) facilities and practices. Propagative procedures should be conducted within a class II biosafety cabinet (BSC) due to the potential for aerosolization. Test loads may not be sufficient to support testing at a local clinical laboratory, and testing can be referred to commercial or public health laboratories. Testing for human diagnostics in the USA should be conducted at laboratories certified for Clinical Laboratory Improvement Amendments testing using established procedures. Personnel should be trained by experienced laboratorians and annual proficiency testing and staff competency assessments should be conducted. Cultivation of agents in the family *Anaplasmataceae* requires use of a BSC and strict aseptic procedures as antibiotics are used sparingly in routine growth.

**5. Safety requirements**—Clinical specimens from patients suspected of having ehrlichiosis or anaplasmosis may be safely tested at BSL-2 facilities using standard precautions. Organisms can be grown within BSL-2 facilities using a class II BSC, although BSL-3 facilities are recommended when high concentrations of the organisms are grown or procedures with high potential for aerosolization are conducted. Prophylactic antibiotics are not recommended for working with these agents. No vaccine is available for laboratorians working with these pathogens.

**6. Nonhuman hosts**—Human diseases caused by members of the *Anaplasmataceae* are zoonotic. *Ehrlichia* spp., *Anaplasma* spp., and "*Neoehrlichia mikurensis*" are maintained in complex ecosystems involving multiple vertebrate animal species. By contrast, *N. sennetsu* is maintained in trematodes that live in aquatic hosts. Typical animal hosts that can serve as reservoirs are provided for each agent listed in the earlier table.

Hard ticks of the family Ixodidae serve as vectors of most species of *Anaplasmataceae*. Tick bites serve as the primary mode of transmission for these species, yet some have been shown to be transmitted through alternate routes such as blood transfusion, organ transplantation, and exposure to blood from infected animals.

*Ehrlichia chaffeensis* and *E. ewingii* are transmitted through the bite of *Amblyomma americanum* in North America, while *Ehrlichia canis* is transmitted by *Rhipicephalus sanguineus. Ehrlichia muris,* and similar organisms have been identified in *Ixodes persulcatus* and *Haemaphysalis flava* ticks in some parts of the world, Eastern Europe and Asia, and in *Ixodes scapularis* in the upper midwestern USA. The vectors of *A. phagocytophilum* are *Ixodes* spp., including *Ixodes scapularis*, *I. ricinus*, *I. pacificus*, and *I. persulcatus* for humans, and these species plus *Ixodes trianguliceps*, *Ixodes spinipalpis* ticks among other animals. "*A. capra*" may be found in Ixodes persulcatus and *Haemaphysalis longicornis* ticks. Neoehrlichiosis is associated with bites of *Ixodes ricinus.*

Sennetsu fever is different from the other organisms described earlier in that it appears to be associated with ingestion of an uncooked trematode-parasitized aquatic host (e.g., fish) with neorickettsiae residing in the trematode.

## Various Laboratory Testing Requirements for Ehrlichiosis and Related Diseases

| Testing Method | Test Strategy | Sensitivity | Specificity | Availability |
|---|---|---|---|---|
| Microscopic examination of blood smears or buffy coat preparations | Screening, presumptive evidence of infection by Anaplasmataceae | 25%–75% for *A. phagocytophilum* 2%–38% for *E. chaffeensis* | Not determined; highly dependent on the skill and experience of the microscopist | Common; clinical laboratories with experienced personnel |

*(Continued)*

## Various Laboratory Testing Requirements for Ehrlichiosis and Related Diseases (Continued)

| Testing Method | Test Strategy | Sensitivity | Specificity | Availability |
|---|---|---|---|---|
| Indirect immunofluorescence assay (IFA) | Screening, confirmatory if tested in acute/convalescent pairs to demonstrate seroconversions (taken to be 4-fold or greater rises in IgG antibodies) | 82%–100% for *A. phagocytophilum* 88%–90% for *E. chaffeensis* IgM: 27%–37% for *A. phagocytophilum* 44% for *E. chaffeensis* | 83%–100% for *A. phagocytophilum*; cross-reactivity noted between *Anaplasma* and *Ehrlichia* spp. False-positives observed with other infections (e.g., Lyme disease, Rocky Mountain spotted fever) and some autoimmune disorders. | Common; commercial laboratories, public health laboratories, universities |
| Enzyme-linked immunosorbent assays (ELISA) | Screening; current commercial kits provide qualitative results; experimental ELISA for the p44 protein would be confirmatory | Not determined | Not determined | Limited; some commercial laboratories, public health laboratories may provide as screening before IFA testing; available for domestic animals |
| Polymerase chain reaction (PCR) assay | Screening; Confirmatory if adequately diverse genes are targeted by specific assays or product is sequenced; best method for pathogens that have not yet been cultivated | 67%–90% for *A. phagocytophilum* 60%–85% for *E. chaffeensis* | Up to 100%; assay-dependent | Limited, but increasing; commercial laboratories; public health laboratories, university research centers; available for domestic animals and ticks. No tests approved or cleared for in vitro diagnostic use by FDA; highly variable performance characteristics. |

*(Continued)*

**Various Laboratory Testing Requirements for Ehrlichiosis and Related Diseases (Continued)**

| Testing Method | Test Strategy | Sensitivity | Specificity | Availability |
|---|---|---|---|---|
| Culture in cell lines | Screening; confirmatory if cultivable strain and sustained isolates are obtained | Highly variable, due to timing and antibiotic treatment; only some of the pathogens have been successfully cultivated in vitro | Variable | Limited; public health laboratories and university research centers; requires prior approval |
| Immunohistochemistry of affected tissues | Screening; confirmatory at group level | Not determined | Variable | Limited; public health laboratories and university research centers; requires prior approval |

**7. Sample/specimen requirements**—Whole blood, serum, or tissue collected from clinically ill patients in the acute stage (within the first week of illness) provides valuable samples for diagnostic testing. Ethylenediaminetetraacetic acid-treated blood is often employed, although other anticoagulants may be suitable for testing. Buffy coats or separated leukocytes may also be employed. Samples for culture should be promptly inoculated into appropriate cell lines. All other samples can be refrigerated until testing. Clinical specimens should be collected early in the illness and before appropriate antibiotic therapy when used for molecular or cultural testing. Convalescent serum samples should be taken 2–4 weeks later for serologic confirmation. Antibodies are not generally detectable until 7–10 days of infection, thus paired analysis provides more diagnostic strength than single-sample determinations.

The preferred specimens for PCR diagnosis are whole blood and buffy coat preparations. Postmortem tissue samples (spleen, liver, lung, and kidney) provide valuable specimens for confirmation of infrequent deaths due to these agents.

All specimens should be refrigerated for transport via overnight shipping services. Freezing tissues or whole blood may limit the available testing options, and may not be recommended for some testing methods. Formalin-fixed, paraffin-embedded tissues for PCR or histopathologic examination and IHC should be shipped at ambient or refrigerated temperatures to avoid damage to the tissue architecture. All samples should be handled using universal/standard precautions in the clinical and laboratory settings.

**8. Testing requirements**—Illnesses due to the *Anaplasmataceae* often present with vague, undifferentiated clinical features, and the most effective testing strategy is to utilize multiple diagnostic methodologies to confirm cases. IgM class antibodies may rise just before or alongside IgG antibodies and may remain elevated for some time (≤2 years in ehrlichiosis and anaplasmosis). This limits their singular use as an indicator of acute infection. Seroconversion in the IgG class is used by public health officials for surveillance purposes, with 4-fold rises in antibody titer providing strong evidence for acute infection. PCR assays are encouraged for diagnosis of acute disease, but sample timing and type are critical for effective use of this method. Whole blood is a rich source of pathogens in the acute stage before antibiotic treatment. After antibiotics are initiated, the ability to detect these pathogens by PCR assays, IHC, or culture progressively and rapidly declines.

Positive and negative controls must be included in all testing runs and performance characteristics of reagents and controls must be documented. Limited reference reagents may be obtained from CDC, but commercial kits and services are increasingly available for these diseases. Serologic cross-reactions may occur across the members of the *Anaplasmataceae*. For instance, *Ehrlichia chaffeensis* and *A. phagocytophilum* may cross-react in up to 20% of cases. Test results should be interpreted in the context of clinical manifestation. As with all clinical testing, proficiency testing should be performed regularly, and the competency of testing personnel should be regularly confirmed.

A summary of the various testing requirements for ehrlichiosis and related diseases is provided in the earlier table.

**9. Reporting requirements**—Cases are nationally notifiable in the USA to public health authorities (see: https://wwwn.cdc.gov/nndss/conditions/notifiable/2018) as ehrlichiosis/anaplasmosis due to the specific agents, or as undetermined ehrlichiosis/anaplasmosis. Cases lacking convalescent serum samples cannot be confirmed by serology and thus will be recorded as probable if they meet the minimum laboratory and clinical criteria. Case reporting is conducted through electronic reports and case report forms to the state health departments, which then report this to the national level. These data are summarized weekly and annually in CDC's published morbidity and mortality reports. Case reporting may be obligatory for the rickettsial diseases including ehrlichiosis in some countries.

CDC accepts deposition of *Anaplasma*, *Ehrlichia*, and other *Anaplasmataceae* isolates into its CDC Rickettsial Isolate Reference Collection (World Data Center for Microorganisms Collection 1093). CDC maintains and distributes strains to researchers globally. Call 1-404-639-1075 for further information on submission requirements. Isolates and purified DNA of select rickettsial organisms may also be available through other microbial resource centers; a full listing of centers is available at: http://www.wdcm.org.

**10. Referral network**—Diagnostic testing is available in the USA through state and national public health laboratories, academic centers, and commercial laboratories. CDC offers testing upon submission by or upon approval of the respective state health departments. Serological tests are available for many of the agents, but some are available only through research centers. Molecular testing is becoming more accessible at commercial and public health laboratories.

**11. Special considerations**—Surveillance case definitions for ehrlichiosis and anaplasmosis for public health surveillance in the USA can be found at: https://wwwn.cdc.gov/nndss/conditions/ehrlichiosis-and-anaplasmosis/case-definition/2008. These diseases may be imported into one state from another or into the USA from other endemic countries, so physicians should solicit information regarding travel histories. Given the potentially life-threatening nature of infection with some agents, empiric treatment with doxycycline is warranted while awaiting laboratory results. Specimens should be taken for laboratory testing prior to administration of antibiotics. Disease often occurs as sporadic cases or in small case clusters. Disease may be recognized in affected pets sharing the same peridomestic space and can act as sentinels for human infection; communication between veterinary and medical professionals can facilitate detection and response.

Additional details on these diseases may be found in *CCDM20* and at: https://www.cdc.gov/mmwr/volumes/65/rr/rr6502a1.htm.

[W. L. Nicholson, B. S. Pritt]

# ENTEROBIASIS

| DISEASE | ICD-10 CODE |
|---|---|
| ENTEROBIASIS | ICD-10 B80 |

**1. Clinical features**—A common intestinal helminthic infection that may range from asymptomatic to recurrently symptomatic. The most common clinical feature is perianal itching which may lead to disturbed sleep, irritability and secondary infection of scratched skin. Other clinical manifestations include vulvovaginitis, salpingitis, and pelvic and liver granulomata. Appendicitis and enuresis have also been reported as possible associated conditions.

**2. Causative agents**—*Enterobius vermicularis*, a small intestinal nematode, commonly known as pinworm. The worm is oviparous, and the adults are found in the lumen of the cecum and appendix and occasionally in ascending colon and ileum. Ectopic migration to the uterus, ovaries, fallopian tubes, liver parenchyma, spleen, lymph nodes, and lungs have been reported.

**3. Laboratory diagnosis**—The diagnosis can be made by demonstrating the presence of worms or their eggs. Adult worms can be seen in the perianal region 2-3 hours after the infected person goes to sleep. Eggs can be demonstrated by applying transparent adhesive tape (i.e., tape swab or pinworm paddle) to the perianal region and examining the tape or paddle microscopically for eggs. xMaterial for examination is best obtained in the morning before bathing or passage of stools. Examination should be repeated 3 or more times before accepting a negative result. Eggs are sometimes found on microscopic stool and urine examination, nail washings, and bed linen, although routine ova and parasite examinations of stool are not reliable, as eggs are not introduced into the fecal stream. Female worms may be found in feces and in the perianal region during rectal or vaginal examinations. Adult worms may also be observed in biopsy specimens processed for routine histology; this is especially true for ectopic cases. There are no serological or molecular tests available for routine diagnosis.

Eggs of *E. vermicularis* measure 50-60 μm long by 20-30 μm wide, oblong and slightly flattened on one side, have a thick, hyaline shell, and are partially embryonated when shed.

Adult female worms are 8-15 mm long, have a long pointed tail, prominent cephalic inflations, and a large bulbous esophagus; mated females will contain eggs in utero. Adult male worms are 2.5 mm long and have a bluntly-rounded tail; prominent cephalic inflations are also visible.

**4. Laboratory capability**—Microscopy should be available. Laboratorians should be trained in the microscopic/morphologic detection of parasites and undergo regular proficiency testing.

**5. Safety requirements**—Clinical specimens should always be collected and handled with universal/standard precautions. *Enterobius vermicularis* is a biosafety level 2 organism. Development to the infectious first stage occurs within 4-6 hours, and eggs in clinical specimens are likely infectious. Paddles and tape preparations should be disposed of as infectious waste.

**6. Nonhuman hosts**—None.

**7. Sample/specimen requirements**—Tape preparations and paddles should be placed in a secure container to prevent contamination during transit and processing. Adult worms should be placed in a liquid preservative such as 10% formalin or 70% laboratory grade ethanol as soon as possible after collection to avoid desiccation and alteration of morphologic features. Specimens in the appropriate preservatives should remain intact indefinitely. To maximize sensitivity, 4–6 tape/paddle preparations should be collected and examined before reporting as negative.

**8. Testing requirements**—Routine examination of both helminth eggs and adults. A calibrated ocular micrometer should be used to measure egg and adult worm size. Diagnosis is confirmatory in specimens meeting morphologic criteria.

**9. Reporting requirements**—*E. vermicularis* is reported at the species level based on the morphology of eggs and adults. Enterobiasis is not nationally reportable in the USA. Report to local health authority; official report justified based on local law or regulation or if the case represents an outbreak in a day care or institutionalized setting.

**10. Referral network**—None.

**11. Special considerations**—Multiple cases in schools and institutions can best be controlled through systematic treatment of all infected individuals and household contacts. Recommended disinfection and washing in hot water of bed linens, toys, and other potentially infected fomites, especially in day cares or institutionalized settings.

[B. Mathison]

# ENTEROVIRUS DISEASES

| DISEASE | ICD-10 CODE |
|---|---|
| ENTEROVIRAL VESICULAR PHARYNGITIS | ICD-10 B08.5 |
| ENTEROVIRAL VESICULAR STOMATITIS WITH EXANTHEM | ICD-10 B08.04 |
| ENTEROVIRAL LYMPHONODULAR PHARYNGITIS | ICD-10 B08.8 |
| MYALGIA, EPIDEMIC | ICD-10 B33.0 |
| VIRAL CARDITIS | ICD-10 B33.2 |
| Enteroviral hemorrhagic conjunctivitis (see "Conjunctivitis/Keratitis") | |
| Meningitis (see "Meningitis") | |
| Poliomyelitis (see "Poliomyelitis") | |

| DISEASE | CAUSATIVE AGENTS |
|---|---|
| ENTEROVIRAL VESICULAR PHARYNGITIS | *Enterovirus A* serotypes CV-A1 to 10, 16, 22, and EV-A71 |
| ENTEROVIRAL VESICULAR STOMATITIS WITH EXANTHEM | Predominantly CV-A16 and EV-A71 but includes other *Enterovirus A* serotypes<br>Less frequently associated with *Enterovirus B* serotypes CV-B2 and CV-B5 |
| ENTEROVIRAL LYMPHONODULAR PHARYNGITIS | *Enterovirus A* serotype CV-A10 |
| MYALGIA, EPIDEMIC | Predominantly associated with *Enterovirus B* serotypes CV-B1 to 3, 5, 6, and E-1, 6<br>Sporadically associated with other *Enterovirus A* and *B* serotypes |
| VIRAL CARDITIS | Primarily *Enterovirus B* serotypes CV-B1 to 5, CV-A9 and CV-A23, but occasionally *Enterovirus A* serotypes CV-A4 and DV-A16, *Enterovirus C* serotype CV-A1, and other enteroviruses |
| Enteroviral hemorrhagic conjunctivitis (see "Conjunctivitis/Keratitis") | |
| Meningitis (see "Meningitis") | |
| Poliomyelitis (see "Poliomyelitis") | |

Enterovirus diseases have multiple clinical manifestations. The clinical features vary accordingly.

**1. Clinical features—**

1) Enteroviral vesicular stomatitis with exanthem (hand, foot, and mouth disease), enteroviral vesicular pharyngitis (herpangina): hand, foot, and mouth disease is a brief, usually mild, febrile illness with papulovesicular rashes over the palms and soles, with or without multiple painful mouth ulcers. Sometimes, the rash may be of maculopapular type without vesicles. It may also involve the buttocks, knees, or elbows, particularly in younger children and infants. In the 2012 CV-A6 outbreaks in North America and Europe, patients typically had perioral and perirectal papules in addition to vesicles on the dorsum of their hands. The skin lesions, which heal spontaneously without scarring, may last for 3–5 days after the onset of illness. Secondary bacterial skin infection is very unusual.

   Herpangina is characterized by a brief, generally mild, febrile illness with multiple painful mouth ulcers that predominantly affect the posterior oral cavity, including the anterior pharyngeal folds, uvula, tonsils, and soft palate. In some children, the ulcers may affect other parts of the mouth, including the buccal mucosa and tongue. The oral lesions may persist for 3–5 days after the onset of illness.

   The most common clinical problems associated with these 2 closely related conditions are odynophagia and dehydration. The odynophagia may be severe in young children and result in inadequate fluid intake and dehydration. Recent epidemics of hand, foot, and mouth disease and herpangina in Asia have shown that infection caused by EV-A71, in contrast to that caused by other enteroviruses, may be associated with central nervous system (CNS) complications, including aseptic meningitis, encephalitis, and acute flaccid paralysis. Children with CNS involvement (encephalitis and acute flaccid paralysis), particularly those aged 5 years or younger, are at risk of acute severe, and sometimes fatal, cardiac dysfunction and pulmonary edema. The warning signs of CNS involvement and systemic complications include persistent fever for more than 48 hours, body temperature higher than 39°C, recurrent vomiting, unexplained irritability, lethargy, myoclonus, focal limb weakness, truncal ataxia, nystagmus, signs of respiratory distress, and skin mottling.

Important differential diagnoses for hand, foot, and mouth disease and herpangina include herpetic gingivostomatitis, aphthous stomatitis, and scabies infestation. Patients with herpetic gingivostomatitis are usually febrile and toxic. The gingiva is typically inflamed and may be bleeding. There may be circumoral ulcers or vesicles without extremity involvement, as well as associated cervical lymphadenopathy. Aphthous stomatitis is characterized by larger, ulcerative lesions of the lips, tongue, and buccal mucosa that are painful but lack constitutional symptoms. It is benign, noncontagious, and commonly affects older children and adults. Recurrence is common. Scabies infestation may sometimes be confused with hand, foot, and mouth disease because it also causes pustules, vesicles, or nodular lesions over the hands and feet. Intense itching and interdigital space involvement are useful clinical clues to the parasitic infestation.

2) Myalgia, epidemic (epidemic pleurodynia, bornholm diseases, devil's grippe): pleurodynia is an uncommon complication of *Enterovirus B* infection. It is characterized by paroxysmal spasmodic pain in the chest or abdomen, which may be intensified by movement, and is usually accompanied by fever and headache. The pain tends to be more abdominal than thoracic in infants and young children, while the reverse applies to older children and adults. Most patients recover within 1 week of onset, but relapses occur; no fatalities have been reported. It is important to differentiate from more serious medical or surgical conditions. Complications occur infrequently and include orchitis, pericarditis, pneumonia, and aseptic meningitis. Localized epidemics are characteristic. During outbreaks of epidemic myalgia, cases of

*Enterovirus B* (serotypes CV-B1 to 5) myocarditis of the newborn have been reported. While myocarditis in adults is a rare complication, the possibility should always be considered.

3) Viral carditis (enteroviral carditis): an acute or subacute viral myocarditis or pericarditis, occurring as a manifestation of infection with enteroviruses, especially *Enterovirus B*. The enteroviruses are commonly identified etiologies of myocarditis. The myocardium is affected, particularly in neonates, in whom fever and lethargy may be followed rapidly by heart failure with pallor, cyanosis, dyspnea, tachycardia, and enlargement of heart and liver. Heart failure may be progressive and fatal, or recovery may take place over a few weeks; some cases run a relapsing course over months and may show residual heart damage (dilated cardiomyopathy). In young adults, pericarditis is the more common manifestation, with acute chest pain, disturbance of heart rate, and often dyspnea. It may mimic myocardial infarction but is frequently associated with pulmonary or pleural manifestations (pleurodynia). The disease may be associated with aseptic meningitis; hepatitis; orchitis; pancreatitis; pneumonia; hand, foot, and mouth disease; rash; or epidemic myalgia (see Myalgia, Epidemic under Clinical Features section in this chapter).

**2. Causative agents**—Coxsackie A viruses, coxsackie B viruses, echoviruses, numbered enteroviruses. The enteroviruses often cocirculate, usually with one predominant serotype, during outbreaks of hand, foot, and mouth disease, and herpangina, and result in clinically indistinguishable skin and mucosal lesions.

The earlier table includes known causative enteroviruses for the various diseases listed; however, the information on enteroviral diseases is constantly expanding both in terms of the discovery of new serotypes and the range of diseases that they can cause, so this listing is not necessarily complete.

**3. Laboratory diagnosis**—To date, more than a 100 different enterovirus serotypes have been described. With such a large number of serotypes and overlapping clinical syndromes, cross-reactivity will confound the interpretation of any results, limiting the usefulness of serology for confirmatory diagnosis. Current diagnostic tools for identification of enteroviruses involve detection of viral ribonucleic acid (RNA) via molecular amplification by the reverse transcription polymerase chain reaction (RT-PCR). These methods (e.g., RT-PCR, multiplex RT-PCR, real-time RT-PCR) typically target the 5' untranslated region (UTR) of the enterovirus genome to identify the genus and 1 or more of the structural genes (VP1 predominantly, VP2, and VP4) for molecular typing (serotyping). Enterovirus detected in a normally sterile site, such as cerebrospinal fluid, confirms causation. There are several widely used commercial and FDA-cleared multiplex PCR assays arranged in panels for diagnosing infections of the respiratory tract, central nervous system, and other organ systems. These often include primers and probes to detect rhinovirus/enterovirus (often called RV/EV in the assay itself). A positive result does not distinguish between them, and further RT-PCR or sequencing is necessary for confirmation. For a confirmatory diagnosis, virus isolation (preferably from the infected site) by cell culture, followed by molecular typing (or direct molecular typing from the clinical specimen) can be performed. Since this may not be possible for most cases, virus isolation or molecular identification from secondary sites (e.g., throat swabs, feces, blood) will provide information on the likely causative agent.

4. **Laboratory capability**—Many clinical laboratories no longer perform cell culture isolation for suspected enterovirus cases in routine diagnostic testing. Molecular testing by real-time RT-PCR may be available in the clinical laboratory of many hospitals and enterovirus real-time RT-PCR is also available in most commercial infectious disease referral laboratories. State or local public health laboratories may also offer enterovirus testing, including both basic detection and typing, but capabilities vary widely by jurisdiction.

5. **Safety requirements**—All human enteroviruses are categorized as biosafety level 2 agents, with universal/standard practices recommended. Additional requirements apply to poliovirus (see "Poliomyelitis").

6. **Nonhuman hosts**—There are a number of enteroviruses that infect animals other than humans. Some enteroviruses of nonhuman primates are related to the human enteroviruses, and human enteroviruses have been detected in certain nonhuman primates, particularly in areas where humans and primates live in close association. However, animal-to-human transmission has not been demonstrated.

7. **Sample/specimen requirements**—Enteroviral infections are very common, especially in childhood. Since most infections are mild or asymptomatic, and virus may be excreted for a prolonged period, detection of enterovirus in a nonsterile site does not necessarily confirm etiology of the illness under investigation. However, it can be highly suggestive if the clinical syndrome is already known to be associated with the detected agent. Enterovirus detected in a normally sterile site or a site directly related to the disease (e.g., in lesion fluid from a hand, foot, and mouth disease case) confirms causation. Virus may be detected in lesion swabs in cases of hand, foot, and mouth disease. Virus may also be recovered from throat swabs up to about 2 weeks after symptom onset and from stool for up to 8 weeks, but detection is most sensitive if swabs are obtained early in the acute phase of the illness. If enterovirus testing is available on-site,

specimens can be kept at 4°C for up to 24 hours prior to testing. If specimens are to be shipped to a reference laboratory, they should be frozen at -20°C or colder and shipped frozen, preferably on dry ice. Fresh tissues should be frozen immediately on liquid nitrogen or dry ice to minimize degradation of virus genome due to nucleases and shipped to the laboratory on dry ice.

**8. Testing requirements**—Traditionally, enterovirus detection and characterization relied on virus isolation in cell culture or suckling mice, followed by typing using serotype-specific antisera. While virus isolation in culture is very sensitive, a number of different cell lines must be used because there is no single cell line that supports growth of all, or even most, enteroviruses, and antisera are not widely available for all enterovirus types. Molecular methods, such as real-time RT-PCR, are now the diagnostic assays of choice and have become the gold standard for enterovirus detection. These assays target conserved sequences in the 5' UTR of the virus genome. The most common molecular typing system is based on RT-PCR and nucleotide sequencing of a portion of the genomic region encoding VP1. The type is inferred by comparison of the partial VP1 sequence with a database containing VP1 sequences for the prototype and variant strains of all human enterovirus types.

**9. Reporting requirements**—Poliovirus infection (either paralytic poliomyelitis or nonparalytic infection with detection of poliovirus) is the only enterovirus infection that is nationally notifiable in the USA (see: https://wwwn.cdc.gov/nndss/conditions/notifiable/2018). Poliovirus infections are also reportable under the International Health Regulations. For further information, see "Poliomyelitis."

**10. Referral network**—Some state or local public health laboratories may offer enterovirus testing, including both basic detection and typing, but capabilities vary widely by jurisdiction. In cases of outbreaks, disease clusters, or unusually severe or fatal disease, public health officials may request specialized enterovirus testing at CDC or the appropriate national reference laboratory.

**11. Special considerations**—None.

[M. S. Oberste]

# ERYTHEMA INFECTIOSUM

(fifth disease parvovirus B19, slapped cheek disease)

| DISEASE | ICD-10 CODE |
|---|---|
| ERYTHEMA INFECTIOSUM | ICD-10 B08.3 |

**1. Clinical features**—A usually mild childhood viral exanthematous disease, with low-grade or no fever, occurring sporadically or in epidemics. Characteristic is a striking erythema of the cheeks (slapped cheek appearance), frequently associated with a lace-like rash on the trunk and extremities, which fades but may recur for 1–3 weeks or longer on exposure to sunlight or heat (e.g., bathing). Itch may occur on the rash-affected skin and on the palmsole. Mild constitutional symptoms may precede onset of rash. In adults, the rash is often atypical or absent, but polyarthropathy (arthralgia or arthritis) may occur. Arthropathy is uncommon in children but occurs in 50% of adults, more commonly in women; distribution is symmetric with involvement of small joints of hands and occasionally ankles, knees, and wrists. Arthropathy may last days to months but then resolves. Twenty-five percent or more of infections may be asymptomatic.

Differentiation from rubella, scarlet fever, dengue fever, and chikungunya fever is necessary. Usually the rash of erythema infectiosum (commonly called fifth disease) does not have raised maculopapular appearance unlike in these diseases. On dark skin the rash is very often missed on examination.

Intrauterine infection in the first half of pregnancy results in hydrops fetalis and fetal death in fewer than 10% of infections, and intrauterine infection infrequently results in fetal anemia that persists in the infant after birth. Infection with human parvovirus B19 (B19V), the cause of erythema infectiosum, may lead to transient aplastic crisis in individuals with hemolytic anemias (e.g., sickle cell disease) as part of the viremic phase of illness (and before the onset of rash illness). Immunosuppressed people may develop severe, chronic anemia. Red cell aplasia has been reported. Several diseases (e.g., rheumatoid arthritis, systemic vasculitis, fulminant hepatitis, and myocarditis) have been reported in association with erythema infectiosum, but no causal link has been established.

**2. Causative agents**—B19V, a 20–25 nm nonencapsidated single-stranded deoxyribonucleic acid (DNA) virus, belonging to the family *Parvoviridae,* genus *Erythroparvovirus.* The virus has a single serotype, but 3 different genotypes. The virus replicates primarily in erythroid precursor cells and cannot be grown in standard tissue culture. B19V is resistant to inactivation by various methods, including heating to 80°C (176°F) for 72 hours.

**3. Laboratory diagnosis**—The diagnosis is usually made based on clinical and epidemiological grounds; however, it can be laboratory confirmed by detection of B19V specific immunoglobulin class M (IgM) antibodies or by a significant rise in IgG antibody levels. IgM levels begin to decline 1–2 months after the onset of symptoms. Diagnosis of B19V infection is ideally made by detecting viral DNA by nucleic acid amplification by quantitative polymerase chain reaction (PCR).

**4. Laboratory capability**—Testing for B19V can be performed by laboratories capable of standard processing of clinical samples and the ability to perform commercial enzyme immunoassays. For confirmation or for diagnosis of transient aplastic crisis, chronic anemia DNA extraction facilities and the ability to perform quantitative PCR are required.

**5. Safety requirements**—B19V is classified as a risk group 2/biosafety level 2 pathogen, and therefore universal/standard laboratory procedures for dealing with human samples should be employed. Samples from patients with transient aplastic crisis or chronic anemia due to B19V may contain very high levels of infectious B19V, and procedures generating aerosols should be performed in a biosafety cabinet.

**6. Nonhuman hosts**—Although some nonhuman primates can be experimentally infected, humans are the only natural hosts.

**7. Sample/specimen requirements**—Serum is the preferred sample for testing and can be used for detection of serological response or detection of viral DNA. For confirmation of intrauterine infection, amniotic fluid or fetal blood can be tested. In rare cases of suspected meningoencephalitis, cerebrospinal fluid should be tested in parallel with a serum sample taken at the same time so that the viral load can be appropriately interpreted.

Tissue samples, including bone marrow samples, may be used for antigen or DNA detection, but results may be difficult to interpret without viral load in a serum sample taken at the same time. Throat/mouth swabs are not suitable for testing as low level B19V DNA can persist and be detected for months to years after infection.

**8. Testing requirements**—Diagnosis of the rash associated with B19V is done by detection of specific IgM by an immunocapture method. Commercial assays using noninfectious viral-like particles as antigen are available. B19V IgM is detectable within 1 day of onset of rash and remains detectable for 2 months. False-positive results can occur, especially in pregnancy or with other viral infections. Confirmation of B19V IgM, if necessary, can be performed by quantitative PCR with an assay calibrated against the WHO B19V DNA standard. Individuals with recent infection will have B19V DNA levels greater than $10^4$ IU/mL.

Evidence of previous B19V infection is by detection of B19V IgG. Samples are positive from 1 day after onset of rash. Antibody remains detectable for life, although there may be some lowering of antibody levels with time.

Diagnosis of patients with transient aplastic crisis, pure red cell aplasia, or chronic anemia due to parvovirus B19 infection is by quantitative PCR on serum or blood samples. In acute infections, viral loads are greater than $10^9$ IU/mL. B19V IgM and/or IgG may be undetectable and are not useful in diagnosis.

B19V DNA can persist at low levels in tissues for months or years following resolution of infection, and therefore detection of low level DNA in tissues may indicate previous infection only. Evidence of active infection can be sought by detection of viral antigen (immunohistochemistry) or B19V-specific viral ribonucleic acid (amplicon across a spliced junction to distinguish from viral DNA), but these are mainly research tools.

There is no role for tissue culture.

**9. Reporting requirements**—Erythema infectiosum or B19V infection is not a reportable infection.

**10. Referral network**—None.

**11. Special considerations**—In addition to fifth disease, erythema infectiosum may also be referred to as parvovirus B19, B19V infection, or slapped cheek disease.

[K. E. Brown]

# EXANTHEMA SUBITUM

(roseola infantum, sixth disease)

| DISEASE | ICD-10 CODE |
|---|---|
| EXANTHEMA SUBITUM | ICD-10 B08.2 |

**1. Clinical features**—Exanthema subitum results from primary infection with a human herpesvirus, particularly the 6B strain (HHV-6B), in children younger than 2 years. It is unusual in children older than this and in adults, where primary infection causes a mild glandular fever-like illness in some individuals. Most infections with HHV-6B are asymptomatic or cause a non-specific fever. Exanthema subitum presents as an acute febrile illness up to 41°C (106°F), which subsides in 3–5 days, followed a few days later by a maculopapular rash on the trunk and later on the remainder of the body, which then fades rapidly. Symptoms are generally mild, but febrile seizures and more severe illness, such as meningoencephalitis or hepatitis, occur in a small proportion.

It may clinically resemble other viral exanthems such as measles, rubella, and parvovirus B19 (erythema infectiosum) infection. However, the mild nature of the illness and the gap between resolution of the fever and onset of the rash are important diagnostic clues.

**2. Causative agents**—HHV-6 (subfamily betaherpesvirus, genus *Roseolovirus*) is found as 2 species, HHV-6A and HHV-6B. Whereas HHV-6A has so far not been associated with any disease, HHV-6B is the most common cause of exanthema subitum. Primary infection with HHV-7, a closely related virus, is an occasional cause of exanthema subitum. Infection with HHV-6B is nearly universal by 2 years of age, with primary HHV-7 infection occurring later up to 5 years old. As with the other herpesviruses, primary infection is followed by lifelong latent infection with the potential for reactivation and sometimes disease. Immunosuppressed individuals may get severe disease due to HHV-6B, including fever, encephalitis, and bone marrow suppression.

**3. Laboratory diagnosis**—The diagnosis of exanthema subitum (also known as roseola infantum or sixth disease) is often made clinically and rarely requires laboratory confirmation as the illness is generally mild and self-limited.

However, if an etiologic diagnosis is required, serologically, primary infection is indicated by immunoglobulin class G (IgG) seroconversion or a rise in IgG over the course of 7–14 days, with detectable IgM appearing 1 week after onset and disappearing by 3–4 weeks.

Virus can also be detected by polymerase chain reaction (PCR) in saliva, peripheral blood, and other sites during primary infection. However, PCR assays are of limited use in the diagnosis of primary infection as the diagnosis of exanthema subitum may be confounded by the phenomenon of chromosomally integrated HHV-6 (ciHHV-6). In about 1% of the human population, HHV-6 has a unique feature whereby the genome of HHV-6A or HHV-6B is integrated into a human chromosome and vertically transmitted. Such germline transmission means that very high levels of viral deoxyribonucleic acid (DNA) will be found continually in every nucleated cell throughout the body. High levels of viral DNA are also found in serum originating from cells damaged before or during separation from clotted blood.

**4. Laboratory capability**—Standard microbiological laboratory with personnel trained to carry out molecular biology techniques, such as PCR, and serological techniques, in particular immunofluorescence testing for IgG and IgM.

**5. Safety requirements**—Biosafety level 2 is required. This implies use of universal/standard microbial practices together with enhanced measures, such as using appropriate personal protective equipment. Personnel working in such laboratories are expected to take care to prevent injuries such as cuts and other breaches of the skin, as well as ingestion and mucous membrane exposures.

**6. Nonhuman hosts**—None.

**7. Sample/specimen requirements**—Laboratory diagnosis of exanthema subitum requires serum or plasma samples, the acute serum taken within the first week of illness and the convalescent serum 10–14 days later.

HHV-6 and HHV-7 DNA can be detected and reproducibly quantified by real-time PCR in a broad range of clinical specimens including whole blood, plasma, serum, and cerebrospinal fluid.

**8. Testing requirements**—Testing for HHV-6B and HHV-7 primary infection is not usually indicated, as exanthema subitum can be diagnosed on the basis of its typical clinical presentation. However, primary infection may not always be accompanied by a rash, and diagnostic testing may be required to establish the cause of serious complications, such as febrile status epilepticus and encephalitis. Quick and accurate diagnosis could also play a role in preventing antibiotic misuse and reducing unnecessary hospitalization. Unfortunately, the current tests have limitations, including general lack of availability in diagnostic laboratories and PCR tests that discriminate between HHV-6A and HHV-6B are often not used.

1) Diagnostic testing using paired sera/plasma: diagnosis of exanthema subitum requires demonstration of HHV-6 or HHV-7 IgG seroconversion; IgM testing has a low accuracy.[1] The gold standard is an indirect immunofluorescence test for IgG antibody. Cells infected with the target reference virus are fixed onto glass slides and incubated with the serum under test. Suitable slides are commercially available. Reading the slide requires a suitable microscope and a trained observer who can take into account the number of fluorescent foci, the intracellular distribution of staining, and possible nonspecific background fluorescence. The sensitivity, specificity, and positive and negative predictive values for the HHV-6 IgG test are 95%, 84%, 91%, and 90% respectively and 95%, 76%, 84%, and 93% for HHV-7 IgG.[2]
2) Confirmatory testing using paired sera/plasma: there is limited cross-reactivity between HHV-6 and HHV-7 antibodies; seroconversion can readily demonstrate primary infection in an HHV-7 seronegative individual and vice versa. However, because primary HHV-6 infection commonly precedes primary HHV-7 infection, difficulty arises because rising titers of antibodies to both viruses may occur. In this situation, antibody avidity can prove very useful as a confirmatory test to distinguish the low avidity IgG response in HHV-7 primary infection from the high avidity HHV-6 response that accompanies it. Dual primary infections may also be differentiated in this way if antibody is detected in a convalescent serum and is found to be of low avidity for both HHV-6 and HHV-7. The antibody test can easily be modified for avidity by including urea in the first incubation step.[3,4]
3) Presumptive testing for primary HHV-6 infection using a single acute serum/plasma: quantitative detection of viral DNA in plasma by PCR is 92% sensitive as compared with virus isolation but

cannot distinguish between active virus replication and ciHHV-6.[5] Confirmation requires a convalescent sample showing HHV-6 IgG seroconversion as compared with the acute.

4) Presumptive testing for primary HHV-7 infection using a single acute serum/plasma: there are few data indicating the sensitivity of an HHV-7 DNA test in plasma for primary HHV-7 infection. However, quantitative PCR is likely to have a similar sensitivity to that of HHV-6, and the results are not complicated by inherited chromosomal integration. Thus, the presence of HHV-7 DNA in an acute sample can be taken as presumptive evidence of primary infection but, as earlier, confirmation requires antibody seroconversion.
5) Presumptive testing for primary HHV-6 and HHV-7 infection using a single convalescent serum/plasma: antibody avidity testing will provide confirmatory evidence if the avidity is low. Determination of avidity enables recent primary infection (within the last 6 weeks) to be differentiated from persistent or recurrent infection.
6) Tests required for exclusion of ciHHV-6: as viremia is short lived in primary HHV-6 infection in children, evidence of persistent high-level DNA in sequential sera or whole blood samples gives presumptive evidence of ciHHV-6. Results from plasma samples should be treated with caution as levels of HHV-6 DNA in ciHHV-6 are highly variable in this type of sample. Confirmatory evidence can be obtained by determining the ratio of HHV-6 DNA to cellular DNA using fluorescence in situ hybridization-confirmed samples.[6] Droplet digital PCR is the method of choice, being the most accurate, as opposed to real time PCR.
7) Limitations of testing:

    - Testing for primary infection should be limited to young children as older children are unlikely to be susceptible to exanthema subitum. Antibody tests have a low sensitivity in older children, adults, and the immunocompromised as antibodies levels are lower than in young children, and the antibody response may be delayed in the immunocompromised.
    - Although testing by indirect immunofluorescence cannot distinguish between antibodies to HHV-6A and HHV-6B due to significant cross-reactivity, recently developed immunoblotting assays appear to have this capability and may prove useful for research purposes.
    - Enzyme immunoassays, using either infected cell lysates or purified virus as antigens, have been developed but their specificity has been repeatedly questioned.

**9. Reporting requirements**—Exanthema subitum is not a reportable disease.

**10. Referral network**—None.

**11. Special considerations**—None.

## References

1. de Oliveira Vianna RA, Siqueira MM, Camacho LA, et al. The accuracy of anti-human herpesvirus 6 IgM detection in children with recent primary infection. *J Virol Methods*. 2008;153(2);273–275.
2. Ward KN, Couto Parada X, Passas J, Thiruchelvam AD. Evaluation of specificity and sensitivity of indirect immunofluorescence tests for IgG to human herpesviruses-6 and-7. *J Virol Methods*. 2002;106(1):107–113.
3. Ward KN, Gray JJ, Fotheringham MW, Sheldon MJ. IgG antibodies to human herpesvirus-6 in young children: changes in avidity of antibody correlate with time after infection. *J Med Virol*. 1993;39(2):131–138.
4. Ward KN, Turner DJ, Couto Parada X, Thiruchelvam AD. Use of immunoglobulin G antibody avidity for differentiation of primary human herpesvirus 6 and 7 infections. *J Clin Microbiol*. 2001;39(3):959–963.
5. Caserta MT, Hall CB, Schnabel K, et al. Diagnostic assays for active infection with human herpesvirus 6 (HHV-6). *J Clin Virol*. 2010;48(1):55–57.
6. Sedlak RH, Cook L, Huang ML, et al. Identification of chromosomally integrated human herpesvirus 6 by droplet digital PCR. *Clin Chem*. 2014;60(5):765–772.

[K. N. Ward]

# FASCIOLIASIS

| DISEASE | ICD-10 CODE |
|---|---|
| FASCIOLIASIS | ICD-10 B66.3 |

**1. Clinical features**—A zoonotic disease caused by *Fasciola* parasites (liver flukes), which predominantly affect the hepatobiliary system. During the acute (early) phase of infection, immature *Fasciola* larvae migrate from the intestine through the abdominal cavity and liver, where they can cause parenchymal damage. The chronic phase begins when the larvae reach the bile ducts, where they mature into adult flukes and start to produce eggs (3–4 months after initial exposure), which are passed from the bile ducts into the intestine (thereafter into feces); the flukes may cause biliary colic or obstructive jaundice. During both phases, clinical features can include fever, malaise, abdominal symptoms (e.g., pain, anorexia, nausea, vomiting, diarrhea, weight loss), eosinophilia (especially during the acute phase), hepatomegaly, and abnormal liver function tests. Ectopic infection, especially by *Fasciola gigantica*, may produce transient or migrating areas of inflammation in the skin over the trunk or other areas of the body.

**2. Causative agents**—The trematodes *Fasciola hepatica* (also known as common liver fluke) and *F. gigantica*.

**3. Laboratory diagnosis**—Based on finding eggs in feces or in biliary or duodenal aspirates during the chronic phase or adults observed in the hepatic ducts via endoscopic retrograde cholangiopancreatogram. Serologic testing (available at CDC within the USA) can be useful (i.e., positive results can provide supportive evidence of the diagnosis) during the acute phase, before eggs are produced; during the chronic phase, in cases with low-level production of eggs; and in cases of ectopic infection. There are no molecular tests available for routine clinical diagnosis of fascioliasis.

Eggs of *F. hepatica* measure 130–150 μm long by 63–90 μm wide, have a thin shell, an inconspicuous operculum lacking defined shoulders, and are unembryonated when shed in feces. Eggs of *F. gigantica* are similar but larger, measuring 160–190 μm long by 70–90 μm wide. Eggs of *F. hepatica* are nearly identical morphologically to the eggs of *Fasciolopsis buski*, a large intestinal trematode. Eggs of *F. hepatica* may also overlap in size with those of *Gastrodiscoides hominis* and some species of *Echinostoma*. When eggs are seen in human stool, additional patient specimens should be requested and tested to rule-out spurious passage following consumption of infected animal livers (pseudofascioliasis).

Adult worms removed via endoscopy are up to 30 mm wide and are flattened and leaf-shaped. The anterior end is distinctly cone-shaped. Eggs may be observed in utero to aid in diagnosis.

A serological immunoblot (i.e., Western blot) assay may aid the diagnosis, especially when eggs are not seen in the stool or even in acute cases. The *F. hepatica* Western blot is based on the observation of a diagnostic band at 38 kDa. In subjects with chronic human fascioliasis, the FhSAP2 immunoblot assay has a sensitivity of 94% and a specificity of 98%. For subjects with acute fascioliasis infection, the assay has a sensitivity of 57% (4 of 7 tests were positive). This assay is currently only available at CDC. There is no information on the performance of the immunoblot on patients infected with *F. gigantica*.

**4. Laboratory capability**—Microscopy and stool concentration/centrifugation capabilities should be available. Laboratorians should be trained in the microscopic/morphologic detection of parasites and undergo regular proficiency testing. Currently, serologic testing for fascioliasis is only available at CDC.

**5. Safety requirements**—Clinical specimens should always be collected and handled with universal/standard precautions. *Fasciola* spp. are biosafety level 2 organisms. Formalin should only be used in a well-ventilated area, preferably in a chemical fume hood. Unpreserved and preserved stools, blood, and sera should be disposed of as infectious waste.

**6. Nonhuman hosts**—The natural definitive hosts for *Fasciola* spp. are ruminants, especially sheep and cattle. The first intermediate host is a freshwater snail, in which cercariae develop. Cercariae are not infective to the human host; instead, cercariae encyst on aquatic vegetation as metacercariae. Humans become infected after ingesting metacercariae on plants.

**7. Sample/specimen requirements**—Stool should be promptly preserved in an appropriate liquid medium, such as 10% buffered formalin or sodium acetate-acetic acid-formalin. Single vial systems for ova and parasites collection are also adequate. Adult worms should also be placed in a liquid preservative such as 10% formalin or 70% laboratory grade ethanol as soon as possible after collection to avoid desiccation and alteration of morphologic features. Specimens in the appropriate preservatives should remain intact indefinitely. Eggs are often shed in low numbers in feces; therefore, to maximize ova and parasite sensitivity, at least 3 stool specimens should be collected.

Serum or plasma separator tubes should be used for collecting specimens for serological testing. A minimum volume of 250 µL of serum is required for testing. Spun serum may be shipped at room temperature; however, whole blood or blood collected in ethylenediaminetetraacetic acid tubes should be shipped chilled.

**8. Testing requirements**—Routine concentration procedures for stool (eggs) and routine examination of gross helminths (adults). A calibrated ocular micrometer should be used to measure egg size. Diagnosis is confirmatory in specimens meeting morphologic criteria.

**9. Reporting requirements**—When eggs are observed in stool, it is common practice to report as *F. hepatica/F. buski* as the eggs of the 2 species are morphologically indistinguishable. More confidence can be given to a species-level identification in cases of *F. gigantica* due to the larger size of the eggs. Adults may be identified to the species level based on morphology and location in the host.

Fascioliasis is not nationally reportable in the USA. Report to local health authority; official report not ordinarily justifiable.

**10. Referral network**—The drug of choice, triclabendazole, is regulated by CDC, so positive results may have to be confirmed by CDC diagnostic laboratories or international laboratories that perform serologic testing before the drug can be released.

**11. Special considerations**—Determine source of infection and identify plants and snails involved in transmission. Prevent eating aquatic plants from contaminated areas.

[B. Mathison]

# FASCIOLOPSIASIS

| DISEASE | ICD-10 CODE |
|---|---|
| FASCIOLOPSIASIS | ICD-10 B66.5 |

**1. Clinical features**—A zoonotic trematode infection of the small intestine, particularly the duodenum. Symptoms result from local inflammation, ulceration of intestinal wall, and systemic toxic effects. Diarrhea usually alternates with constipation; vomiting and anorexia are frequent. Large numbers of flukes may produce acute intestinal obstruction. Patients may show edema of the face, abdominal wall, and legs within 20 days after massive infection; ascites is common. Eosinophilia is usual. Secondary anemia may occur. Death is rare; light infections are usually asymptomatic.

**2. Causative agents**—*Fasciolopsis buski*, a large intestinal trematode distributed in Southeast Asia and the Indian subcontinent.

**3. Laboratory diagnosis**—Through detection of the large flukes via endoscopy or characteristic eggs in stool or vomitus. There are no serologic nor molecular tests available for routine clinical diagnosis of fasciolopsiasis.

Eggs of *F. buski* measure 130–150 µm long by 63–90 µm wide, have a thin shell, have an inconspicuous operculum lacking defined shoulders, and are unembryonated when shed in feces. Eggs of *F. buski* are nearly identical morphologically to the eggs of *Fasciola hepatica*, a large hepatic trematode.

Adults are large, flat, and leaf-shaped, measuring 20–75 mm in length. The anterior end is rounded and not distinctly cone-shaped as seen with *F. hepatica*.

**4. Laboratory capability**—Microscopy and stool concentration/centrifugation capabilities should be available. Laboratorians should be trained in the microscopic/morphologic detection of parasites and undergo regular proficiency testing.

**5. Safety requirements**—Clinical specimens should always be collected and handled with universal/standard precautions. *F. buski* is a biosafety level 2 organism. Formalin should only be used in a well-ventilated area, preferably in a chemical fume hood. Unpreserved and preserved stools should be disposed of as infectious waste.

**6. Nonhuman hosts**—The natural definitive hosts for *F. buski* are usually pigs. The first intermediate host is a freshwater snail, in which cercariae develop. Cercariae are not infective to the human host; instead, cercariae encyst on aquatic vegetation as metacercariae. Humans become infected after ingesting metacercariae on plants.

**7. Sample/specimen requirements**—Stool should be promptly preserved in an appropriate liquid medium, such as 10% buffered formalin or sodium acetate-acetic acid-formalin. Single vial systems for ova and parasite (O&P) collection are also adequate. Adult worms should also be placed in a liquid preservative such as 10% formalin or 70% laboratory grade ethanol as soon as possible after collection to avoid desiccation and alteration of morphologic features. Specimens in the appropriate preservatives should remain intact indefinitely. Eggs are often shed in low numbers in feces, and so to maximize O&P sensitivity, at least 3 stool specimens on successive days should be collected.

**8. Testing requirements**—Routine concentration procedures for stool (eggs) and routine examination of gross helminths (adults). A calibrated ocular micrometer should be used to measure egg size. Diagnosis is confirmatory in specimens meeting morphologic criteria.

**9. Reporting requirements**—When eggs are observed in stool, it is common practice to report as *F. hepatica/F. buski*, as the eggs of the 2 species are morphologically indistinguishable. Adults may be identified to the species level based on morphology and location in the host.

Fasciolopsiasis is not nationally reportable in the USA. Report to local health authority; case report to local health authority may be required in some endemic areas.

**10. Referral network**—None.

**11. Special considerations**—None.

[B. Mathison]

# FILARIASIS

| DISEASE | ICD-10 CODE |
|---|---|
| BANCROFTIAN FILARIASIS | ICD-10 B74.0 |
| MALAYAN FILARIASIS | ICD-10 B74.1 |
| TIMOREAN FILARIASIS | ICD-10 B74.2 |
| DIROFILARIASIS | ICD-10 B74.8 |
| MANSONELLOSIS | ICD-10 B74.4 |
| OTHER NEMATODES PRODUCING MICROFILARIAE IN HUMANS | |
| Loiasis (see "Loiasis") | |
| Onchocerciasis (see "Onchocerciasis") | |

# I. BANCROFTIAN FILARIASIS, MALAYAN FILARIASIS (Brugian filariasis), TIMOREAN FILARIASIS

**1. Clinical features**—Bancroftian filariasis occurs in 2 biologically different forms. In one, the microfilariae circulate in the peripheral blood at night (nocturnal periodicity) with greatest concentrations between 10 PM and 2 AM; in the other, microfilariae circulate continuously in the peripheral blood but occur in greater concentration in the daytime (diurnal subperiodicity). Adult parasites primarily cause lymphatic damage; the subsequent lymphoedema and its progression are due to secondary bacterial infections. Clinical manifestations in regions of endemic filariasis include (a) a symptomatic and parasitologically negative form; (b) asymptomatic microfilaremia; (c) filarial fevers manifested by high fever, acute recurrent lymphadenitis, and retrograde lymphangitis with or without microfilaremia; (d) lymphostasis associated with chronic signs, including hydrocele, chyluria, lymphoedema and elephantiasis of the limbs, breasts and genitalia, with low-level or undetectable microfilaremia; and (e) tropical pulmonary eosinophilic syndrome, manifested by paroxysmal nocturnal asthma, chronic interstitial lung disease, recurrent low-grade fever, profound eosinophilia, and degenerating microfilariae in lung tissues but not in the bloodstream (occult filariasis).

Brugian and Timorean filariasis have clinical manifestations similar to those of Bancroftian filariasis, except that the recurrent acute attacks of adenitis and retrograde lymphangitis associated with fever are more severe, while chyluria is uncommon and elephantiasis is usually confined to the distal extremities, most frequently to the legs below the knees. Hydrocele and breast lymphoedema are rarely if ever seen.

**2. Causative agents**—*Wuchereria bancrofti, Brugia malayi, and Brugia timori*; filarial nematodes that reside in the lymphatic system. *W. bancrofti* occurs nearly worldwide in the tropics and subtropics. *B. malayi* occurs in Southeast Asia west to the Indian subcontinent. *B. timori* is restricted to the Lesser Sunda Islands in Indonesia and in Timor-Leste where it replaces *B. malayi*.

**3. Laboratory diagnosis**—Microfilariae are best detected during periods of maximal microfilaremia. Live microfilariae can be seen under low power in a drop of peripheral blood (finger prick) on a microscope slide or in hemolyzed blood in a counting chamber. Thick and thin smears stained with Giemsa, Wright-Giemsa, or hematoxylin permit species identification. Microfilariae may be concentrated by filtration of anticoagulated blood through a Nuclepore filter (2–5 mm pore size), in a Swinnex adapter, or by the Knott technique (i.e., centrifugal sedimentation of 2 mL of anticoagulated blood mixed with 10 mL of 2% formalin).

Microfilariae of *W. bancrofti* are 244–296 µm long by 7.5–10.0 µm wide in stained blood films. They possess a relatively short head space, and the tail is anucleate and tapers to a point. In general, the nuclear column is relatively loose, and individual nuclei can be visualized throughout the column. In specimens preserved in a timely manner, a sheath is usually present and does not stain pink with Giemsa at an appropriate pH 6.8–7.2. Microfilariae of *B. malayi* are 177–230 μm long by 5–6 μm wide in stained blood films. They possess a longer head space and a more compact nuclear column. The tail tapers to a point and possesses both a terminal nucleus and a subterminal nucleus, with significant gaps between these nuclei and the nuclear column. In properly preserved specimens, a sheath is usually present that stains bright pink with Giemsa at an appropriate pH 6.8–7.2. Microfilariae of *B. timori* are similar to those of *B. malayi* but are larger, having a mean length of 310 μm and a width of 6–7 μm. The long head space and arrangement of tail nuclei is similar between the 2 species. Unlike with *B. malayi*, the sheath of *B. timori* does not stain bright pink with Giemsa at a pH of 6.8–7.2.

Antibody detection is available commercially and at CDC, WHO, and NIH for immunoglobulin class G (IgG) or IgG4 responses against crude extracts from Brugia spp. There is cross-reactivity to other nematode infections and the tests cannot distinguish between past and present infections. There are 2 Wb123 antigen assays specific for W. bancrofti infection: Filaria Detect IgG4 ELISA (Inbios, Seattle, WA) and SD Bioline Lymphatic Filariasis IgG4 Rapid Test (Stanford Diagnostics, Seoul, South Korea); sensitivities for both are 70%–80% and specificities greater than 97%. Antigen detection tests for W. bancrofti include Tropbio Filariasis Antigen II ELISA (Celllabs, Queensland, Australia), BinaxNOW Filariasis immunochromatographic (ICT) card assay (Alere International, Waltham, MA), and Alere Filariasis Test Strip ICT assay (Alere International) with sensitivities of 96%–100% and 98% specificity. No antigen tests currently are FDA-approved in the USA. There are currently no commercial assays available for antigen detection of Brugia infections.

**4. Laboratory capability**—Microscopy and serologic capabilities (ELISA) should be available. Laboratorians should be trained in the microscopic/morphologic detection of parasites and undergo regular proficiency testing. Serologic testing for parasitic diseases is usually performed at specialized reference laboratories.

**5. Safety requirements**—Clinical specimens should always be collected and handled with universal precautions. Filarial nematodes are biosafety level 2 organisms. Blood and sera should be disposed of as infectious waste.

**6. Nonhuman hosts**—All 3 species are transmitted by mosquitoes. *Wuchereria bancrofti* is transmitted by many species, the most important being *Culex quinquefasciatus*, *Anopheles gambiae*, *Anopheles funestus*, *Aedes polynesiensis*, *Aedes scapularis*, and *Aedes pseudoscutellaris*. *B. malayi* is transmitted by various species of *Mansonia*, *Anopheles*, and *Aedes*. *B. timori* is transmitted by *Anopheles barbirostris*.

**7. Sample/specimen requirements**—The ideal blood specimen for morphology is a finger prick; however, venous blood collected in ethylenediaminetetraacetic acid (EDTA) is sufficient. For maximum sensitivity, blood should be collected between 10 PM and 2 AM when the microfilariae are likely to be circulating in peripheral blood.

Serology may be performed on serum or plasma derived from EDTA-preserved blood. A minimum of 500 μL of serum should be submitted for serologic testing.

**8. Testing requirements**—Routine staining procedures for blood parasitology (i.e., Giemsa, Wright-Giemsa, hematoxylin) and concentration procedures (i.e., Knott's). A calibrated ocular micrometer should be used to measure microfilariae. Diagnosis is confirmatory in specimens meeting morphologic criteria.

Plate readers used for ELISA should have annual maintenance performed. Known positive and negative controls should be tested with each run. Laboratories should participate in external quality assessment at least annually.

**9. Reporting requirements**—Positive cases from humans may be reported at the species level based on the morphology of the microfilariae.

ELISA results are positive at greater than or equal to 12.4 units/μL; the presence of immunoglobulin class G4 significantly above the cutoff value may indicate infection with filarial species at some indeterminate time.

Reporting may be required in some endemic regions; reporting of cases with demonstrated microfilariae or circulating filarial antigen provides information on areas of transmission.

**10. Referral network**—None.

**11. Special considerations**—WHO has launched a global program for the elimination of lymphatic filariasis as a public health problem through an alliance of endemic countries and partners from the public and private sectors. For further information, see:

- http://www.filariasis.org
- http://www.cdc.gov/parasites/lymphaticfilariasis
- http://www.who.int/tdr/diseases-topics/lymphatic-filariasis/en

## II. DIROFILARIASIS (zoonotic filariasis)

**1. Clinical features**—*Dirofilaria immitis* lodges in a pulmonary artery, where it may form the nidus of a thrombus; this can then lead to vascular occlusion, coagulation, necrosis, and fibrosis. Symptoms are chest pain, cough, and hemoptysis. Eosinophilia is infrequent. A fibrotic nodule, 1–3 cm in diameter, which is most commonly asymptomatic, is recognizable by X-ray as a coin lesion.

Various species of *Dirofilaria* other than *D. immitis* cause subcutaneous lesions. The worms develop in or migrate to the conjunctivae and the subcutaneous tissues of the scrotum, breasts, arms, and legs, but microfilaremia is rare.

**2. Causative agents**—Zoonotic filarial nematodes in the genus *Dirofilaria*, including *D. immitis* (the dog heartworm, cosmopolitan), *Dirofilaria repens* (Old World), *Dirofilaria tenuis* (North America), *Dirofilaria striata* (North and South America), and *Dirofilaria ursi* (northern North America).

**3. Laboratory diagnosis**—Diagnosis of *D. immitis* infection is usually made by clinical presentation and characteristic coin lesion on X-rays; larvae and young adults may be observed in pulmonary biopsy specimens.

Diagnosis of non-*immitis* species is usually made by the finding of adult worms in biopsy specimens or recovered from the eye. Recognition of *Dirofilaria* is usually based on observing specific morphologic features including longitudinal external cuticular ridges and an internal cuticular ridge that runs along the base of the lateral chords and tall, polymyarian musculature.

**4. Laboratory capability**—Microscopy should be available. As dirofilariasis is usually diagnosed by observing worms in biopsy specimens, identification is often performed by pathologists and parasitologists in specialized reference laboratories. Laboratorians should be trained in the microscopic/morphologic detection of parasites and undergo regular proficiency testing.

**5. Safety requirements**—Clinical specimens should always be collected and handled with universal precautions. Filarial nematodes are biosafety level 2 organisms. Formalin should only be used in a well-ventilated area, preferably in a chemical fume hood. Biopsy specimens and whole worms should be disposed of as infectious waste.

**6. Nonhuman hosts**—Carnivores are normal definitive hosts for *Dirofilaria* sp., including dogs (*D. immitis*, *D. repens*), cats (*D. repens*, *D. striata*), raccoons (*D. tenuis*), and bears (*D. ursi*). All species are transmitted by mosquitoes, except for *D. ursi* that is transmitted by black flies.

**7. Sample/specimen requirements**—For non-*immitis* spp. in subcutaneous lesions, biopsy specimens should be collected and processed per standard histological procedures. Whole worms removed from lesions should be promptly placed in a liquid preservative such as 70% ethanol or 10% buffered formalin.

**8. Testing requirements**—Tissue parasitology. Diagnosis is confirmatory in specimens meeting morphologic criteria.

**9. Reporting requirements**—A degenerating nematode within an artery in a pulmonary infarct permits a presumptive diagnosis of *D. immitis*. Positive cases of non-*immitis* spp. from humans are usually reported at the genus level. Dirofilariasis is not nationally reportable in the USA. Report to local health authority; official report not ordinarily justifiable.

**10. Referral network**—None.

**11. Special considerations**—None.

## III. MANSONELLOSIS

**1. Clinical features**—*Mansonella perstans* is usually asymptomatic, but eye infection from immature stages has been reported. *Mansonella streptocerca* is suspected of causing cutaneous edema and thickening of the skin, hypopigmented macules, pruritus, and papules. *Mansonella ozzardi* infection is generally asymptomatic but may be associated with allergic manifestations such as arthralgia, pruritus, headaches, and lymphadenopathy.

**2. Causative agents**—Filarial nematodes in the genus *Mansonella*, including *M. perstans* (western Africa, northeastern South America), *Mansonella streptocerca* (western and central Africa), and *Mansonella ozzardi* (Central and South America, West Indies).

**3. Laboratory diagnosis**—Diagnosis of *M. perstans* and *M. ozzardi* is made by the finding of microfilariae in circulating blood; neither species exhibits specific periodicity. Diagnosis of *M. streptocerca* is made by finding of microfilariae in skin snips. There are no serologic nor molecular tests available for routine clinical diagnosis.

Microfilariae of *M. perstans* measure 190–200 μm in stained blood films. Microfilariae lack a sheath and are aperiodic. They possess a compact nuclear column that contains nuclei to the tip of the bluntly rounded tail.

Microfilariae of *M. ozzardi* are 163–230 μm long and always lack a sheath. They have a dense nuclear column that falls well short of the slender, pointed tail.

Microfilariae of *M. streptocerca* are unsheathed, measuring 180–240 μm in length. Nuclei extend to the tip of the tail, which is usually bent into a hook-like shape.

**4. Laboratory capability**—Microscopy should be available. Laboratorians should be trained in the microscopic/morphologic detection of parasites and undergo regular proficiency testing.

**5. Safety requirements**—Clinical specimens should always be collected and handled with universal precautions. Filarial nematodes are biosafety level 2 organisms. Formalin should only be used in a well-ventilated area, preferably in a chemical fume hood. Blood and skin snips should be disposed of as infectious waste.

**6. Nonhuman hosts**—Biting midges in the genus *Culicoides* are vectors for all 3 species; in the Caribbean, *M. ozzardi* is also transmitted by black flies.

**7. Sample/specimen requirements**—For *M. perstans* and *M. ozzardi*, the ideal blood specimen for morphology is a finger prick; however, blood collected in EDTA is sufficient. As these organisms do not exhibit specific periodicity, blood does not need to be collected at a specific time.

For *M. streptocerca*, skin snips should be collected from selected sites on the body; common locations include the hip, scapular area, and lower calf. Surveys have demonstrated that when the microfilarial density is high, 2 snips can be adequate, but if the density is low, 4 snips at multiple sites improves the sensitivity. Skin snips should be placed in physiological saline or water at room temperature for 30 minutes to 3 hours before microscopy; if still negative, hold overnight at 37°C. After incubation, the liquid may be placed in alcohol or formalin to preserve microfilariae.

**8. Testing requirements**—Routine staining procedures for blood parasitology (i.e., Giemsa, Wright-Giemsa, hematoxylin). A calibrated ocular micrometer should be used to measure microfilariae. Diagnosis is confirmatory in specimens meeting morphologic criteria.

**9. Reporting requirements**—Positive cases from humans may be reported at the genus or species level based on the morphology of the microfilariae. Mansonellosis is not nationally reportable in the USA. Report to local health authority; official report not ordinarily justifiable.

**10. Referral network**—None.

**11. Special considerations**—None.

[B. Mathison]

# FOODBORNE INTOXICATIONS

| DISEASE | ICD-10 CODE |
|---|---|
| FOODBORNE STAPHYLOCOCCAL INTOXICATION | ICD-10 A05.0 |
| FOODBORNE *CLOSTRIDIUM PERFRINGENS* INTOXICATION | ICD-10 A05.2 |
| FOODBORNE *BACILLUS CEREUS* INTOXICATION | ICD-10 A05.4 |
| SEAFOOD POISONING | |
| SCROMBOID FISH POISONING | ICD-10 T61.1 |
| CIGUATERA FISH POISONING | ICD-10 T61.0 |
| PARALYTIC SHELLFISH POISONING | ICD-10 T61.2 |
| NEUROTOXIC SHELLFISH POISONING | |
| DIARRHETIC SHELLFISH POISONING | ICD-10 T61.2 |
| AMNESIC SHELLFISH POISONING | ICD-10 T61.2 |
| PUFFER FISH POISONING (TETRODOTOXIN) | ICD-10 T61.2 |
| AZASPIRACID POISONING | ICD-10 T61.2 |

# I. FOODBORNE STAPHYLOCOCCAL INTOXICATION

**1. Clinical features**—Intoxication (not an infection) of abrupt and sometimes violent onset, with severe nausea, cramps, vomiting, and prostration, often accompanied by diarrhea and sometimes with subnormal temperature and lowered blood pressure. Deaths are rare. Illness commonly lasts only 1–2 days but can take longer in severe cases. In rare cases, the intensity of symptoms may require hospitalization, and unnecessary surgical exploration has sometimes been done in pursuit of a diagnosis.

**2. Causative agents**—Staphylococci multiply in food and produce the toxins even when water activity is too low for the growth of many other competing bacteria. However, the level of enterotoxin only reaches dangerous levels when a relatively high (e.g., >1,000/g) concentration of staphylococci is reached in the food. Therefore, low levels of staphylococci are typically accepted in certain foods in national legislation. It should be noted that several enterotoxins of *Staphylococcus aureus* are stable at boiling point and resist some thermal processing procedures; therefore, in outbreak investigations, detection of enterotoxin is more reliable than enumeration of staphylococci.

**3. Laboratory diagnosis**—Clinical diagnosis is easier when a group of cases present with the characteristic acute, predominantly upper gastrointestinal symptoms and a short interval between eating a common food item and the onset of symptoms (usually within 4 hours). Differential diagnosis includes other recognized forms of food poisoning as well as chemical poisons.

With regard to a laboratory diagnosis in the outbreak setting, recovery of large numbers of staphylococci ($\geq 10^5$ organisms/g of food), or detection of enterotoxin from an epidemiologically implicated food item, confirms the diagnosis. In heat treated food it may be possible to identify enterotoxin in the food in the absence of viable organisms. Recovery of large numbers of enterotoxin-producing staphylococci from stool or vomitus from a single person supports the diagnosis. In outbreak settings, pulsed field gel electrophoresis (PFGE) may be useful in subtyping strains, as might whole genome sequencing (WGS).

**4. Laboratory capability**—Biosafety level 2 (BSL-2) with the capability to culture/enumerate microorganisms and to perform serological or molecular tests. Personnel working with infectious agents or potentially infected materials must be fully trained and proficient in the practices and techniques required for handling such material safely.

**5. Safety requirements**—Staphylococcal enterotoxins are highly toxic. Safety equipment such as biosafety cabinets (BSC), enclosed containers, and other engineering controls should be employed to avoid exposures to hazardous biological materials. The appropriate personal protective equipment (PPE), such as laboratory coat, safety glasses, and gloves, should be worn. All nondisposable materials that have been in contact with staphylococcal enterotoxins should be decontaminated by steam autoclave or with more than 0.5% NaOCl or more than 0.25% NaOH for 30 minutes.[1]

**6. Nonhuman hosts**—*S. aureus* is the normal flora commonly found on the skin and mucous membranes in a wide variety of mammals and birds. The bacterium can be disseminated in the environment and survive for long periods.

**7. Sample/specimen requirements**—Vomitus or fresh stool/rectal swab specimens from ill patients should be collected as soon as possible since delay may impede identification of the causative agent. Enclose the specimens in a secure container and label clearly. Place the container in a waterproof bag with tissue, towels, or other blotting material to absorb any leakage. Ship the sample in a well-insulated box with frozen refrigerant packs. If not shipped immediately, hold specimens refrigerated. Implicated food samples should be collected aseptically and in their original container. Put them in a sterile bag to avoid any cross-contamination. Check original packages or containers for code numbers that can be used in trace-back analysis. Due to the perishable nature of fresh produce, it is important that analyses start immediately upon arrival of samples to the laboratories. Samples should not be frozen at any time prior to analysis. For outbreak investigations, maintain chain of custody of the samples/specimens. Keep all packages not sent for laboratory examination until the end of the investigation.

**8. Testing requirements**—Isolation and enumeration of *S. aureus* is usually done using microbiological techniques with dedicated media such as Baird Parker or rabbit plasma fibrinogen agar. Recovery of at least $10^5$ *S. aureus* $g^{-1}$ from vomitus/stool or food samples generally confirms *S. aureus* as the causative agent for the outbreak. In some cases, confirmation of staphylococcal food poisoning (SFP) by isolation of *S. aureus* is difficult in thermal processed foods because *S. aureus* is heat sensitive.

Detection of classical staphylococcal enterotoxins (SEs)—serological groups A to E—by immunological assays is commonly used to screen and confirm SFP. Currently several commercial test kits are available. The SET-RPLA kit (Thermo Fisher Scientific, Waltham, MA) detects staphylococcal enterotoxins A, B, C, and D in foods by reverse passive latex agglutination (RPLA). The assay is semiquantitative and can be completed within 24 hours. Transia immunoenzymatic test (Diffchamb SA, Lyon, France) is designed for the detection and differentiation of the 5 different serological groups (A–E) in food samples and cultural supernatants. The results could be obtained in less than 2 hours. VIDAS Staph enterotoxin 2 (SET2; bioMérieux, Durham, NC) utilizes the enzyme-linked fluorescent assay techniques and provides quantitative testing for the detection of staphylococcal enterotoxins A, B, C1, C2, C3, D, and E on the VIDAS automated immunoanalyzer. Owing to the low amount of SEs present in food it is crucial to concentrate the extract before performing detection assays. Bio-Detect Test strip (Alexeter Technologies, Wheeling, IL) can be used to screen specifically staphylococcal enterotoxin B with a detection limit of 0.1 μg/ml. Results obtained by the test trip should be confirmed by additional method due to possible cross-reactivity with other compounds.

Molecular biology methods such as polymerase chain reaction (PCR) have been employed to rapidly screen *S. aureus* strains for SE-encoding genes in foods. The PCR approach may also detect previously unidentified SE genes. However, the PCR cannot be the sole test for confirming *S. aureus* as causative agent in an outbreak.

Identification by PFGE or WGS of the same subtype of *S. aureus* from the stool or vomitus of 2 or more ill people also confirms the diagnosis.

During outbreak investigations it is critical to maintain the chain of custody of samples and ensure the integrity of analytical data.

**9. Reporting requirements**—Staphylococcal food poisoning outbreaks are reportable in the USA, and EU member states laboratories within other settings should determine the reporting requirements within their respective jurisdictions.

**10. Referral network**—Specialty laboratories or state and national reference laboratories should be consulted when the primary testing laboratory is unfamiliar with staphylococcal enterotoxin testing.

**11. Special considerations**—Staphylococcal toxins could be used as a biological agent either by contamination of food or by aerosolization (using pressure to produce a fine mist)[2] and are on the Select Agents and Toxins list.[3] Laboratory exposures of staphylococcal enterotoxin B causing conjunctivitis and gastrointestinal symptoms have been reported.[4] Personal protective measures are paramount when working with SEs.

## II. FOODBORNE CLOSTRIDIUM PERFRINGENS INTOXICATION (enteritis necroticans, pigbel)

**1. Clinical features**—An intestinal disorder characterized by sudden onset of colic followed by diarrhea; nausea is common, but vomiting and fever are usually absent. Generally, a mild disease of short duration—1 day or less—and rarely fatal in previously healthy people. Outbreaks of severe disease with high case-fatality rates associated with necrotizing enteritis have been documented in postwar Germany and in Papua New Guinea (pigbel).

**2. Causative agents**—Type A strains of *Clostridium perfringens* cause typical food poisoning outbreaks through production of *C. perfringens* enterotoxin (CPE) in the ileum. Type C strains cause necrotizing enteritis through production of the beta toxin.

**3. Laboratory diagnosis**—In the outbreak setting, diagnosis is confirmed by demonstration of *C. perfringens* in semiquantitative anaerobic cultures of food ($\geq 10^5$/g) or patients' stool ($\geq 10^6$/g), in addition to clinical and epidemiological evidence. Detection of CPE in patients' stool also confirms the diagnosis. Genomic typing, including PFGE and WGS, can help in comparing food and patient strains.

**4. Laboratory capability**—BSL-2 facility with the ability to culture anaerobic microorganisms and to perform serological or molecular tests. Personnel working with infectious agents or potentially infected materials must be fully trained and proficient in the practices and techniques required for handling such material safely.

**5. Safety requirements**—Safety equipment such as BSCs, enclosed containers, and other engineering controls should be employed to avoid exposures to hazardous biological materials. Proper PPE should be worn.

**6. Nonhuman hosts**—*C. perfringens* can be found in the gastrointestinal tract of healthy people and animals (cattle, fish, pigs, and poultry). Spores of the organism can survive in soil for years.

**7. Sample/specimen requirements**—For optimal recovery of *C. perfringens*, stool specimens should be obtained, transported in ice packs, and processed within 24 hours of collection. Swab specimens are inadequate for the toxin assay due to insufficient sample volume. Suspected food can also be collected in outbreaks. In suspected enteritis necroticans (*C. perfringens* Type C), 3 blood cultures from 3 different venipuncture sites, stool (> 25 g), and bowel luminal contents should be collected.

**8. Testing requirements**—Assays available for the detection of CPE include antigen-based immunological methods. Microplate enzyme-linked immunosorbent assay (ELISA) test kit (Techlab, Blacksburg, VA), a quantitative method for investigational use only, can detect 5 ng/g CPE in fecal specimens in less than 2.5 hours.

The RPLA assay (Oxoid) is more sensitive than ELISA but produces some nonspecific reactions. Most fecal specimens from food poisoning incidents have enterotoxin concentrations exceeding 1 μg/g feces. Therefore, the less-sensitive assay system would be adequate for laboratory confirmation of *C. perfringens* food poisoning in outbreaks.[5,6] When there is a low-titer positive sample, both ELISA and RPLA tests should be performed to rule out false-positive/negative results.

Culture of *C. perfringens* from patient fecal specimens lacks clinical usefulness because of the high prevalence of the organism in both healthy people and diarrheic patients. Multiplex PCR has been utilized to characterize *C. perfringens* toxin genes but with limited diagnostic utility when used alone. When in conjunction with immunological assay, PCR has been used to rule out *C. perfringens* Type C infection based on the absence of β-toxin genes in the isolates.[7] *C. perfringens* Type A produces α-toxin, not β-toxin, while *C. perfringens* type C produces both α-toxin and β-toxin.[8]

PFGE and WGS are effective means to analyze the genetic diversity among *C. perfringens* isolates.

**9. Reporting requirements**—Illness attributed to *C. perfringens* toxin is generally reportable. Laboratories should determine reporting requirements within their respective jurisdictions.

**10. Referral network**—*C. perfringens* serotyping is available in only a few laboratories worldwide.

**11. Special considerations**—This organism loses viability rapidly in foods that have been stored refrigerated, and fecal counts can still be high in elderly people in the absence of illness.

## III. FOODBORNE BACILLUS CEREUS INTOXICATION

**1. Clinical features**—Intoxication characterized in some cases by sudden onset of nausea and vomiting, and in others by colic and diarrhea. Illness generally persists no longer than 24 hours and is rarely fatal. Very rare fatal cases seem to be related to liver failure.

**2. Causative agents**—*Bacillus cereus*, an aerobic spore former. Two enterotoxins have been identified: a heat stable emetic toxin cereulide causing vomiting is produced in food when *B. cereus* levels reach $10^5$ colony-forming units per gram of food; and several heat labile toxins, causing diarrhea, which are formed during vegetative growth of *B. cereus* in the small intestine of the patient.

**3. Laboratory diagnosis**—In outbreak settings, diagnosis is confirmed through quantitative cultures on selective media to estimate the number of organisms present in the suspected food (generally $>10^5$–$10^6$ organisms/g of the incriminated food are required). Isolation of organisms from the stool of 2 or more ill persons and not from stools of controls also confirms the diagnosis. Enterotoxin testing is valuable but may not be widely available.

**4. Laboratory capability**—BSL-2 facility with the ability to culture microorganisms and to perform serological or molecular tests. Personnel working with infectious agents or potentially infected materials must be fully trained and proficient in the practices and techniques required for handling such material safely.

**5. Safety requirements**—Clinical or food samples for isolation of *B. cereus* can be handled safely on the open bench without special precautions. Efforts should be made to avoid manipulations that produce aerosols. Any procedures that have the potential to generate aerosols should be done in a BSC. Eye protection must be used where there is a known or potential risk of exposure to splashes.

**6. Nonhuman hosts**—The natural environmental reservoir for *B. cereus* consists of decaying organic matter, fresh and marine waters, vegetables and fomites, and the intestinal tract of invertebrates.

**7. Sample/specimen requirements**—Vomitus or fresh stool/rectal swab specimens from ill patients should be collected as soon as possible since delay may impede identification of the causative agent. Enclose the specimens in a secure container and label clearly. Place the container in a waterproof bag with tissue, towels, or other blotting material to absorb any leakage. Ship the sample in a well-insulated box with frozen refrigerant packs. If not shipped immediately, hold specimens refrigerated. Implicated food samples should be collected aseptically and in their original container, if available. Put them in a sterile bag to avoid any cross-contamination. Check original packages or containers for code numbers that can be used to trace back analysis. Samples should not be frozen at any time prior to analysis. For outbreak investigations, maintain chain of custody of the samples/specimens. Keep all packages not sent for laboratory examination until the end of the investigation.

**8. Testing requirements**—Confirmation of an outbreak relies on the isolation of *B. cereus* from food and the detection of *B. cereus* in the feces and/or vomitus of the affected persons. Chromogenic selective and differential agar is often used to promote the growth and identification of *B. cereus* in foods.

*B. cereus* enterotoxins (BDE) cause emetic and/or diarrheic food poisoning. Two enterotoxin complexes, hemolysin BL (Hbl) and the nonhemolytic (Nhe), as well as a protein (Cytotoxin K1) have been identified as causative agents for the diarrheal.[9–12] For the detection of Hbl and Nhe, 3 commercial kits, the *Bacillus* diarrheal enterotoxin visual immunoassay (BDE VIA, Tecra, Austin, TX), *B. cereus* enterotoxin (BCE-RPLA, Oxoid), and the Duopath Cereus Enterotoxins (Merck, Washington, DC) are available and frequently used for the analysis of enterotoxin production by *B. cereus*. The BCE-RPLA detects mainly the Hbl component and BDE VIA recognizes Nhe, while Duopath detects both Hbl and Nhe. Comparison of the 3 kits indicate that BCE-RPLA assay is more sensitive than the Duopath kit in the detection of Hbl, and Duopath is more sensitive than BDE VIA in the detection of Nhe.[13]

Liquid chromatography coupled with mass spectrometry (LC-MS) was reported to detect *B. cereus* emetic toxin.[14] LC-MS is highly specific and sensitive. The main drawbacks, however, are the labor-intensive sample preparation, high upfront investment, and preventive maintenance costs. Therefore, it is not suitable for routine diagnostic tests.

It is recommended to test for both Hbl and Nhe enterotoxins in foods because either alone can cause illness.

**9. Reporting requirements**—Only when associated with an outbreak.

**10. Referral network**—Reference or national laboratories.

**11. Special considerations**—Studies indicated that preformed enterotoxins do not contribute significantly to diarrheal food poisoning[15,16] as they did not withstand gastrointestinal passage under the simulated conditions. Thus, infective dose does not necessarily correspond with the ingested dose.

## IV. SCOMBROID FISH POISONING (histamine poisoning)

**1. Clinical features**—A syndrome of tingling and burning sensations around the mouth, facial flushing and sweating, nausea and vomiting, headache, palpitations, dizziness, and rash. Histamine poisoning (scombroid poisoning) is a worldwide problem that occurs after the consumption of food containing biogenic amines, particularly histamine at concentrations higher than 500 ppm. Symptoms occur within a few hours after eating food containing high levels of free histamine; biogenic amines are typically formed through microbial decarboxylation of amino acids in the food in question, and these substances are heat stable. Histamine poisoning is often caused by fish products, often from the Scombroidea fish group (e.g., mackerel and tuna), and any foods that contain the appropriate amino acids can undergo certain bacterial growth and may lead to scombroid poisoning, when ingested. Symptoms resolve spontaneously within 12 hours and there are no long-term sequelae. In severe cases, antihistamines, either through inhalators or intravenously, may be effective in relieving symptoms.

**2. Causative agents**—Occurrence is worldwide. Histamine is produced in fish due to product mishandling resulting in bacterial conversion of histidine to histamine in temperature abused, dark-flesh fish.

**3. Laboratory diagnosis**—Detection of histamine in epidemiologically implicated food confirms the diagnosis. Good hygiene and rapid refrigeration prevents microbial spoilage and decarboxylation. Symptoms may be markedly worse in patients taking isoniazid or other drugs interfering with histamine metabolism.

**4. Laboratory capability**—Chemistry laboratory facilities equipped for fluorescence spectrometry, high performance liquid chromatography (HPLC), or immunoassay instrumentation.

**5. Safety requirements**—BSL-1 using good laboratory practices.

**6. Nonhuman hosts**—Not applicable.

**7. Sample/specimen requirements**—Samples for testing are nonclinical such as unconsumed portions of fish implicated in outbreaks. Variability in histamine levels between fish in a given lot can be high.

**8. Testing requirements**—Histamine in fish can be assessed using various immunoassays and enzymatic test kits capable of detecting histamine at the 50 mg/kg action level. Confirmation in the USA requires use of a fluorescence spectrometer, while Europe requires HPLC methods for confirmation.

**9. Reporting requirements**—Scombroid fish poisoning is reportable to the health authorities in various states in the USA. Laboratories should determine reporting requirements within their respective jurisdictions. If confirmation test is needed, a frozen reserve sample should be held for further testing.

**10. Referral network**—No known referral laboratory networks. Laboratory testing capability exists in many government regulatory laboratories including FDA.

**11. Special considerations**—None.

## V. CIGUATERA FISH POISONING

**1. Clinical features**—A characteristic gastrointestinal and neurological syndrome may occur within 1 hour after eating tropical reef fish. Gastrointestinal symptoms (diarrhea, vomiting, abdominal pain) occur first, usually within 24 hours of consumption. In severe cases, patients may also become hypotensive, with a paradoxical bradycardia. Neurological symptoms, including pain and weakness in the lower extremities and circumoral and peripheral paresthesias, may occur at the same time as the acute symptoms or follow 1–2 days later; they may persist for weeks or months. Symptoms such as temperature reversal (ice cream tastes hot, hot coffee seems cold) and aching teeth are frequently reported. In very severe cases, neurological symptoms may progress to coma and respiratory arrest within the first 24 hours of illness. Most patients recover completely within a few weeks; intermittent recrudescence of symptoms can occur over a period of months to years.

**2. Causative agents**—This syndrome is caused by the presence in the fish of heat stable toxins elaborated by the dinoflagellate *Gambierdiscus toxicus*, an algae growing on underwater reefs. Fish eating the algae become toxic, and the effect is magnified through the food chain so that large predatory fish become the most toxic; this occurs worldwide in tropical areas. CDC reports that ciguatera poisoning accounts for over 25% of marine biotoxin foodborne illness outbreaks and has 5 times the reported incidence of paralytic shellfish poisoning (PSP) and neurotoxic shellfish poisoning (NSP) combined.

**3. Laboratory diagnosis**—There is no diagnostic test available for detecting the toxins in human specimens. The diagnosis is based on clinical symptoms.

**4. Laboratory capability**—Although diagnostic methods for detecting the toxins are still under development, laboratory tests for detecting the toxins in samples of the implicated fish have been developed. Chemistry laboratory equipped for routine testing is adequate for screening by immunoassays, enzyme inhibition assays, cytotoxity in cultured cell lines, and/or mouse bioassay. Specialized training in liquid chromatography-tandem mass spectrometry (LC-MS/MS) detection of ciguatera toxin.

**5. Safety requirements**—BSL-1 using good laboratory practices.

**6. Nonhuman hosts**—Large predatory fish in warm waters such as barracuda, grouper, amberjack, and others bio-accumulate the toxins in their flesh, with highest levels found in the liver.

**7. Sample/specimen requirements**—Samples for testing are nonclinical such as unconsumed portions of fish implicated in outbreaks. The samples should be stored and transported frozen.

**8. Testing requirements**—Testing is severely limited by the lack of commercially available analytical standards for the ciguatoxins. A mouse bioassay has traditionally been the primary method of screening. A cytotoxicity-based method that uses cultured mouse neuroblastomas (Neuro-2a cell line, American Type Culture Collection CCL-131, Manassas, VA) is available and has the required sensitivity for screening (0.01 μg/kg for Pacific ciguatoxins and for Caribbean exposures 0.1 μg/kg per FDA advisory levels).[17] LC-MS/MS methods exist for confirmation, but the limit of detection is above the advisory level for Pacific ciguatoxins.

**9. Reporting requirements**—Ciguatera fish poisoning is reportable to health authorities in various states in the USA. Laboratories should determine reporting requirements within their respective jurisdictions. If confirmation test is needed, a reserve sample should be held frozen if available for further testing.

**10. Referral network**—No referral networks exist. Testing capability is limited to a few research and regulatory laboratories.

**11. Special considerations**—None.

## VI. PARALYTIC SHELLFISH POISONING

**1. Clinical features**—PSP is a characteristic syndrome, predominantly neurological, starting within minutes to several hours after eating bivalve mollusks. Initial symptoms can begin from 15 minutes to 10 hours after eating and include paresthesias of the mouth and extremities accompanied by gastrointestinal symptoms. In severe cases, ataxia, dysphonia, dysphagia, and muscle paralysis with respiratory arrest and death may occur within 12 hours. Symptoms usually resolve completely within hours to days after shellfish ingestion.

**2. Causative agents**—This syndrome is caused by the presence in shellfish of saxitoxins or other toxins produced by *Alexandrium* spp. and other dinoflagellates. Concentration of these toxins occurs during massive algal blooms known as red tides but also in the absence of recognizable algal bloom. PSP is common in shellfish harvested from colder waters above 30°N and below 30°S latitude but may also occur in tropical waters. In North America, PSP is primarily a problem in northern latitudes. Blooms of the causative *Alexandrium* spp. occur several times each year, in the Northern hemisphere primarily from April through October. Shellfish remain toxic for several weeks after the bloom subsides. Most cases occur in individuals or small groups who gather shellfish for personal consumption.

**3. Laboratory diagnosis**—Diagnosis is based on clinical symptoms, epidemiological findings, and indirectly by shellfish testing. Detection of toxin in epidemiologically implicated food confirms the diagnosis. Standard methods include a mouse bioassay, immunoassay, and competitive binding assay.

**4. Laboratory capability**—Laboratory equipped for mouse bioassay or for receptor binding assay a facility for handling radionuclides.

**5. Safety requirements**—BSL-1 using good laboratory practices.

**6. Nonhuman hosts:**—Although humans are primarily exposed to saxitoxins by ingesting contaminated shellfish, there have been documented intoxications implicating puffer fish in the eastern USA. Saxitoxins have also been found in low levels in the GI tract of mackerel. The toxins likely have an adverse impact on a wide array of mammals and have been blamed for illness and deaths in marine mammals.

**7. Sample/specimen requirements**—Samples for testing are non-clinical such as unconsumed portions of shellfish implicated in outbreaks. The samples should be stored and transported frozen.

**8. Testing requirements**—In the USA testing is primarily by mouse bioassay; however, more contemporary official methods with better detectability are now approved for official use and are based on a receptor binding assay or HPLC. The quarantine level for molluscan shellfish is 800 μg/kg saxitoxin equivalents.

**9. Reporting requirements**—Paralytic shellfish poisoning is reportable to the health authorities in various states in the USA. Laboratories should determine reporting requirements within their respective jurisdictions. If confirmation test is needed, a reserve sample should be held frozen if available for further testing.

**10. Referral network**—Shellfish-producing states in the USA routinely test for paralytic shellfish toxins. This testing supports monitoring programs under the Interstate Shellfish Sanitation Conference with federal oversight by the National Shellfish Sanitation Program (primarily FDA).[17]

**11. Special considerations**—None.

## VII. NEUROTOXIC SHELLFISH POISONING

**1. Clinical features**—Neurotoxic shellfish poisoning is associated with algal blooms (red tides) of *Karenia brevis*, which produce brevetoxin. Red tides have long occurred along the Florida coast, where the syndrome has been most studied, with associated mortality in fish, seabirds, and marine mammals. Symptoms after eating toxic shellfish—including circumoral paresthesias and paresthesias of the extremities, dizziness and ataxia, myalgia, and gastrointestinal symptoms—tend to be mild and resolve quickly and completely. Respiratory and eye irritation can also occur, apparently through aerosolization of the toxin through wind and wave action.

**2. Causative agents**—Algal blooms (red tides) of *Karenia brevis*, which produce brevetoxin.

**3. Laboratory diagnosis**—Based on clinical symptoms. There is no diagnostic test available for detecting the toxins in human specimens.

**4. Laboratory capability**—Chemistry laboratory equipped for routine testing is adequate for screening by immunoassays and enzyme inhibition for toxins in implicated fish samples. Confirmation requires specialized training in LC-MS/MS. Traditional methods include a mouse bioassay, which has specific requirements for animal housing and handling.

**5. Safety requirements**—BSL-1 using good laboratory practices.

**6. Nonhuman hosts**—Although humans are primarily exposed to brevetoxins by ingesting contaminated shellfish, there have been many documented intoxications due to inhaling toxic aerosols. The toxins likely have an adverse impact on a wide array of mammals and have been blamed for illness and deaths in marine mammal.

**7. Sample/specimen requirements**—Samples for testing are non-clinical such as unconsumed portions of shellfish implicated in outbreaks. Variability between shellfish in a given area can be high. The samples should be stored and transported frozen.

**8. Testing requirements**—In the USA, testing is primarily by mouse bioassay. ELISA kits are commercially available, and LC-MS/MS methods are available for confirmation. The advisory level is 800 μg/kg brevetoxin-2.

**9. Reporting requirements**—Neurotoxic shellfish poisoning is reportable to health authorities in various states in the USA. Laboratories should determine reporting requirements within their respective jurisdictions. If confirmation test is needed, a reserve sample should be held frozen if available for further testing.

**10. Referral network**—In the USA there is a national monitoring program using state laboratories under the Interstate Shellfish Sanitation Conference with federal oversight by the National Shellfish Sanitation Program. Federal oversight and management is by the FDA.[17]

**11. Special considerations**—None.

## VIII. DIARRHETIC SHELLFISH POISONING

**1. Clinical features**—Diarrhetic shellfish poisoning (DSP) results from eating mussels, scallops, or clams that have fed on *Dinophysis* spp. dinoflaggelates. These algae can produce okadaic acid and a number of derivative toxins. Symptoms include diarrhea, nausea, vomiting, and abdominal pain.

**2. Causative agents**—Okadaic acid produced by algal dinoflaggelates from *Dinophysis* spp.

**3. Laboratory diagnosis**—Methods of detection of DSP in shellfish include mouse bioassay, ELISA, and liquid chromatographymass spectrometry.[18,19] Presence of total DSP toxins in epidemiologically implicated shellfish is the primary method for diagnosing this intoxication.

**4. Laboratory capability**—Chemistry laboratory equipped for screening by immunoassay or enzyme inhibition. LC-MS/MS confirmation methods exist.

**5. Safety requirements**—BSL-1 using good laboratory practices.

**6. Nonhuman hosts**—Humans are exposed to the DSP toxins by ingesting contaminated shellfish.

**7. Sample/specimen requirements**—Samples for testing are nonclinical such as unconsumed portions of shellfish implicated in outbreaks. Variability between shellfish in a given area can be high. Samples should be held and shipped frozen.

**8. Testing requirements**—Chemistry laboratory equipped for routine testing is adequate for screening by immunoassays and enzyme inhibition. Confirmation requires specialized training in LC-MS/MS. Screening for the DSP toxins can be achieved using commercial kits based on immunoassay or phosphatase inhibition. The USA advisory level is 160 μg/kg,[17] based on total toxin concentrations following alkaline hydrolysis.

**9. Reporting requirements**—Diarrhetic shellfish poisoning is reportable to health authorities in various states in the USA. Laboratories should determine reporting requirements within their respective jurisdictions. If confirmation test is needed, a reserve sample should be held frozen if available for further testing.

**10. Referral network**—In the USA, DSP is an emerging problem, and only a few laboratories routinely test for diarrhetic shellfish toxins. Testing is done in support of monitoring programs under the Interstate Shellfish Sanitation Conference with federal oversight by the National Shellfish Sanitation Program managed by the FDA.[17]

**11. Special considerations**—None.

## IX. AMNESIC SHELLFISH POISONING

**1. Clinical features**—Vomiting, abdominal cramps, diarrhea, headache, and short-term memory loss. Acute intoxication in some patients results in antegrade memory deficits with relative preservation of other cognitive functions together with clinical and electromyographical evidence of pure motor or sensorimotor neuropathy and axonopathy.

**2. Causative agents**—Ingestion of shellfish containing domoic acid produced by the diatom *Pseudonitzschia pungens*.

**3. Laboratory diagnosis**—Presence of domoic acid above 20 ppm in epidemiologically implicated shellfish.

**4. Laboratory capability**—Chemistry laboratory equipped for screening by immunoassays and liquid chromatography with ultraviolet detection (LC-UV) for confirmation.

**5. Safety requirements**—BSL-1 using good laboratory practices.

**6. Nonhuman hosts**—Humans are exposed to domoic acid by ingesting contaminated shellfish.

**7. Sample/specimen requirements**—Samples for testing are non-clinical such as unconsumed portions of shellfish implicated in outbreaks. Variability between shellfish in a given area can be high. Samples should be held and shipped frozen.

**8. Testing requirements**—Commercial immunoassays are available but high-performance LC-UV is the officially accepted method in the USA. LC-MS/MS methods are also available.

**9. Reporting requirements**—Amnesic shellfish poisoning is reportable to health authorities in various states in the USA. Laboratories should determine reporting requirements within their respective jurisdictions. If confirmation test is needed, a reserve sample should be held frozen if available for further testing.

**10. Referral network**—Shellfish producing states of the USA have monitoring programs under the Interstate Shellfish Sanitation Conference with federal oversight by the National Shellfish Sanitation Program managed by FDA.

**11. Special considerations**—None.

## X. PUFFER FISH POISONING (TETRODOTOXIN)

**1. Clinical features**—Rapid onset of paresthesias, dizziness, gastrointestinal symptoms, and ataxia, often progressing to paralysis, including of the diaphragm muscles, leading to death within several hours after eating. Case-fatality rates from 10%-60% have been reported.

**2. Causative agents**—Tetrodotoxin, a heat stable, nonprotein neurotoxin, thought to be produced by bacteria in the gut, then concentrated in the skin and viscera of puffer fish, porcupine fish, ocean sunfish, and species of newts and salamanders.

**3. Laboratory diagnosis**—Based on clinical symptoms. There is no diagnostic test available although methods exist to detect toxin in blood or urine using LC-MS/MS.

**4. Laboratory capability**—Chemistry laboratory equipped for screening by immunoassays and enzyme inhibition. For mouse bioassay, animal handling facilities are required. Confirmation requires specialized training in LC-MS/MS.

**5. Safety requirements**—BSL-1 using good laboratory practices.

**6. Nonhuman hosts**—Humans are exposed to tetrodotoxins by ingesting contaminated fish or shellfish, although there have been rare cases where ingestion of toxic amphibians (newts) or exposure to tropical octopus resulted in illness.

**7. Sample/specimen requirements**—Samples for testing are nonclinical such as unconsumed portions of seafood implicated in outbreaks. Samples should be held and shipped frozen.

**8. Testing requirements**—Laboratory capability for screening and confirmation is very limited due to the rarity of this illness.

**9. Reporting requirements**—Puffer fish poisoning is reportable to the health authorities in various states in the USA. Laboratories should determine reporting requirements within their respective jurisdictions. If confirmation test is needed, a reserve sample should be held frozen if available for further testing.

**10. Referral network**—None.

**11. Special considerations**—None.

## XI. AZASPIRACID POISONING

**1. Clinical features**—Severe diarrhea and vomiting with abdominal pain and occasional nausea, chills, headaches, and stomach cramps. Symptoms occur 12–24 hours after consumption and persist for up to 5 days.

**2. Causative agents**—Azaspiracid (AZA), a toxin that concentrates in a variety of shellfish.

**3. Laboratory diagnosis**—A regulatory limit of 160 µg AZA/kg whole shellfish flesh has been established by the EU.

**4. Laboratory capability**—Chemistry laboratory equipped for screening by immunoassays and enzyme inhibition. Confirmation requires specialized training in LC-MS/MS.

**5. Safety requirements**—BSL-1 using good laboratory practices.

**6. Nonhuman hosts**—Humans are exposed to AZA by ingesting contaminated shellfish.

**7. Sample/specimen requirements**—Samples for testing are nonclinical such as unconsumed portions of shellfish implicated in outbreaks. Variability between shellfish in a given area can be high. Samples should be held and shipped frozen.

**8. Testing requirements**—Specific training in LC-MS/MS confirmation methods.

**9. Reporting requirements**—None.

**10. Referral network**—None.

**11. Special considerations**—None.

## References


1. Wilson D, Chosewood L, eds. *Biosafety in Microbiological and Biomedical Laboratories (BMBL)*. 5th ed. Washington, DC: US Department of Health and Human Services; 2009:390-391.
2. Anderson PD. Bioterrorism: toxins as weapons. *J Pharm Pract*. 2012;25(2):121-129.
3. Centers for Disease Control and Prevention. Possession, use, and transfer of select agents and toxins; biennial review. Final rule. *Fed Regist*. 2012;77(194):61083.
4. Rusnak JM, Kortepeter M, Ulrich R, Poli M, Boudreau E. Laboratory Exposures to Staphylococcal Enterotoxin B. *Emerg Infect Dis*. 2004;10(9):1544-1549.
5. Bartholomew BA, Stringer MF, Watson GN, Gilbert RJ. Development and application of an enzyme linked immunosorbent assay for Clostridium perfringens type A enterotoxin. *J Clin Pathol*. 1985;38(2):222-228.
6. Berry PR, Rodhouse JC, Hughes S, Bartholomew BA, Gilbert RJ. Evaluation of ELISA, RPLA, and Vero cell assays for detecting Clostridium perfringens enterotoxin in faecal specimens. *J Clin Pathol*. 1988;41(4):458-461.
7. Centers for Disease Control and Prevention. Fatal foodborne Clostridium perfringens illness at a state psychiatric hospital—Louisiana, 2010. *MMWR*. 2012;61(32):605.
8. Brynestad S, Granum PE. Clostridium perfringens and foodborne infections. *Int J Food Microbiol*. 2002;74(3):195-202.
9. Beecher DJ, Schoeni JL, Wong AC. Enterotoxic activity of hemolysin BL from Bacillus cereus. *Infect Immun*. 1995;63(11):4423-4428.
10. Lund T, Granum PE. Characterisation of a non-haemolytic enterotoxin complex from Bacillus cereus isolated after a foodborne outbreak. *FEMS Microbiol Lett*. 1996;141(2-3):151-156.
11. Granum PE, O'Sullivan K, Lund T. The sequence of the non-haemolytic enterotoxin operon from Bacillus cereus. *FEMS Microbiol Lett*. 1999;177(2):225-229.
12. Lund T, De Buyser ML, Granum PE. A new cytotoxin from Bacillus cereus that may cause necrotic enteritis. *Mol Microbiol*. 2000;38(2):254-261.
13. Ceuppens S, Rajkovic A, Hamelink S, Van de Wiele T, Boon N, Uyttendaele M. Enterotoxin production by Bacillus cereus under gastrointestinal conditions and their immunological detection by commercially available kits. *Foodborne Pathog Dis*. 2012;9(12):1130-1136.
14. Delbrassinne L, Andjelkovic M, Rajkovic A, Bottledoorn N, Mahillon J, Van Loco J. Follow-up of the Bacillus cereus emetic toxin production in penne pasta under household conditions using liquid chromatography coupled with mass spectrometry. *Food microbiol*. 2011;28(5):1105-1109.
15. Granum PE, Brynestad S, Kramer JM. Analysis of enterotoxin production by Bacillus cereus from dairy products, food poisoning incidents and non-gastrointestinal infections. *Int J Food Microbiol*. 1993;17(4):269-279.

16. Turnbull PC, Jørgensen K, Kramer JM, Gilbert RJ, Parry JM. Severe clinical conditions associated with Bacillus cereus and the apparent involvement of exotoxins. *J Clin Pathol*. 1979;32(3):289–293.
17. US Food and Drug Administration. Chapter 6: natural toxins. Available at: https://www.fda.gov/downloads/food/guidanceregulation/ucm252395.pdf. Accessed September 30, 2018.
18. US Food and Drug Administration. *Bad Bug Book*. Available at: https://www.fda.gov/downloads/food/foodsafety/foodborneillness/foodborneillnessfoodbornepathogensnaturaltoxins/badbugbook/ucm297627.pdf. Accessed September 30, 2018.
19. Lloyd JK, Duchin JS, Borchert J, Quintana HF, Robertson A. Diarrhetic shellfish poisoning, Washington, USA, 2011. *Emerg Infect Dis*. 2013;19(8):1314–1316.

[J. Hu, D. Rice]

# FUNGAL DISEASES OF THE SKIN, HAIR, AND NAILS

(tinea, ringworm, dermatophytosis, dermatomycosis, epidermophytosis, trichophytosis, microsporosis)

| DISEASE | ICD-10 CODE |
|---|---|
| TINEA BARBAE<br>TINEA CAPITIS | ICD-10 B35.0 |
| BLACK PIEDRA<br>WHITE PIEDRA | ICD-10 B36.3 |
| TINEA CRURIS<br>TINEA CORPORIS | ICD-10 B35.6 |
| TINEA PEDIS | ICD-10 B35.3 |
| ONCHOMYCOSIS DUE TO DERMATOPHYTES | ICD-10 B35.1 |

Fungal diseases of the skin, hair, and nails can be split into those caused by dermatophyte fungi, specialist parasites of keratin (previously classified in the 3 genera *Epidermophyton, Microsporum*, and *Trichophyton*, but now also includes *Nannizzia*, *Arthroderma*, *Lophophyton*, *Paraphyton*), and those caused by other dermatomycotic molds and commensal yeast species. Most skin infections are confined to the stratum corneum, although if a hair follicle becomes infected, an infection may extend down to the dermis. There are also some disseminated yeast and mold infections, which can present with cutaneous lesions as a result of hematogenous dissemination.

The most common dermatophyte infection, suffered by about 10% of the adult population, is tinea pedis or athlete's foot, an infection of the interdigital skin of the toe web characterized by itching, flaking, scaling, or cracking of the skin or by a diffuse scaling over the sole and sides of the foot known as moccasin type athlete's foot. A similar infection with diffuse, fine scaling affecting the palms of the hands is known as tinea manuum. This latter type of infection of the hands and feet can be caused by the mold *Neoscytalidium dimidiatum,* which is one of the few nondermatophyte molds able to cause infection of the skin and nails. Another nondermatophyte mold, *Hortea werneckii,* causes an infection known as tinea nigra, which has a distinctive brown coffee-stain appearance usually on the palm of the hand or plantar area of the foot.

Dermatophyte infection of the smooth skin of the trunk and limbs—tinea corporis—characteristically produces 1 or more spreading, erythematous ring-shaped lesions, from which the disease name "ringworm" was derived. The periphery is often raised and vesicular or pustular and is usually dry and scaly, often with clearing of the central area. Lesions caused by zoophilic species, which are less well adapted to their human hosts, often illicit more inflammation and intense itching. *Malassezia furfur* is a commensal yeast species that causes pityriasis versicolor, a skin condition characterized by the appearance of an asymptomatic, scaly, hypo- or hyper-pigmented rash usually on the upper trunk and back. *Malassezia* spp. can also cause a folliculitis in which itchy papules and pustules appear widely scattered on the shoulders and back, particularly in teenagers and young adults. Both conditions appear to be exacerbated by sun exposure.

Dermatophyte infection of the skin of the groin area is known as tinea cruris and is more common in humid environments. The infection is generally bilateral and may involve the upper surface of the thigh and the perineum. This presents with erythematous scaling often with a raised margin. Yeast species may cause a similar infection of warm, moist body sites, typically groin, axilla, and sub-mammary skin folds. Known as candida intertrigo or nappy dermatitis, such infections can often be distinguished clinically by the appearance of satellite pustules and papules formed outside the border of infection.

Dermatophyte onychomycosis, known as tinea unguium, is an infection of the nail plate usually caused by anthropophilic dermatophytes, notably *Trichophyton rubrum.* Nails are often thickened and discolored and may be crumbly with infection starting in the distal and lateral margins. Few nondermatophyte molds can infect otherwise healthy nails but can become established once a nail is damaged by infection with a dermatophyte or by some physical trauma. This often results in greatly discolored, thickened nails (see later table for a list of the most common nondermatophyte mold and yeast species that cause infection). Yeast nail infection is seen most often in fingernails in individuals whose hands remain moist for long periods. It is usually accompanied by paronychia, with swelling of the nail fold, pain, and occasional discharge of pus.

**Nondermatophyte Causes of Skin, Nail, and Hair Infection**

| **Mold Species** | **Usual Site of Infection** |
|---|---|
| *Alternaria* spp. | skin, nail |
| *Aspergillus niger*, *Aspergillus flavus* | ear (otitis) |
| *Aspergillus versicolor/sydowii* | nail |
| *Chrysosporium* spp. | skin |
| *Fusarium* spp. | nail |
| *Neoscytalidium dimidiatum/hyalinum* | nail and skin of hands and feet |
| *Onychocola canadensis* | nail |
| *Hortea werneckii* | skin (tinea nigra) |
| *Piedraia hortae* | hair shaft (black piedra) |
| *Sarocladium* spp. | nail |
| *Scopulariopsis* spp. | nail |
| **Yeast Species** | |
| *Candida* spp. | skin, nail |
| *Malassezia* spp. | skin, scalp |
| *Trichosporon* spp. | hair shaft (white piedra), skin |
| *Cryptococcus* spp. | skin |

Scalp infection, tinea capitis, is most often seen in children and presents with patches of scalp-hair loss and scaling. Infected hairs may become brittle and break off easily. They often leave a characteristic black dot appearance, especially with those species causing infection in the hair shaft (endothrix infection). Sometimes, and especially with animal-derived infections, there is a much more inflammatory reaction, with the formation of a crusting, suppurative area known as a kerion. Favus is a rare scalp infection, seen in small endemic foci, caused by *Trichophyton schoenleinii*, in which yellowish, crusty lesions with a mousy aroma (scutula) form a mat on the scalp surface. This is the only form in which hair loss is likely to be permanent.

Other scalp infections caused by fungi include black piedra, in which black, hard nodules formed by the mold *Piedraia hortae* occur along the hair shaft and white piedra caused by the yeasts of the genus *Trichosporon*, which white, pasty nodules form along the hair shaft. White piedra is most often seen on the genital hairs but also affects hairs of the axilla and scalp. *Malassezia* spp. may also have a role in the formation of dandruff and in seborrheic dermatitis.

**1. Clinical features—**

1) Tinea barbae and tinea capitis (ringworm of the beard and scalp, kerion, favus), black piedra, white piedra: a fungal disease that

begins as a small area of erythema and/or scaling and spreads peripherally, leaving scaly patches of temporary baldness. Infected hairs become brittle and break off easily. Occasionally, boggy, raised suppurative lesions develop, called kerions. Favus of the scalp, a variety of tinea capitis, is characterized by a mousy smell and by the formation of small, yellowish, cuplike crusts that amalgamate to form a pale or yellow visible mat on the scalp surface. Affected hairs of a favus do not break off but become grey and lusterless, eventually falling out and leaving baldness that may be permanent. Tinea capitis is easily distinguished from black piedra. Black piedra is characterized by black, hard, gritty nodules on hair shafts, caused by *P. hortai*. White piedra is caused by *Trichosporon* spp., particularly *Trichosporon ovoides* or *Trichosporon inkin*, which produce white, soft, pasty nodules. Infections are usually seen on the scalp but may also be seen on armpit, facial, or pubic hair.

2) Tinea cruris (ringworm of groin and perianal region), tinea corporis (ringworm of the body): a fungal disease of the skin other than of the scalp, bearded areas, and feet, characteristically appearing as flat, spreading, ring-shaped, or circular lesion with a characteristic raised edge around all or part of the lesion. This periphery is usually reddish, vesicular, or pustular, and may be dry and scaly or moist and crusted. As the lesion progresses peripherally, the central area often clears, leaving apparently normal skin. Differentiation from inguinal candidiasis, often distinguished by the presence of satellite pustules outside the lesion margins, is necessary because treatment differs. Lesions are aggravated by friction and excessive perspiration in axillary and inguinal regions and when environmental temperatures and humidity are high. All ages are susceptible.
3) Tinea pedis (ringworm of the foot, athlete's foot): presents with characteristic scaling or cracking of the skin, especially between the toes (interdigital), diffuse scaling over the sole of the foot (dry type), or blisters containing a thin watery fluid; commonly called athlete's foot. In severe cases, vesicular lesions appear on various parts of the body, especially the hands; these dermatophytids do not contain the fungus but are an allergic reaction to fungus products. Itching is often a clue that dermatophyte fungi are present. *Scytalidium* can also cause similar dry lesions on the sole. Note that bacteria, including Gram-negative organisms and coryneforms, as well as *Candida* and *Scytalidium* spp., may produce similar lesions.
4) Onychomycosis due to dermatophytes (tinea unguium, ringworm of the nails, onychomycosis): a chronic fungal disease involving

1 or more nails of the hands or feet. The nail gradually becomes detached from the nail bed, thickens, and becomes discolored and brittle; an accumulation of soft keratinous material forms beneath the nail or the nail becomes chalky and disintegrates.

**2. Causative agents**—Most infections of the feet, smooth skin, groin, axilla and nails are caused by the anthropophilic dermatophytes *T. rubrum*, *Trichophyton interdigitale*, and *Epidermophyton floccosum*. Zoophilic and geophilic species are more likely to cause infection of exposed body sites such as the hands, limbs, face, and scalp. See the later table for a list of the most common dermatophyte species and their usual habitat.

**Dermatophyte Species and Their Usual Habitat**

| **Anthropophilic Dermatophyte Species** | **Usual Host Animal or Habitat** |
|---|---|
| *Epidermophyton floccosum* | human: groin, feet |
| *Microsporum audouinii* | human: scalp |
| *Trichophyton interdigitale* | human: feet, nails |
| *Trichophyton rubrum* | human: feet, nails, groin, trunk |
| *Trichophyton schoenleinii* | human: scalp |
| *Trichophyton tonsurans* | human: scalp, face, trunk, limbs |
| *Trichophyton violaceum* | human: scalp, face, trunk, limbs |
| **Zoophilic Dermatophyte Species** | |
| *Microsporum canis* | cat, dog |
| *Microsporum equinum* | horse |
| *Microsporum gallinae* | chicken |
| *Microsporum nanum* | pig |
| *Microsporum persicolor* | rodents |
| *Trichophyton erinacei* | hedgehog |
| *Trichophyton mentagrophytes* | rodents |
| *Trichophyton verrucosum* | cattle |
| **Geophilic Dermatophyte Species** | |
| *Microsporum fulvum* | soil |
| *Microsporum gypseum* | soil |

**3. Laboratory diagnosis**—Some preliminary diagnostic information can be obtained by looking for fluorescence of the lesions under a special filtered ultra-violet light known as a Wood's light. Under such a light, infections with *Microsporum*, but not *Trichophyton,* display a green fluorescence, whereas favus and pityriasis versicolor display pale yellow fluorescence.

Fluorescence can help in selecting the best hairs to pluck or skin to scrape to send to the laboratory.

To diagnose an infection, an appropriate and representative sample of skin, hair, and/or nail should be taken from the site of infection after wiping the area with 70% alcohol. For lesions of the skin and nail, it is important to try to obtain samples from the advancing edge of the infection. For scalp infection, plucked hairs are required in addition to any loose skin scale, as it is the hair root that is important for microscopy and culture. If it is difficult to obtain samples, a soft-bristle toothbrush may be rubbed over the surface to pick up infected skin squames.

On arrival in the laboratory, the sample should be examined microscopically and cultured on selective media incubated at 28°C for a minimum of 2 weeks. Microscopic examination of the test sample follows presoftening in 10% potassium hydroxide; this is enhanced by the application of optical brighteners such as blankophor or calcofluor and examination under a fluorescence microscope. Any fungal elements seen should be recorded as branching hyphae, arthrospores, budding yeast cells, filamentous yeast, etc. When infected hairs are examined, it is important to note whether fungal spores are predominantly within the hair shaft as in endothrix infection, around the hair shaft as in ectothrix infection, or favic, in which hyphae and spores can be seen within the hair shaft. The orientation of the infection provides a strong indication of the likely infecting species.

As cutaneous specimens are often contaminated with bacteria, it is important to use a selective medium containing chloramphenicol and also cycloheximide to inhibit growth of nondermatophyte molds. For nail samples, and for some rare skin and hair infections, the pathogen may be a nondermatophyte mold such as *N. dimidiatum, Scopulariopsis brevicaulis, Fusarium* spp., or yeast such as *Trichosporon* spp.; therefore, a second agar omitting cycloheximide, which would be inhibitory to these fungi, should also be employed. Molds other than *Neoscytalidium* isolated from nail samples should not be reported unless they are grown in pure culture from the majority of the inoculum points and appropriate hyphae have been seen on direct microscopic examination. *M. furfur,* the causative yeast of the skin condition pityriasis versicolor, will not grow on agar unless there is a lipid source. However, most infections are diagnosed by the typical microscopic appearance of budding yeast and short, nonbranching hyphae; therefore, culture is not usually required.

Cultures can usually be identified by their macroscopic and microscopic phenotypic morphology, but occasionally polymerase chain reaction (PCR) amplification of the isolate's deoxyribonucleic acid using internal transcribed spacer and D1-D2 primers followed by sequencing and comparison with published databases may be required.

**4. Laboratory capability**—Local microbiology laboratories should be capable of providing an isolation and identification service for fungal isolates from the skin, hair, and nails. Microbiologists trained in mycology are required for definitive identification.

**5. Safety requirements**—In the UK, the Advisory Committee on Dangerous Pathogens lists the dermatophyte agents and most other yeast and molds causing cutaneous lesions as hazard group 2 organisms; therefore, biosafety level 2 laboratory practices are sufficient for handling the agents. However, there are some endemic dimorphic mycoses that may present with cutaneous lesions, and cultures of the causative agents of these infections would be classed as hazard group 3 organisms; therefore, clinical specimens of unknown etiology from patients from endemic areas should be handled in accordance with local risk assessment for other potential agents. In the USA, mycology work should be conducted in a certified class II laminar-airflow biosafety cabinet.

**6. Nonhuman hosts**—The anthropophilic and zoophilic dermatophyte species, affecting humans and animals respectively, are closely related to geophilic species found in the soil. These environmental strains can cause infections in persons, such as garden center workers who have close contact with the soil. Dermatophyte species often adapted to a particular host animal are able to cause zoonoses in animal handlers that come into close contact with them or their fomites. Zoonoses range from *Microsporum canis* infections from companion animals such as cats and dogs to *Trichophyton mentagrophytes* from rodents and *Trichophyton verrucosum* from cattle. The body sites most commonly affected by zoophilic and geophilic dermatophytes are the scalp, face, trunk, and limbs (see earlier table).

**7. Sample/specimen requirements**—To diagnose an infection an appropriate and representative sample of skin, hair, and/or nail should be taken from the advancing edge of the site of infection after wiping the area with 70% alcohol. For scalp infection, plucked hairs are required in addition to any loose skin scale as it is the hair root that is important for microscopy and culture. These should be transported to the laboratory at ambient temperature, ideally wrapped in black paper or a paper envelope to keep the specimen dry. Sterile plastic containers may be used for nail samples, and disposable soft-bristle toothbrush samples may be used for scalp infections in addition to plucked hairs. Samples should not be refrigerated as this may reduce the viability of some dermatophyte pathogens.

**8. Testing requirements**—On arrival in the laboratory, the sample should be examined microscopically following presoftening in 10% potassium hydroxide; this is enhanced by the application of optical brighteners such as blankophor or calcofluor and examination under a fluorescence microscope. Fungal elements seen at this stage are diagnostic for fungal infection. Some fungal infections are so distinctive on microscopy that definitive identification is possible, but culture at 28°C–30°C on selective agar is usually necessary to identify the involved pathogen. Cultures, particularly of nail samples, may fail to grow despite the positive direct microscopy. Some laboratories now carry out PCR tests directly on samples and can immediately report the pathogen identity.

**9. Reporting requirements**—Local laboratories should be providing an isolation and identification service for fungal isolates from the skin, hair, and nails. Reporting of outbreaks to the local health authority is obligatory in some countries. Outbreaks in schools or other institutions should also be reported.

**10. Referral network**—Isolates that are unusual or difficult to identify should be referred to specialist mycology reference laboratories.

**11. Special considerations**—Epidemiological analysis is important for animal-acquired infections to link cases and identify any potential clusters or outbreaks. This also applies to anthropophilic infections of the scalp particularly seen among young children in schools, or sometimes causing outbreaks in institutions, where identification of the infecting organism and tracing of infected individuals is important to limit the spread. This is particularly true of *Trichophyton tonsurans*, which can readily spread from person to person. A carrier state has also been recognized for this species; therefore, sampling should be extended to close contacts even if they are not symptomatic.

[E. M. Johnson]

# GIARDIASIS

(*Giardia* enteritis)

| DISEASE | ICD-10 CODE |
|---|---|
| GIARDIASIS | ICD-10 A07.1 |

**1. Clinical features**—A protozoan infection, principally of the upper small intestine. It can remain asymptomatic; cause acute diarrhea; be self-limited in 2–4 weeks; and lead to intestinal symptoms such as chronic diarrhea, steatorrhea, abdominal cramps, bloating, frequent loose and pale greasy stools, fatigue, malabsorption (of fats and fat-soluble vitamins), and weight loss. There is usually no extraintestinal invasion, but reactive arthritis and, in severe giardiasis, damage to duodenal and jejunal mucosal cells may occur.

**2. Causative agents**—*Giardia duodenalis* (*Giardia lamblia*, *Giardia intestinalis*), a flagellate protozoan.

**3. Laboratory diagnosis**—*G. duodenalis* is identified by the finding of trophozoites and/or cysts in feces, duodenal aspirates, or duodenal string test processed for routine ova and parasite (O&P) examination. Because *Giardia* infection is often asymptomatic, the presence of *G. duodenalis* (in stool or duodenal aspirates) does not necessarily indicate that *Giardia* is the cause of illness. O&P testing is typically 2-tiered, where wet mount microscopical examination of unstained stool concentrate precedes microscopy of stained stool concentrate (e.g., trichrome staining).

Trophozoites of *G. duodenalis* are 10–20 μm in length and pyriform in shape. There are 2 nuclei that are not visible in unstained preparations, a pair of curved median bodies, and a large bowl-shaped sucking disk that covers most of the anterior half of the ventral surface. There are 8 flagella: 4 lateral, 2 ventral, and 2 directed posteriorly. Flagella are not always visible in permanent stained preparations, although in living trophozoites the movement of the flagella is evident. In direct wet mounts, *G. duodenalis* is described as having falling-leaf motility. Cysts are oval in shape and measure 8–19 μm in length. Mature cysts have 4 nuclei, while immature cysts usually have 2 nuclei. Intracytoplasmic fibrils are visible in iodine-stained wet mounts and permanent stains. Microscopy is considered the gold standard for diagnosis of giardiasis.

There are also many commercially available antigen detection-based assays including enzyme immunoassays/enzyme-linked immunosorbent assays (EIA/ELISA), immunochromatographic assays (widely known as rapid diagnostic tests or point-of-care tests), and microscopical immunofluorescent assays targeting cysts. Nucleic acid-based tests, such as polymerase chain reaction (PCR), are increasingly being used to detect *G. duodenalis* and are incorporated in commercial multipathogen panels (e.g., FilmArray Gastrointestinal Panel, BioFire Diagnostics, Salt Lake City, UT).

There are no serologic assays (i.e., antibody detection) for routine clinical diagnosis of giardiasis. Noncommercial, research laboratory serological assays are available to support epidemiological studies.

**4. Laboratory capability**—Microscopy, stool concentration/centrifugation (minimally achieving 1,000 *g* and accommodating 15 mL screw-cap tubes), and permanent slide staining capabilities should be available in most clinical and public health laboratories. Laboratorians should be trained in the microscopic/morphologic detection of parasites and undergo regular proficiency testing. Laboratories that perform immunofluorescence assays typically use common filter sets for visualizing targets labeled with fluorescent dyes (e.g., fluorescein [green], rhodamine [red], or similar). Commercial assays may require specialized equipment including microplate readers (ELISA), fluorescent microscopes, thermocycler systems (PCR), or custom hardware platforms that will require routine maintenance.

Laboratorians trained in performing nucleic acid-based diagnostic assays are needed for molecular detection of giardiasis. Specific equipment required will depend on the type of assay selected (standard thermocycler, real-time PCR thermocycler, or multiplex molecular platform). Deoxyribonucleic acid (DNA) extraction processes should include a step for mechanical disruption (e.g., bead beating) of the cysts to ensure release of the DNA. A unidirectional workflow should be implemented to reduce risk of false-positive results because of amplicon contamination.

**5. Safety requirements**—Clinical specimens should always be collected and handled with standard precautions. *G. duodenalis* is a biosafety level 2 organism. Cysts are immediately infective when shed in human feces. Formalin, as a stool fixative, should only be used in a well-ventilated area, preferably in a chemical fume hood. Scant data are available for the persistence of cyst infectivity in standard stool fixative/preservatives; consequently, unpreserved and preserved stools should be disposed of as infectious waste. Reagent and stain disposal should follow manufacturer safety data sheet guidelines or follow local institutional hazardous waste guidelines.

**6. Nonhuman hosts**—Through molecular subtyping, *G. duodenalis* has been divided into multiple assemblages or genotypes. Several of these are more prevalent in humans, while others are more prevalent in nonhuman animals such as dogs, cats, rodents, and ruminants. Some genotypes have been detected in both human and nonhuman mammals.

**7. Sample/specimen requirements**—Stool should be promptly preserved in a liquid medium appropriate for microscopical examination or for antigen detection (e.g., EIA/ELISA or immunochromatographic assays). Formalin-based fixatives are suitable for microscopical assays. Single vial alcohol-based systems for O&P collection are also appropriate (e.g., EcoFix, Meridian Bioscience, Cincinnati, OH; TotalFix, Medical Chemical Corporation, Torrance, CA). If nucleic acid-based assays are to be utilized, stool should be left unpreserved or placed in a medium that is acceptable for molecular detection (i.e., lacking formalin or mercury). To maximize microscopy sensitivity, up to 3 separate stool specimens should be collected on different days.

**8. Testing requirements**—Diagnostic assays are based on identification of the parasite (whole organism, antigen, or nucleic acids) in stool, as culture methods for clinical isolates are variably successful and are not used in diagnosis. Microscopical assays typically include routine concentration procedures (e.g., formalin ethyl acetate sedimentation) and permanent staining of stool. A calibrated ocular micrometer should be used to measure cyst and trophozoite sizes. Diagnosis is confirmatory in specimens meeting morphologic criteria in laboratories with appropriate training; however, antigen or nucleic acid-based assays are more suitable for confirmation of diagnosis.

Molecular diagnosis can be useful for clarification of suspicious microscopy findings and for providing a more sensitive detection compared with bright-field microscopy. For in-house assays, cutoff values for what should be considered a positive result should be established based on a laboratory-specific validation using known positives and negatives.

Assay sensitivity and specificity follows this general pattern: microscopy is considered the gold standard for diagnosing giardiasis, but its performance is linked to the training and skills of the microscopist and repeated stool testing (until $\geq 3$ negative). Antigen detection assays generally demonstrate a performance range between 50%–100% sensitive and 90%–100% specific. Rapid tests generally show lower sensitivities, while ELISAs are typically greater than 95% sensitive. Immunofluorescent microscopy is typically greater than 99% sensitive and specific, and nucleic acid-based assays (e.g., PCR) are essentially 100% sensitive and specific. Specificity can vary considerably for nonspecific staining methods, depending on microscopist skills, but antigen and nucleic acid-based assays show high specificity, approaching 100%, especially when used as confirmation of positive results.

Serology is not available for routine clinical diagnosis.

**9. Reporting requirements**—Reporting requirements/criteria vary by country and local jurisdiction. In jurisdictions where formal reporting mechanisms are not yet established, clinicians and laboratory workers who identify cases of giardiasis are encouraged to inform the appropriate health departments. In the USA, giardiasis (confirmed and probable) is included in the National Notifiable Diseases Surveillance System. Positive cases from humans may be reported as *G. duodenalis* identified.

**10. Referral network**—None.

**11. Special considerations**—Institute an epidemiological investigation of clustered cases in an area or institution to determine source of infection and mode of transmission. A common vehicle, such as water, food, or association with a day care center or recreational area must be investigated; institute applicable preventive or control measures. Control of person-to-person transmission requires special emphasis on personal cleanliness and sanitary disposal of feces.

[M. J. Arrowood, B. Mathison]

# GONOCOCCAL INFECTIONS

| DISEASE | ICD-10 CODE |
|---|---|
| GENITOURINARY GONOCOCCAL INFECTION | ICD-10 A54.0–A54.2 |
| GONOCCOCAL OPHTHALMIA NEONATORUM | ICD-10 A54.3 |

**1. Clinical features—**

1) Genitourinary gonococcal infection (gonorrhea, gonococcal urethritis, gonococcal vulvovaginitis, gonococcal cervicitis, gonococcal bartholinitis, clap, strain, gleet, dose, GC): a bacterial disease limited to noncornified columnar and cuboidal epithelium, which differs in males and females in course, severity, and ease of recognition. In males, gonococcal infection generally presents as an acute purulent discharge from the anterior urethra with dysuria within 2–7 days after exposure. A minority of gonococcal infections in males are asymptomatic. In females, infection is followed by the development of mucopurulent cervicitis, often asymptomatic, although some women with infection have abnormal vaginal discharge and vaginal bleeding after intercourse. In 10%–20%, there is also uterine invasion, often timed with menstruation, with resultant endometritis, salpingitis, or pelvic peritonitis, and subsequent risk of infertility and ectopic pregnancy.

In females and males who have sex with men, pharyngeal and anorectal infections also occur. While infection of the pharynx and rectum often are asymptomatic, anorectal infections may cause pruritis, tenesmus, and discharge. Conjunctivitis occurs in newborns born to infected mothers with resultant blindness if not rapidly and adequately treated.

Septicemia (also known as disseminated gonococcal infection) may occur in 0.5%–3% of untreated gonococcal infections and can result in arthritis, skin lesions, and (rarely) endocarditis and meningitis. Arthritis can produce permanent joint damage if appropriate antibiotics are not used. Death is rare except among persons with endocarditis and underlying health conditions such as complement deficiency.

Nongonococcal urethritis (NGU) and mucopurulent cervicitis are caused by other sexually transmitted agents and seriously complicate the clinical diagnosis of gonorrhea; the organisms that cause these diseases often coexist with gonococcal infections. In many populations, the incidence of NGU exceeds that of gonorrhea.

*Chlamydia trachomatis* (see "Chlamydial Infections") causes about 30%–40% of NGU in most industrialized countries.

2) Gonococcal opthalmia neonaturum: acute redness and swelling of conjunctiva in one or both eyes, with mucopurulent or purulent discharge, typically occurring within 1–5 days of birth. Corneal ulcer, perforation, and blindness may occur if antimicrobial treatment is not given promptly. The gonococcus is the most serious but not the most frequent infectious cause of opthalmia neonatorum. The most common infectious cause is *C. trachomatis*, which produces inclusion conjunctivitis that tends to be less acute than gonococcal conjunctivitis and usually appears 5–14 days after birth (see "Chlamydial Infections"). Any purulent neonatal conjunctivitis should be considered gonococcal until proven otherwise.

**2. Causative agents**—*Neisseria gonorrhoeae*, the gonococcus.

**3. Laboratory diagnosis**—Made by Gram stain of discharge, bacteriological culture on selective media (e.g., modified Thayer-Martin agar), or tests that detect gonococcal nucleic acid. Typical Gram-negative, intracellular diplococci can be considered diagnostic in male urethral smears, but Gram stain is not recommended to diagnose *N. gonorrhoeae* infection in women. Cultures on selective media, plus presumptive identification based on both macroscopic and microscopic examination, and biochemical testing are sensitive and specific, as are nucleic acid amplification tests. However, culture is highly dependent on adequate specimen collection, optimal transport conditions, and proficient laboratory procedures. Nucleic acid amplification tests (NAATs) are more sensitive than culture since viable bacteria are not required and additional specimen types can be utilized. In cases with potential legal implications, specimens should be cultured and isolates confirmed as *N. gonorrhoeae* by biochemical as well as enzymatic tests and preserved to enable additional or repeated testing. Because of decreased susceptibility to a number of antibiotics, including third generation cephalosporins, intermittent regional (supranational) surveillance for antimicrobial susceptibility of *N. gonorrhoeae* should be undertaken.

**4. Laboratory capability**—Culture isolation and identification requires a microbiology laboratory with personnel trained in aseptic technique. More stringent environments involving unidirectional workflow from specimen processing to testing and highly skilled technical staff are required for laboratories using open NAATs. By contrast, enclosed NAATs may be performed by personnel with minimal training and in basic environments.

**5. Safety requirements**—Biosafety level 2; all specimens, microbial cultures and inoculated products should be considered infectious and handled appropriately. Aseptic technique and universal/standard precautions for handling the bacterial group studied should be observed throughout this procedure.

**6. Nonhuman hosts**—Humans are the only known reservoir for *N. gonorrhoeae*. A murine model to investigate pathogenesis has been described but not widely used.

**7. Sample/specimen requirements**—Specimens collected for gonorrhea culture should be obtained by using swabs with plastic or wire shafts and rayon, Dacron, or calcium alginate tips. Other swab material such as wood shafts and cotton tips might be inhibitory or toxic to the organism and should be avoided. Several nonnutritive swab transport systems are available, and some studies suggest that these transport systems might maintain gonococcal viability for up to 48 hours in ambient temperatures. However, environmental conditions might vary by location and season, which could affect the viability of gonorrhea in these transport systems; thus, additional local validation of transport conditions might be needed. Culture medium transport systems are preferred because there are some advantages over swab transport systems (e.g., extended shelf life and better recovery because cultivated isolates are being transported rather than a clinical specimen). Culture medium is inoculated with the swab specimen and then placed immediately into a $CO_2$-enriched atmosphere for transportation to the laboratory. Because *N. gonorrhoeae* has demanding nutritional and environmental growth requirements, optimal recovery rates are achieved when specimens are inoculated directly and when the growth medium is incubated in an increased $CO_2$ environment as soon as possible. Swab and urine specimens can be used to test for *N. gonorrhoeae* by NAATs. Vaginal swabs can be collected by either the patient or health care provider. More invasive cervical and urethral swabs must be collected by a health care provider. These specimens can be stored frozen or at temperatures up to 25°C for several months prior to testing according to product inserts.

**8. Testing requirements**—NAATs are recommended for detection of urogenital, rectal, and oropharyngeal infections caused by *N. gonorrhoeae* infections in women and men with and without symptoms. The sensitivity of NAATs range from 90%–100% and the specificity exceeds 97% across all specimens and tests. Because NAATs are so sensitive, efforts are warranted to prevent contamination of specimens in the clinic or spread of environmental amplicon in the laboratory. Laboratories should follow standard molecular method techniques, clean workspaces and equipment frequently, include multiple negative controls in each run, and monitor the rate of indeterminate and positive results, as a change in monthly trends might indicate a need to investigate the accuracy of the results. Environmental monitoring might be required as recommended by the manufacturer. If environmental amplicons are found, robust cleaning of the laboratory is needed until negative results are obtained. Steps to prevent cross-contamination include proper testing of laboratory workflow design and strict adherence to testing and quality assurance protocols.

Assessing *N. gonorrhoeae* isolates for antibiotic susceptibility requires viable isolates because accurate genetic markers of antibiotic resistance to recommended therapies remain to be documented. Isolates recovered from a genital specimen on selective medium that are Gram-negative diplococcus and oxidase-positive might be presumptively identified as *N. gonorrhoeae*. A presumptive identification indicates only that a Gram-negative, oxidase-positive diplococcus (e.g., other *Neisseria* spp. or *Branhamella catarrhalis*) might be isolated from such specimens. Certain coccobacilli, including *Kingella denitrificans*, might appear to be Gram-negative diplococci in Gram-stained smears. A confirmed laboratory diagnosis of *N. gonorrhoeae* requires additional biochemical tests such as acid production from glucose, maltose, lactose, sucrose, and fructose; superoxol production; reduction of nitrate; polysaccharide production from sucrose; and tributyrin hydrolysis. A presumptive test result is sufficient to initiate antimicrobial therapy, but additional tests must be performed to confirm the identity of an isolate as *N. gonorrhoeae*. Agar plate dilution testing that provides minimum inhibitory concentration values of tested antibiotics is the preferred method for testing the susceptibility of *N. gonorrhoeae* but might be too difficult to perform in laboratories with limited capacity and low testing volumes. Etest is a simpler method for determining minimal inhibitory susceptibilities of gonococcal isolates, but it is more costly when testing a large number of isolates. The easiest antimicrobial susceptibility method is disk diffusion, but it is limited by the lack of interpretive clinical breakpoint criteria.

**9. Reporting requirements**—Results should be reported based on bacterial identification or NAATs. Minimal inhibitory concentration values are preferred when reporting antimicrobial susceptibility results given the lack of clinical breakpoint data for relevant therapeutic agents. Gonorrhea is a communicable disease of public health significance and is notifiable in many countries. Laboratories should verify their obligation to report positive findings.

**10. Referral network**—No specific referral networks exist but laboratorians are encouraged to contact CDC if *N. gonorrhoeae* is isolated from patients suspected to have failed CDC recommended treatment or if culture isolates display decreased susceptibility to front line antimicrobial agents.

**11. Special considerations**—WHO and CDC consider the emergence of antimicrobial resistant *N. gonorrhoeae* a global health concern due to the limited treatment options.

[J. R. Papp]

# GRANULOMA INGUINALE

(donovanosis)

| DISEASE | ICD-10 CODE |
|---|---|
| GRANULOMA INGUINALE | ICD-10 A.58 |

**1. Clinical features**—A chronic and progressively destructive but poorly communicable bacterial disease of the skin and mucous membranes of the external genitalia, inguinal, and anal regions. One or more indurated nodules or papules lead to slowly spreading, necrotic, hypertrophic, granulomatous, ulcerative, or sclerotic lesions. The lesions are characteristically nonfriable, beefy red granulomas, and extend peripherally with characteristic rolled edges to eventually form fibrous tissue. Lesions occur most common on warm, moist surfaces, such as the folds between the thighs, the perianal area, the scrotum, or the vulvar labia and vagina. The genitalia are involved in close to 50% of cases, the inguinal region in close to 10%, the anal region in 5%–10%, and distant sites in 1%–5%. If neglected, the process may result in extensive destruction of genital organs and may spread by autoinoculation to other parts of the body.

**2. Causative agents**—The causative agent is *Klebsiella granulomatis* (*Donovania granulomatis*, *Calymmatobacterium granulomatis*), a Gram-negative bacillus.

**3. Laboratory diagnosis**—Laboratory diagnosis is based on demonstration of intracytoplasmic Gram-negative, rod-shaped organisms (Donovan bodies) in Wright- or Giemsa-stained smears of granulation tissue or biopsy specimens. The presence of large infected mononuclear cells filled with deeply staining Donovan bodies is pathognomonic. Culture is not routinely available. Serological tests are unreliable, and polymerase chain reaction is available only in research settings. *Haemophilus ducreyi* should be excluded by culture on appropriate selective media.

**4. Laboratory capability**—The laboratory must be skilled in histopathology, cytopathology, and microscopy to provide primary diagnostic support. Culture isolation is extremely difficult given the lack of artificial media. Cell culture is rarely used for isolation but can be performed using fresh human monocytes or Hep-2 cell lines. There are no commercial nucleic acid amplification tests to detect *K. granulomatis*, though research laboratories may have developed in-house assays. Serologic testing by complement fixation or indirect immunofluorescence has been reported but has not been adopted for routine diagnostic practice.

**5. Safety requirements**—Biosafety level 2; all specimens, microbial cultures and inoculated products should be considered infectious and handled appropriately. Aseptic technique and universal/standard precautions for handling the bacterial group studied should be observed throughout this procedure.

**6. Nonhuman hosts**—Humans are the only known reservoir for *K. granulomatis*.

**7. Sample/specimen requirements**—A cotton-tipped swab should be gently rolled across the lesion to remove excess exudate prior to specimen collection. Roll a second swab across the base of the lesion, which has the greatest likelihood of containing Donovan bodies, and then roll it onto a glass slide. Allow the glass slide to air-dry before transport to the laboratory at ambient temperature. Punch (3–5 mm diameter) or snip biopsies can be collected from the lesion periphery and fixed in 10% formalin for histopathology or directly smeared onto a glass slide.

**8. Testing requirements**—Giemsa staining is typically used to microscopically visualize Donovan bodies in direct lesion smears. A modified Giemsa method that involves dipping the slide 5 times in a fixative such as methanol, 6 times in eosin solution, 6 times in a thiazide dye mixture, and then rinsed with phosphate buffer, pH 6.8, has been successfully used. Alternatively, slides fixed in methanol can be stained for 30 minutes with 10% Giemsa and rinsed with buffered water or phosphate-buffered saline, pH 7.0–7.2. Slides are allowed to air-dry and then examined under oil immersion (1000x magnification) with a light microscope. Bi-polar stained bodies that resemble closed safety pins within vacuoles in the cytoplasm of large histiocytes and, less frequently, in plasma cells and polymorphonuclear leukocytes are characteristic of Donovan bodies. Other stains such as Wright and Leishman can be used with comparable sensitivity to Giemsa. Silver staining may be slightly more sensitive.

Formalin-fixed biopsy specimens should be stained with Giemsa. Hematoxylin and eosin stained specimen slides may fail to distinguish Donovan bodies unless present in large numbers but would be sufficient in identifying acute and chronic inflammation with granulation tissue.

**9. Reporting requirements**—Results should be reported based on microscopic examination of lesion material. Granuloma inguinale is a communicable disease of public health significance and is required to be reported to the public health authorities in a number of countries. Laboratory directors should determine if it is a laboratory-reportable disease in their specific setting.

**10. Referral network**—No specific referral networks exist.

**11. Special considerations**—None.

[J. R. Papp]

# HANTAVIRAL DISEASES

| DISEASE | ICD-10 CODE |
|---|---|
| HEMORRHAGIC FEVER WITH RENAL SYNDROME | ICD-10 A98.5 |
| HANTAVIRUS PULMONARY SYNDROME | ICD-10 B33.4 |

HEMORRHAGIC FEVER WITH RENAL SYNDROME (epidemic hemorrhagic fever, Korean hemorrhagic fever, Nephropathia epidemica, hemorrhagic nephroso-nephritis, HFRS); HANTAVIRUS PULMONARY SYNDROME (hantavirus adult respiratory distress syndrome, hantavirus cardiopulmonary syndrome, HPS, HCPS)

**1. Clinical features**—An acute zoonotic disease with 2 similar syndromes, featuring febrile prodrome, thrombocytopenia, leukocytosis and capillary leakage.

1) Hemorrhagic fever with renal syndrome (HFRS): characterized by abrupt onset of fever, lower back pain, varying degrees of hemorrhagic manifestations, and renal involvement. Severe illness is associated with Hantaan and Seoul viruses (primarily in Asia) and Dobrava virus (in the Balkans). Disease is characterized by 5 clinical phases that frequently overlap: febrile, hypotensive, oliguric, diuretic, and convalescent.

   The febrile phase, which lasts 3–7 days, is characterized by high fever, headache, malaise, and anorexia, followed by severe abdominal or lower back pain, and often accompanied by nausea and vomiting, facial flushing, petechiae, and conjunctival injection. Most cases show an elevated hematocrit, thrombocytopenia, and creatinine. The hypotensive phase lasts from several hours to 3 days and is characterized by defervescence and abrupt onset of hypotension, which may progress to shock and more apparent hemorrhagic manifestations. Blood pressure returns to normal or is high in the oliguric phase (3–7 days), nausea and vomiting may persist, severe hemorrhage may occur, and urinary output falls dramatically.

   The case-fatality rate ranges from 5%–15%, and the majority of deaths occur during the hypotensive and oliguric phases. Diuresis heralds the onset of recovery in most cases, with polyuria of 3–6 L per day. Convalescence takes weeks to months. Infections caused by Seoul virus, carried by Norway and Black rats, are clinically milder, although severe disease may occur with this strain. They show less clear distinction between clinical phases.

Less severe illnesses (case-fatality rate < 1%) are caused by Puumala virus, referred to as nephropathia epidemica and Saaremaa viruses.

2) Hantavirus pulmonary syndrome (HPS): characterized by fever, myalgias, and gastrointestinal complaints, followed by the abrupt onset of respiratory distress and hypotension. The illness progresses rapidly to severe respiratory failure and shock. Most cases show an elevated hematocrit, hypoalbuminemia, and thrombocytopenia. The fatality rate can be as high as 35%–50%. In survivors, recovery from acute illness is rapid, but full convalescence may require weeks to months. Restoration of normal lung function generally occurs, but pulmonary function abnormalities may persist in some individuals. Renal and hemorrhagic manifestations are usually absent, except in some severe cases. No unapparent infections have been documented, but milder infections without frank pulmonary edema have occurred, and antibody prevalence studies, especially in South America, have detected serological-positive people with no recollection of the typical disease.

**2. Causative agents**—Hantaviruses (genus *Orthohantavirus* of the family *Hantaviridae*: 3-segmented ribonucleic acid [RNA] viruses with spherical to oval particles, 95–110 nm in diameter). More than 25 antigenically distinguishable viral species exist, each associated primarily with a single rodent species. However, very few virus isolates from human or rodents exist.

1) HFRS: Hantaan, Dobrava, Puumala, Saaremaa, Seoul viruses.
2) HPS: Andes (Argentina, Chile), Laguna Negra (Bolivia, Paraguay), Juquitiba (Brazil), Black Creek Canal and Bayou (southeastern USA), New York-1 and Monongahela (eastern USA); Sin Nombre (North America).

**3. Laboratory diagnosis**—In very early samples, conventional or real-time polymerase chain reaction (PCR) could be used on blood clot rather than serum; autopsy or biopsy samples could also be tested by molecular assays. Almost all patients have immunoglobulin class M (IgM), and most even have IgG antibodies detectable by enzyme-linked immunosorbent assay (ELISA), Western blot, or strip immunoblot techniques at the time of hospitalization, and virus cannot be isolated. Immunohistochemistry on formalin-fixed tissues is an excellent method of diagnosis when no other samples are available in fatal human cases.

**4. Laboratory capability**—In some countries, commercial assays are available, and clinical and public health laboratories are capable of testing for hantaviral disease. In most countries, however, testing may have to be referred to a higher-level testing facility. Clinical specimens from suspect patients should always be collected and handled with universal/standard precautions. Molecular and serological techniques are needed for identification of cases.

Commercial assays are available in different areas of the world and some states and government laboratories are providing diagnostic assays.

**5. Safety requirements**—Hantaviruses are biosafety level 2 (BSL-2) and BSL-3 agents. No human vaccines are currently available for HPS. Chinese and Korean manufacturers are producing vaccines against HFRS associated with Hantaan and Seoul viruses. Collection and handling of infectious or suspected infectious clinical specimens should be performed by trained personnel using universal protective equipment. Procedures generating aerosols (e.g., centrifugation) should be minimized. People working with potentially infected rodents during ecological studies should wear appropriate protective equipment based on risk assessment.

**6. Nonhuman hosts**—Each hantavirus species is generally associated with 1 rodent species, but there is evidence for host-switches without epidemiological implications. Recently, hantaviruses have been detected in other mammal groups including of the orders Eulipyphla and Chiroptera but without any evidence of human-associated diseases. Humans are incidental hosts.

1) HFRS: field rodents (*Apodemus* spp. for Hantaan, Dobrava, and Saaremaa viruses in Asia and the central European areas; *Myodes* (formerly *Clethrionomys*) spp. for Puumala in Western Europe and Scandinavia; *Rattus* spp. for Seoul virus (worldwide).
2) HPS: in North America, the major reservoir of Sin Nombre virus appears to be the deer mouse, *Peromyscus maniculatus*. Antibodies have also been found in other *Peromyscus* spp., pack rats, the chipmunk, and other rodents. In other regions, hantavirus strains have been associated mainly with other rodent species of the subfamily *Sigmodontinae*.

**7. Sample/specimen requirements**—Diagnosis requires samples (i.e., serum, heparinized plasma, or whole blood) collected during acute febrile stage of disease, or early convalescence for serology (IgM and IgG). Viral RNA can be detected in blood collected in the early stage of the disease. Diagnostic samples should be shipped at 4°C for serology or in dry ice for PCR assays and kept at -80°C for long-term storage. From tissues collected during autopsies or from biopsies, viral antigens can be detected by immunohistochemistry; formaldehyde-fixed tissue and paraffin-embedded blocks should be stored and shipped at room temperature.

**8. Testing requirements**—Hantaviruses infections are rare but there are commercially available assays in different parts of the world. Additionally, diagnostic reagents are available in some state and governmental laboratories. As for other infectious diseases, the diagnosis should always be based on the results of a combination of clinical and laboratory data. During acute febrile stages of disease, virus DNA can sometimes be detected by conventional or real-time

PCR, followed by sequencing. In general, IgM and even IgG antibodies can be detected by ELISA very early in the clinical phase of the disease. Virus antigens can be detected by immunohistochemistry in tissues samples collected post-mortem or in lung biopsies. Direct detection of IgM, or IgM and IgG antibodies in an individual with a clinically compatible illness constitutes a confirmed disease case.

**9. Reporting requirements**—Hantavirus pulmonary syndrome in the USA is reportable by guidelines of the Council of State and Territorial Epidemiologists. Suspected cases should be reported to state health authorities, and, if confirmed, to CDC through the National Notifiable Diseases Surveillance System. If hantavirus infection is suspected, contact the CDC Viral Special Pathogens Branch by phone (470-312-0094 or 404-639-1115; after hours: 770-488-7100) or e-mail (spather@cdc.gov).

**10. Referral network**—Testing can be performed commercially or at select reference laboratories. Laboratory-confirmed clinical human cases should be reported to local authorities (see Reporting Requirements section in this chapter).

**11. Special considerations**—Occurrence of hantavirus infections does not constitute an International Health Regulations reportable event to WHO. Isolation of hantaviruses is not reportable to the Federal Select Agent Program in the USA.

[P. E. Rollin, S. Nichol]

# HELICOBACTER PYLORI INFECTION

| DISEASE | ICD-10 CODE |
|---|---|
| HELICOBACTER PYLORI INFECTION | ICD-10 K29 |

**1. Clinical features**—A bacterial infection by *Helicobacter pylori* causing acute and chronic gastritis, primarily in the antrum of the stomach, and peptic ulcer disease. *H. pylori* colonizes humans and is found to colonize more than 50% of the human population worldwide. Most of those infected with *H. pylori* remain asymptomatic, and without treatment infection is often lifelong. The key pathophysiological event in *H. pylori* infection is initiation and continuance of an inflammatory response. Development of atrophy and intestinal metaplasia of the gastric mucosa are strongly associated with *H. pylori* infection. Infection with *H. pylori* is epidemiologically associated with development of gastric adenocarcinoma and gastric mucosa-associated lymphoid tissue (MALT)–type lymphoma. Oxidative and nitrosative stress in combination with inflammation plays an important role in gastric carcinogenesis. Thus *H. pylori* infection has been found to be the major risk factor for gastric carcinogenesis, with environmental factors (e.g., high saline- or nitrosamine-containing food) and genetic susceptibility being additional contributing risk factors for development of gastric cancer.

Dyspepsia is a common and complex condition consisting of chronic upper gastrointestinal symptoms. Patients with alarm symptoms should be referred for prompt endoscopy and without alarm symptoms can be tested for *H. pylori*, and if positive, treated.

**2. Causative agents**—Characterized in 1983, *H. pylori* is a helical-shaped, Gram-negative bacterium whose motility, which is key to its ability to penetrate the mucus layer and reach the epithelial cells, is facilitated by 4–8 unipolar flagella. It is positive for the catalase, oxidase, and urease tests. In the laboratory the bacterium can be cultured at 34°C–40°C under microaerophilic conditions; with optimal growth at oxygen levels of 2%–5%, supplemented with 5% to 10% carbon dioxide and high humidity.

**3. Laboratory diagnosis**—The laboratory can serve as an adjunct to clinical diagnostic procedures. Diagnostic methods are categorized according to whether or not an endoscopy is necessary and whether the diagnosis is to be set before or after an eradication treatment. Biopsy-based tests include histological evaluation, culture, polymerase chain reaction (PCR), and the rapid urease test, all of which are performed on tissue obtained during endoscopy. Alternatively, the urea breath test, serology, and stool antigen test can be performed as noninvasive procedures. Serum antibody tests may remain positive for months after treatment. The sensitivity and specificity of different tests depend on the age of the patients and the disease they present. Testing for *H. pylori* infection is indicated in patients with dyspeptic symptoms, a past history of documented peptic ulcer disease, gastric cancer, or gastric MALT lymphoma.

**4. Laboratory capability**—A contained, purpose-built, microbiological facility is required to handle this pathogen with the capacity to autoclave microbiological waste. Staff should be trained and shown to be competent to handle potentially hazardous biological agents and should be able to carry out basic phenotypic techniques.

**5. Safety requirements**—Employers have a responsibility to protect their workers from the risks related to exposure to hazardous biological agents.[1] *H. pylori* is a hazard group 2 bacterium and should be handled within a biosafety level 2 laboratory. Gloves and other personal protective equipment should be worn, including laboratory coat and laboratory safety glasses. Finally, although not essential, it is recommended to use a class I or II microbiological biosafety cabinet when handling this pathogen.

**6. Nonhuman hosts**—Humans are the main natural reservoir for *H. pylori*, and in untreated individuals, it can persist for years or even decades. In rare occasions, *H. pylori* has been found in some primates and domestic pets. Due to its fastidious growth requirement, *H. pylori* does not easily survive in other environments.

**7. Sample/specimen requirements**—A stool specimen is required for stool antigen testing. Gastric biopsies are required for culture of *H. pylori*. Biopsies should be collected directly following a treatment-free interval of 2 weeks without proton pump inhibitor and 4 weeks without antibiotics. Additionally, biopsies should be collected from multiple sites; at least 2 from the antrum and 2 from the anterior and posterior corpus, respectively. All biopsy specimens should be taken with sterile instruments and before histology specimens are collected, to reduce risk of contamination. Culture of *H. pylori* from biopsy material should be performed without delay, preferably within 24 hours of collection. If it is necessary to transport biopsies to a centralized specialist microbiology laboratory for culture and isolation of the organism, then a suitable transport medium (e.g., Dents medium) should be used.

A pure culture of *H. pylori* is required to perform phenotypic antimicrobial sensitivity testing. Both the European Committee on Antimicrobial Susceptibility Testing and the British Society for Antimicrobial Chemotherapy recommend the use of Etest strips (bioMérieux, Durham, NC) for *H. pylori* culture-based antimicrobial susceptibility testing.

**8. Testing requirements**—Testing facilities must adhere to the quality standards of their accreditation body, and diagnostic laboratories must follow the manufacturer's instructions for any assay being performed. Diagnosis of infection may be established using a variety of invasive and noninvasive techniques; the selection of which is often determined based on whether or not eradication treatment has commenced.

Invasive techniques used to determine an infection typically rely on the collection of gastric biopsies and, while histological examination of multiple biopsies can be used for diagnosis, bacterial culture from these biopsies is the most specific method. Culture-based methods have added advantages over histological as further characterization of the causative organism, such as antimicrobial susceptibility testing, can be carried out. These techniques can be limited in their deployment as they are expensive and require experienced, qualified staff and appropriate laboratory facilities. A cheaper alternative is the rapid urease test, which can be applied directly to biopsy specimens. Alternatively, serology may also be used for diagnosis of *H. pylori* colonization. Although they are considered relatively inexpensive and readily available, care must be taken when interpreting *H. pylori* serology results as the method does not discriminate between a current infection and recent exposure.

Noninvasive techniques such as the urea breath test, which utilize the organism's ability to release carbon dioxide from urea, and stool antigen testing can be applied to monitor the eradication of an infection.

PCR has also been used to detect *H. pylori* directly in deoxyribonucleic acid extracts from clinical specimens and has been applied to both biopsy and fecal sample types. However, caution must be taken since the technique does not distinguish between viable and nonviable organisms.

**9. Reporting requirements**—Notification of *H. pylori* infections is not required. The prevalence of *H. pylori* antibiotic resistance varies significantly from country to country and even between regions within the same country. National surveillance of *H. pylori* antimicrobial resistance to clarithromycin, amoxicillin, and metronidazole helps to inform potential success of the front line triple therapy.

**10. Referral network**—Biopsy specimens may be sent to specialized reference laboratories for isolation and phenotypic susceptibility testing. A multilocus sequence typing scheme is available and may be performed for strain discrimination.

**11. Special considerations**—None.

## References

1. EUR-Lex. Directive 2000/54/EC of the European Parliament and of the Council of 18 September 2000. Available at: https://eur-lex.europa.eu/legal-content/EN/ALL/?uri=CELEX%3A32000L0054. Accessed February 15, 2019.

[D. Ready, C. Swift]

# HEPATITIS, VIRAL

(viral hepatitis A, viral hepatitis B, viral hepatitis C, viral hepatitis D, viral hepatitis E)

| DISEASE | ICD-10 CODE |
|---|---|
| HEPATITIS A | ICD-10 B15 |
| HEPATITIS B | ICD-10 B16 |
| HEPATITIS C | ICD-10 B17.1 |
| HEPATITIS D | ICD-10 B17.0 |
| HEPATITIS E | ICD-10 B17.2 |
| HEPATOCELLULAR CARCINOMA | ICD-10 C22.0 |

Viral hepatitis is etiologically linked to 5 hepatotropic viruses: hepatitis A virus (HAV), hepatitis B virus (HBV), hepatitis C virus (HCV), hepatitis D virus (HDV), and hepatitis E virus (HEV). The diseases caused by these viruses have similar clinical presentations but have variations in epidemiological, immunological, clinical, and pathological characteristics. The clinical case definition for acute viral hepatitis is discrete onset of symptoms consistent with hepatitis (e.g., fever, fatigue, dark urine, nausea, abdominal pain, and anorexia) and either jaundice or elevated serum aminotransferase levels. The laboratory diagnostic, prevention, and control of different viral hepatitides vary greatly. Each is presented later in separate sections.

## I. HEPATITIS A (viral hepatitis A, HAV infection; historically also designated as follows: infectious hepatitis, epidemic hepatitis, epidemic jaundice, catarrhal jaundice, type A hepatitis, HA)

**1. Clinical features**—The disease varies in clinical severity from asymptomatic illness to a severely disabling disease lasting several months. In most developing countries, infection manifests as an asymptomatic or mild illness in childhood. Onset of illness in adults in nonendemic areas is usually abrupt, with fever, malaise, anorexia, nausea, and abdominal discomfort, followed within a few days by jaundice. Prolonged, relapsing hepatitis for up to 1 year occurs in 15% of cases; no chronic infection is known to occur. Convalescence is often prolonged. In general, severity increases with age, but complete recovery without sequelae or recurrences is the rule. Reported case-fatality is normally low, 0.1%–0.3%; it can reach 1.8% for adults older than 50 years.

**2. Causative agents**—HAV is a 27 nm positive-strand ribonucleic acid (RNA) virus classified as a member of the family *Picornaviridae*. There are 6 genotypes, according to the classification based on sequences derived from the complete VP1 region. HAV genotypes I, II, and III infect humans and are further divided into subtypes A and B; subtype C was proposed in genotype I. Most of the strains infecting humans belong to genotype I. Geographic distribution of HAV genotypes and subtypes is distinctive, a feature helpful in identifying the source during hepatitis A outbreak investigations. HAV genotype IA is prevalent in South America, North America, Europe, Asia, and Africa; genotype IB, mostly endemic in the Middle East and South Africa, also became prevalent in the USA since 2016, causing outbreaks among people reporting drug use and/or homelessness. Generally, clinical presentation of infections with different HAV genotypes is similar. However, among severe cases with acute liver failure, HAV genotype IB was found more frequently than among the nonliver-failure cases. Regardless of its genetic heterogeneity, only a single serotype of HAV has been identified.

**3. Laboratory diagnosis**—Mild infections may be detectable only through laboratory tests of liver function. Serologic testing is required to confirm the hepatitis A diagnosis. Detection of immunoglobulin class M (IgM) antibodies against HAV (IgM anti-HAV) in the serum of acutely or recently ill patients indicates acute infection.

IgM anti-HAV is detectable early at the onset of clinical symptoms and remains detectable for up to 6 months. Symptom onset ranges from 15–50 days, with a median onset of 28 days. In the absence of laboratory testing, clinical features combined with epidemiologic evidence (e.g., onset of illness in a household or sexual contact of an infected person during the 15–50 days before the onset of symptoms) may provide support for the diagnosis.

IgG antibodies against HAV (IgG anti-HAV) in the serum begin to rise right before or at the time of symptom onset and persist to provide lifelong immunity. IgG anti-HAV is also produced following the immunization with hepatitis A vaccine. Some commercial diagnostic tests measure total (IgM and IgG) anti-HAV. Serologic tests for IgG anti-HAV or total anti-HAV may be used to determine whether a patient has been exposed to HAV in the past or remains susceptible to infection, but these findings are not helpful in diagnosing acute hepatitis A.

HAV RNA can be detected through nucleic acid amplification tests (NAT) in blood and stools of most persons soon after the infection, at least 2 weeks prior to onset of clinical illness, and persists through the peak period of liver enzyme elevation. Sequencing the VP1-P2A junction of the HAV genome allows for the identification of HAV genotypes and determines links of transmission between hepatitis A–infected individuals in an outbreak setting.

**4. Laboratory capability**—Clinical specimens from unknown patients suspected of having viral hepatitis infection should always be collected and handled according to standard safety precautions. Equipment and standard operating procedures (SOPs) should be in place before initiating any routine preanalytic, analytic, and postanalytic diagnostic activities including processing and aliquoting of clinical specimens. Testing of human samples for diagnostic purposes should occur in an International Standard Organization (ISO)–accredited or Clinical Laboratory Improvement Amendments (CLIA)–regulated laboratory that routinely performs proficiency testing (PT) and competency assessments (CA) of laboratory personnel in the established techniques. All non–FDA-approved assays, including commercial and laboratory-developed tests (LDTs), must be validated to establish performance characteristics; SOPs must be approved by authorized, qualified personnel and the laboratory quality manager. Facilities should be equipped with a validated method for decontaminating all laboratory waste (e.g., autoclaving or chemical disinfection).

**5. Safety requirements**—HAV is a biosafety level 2 (BSL-2) agent. Any material of human origin should always be considered as potentially infectious and treated as such. Standard safety precautions are recommended during preanalytic, analytic, and postanalytic processing of clinical specimens and handling of diagnostic kits. Specimens and assay components should be handled, stored, and disposed of in accordance with the procedures defined by the appropriate national biohazard safety guideline or regulation (e.g., see *Biosafety in Microbiological and Biomedical Laboratories*, 5th Edition available at: https://www.cdc.gov/biosafety/publications/bmbl5).

Consistent adherence to universal and standard precautions is required, with special attention paid to procedures that have the potential to generate aerosols. Aliquoting blood, plasma, serum, or stool samples should occur in a class II biological safety cabinet (BSC). All laboratory supervisors are responsible for establishing and documenting specific entry requirements (e.g., baseline serum and immunizations) and any required *Picornaviridae* and medical surveillance programs in their laboratories.

For pre- and postexposure hepatitis A prophylaxis, there are effective hepatitis A vaccines recommended for laboratory personnel working in the laboratories handling clinical specimens; these vaccines can be used before and after a potential exposure. For preexposure immunization against hepatitis A, 2 single-antigen hepatitis A vaccines (VAQTA, Merck, Kenilworth, NJ; HAVRIX, GlaxoSmithKline, Middlesex, UK) and 1 combination vaccine (TWINRIX, GlaxoSmithKline) are currently licensed in the USA for use in persons aged 1 year or older. All are inactivated, highly immunogenic vaccines, generating long-lasting protection against HAV after vaccination with the full, 2-dose series. Both the VAQTA and HAVRIX vaccines are licensed in 2 formulations, which differ according to age of vaccinee: TWINRIX is licensed for use in persons older than 18 years.

To protect persons after a potential exposure to hepatitis A, hepatitis A vaccine should be given as soon as possible, but no later than 2 weeks after exposure. If vaccine is not available, or in persons for whom vaccine is contraindicated, immune globulin can provide short-term protection against hepatitis A both pre- and postexposure. Immune globulin must be administered within 2 weeks after exposure for maximum protection. Because hepatitis A cannot be reliably diagnosed on clinical presentation alone, serological confirmation of HAV infection by IgM anti-HAV testing in the specimens from index patients should be obtained before the administration of postexposure prophylaxis.

Additional guidance on prevention of hepatitis A through active or passive immunization is available at: https://www.cdc.gov/mmwr/preview/mmwrhtml/rr5507a1.htm. Additional guidance on updated dosing instructions for immune globulin (human) GamaSTAN S/D for hepatitis A virus prophylaxis is available at: https://www.cdc.gov/mmwr/volumes/66/wr/mm6636a5.htm?s_cid=mm6636a5_e. The Advisory Committee on Immunization Practices (ACIP) provides advice and guidance to CDC regarding use of vaccines and related agents for control of vaccine-preventable diseases in the US civilian population. Updated hepatitis A ACIP vaccine recommendations are available at: https://www.cdc.gov/vaccines/hcp/acip-recs/vacc-specific/hepa.html.

**6. Nonhuman hosts**—HAV infects primates. There are several reports of isolation of HAV-related viruses from Old World monkeys in the wild, several of which have significant sequence variation and minor antigenic differences when compared with human HAV. Experimental infection in guinea pigs resulted in virus replication in the absence of clinical disease. No other rodent laboratory animal model has been shown to be susceptible to HAV. This virus is usually difficult to adapt and grow in vitro. Chimpanzees, tamarins, and marmosets have been used as animal models of HAV infection. The simian virus isolated from an African green monkey caused severe hepatitis in African green monkeys, rhesus macaques, and tamarins, but not in chimpanzees.

**7. Sample/specimen requirements**—Collection of specimens is recommended from all patients with clinical features compatible with viral hepatitis. Blood or stool sample should be collected as soon as the disease is suspected, and serum or plasma should be separated promptly. The accuracy of either serologic or molecular virology technique is dependent upon the quality of the sample that is used. Therefore, blood, serum/plasma, and stool specimens should be handled aseptically to minimize the probability of contamination.

Serum, plasma, and stool are best stored frozen, and multiple freeze-thaw cycles should be avoided. Storage at 3°C–8°C for 48 hours is acceptable for serology, but not for molecular techniques. Storage above 15°C for more than a few hours should be avoided. Maintaining a storage history can provide valuable study data, particularly if samples are subjected to storage for a long time under suboptimal conditions. Specimens should be submitted for testing using accompanying documents. Those being sent to a reference laboratory should be packed by trained personnel with sufficient amounts of dry ice to prevent thawing en route, labeled "Clinical Specimens Category B," and shipped using overnight express.

**8. Testing requirements**—Initial laboratory evaluation for HAV infection includes a biochemical liver panel, complete blood count (CBC), and International Normalized Ratio (INR). However, acute viral hepatitis caused by any of the 5 hepatitis viruses cannot be distinguished clinically or biochemically; HAV superinfection of patients with chronic HBV and HCV infections can ensue. Therefore, differential diagnosis employs serologic tests for acute viral hepatitis profile (IgM anti-HAV, hepatitis B surface antigen [HBsAg], IgM antibodies to the hepatitis B core antigen [IgM anti-HBcAg], and antibodies to HCV [anti-HCV]). If IgM anti-HAV is detected, HAV RNA can be tested by NAT, and if positive, sequencing can determine HAV genotype.

**9. Reporting requirements**—Acute hepatitis A is a nationally notifiable disease in the USA. The case definition for acute hepatitis A is available at: https://wwwn.cdc.gov/nndss/conditions/hepatitis-a-acute/case-definition/2019. Laboratories operating in other countries should determine whether hepatitis A cases are reportable within their respective jurisdiction.

**10. Referral network**—CDC's Division of Viral Hepatitis serves as a WHO Collaborating Centre for Reference and Research on Viral Hepatitis. The CDC laboratory can provide technical assistance with diagnostic support and characterization of HAV isolates.

**11. Special considerations**—Additional guidance on viral hepatitis surveillance and case management is available at: https://www.cdc.gov/hepatitis/statistics/surveillanceguidelines.htm. For further information on hepatitis A serology, see: https://www.cdc.gov/hepatitis/resources/professionals/training/serology/training.htm.

## II. HEPATITIS B (viral hepatitis B, HBV infection; historically also designated as follows: type B hepatitis, serum hepatitis, homologous serum jaundice, Australia antigen hepatitis, HB)

**1. Clinical features**—Fewer than 10% of children and 30%–50% of adults with acute HBV infection show icteric illness: disease is often milder and anicteric in children; in infants it is usually asymptomatic. In those with clinical illness, the onset is usually insidious, with anorexia, vague abdominal discomfort, nausea, and vomiting, sometimes arthralgia and rash, often progressing to jaundice. Fever may be absent or mild. Severity ranges from unapparent cases detectable only by liver function tests to fulminating, fatal cases of acute hepatic necrosis. The case-fatality rate is about 1%; higher in those older than 40 years of age. Fulminant HBV infection also may occur during pregnancy and among newborns of infected mothers.

After acute HBV infection, the risk of developing chronic infection varies inversely with age; chronic HBV infection occurs among about 90% of infants infected at birth, 20%–50% of children infected from ages 1–5 years, and 1%–10% of persons infected as older children and adults. Chronic HBV infection is also common in persons with immunodeficiency. Persons with chronic infection may or may not have a history of clinical hepatitis. Those with active chronic HBV infection have elevated aminotransferases; biopsy findings range from normal to severe necro-inflammatory hepatitis, with or without cirrhosis. An estimated 15%–25% of persons with chronic HBV infection die prematurely of either cirrhosis or hepatocellular carcinoma (HCC). Approximately 50% of HCC cases globally are attributable to chronic HBV infection.

**2. Causative agents**—HBV is a spherical *orthohepadnavirus* with a diameter of approximately 42 nm belonging to the family *Hepadnaviridae*. The viral genome is represented by a single copy of a partially double-stranded deoxyribonucleic acid (DNA). The genome is enclosed into a 22–27 nm nucleocapsid core, which is surrounded by an outer lipoprotein membrane consisting of 3 forms of viral envelope protein: large (L), middle (M), and small (S), designated as HBsAg. HBsAg is antigenically heterogeneous, with a common determinant (a) and 2 pairs of mutually exclusive determinants (d, y, w, and r), resulting in 4 major serologic subtypes: *adw*, *ayw*, *adr*, and *ayr*. The distribution of these subtypes varies geographically; because of the conserved "a" determinant region, protection against 1 subtype appears to confer protection against the other subtypes, and no differences in clinical features have been related to subtype. The "a" determinant plays a key role in the serologic diagnostic of HBV; mutations in the S-gene region encoding this determinant can lead to expression of HBsAg that is undetectable by antibodies used in some commercial diagnostic assays. HBV is classified into 9 main genotypes (A–I). HBV genotypes are associated with risk for certain outcomes of chronic infection, such as cirrhosis and HCC. In the North American Arctic, HBV genotype F is associated with HCC in young children as well as adults aged younger than 30 years. In Asia and the Arctic, HBV genotype C has also been associated with a significantly higher risk of HCC than other genotypes.

**3. Laboratory diagnosis**—Mild infections may be detectable only through laboratory tests of liver function. Hepatitis B cannot be distinguished from other types of viral hepatitis on the basis of clinical or epidemiologic features alone. Serologic testing is required to confirm the diagnosis.

Demonstration in serum of specific viral antigens and/or antibodies confirms diagnosis. The following antigen and antibody detection assays are useful for the laboratory diagnostic of HBV infection:

1) HBsAg and antibody to HBsAg (anti-HBs)
2) IgM and IgG antibody to HBcAg (total anti-HBc and IgM anti-HBc)
3) Hepatitis B e antigen (HBeAg) and antibody to HBeAg (anti-HBe)
4) Commercial, FDA-approved kits are available for all markers except HBcAg

Evidence of active HBV infection is demonstrated by HBsAg, which can be detected in serum from several weeks before onset of symptoms to weeks or months after onset. This serologic marker is present in serum during acute infections and persists in chronic infections. The presence of HBsAg indicates that the person is infectious.

Total anti-HBc appears at the onset of illness and persists indefinitely. Demonstration of total anti-HBc in serum indicates exposure to HBV. High titers of IgM anti-HBc are detected during acute infection and usually disappear within 6 months, although they can persist at low levels during exacerbations of chronic hepatitis B.

HBeAg can be found in serum during the transient infection, as well as in patients with chronic HBV infection during the high viral replicative phase. The presence of HBeAg is generally associated with relatively high infectivity. Anti-HBe seroconversion occurs during the resolution of acute infection.

Protective immunity follows infection if anti-HBs develop and HBsAg becomes negative.

HBV DNA can be detected in blood of patients during the acute phase of infection among inactive HBsAg-carriers and in patients with chronic hepatitis B. In low titers, HBV DNA can be found in patients who are HBsAg-negative and anti-HBc-positive due to loss of HBsAg in serum after transient infection, either with or without seroconversion to anti-HBs. Occult hepatitis B, a form of chronic HBV infection found in up to 30% of patients with liver disease of unknown etiology (also characterized by HBsAg-negative/anti-HBc-positive serologic results) can be diagnosed only by testing for HBV DNA. FDA-approved, NAT methodologies can detect HBV DNA at levels as low as 10 IU/mL. These assays can be used both for diagnosis and management of patients on antiviral therapy.

LDTs for viral genome sequencing can be used to determine the HBV genotype, mutations associated with resistance to antiviral therapy, and links of transmission that are helpful for the investigation of hepatitis B outbreaks. LDTs are for research use only and therefore are not recommended for diagnostic purposes.

The following are uniform laboratory-testing criteria for the diagnosis and reporting of nationally notifiable infectious diseases:

1) Acute hepatitis B: HBsAg positive and IgM anti-HBc positive (if done).
2) Chronic hepatitis B: IgM anti-HBc negative and a positive result on 1 of the following tests—HBsAg, HBeAg, or HBV DNA—or HBsAg positive, HBV DNA positive, or HBeAg positive 2 times at least 6 months apart (any combination of these tests performed 6 months apart is acceptable).
3) Perinatal hepatitis B (acquired in the USA or US territories): laboratory evidence of HBV infection in an infant born to a HBV-infected mother consists of 1 or more of the following:
    - positive HBsAg test (only if at least 4 weeks after last dose of hepatitis B vaccine)
    - positive HBeAg test
    - detectable HBV DNA

**4. Laboratory capability**—Clinical specimens from unknown patients suspected of having viral hepatitis infection should always be collected and handled according to standard/universal safety precautions. Equipment and SOPs should be in place before initiating any routine preanalytic, analytic, and postanalytic diagnostic activities, including processing and aliquoting of clinical specimens. Testing of human samples for diagnostic purposes should occur in an ISO-accredited or CLIA-regulated laboratory that routinely performs PT and CA of laboratory personnel in the established techniques. All non-FDA-approved assays including commercial and LDTs must be validated to establish performance characteristics; SOPs must be approved by authorized, qualified personnel and the laboratory quality manager. Facilities should be equipped with a validated method for decontaminating all laboratory waste (e.g., autoclaving or chemical disinfection).

**5. Safety requirements**—HBV is a BSL-2 agent. Any material of human origin should always be considered as potentially infectious and treated as such. Standard and universal safety precautions are recommended during preanalytic, analytic, and postanalytic processing of clinical specimens and handling of diagnostic kits. Specimens and assay components should be handled, stored, and disposed of in accordance with the procedures defined by the appropriate national biohazard safety guideline or regulation (e.g., see *Biosafety in Microbiological and Biomedical Laboratories*, 5th Edition available at: https://www.cdc.gov/biosafety/publications/bmbl5).

Consistent adherence to universal precautions is required, with special attention paid to procedures that have the potential to generate aerosols. Aliquoting of blood, plasma, or serum samples should occur in a class II BSC. All laboratory supervisors are responsible for establishing and documenting specific entry requirements (e.g., baseline serum and immunizations) and any required personal protective equipment (PPE) and medical surveillance programs in their laboratories.

Pre- and postexposure hepatitis B prophylaxis: 3 effective single-antigen hepatitis B vaccines and 2 combination vaccines are currently licensed in the USA. Single-antigen (Engerix-B, GlaxoSmithKline; Recombivax HB, Merck; HEPLISAV-B, Dynavax) and combined hepatitis A and hepatitis B (TWINRIX, GlaxoSmithKline) vaccines are recommended for persons older than 18 years who are at increased occupational risk (e.g., laboratory personnel handling clinical specimen, health care workers, and public safety workers at risk for exposure to blood or blood-contaminated body fluids).

Laboratory personnel with anti-HBs greater than or equal to 10 mIU/mL after receipt of the primary vaccine series are considered immune; those with anti-HBs less than 10 mIU/mL after receipt of the primary series should be revaccinated. Immunocompetent persons are considered to have long-term protection and may not need further periodic testing to assess anti-HBs levels.

After percutaneous (e.g., needle-stick) or mucous membrane exposures to blood that might contain HBV, wounds and skin sites that have been in contact with blood or body fluids should be washed with soap and water; mucous membranes should be flushed with water. For vaccinated personnel with subsequent documented anti-HBs greater than 10 mIU/mL, no postexposure prophylaxis is necessary regardless of the source patient's HBsAg status.

For vaccinated personnel with anti-HBs less than 10 mIU/mL and previously unimmunized personnel, an additional single hepatitis B vaccine dose should be given as soon as possible but preferably within 24 hours when the source patient is HBsAg-negative. When the source patient is HBsAg-positive or the status is unknown, administration of hepatitis B immunoglobulin

(HBIG) is recommended; a complete series of hepatitis B vaccination should be started simultaneously. Two HBIG products are licensed for use in the USA: HepaGam B (Aptevo Bio Therapeutics, Seattle, WA) and Nabi-HB (Biotest Pharmaceuticals Corporation, Boca Raton, FL).

Hotline providing clinicians with 24-hour guidance on managing occupational exposures to HIV, viral hepatitis, and other bloodborne pathogens can be found at: http://nccc.ucsf.edu/clinician-consultation/pep-post-exposure-prophylaxis. Information on recommended schedules for hepatitis B vaccination, including adult immunization schedule can be found at: https://www.cdc.gov/hepatitis/hbv/hbvfaq.htm#D15. The ACIP provides advice and guidance to the CDC director regarding use of vaccines and related agents for control of vaccine-preventable diseases in the civilian population of the USA. Updated hepatitis B ACIP vaccine recommendations are available at: https://www.cdc.gov/vaccines/hcp/acip-recs/vacc-specific/hepb.html.

**6. Nonhuman hosts**—In nature, *orthohepadnaviruses* infects higher primates, woodchucks, ground squirrels, and ducks. In early studies, presence of HBsAg, formerly known as Australia antigen, and evidence of chronic infection were found in the serum of captive chimpanzees; these primates were employed periodically to study virus transmission, host response, and vaccination. Early studies of Woodchuck Hepatitis Virus (WHV) established a correlation between chronic WHV and HCC, confirming that *orthohepadnavirus* infection was a cause of liver cancer. The first avian virus representing the *Hepadnaviridae* family (genus *avihepadnavirus)* was discovered in the domestic duck. In domestic flocks, duck HBV (DHBV) is widely distributed, persisting as chronic infection in approximately 10% of birds. Ducks were used for comprehensive study of virus replication. More recently, more cost-effective and sustainable laboratory models have been developed using chimeric mice and *Tupaia* (treeshrew).

**7. Sample/specimen requirements**—Collection of specimens is recommended from all patients with clinical features compatible with viral hepatitis. Blood samples should be collected as soon as the disease is suspected, and serum should be separated promptly. The accuracy of any serologic or molecular virology technique is dependent upon the condition of the sample that is used. Therefore, both blood and serum or plasma specimens should be handled aseptically to minimize the probability of contamination.

Serum and plasma are best stored frozen, and multiple freeze-thaw cycles should be avoided. Storage at 3°C–8°C for 48 hours is acceptable for serology but not for molecular techniques. Storage above 15°C for more than a few hours should be avoided. Maintaining a storage history can provide valuable study data, particularly if samples are subjected to storage for a long time under suboptimal conditions. Specimens should be submitted for testing using accompanying documents. Those being sent to a reference laboratory should be packed by trained personnel with sufficient amounts of dry ice to prevent thawing en route, labeled with "Clinical Specimens Category B," and shipped using overnight express.

**8. Testing requirements**—The initial laboratory evaluation includes a biochemical liver panel, CBC, and INR. However, acute hepatitis caused by any of the 5 hepatitis viruses cannot be distinguished clinically nor biochemically; HBV superinfection of patients with chronic hepatitis C can ensue. Therefore, differential diagnosis employs serologic tests for acute viral hepatitis profile (IgM anti-HAV, HBsAg, IgM anti-HBc, and anti-HCV). If HBsAg is detected, further laboratory diagnosis and staging of HBV infection is recommended by employing a testing algorithm, which may include both serologic and NATs to detect HBV DNA.

**9. Reporting requirements**—Acute, chronic and perinatally transmitted hepatitis B is nationally notifiable disease in the USA.

The case definitions for acute, chronic, and perinatal hepatitis B are available at: https://wwwn.cdc.gov/nndss/conditions/hepatitis-b. Hepatitis B is a reportable disease in most countries. Laboratories should determine whether hepatitis B cases are reportable within their respective jurisdiction.

**10. Referral network**—CDC's DVH serves as a WHO Collaborating Centre for Reference and Research on Viral Hepatitis. The CDC laboratory can provide technical assistance with diagnostic support and characterization of HBV isolates.

**11. Special considerations**—Additional guidance on viral hepatitis surveillance and case management is available at: https://www.cdc.gov/hepatitis/SurveillanceGuidelines.htm.

Information on the training in hepatitis B laboratory testing and interpretation of results can be found at: https://www.cdc.gov/hepatitis/hbv/index.htm. Information on the investigation and management of hepatitis B outbreaks in particular settings and populations can be found at: https://www.cdc.gov/hepatitis/outbreaks/index.htm

## III. HEPATITIS C (viral hepatitis C, HCV infection; historically also designated as follows: type C hepatitis; non-A, non-B hepatitis)

**1. Clinical features**—Onset is usually insidious, with anorexia, vague abdominal discomfort, nausea, and vomiting; progression to jaundice is less frequent than with hepatitis B. While only 20%–30% of acute infections are symptomatic, 75%–85% of acute infections become chronic. Reinfection may occur among persons with previous, resolved infections and among those with chronic infection. Of chronically infected persons about 5%–20%

develop cirrhosis over a period of 20–30 years, and 1%–5% will die from the consequence of chronic infection (i.e., from cirrhosis and hepatocellular carcinoma).

**2. Causative agents**—HCV is an enveloped RNA virus classified as a separate genus (*Hepacivirus*) in the *Flaviviridae* family. Seven HCV genotypes (1–7) and approximately 100 subtypes, designated with small letters of the Latin alphabet (e.g., a, b, k) have been described so far. Coinfection with different genotypes and subtypes has been documented in at-risk populations; sometime intergenotypic recombination may occur, resulting in circulating recombinant forms (e.g., 2k/1b). Evidence is limited regarding differences in clinical features, disease outcome, or progression to cirrhosis or HCC among persons with different genotypes.

**3. Laboratory diagnosis**—Hepatitis C cannot be distinguished from other types of viral hepatitis on the basis of clinical or epidemiologic features alone. Acute hepatitis C is usually asymptomatic and may remain undiagnosed.

Mild infections may be detectable through laboratory liver function tests. To confirm the diagnosis in persons with elevated alanine aminotransferase (ALT) levels, screening for anti-HCV and, if positive, reflex to HCV RNA should be performed as outlined in this recommended testing sequence for identifying current HCV infection: https://www.cdc.gov/hepatitis/hcv/pdfs/hcv_flow.pdf.

Alternatively, presence of viremia could be determined by a positive test for hepatitis C core antigen (HCVcAg), a test commercially available in many countries in Europe and Asia but not in the USA.

Tests that detect antibodies include the rapid diagnostic test (RDT), enzyme immunoassay (EIA), the enhanced chemiluminescence immunoassay (CIA), and the recombinant immunoblot assay. These tests do not distinguish between acute, chronic, or resolved infections. RDT, EIA, and CIA tests for anti-HCV detection are suitable for screening populations. A negative anti-HCV test suffices to exclude a diagnosis of chronic HCV infection in immunocompetent patients. For anti-HCV-negative persons who might have been exposed to HCV within the past 6 months, testing for HCV RNA or follow-up testing for HCV antibody is recommended. For persons who are immunocompromised, testing for HCV RNA can be considered. To differentiate past, resolved HCV infection from false-positive anti-HCV result, testing with another HCV antibody assay can be considered. Immunoblot is sometimes used as a supplemental assay in persons with a screening positive anti-HCV who test negative for HCV RNA. Supplemental immunoblot tests are not commercially available in the USA; however, such tests are available in Europe and other countries.

Acute or chronic HCV infection in a patient with a screening positive anti-HCV test should be confirmed by detection of HCV RNA in serum. Target amplification techniques using real-time, or quantitative, polymerase chain reaction (qPCR), transcription-mediated amplification (TMA), and signal amplification techniques (branched DNA) may be used to measure HCV RNA levels. These levels are reported in IU/mL. Among persons with recent HCV exposure, a single HCV RNA positive test confirms active HCV replication, but a single negative test result does not exclude viremia and may reflect either early phase of infection or transient decline in viral level below the analytical sensitivity of the assay used. A follow-up HCV RNA testing with an assay of the same or higher sensitivity should be performed to confirm the presence or absence of active HCV replication in such persons. Among persons without suspicion of recent exposure who are undergoing routine screening, a single negative HCV RNA test may be sufficient to exclude chronic infection. HCV RNA levels and HCV genotype help determine the likelihood of response to treatment among patients undergoing antiviral therapy. Point-of-care (POC) assays for HCV RNA can provide results in less than 2 hours. HCVcAg is a serologic test for detection of HCV core antigen and can be used to establish the status of current HCV infection in persons who test positive for anti-HCV. It is available in high-throughput immunodiagnostic systems and is optimal for centralized testing. Neither POC HCV RNA nor HCVcAg tests are commercially available in the USA; however, they are being used by some countries that have implemented hepatitis C elimination programs.

To determine need for biopsy, patient's age and noninvasive serum markers (e.g., platelet count and aspartate aminotransferase-to-platelet ratio index) may sometimes be used to provide an indirect histological assessment of liver fibrosis (FIB-4) in HCV patients using the following Web-based tool: https://www.mdcalc.com/fibrosis-4-fib-4-index-liver-fibrosis.

Persons with low fibrosis scores may be appropriate candidates for medical management and may not require liver biopsy if their FIB-4 scores remain low. Persons with high fibrosis/cirrhosis scores may need liver biopsy for confirmation of cirrhosis unless other clinical or imaging signs of progression to end-stage liver disease are present. Liver biopsy can provide direct histological assessment of liver injury due to HCV infection but cannot be used to diagnose HCV infection.

4. **Laboratory capability**—Clinical specimens from unknown patients suspected of having viral hepatitis infection should always be collected and handled according to standard safety precautions. Equipment and SOPs should be in place before initiating any routine preanalytic, analytic, and postanalytic diagnostic activities, including processing and aliquoting of clinical specimens. Testing of human samples for diagnostic purposes should occur in an ISO-accredited or CLIA-regulated laboratory that routinely performs PT and CA of laboratory personnel in the established techniques. All non–FDA-approved assays, including commercial and LDTs, must be validated to establish performance characteristics; SOPs must be approved by authorized, qualified personnel and the laboratory quality manager. Facilities should be equipped with a validated method for decontaminating all laboratory waste (e.g., autoclaving or chemical disinfection).

**5. Safety requirements**—HCV is a BSL-2 agent. Any material of human origin should always be considered potentially infectious and treated as such. Standard safety precautions are recommended during preanalytic, analytic, and postanalytic processing of clinical specimens and handling of diagnostic kits. Specimens and assay components should be handled, stored, and disposed of in accordance with the procedures defined by the appropriate national biohazard safety guideline or regulation (e.g., see *Biosafety in Microbiological and Biomedical Laboratories*, 5th Edition available at: https://www.cdc.gov/biosafety/publications/bmbl5).

Consistent adherence to universal/standard precautions is required, with special attention paid to procedures that have the potential to generate aerosols. Aliquoting of blood, plasma, or serum samples should occur in a class II BSC. All laboratory supervisors are responsible for establishing and documenting specific entry requirements (e.g., baseline serum) and any required PPE and medical surveillance programs in their laboratories.

Neither passive (immunoglobulin) nor active (vaccine) immunization is available to prevent HCV infection. Routine virus inactivation of plasma-derived products, risk-reduction counseling for persons uninfected but at high risk (e.g., injecting drug users and health care workers), and nosocomial control activities must be maintained.

A hotline providing clinicians with 24-hour guidance on managing occupational exposures to HIV, viral hepatitis, and other bloodborne pathogens can be found at: http://nccc.ucsf.edu/clinician-consultation/pep-post-exposure-prophylaxis.

**6. Nonhuman hosts**—The chimpanzee has been the only animal model for HCV infection. Recently, other models, which include transgenic mouse models, subgenomic replicon, and other tissue culture systems are being used for studying HCV biology and development of antiviral drugs.

**7. Sample/specimen requirements**—Collection of specimens is recommended from all patients with clinical features compatible with viral hepatitis. Blood samples should be collected as soon as the disease is suspected, and serum should be separated promptly. The accuracy of any serologic or molecular virology technique is dependent upon the quality of the sample used. Therefore, both blood and serum or plasma specimens should be handled aseptically to minimize the probability of contamination.

Serum and plasma are best stored frozen, and multiple freeze-thaw cycles should be avoided. Storage at 3°C–8°C for 48 hours is acceptable for serology but not for molecular techniques. Storage above 15°C for more than a few hours should be avoided. Maintaining a storage history can provide valuable study data, particularly if samples are subjected to storage for a long time under suboptimal conditions. Specimens should be submitted for testing using accompanying documents. Those being sent to a reference laboratory should be packed by trained personnel with sufficient amounts of dry ice to prevent thawing en route, labeled "Clinical Specimens Category B," and shipped using overnight express.

**8. Testing requirements**—The initial laboratory evaluation includes a biochemical liver panel, CBC, and INR. However, acute hepatitis caused by any of the 5 hepatitis viruses cannot be distinguished clinically nor biochemically; HCV superinfection of patients with chronic HBV infection can ensue. Therefore, differential diagnosis employs serologic tests for acute viral hepatitis profile (IgM anti-HAV, HBsAg, IgM anti-HBc, and anti-HCV). If anti-HCV is detected, reflex testing for HCV RNA is done according to the following publication available at: https://www.cdc.gov/mmwr/pdf/wk/mm62e0507a2.pdf.

**9. Reporting requirements**—Acute, chronic, and perinatally transmitted hepatitis C is a nationally notifiable disease in the USA. Case definitions for acute, chronic, and perinatal hepatitis C are available at: https://wwwn.cdc.gov/nndss/conditions/hepatitis-c. Hepatitis C is a reportable disease in most countries. Laboratories should determine whether hepatitis C cases are reportable within their respective jurisdiction.

**10. Referral network**—CDC's DVH serves as a WHO Collaborating Centre for Reference and Research on Viral Hepatitis. The CDC laboratory can provide technical assistance with diagnostic support and characterization of HCV isolates, as well as bioinformatics support to determine patterns of disease transmission using the laboratory-developed, state-of-the-art Global Hepatitis Outbreak and Surveillance Technology (GHOST) platform.

**11. Special considerations**—Additional guidance on viral hepatitis surveillance and case management is available at: https://www.cdc.gov/hepatitis/SurveillanceGuidelines.htm.

Information on the training in hepatitis C laboratory testing and interpretation of result is available at: https://www.cdc.gov/hepatitis/hcv/index.htm. Information on the investigation and management of hepatitis C outbreaks in particular settings and populations is available at: https://www.cdc.gov/hepatitis/outbreaks/index.htm. For further information on hepatitis C outbreak investigations using CDC's Global Hepatitis Outbreak and Surveillance Technology, see: https://www.cdc.gov/amd/project-summaries/ghost-hep-c.html.

## IV. HEPATITIS D (viral hepatitis D; hepatitis delta virus; delta agent hepatitis; delta-associated hepatitis; HDV infection)

**1. Clinical features**—The onset of HDV infection is usually abrupt, with signs and symptoms resembling those of HBV; infection may be severe and is always associated with a coexistent HBV infection, either as acute coinfection or as superinfection among persons with chronic HBV infection. In the former case, the infection is usually self-limited; in the latter, it usually progresses to chronic hepatitis. Acute HDV can be misdiagnosed as an exacerbation of chronic HBV. As the outcome of HDV infection is associated with the host immune response to HBV, children with acute coinfection may have a severe clinical course with greater likelihood of progression to chronic hepatitis. In studies throughout Europe and the USA, 25%–50% of fulminant hepatitis cases thought to be caused by HBV were associated with concurrent HDV infection.

**2. Causative agents**—HDV virion measures 35–37 nm consisting of a coat of HBsAg and a unique internal antigen known as the delta antigen. Encapsulated with the delta antigen is the genome: a single-stranded, 1672–1697 nucleotide long circular conformation RNA, which can fold on itself to form an unbranched, rod-like structure. HDV is unable to infect an individual by itself and requires coinfection with HBV to undergo a complete replication cycle. Synthesis of HDV in turn results in temporary suppression of synthesis of HBV components. About 70%–90% of patients with HDV coinfection are HBeAg negative, and most have low levels of serum HBV DNA. HDV is best considered a defective RNA virus that is related more to plant viroids than to other human pathogens; it is classified in a separate genus *Deltavirus*. Eight genotypes (1–8) and 2 subtypes (1a and 1b) of HDV have been identified.

**3. Laboratory diagnosis**—The laboratory diagnosis of HDV infection includes simultaneous detection of various HBV and HDV serologic markers among persons positive for HBsAg; testing of HBV-uninfected individuals is not required. Detection of total antibody (IgG and IgM) to HDV (anti-HDV) by EIA indicates current or acute, chronic, or past HDV infection; it does not differentiate between coinfection and superinfection.

For differential diagnosis, evaluation of IgM anti-HBc test results, in combination with the total anti-HDV-positive result, is sufficient. Presence of IgM anti-HBc indicates acute HDV infection; a negative test for IgM anti-HBc suggests HDV superinfection of an HBsAg carrier. Viremia, occurring with both acute and chronic HDV infection, can be determined by testing for HDV RNA. HDV antigen is also used as a marker for viremia. In coinfection, which is usually self-limited, the markers of viremia are transient. Chronic HDV can be diagnosed by determining the persistence of viremia beyond 6 months from onset. Quantitative assays can be used for the monitoring of antiviral therapy; HDV genotype can be determined by sequencing.

**4. Laboratory capability**—Clinical specimens from unknown patients suspected of having viral hepatitis infection should always be collected and handled according to standard safety precautions. Equipment and SOPs should be in place before initiating any routine preanalytic, analytic, and postanalytic diagnostic activities including processing and aliquoting of clinical specimens. Testing of human samples for diagnostic purposes should occur in an ISO-accredited or CLIA-regulated laboratory that routinely performs PT and CA of laboratory personnel in the established techniques. All non–FDA-approved assays, including commercial and LDTs, must be validated to establish performance characteristics; SOPs must be approved by authorized, qualified personnel and the laboratory quality manager. Facilities should be equipped with a validated method for decontaminating all laboratory waste (e.g., autoclaving or chemical disinfection).

**5. Safety requirements**—HDV is a BSL-2 agent. Any material of human origin should always be considered potentially infectious and treated as such. Standard safety precautions are recommended during preanalytic, analytic, and postanalytic processing of clinical specimens and handling of diagnostic kits. Specimens and assay components should be handled, stored, and disposed of in accordance with the procedures defined by the appropriate national biohazard safety guideline or regulation (e.g., see *Biosafety in Microbiological and Biomedical Laboratories*, 5th Edition available at: https://www.cdc.gov/biosafety/publications/bmbl5).

Consistent adherence to universal precautions is required, with special attention to procedures with potential to generate aerosols. Aliquoting of blood, plasma, or serum samples should occur in a class II BSC. All laboratory supervisors are responsible for establishing and documenting specific entry requirements (e.g., baseline serum and immunizations) and any required PPE and medical surveillance programs in their laboratories.

Potentially, all HBsAg-positive carriers are susceptible to infection with HDV. These persons should be counseled about the health risk posed by HDV superinfection and ways to control and prevent transmission. The only effective measure for persons infected with HBV is avoidance of exposure to any potential source of HDV. For HBV-naïve individuals, HBV vaccination also prevents HDV infection and is recommended for laboratory personnel who handle clinical specimens, health care workers, and public safety workers at risk for exposure to blood or blood-contaminated body fluids.

**6. Nonhuman hosts**—HDV can be transmitted experimentally to chimpanzees and to woodchucks infected with HBV and woodchuck hepatitis virus, respectively. Transgenic mice carrying a replication-competent HDV genome have also been developed for studying HDV replication in vivo.

**7. Sample/specimen requirements**—Specimen collection is recommended only for patients with clinical features compatible with viral hepatitis who test positive for HBsAg. Blood samples should be collected as soon as the disease is suspected, and serum should be separated promptly. The accuracy of any serologic or molecular virology technique depends on the quality of the sample that is used. Therefore, blood, serum, and plasma specimens should be handled aseptically to minimize the probability of contamination.

Serum and plasma are best stored frozen, and multiple freeze-thaw cycles should be avoided. Storage at 3°C–8°C for 48 hours is acceptable for serology, but not for molecular techniques. Storage above 15°C for more than a few hours should be avoided. Specimens should be submitted for testing using accompanying documents. Those being sent to a reference laboratory should be packed by trained personnel with sufficient amounts of dry ice to prevent thawing en route, labeled "Clinical Specimens Category B," and shipped using overnight express.

**8. Testing requirements**—The initial laboratory evaluation includes a biochemical liver panel, CBC, and INR. However, acute hepatitis caused by any of the 5 known hepatitis viruses cannot be distinguished clinically nor biochemically. Therefore, differential diagnosis employs serologic tests for acute viral hepatitis profile (IgM anti-HAV, HBsAg, IgM anti-HBc, and anti-HCV). If HBsAg is detected, further laboratory diagnosis and staging of HDV infection is recommended by employing a testing algorithm, which may include both serologic and molecular virology tests.

**9. Reporting requirements**—HDV is not a reportable disease in the USA. Laboratories in other countries should determine reporting requirements within their respective jurisdictions.

**10. Referral network**—CDC's DVH serves as a WHO Collaborating Centre for Reference and Research on Viral Hepatitis. The CDC laboratory can provide technical assistance with diagnostic support and characterization of HDV isolates.

**11. Special considerations**—Information on training in hepatitis D serology and laboratory testing requests can be found at: https://www.cdc.gov/hepatitis/hdv/index.htm.

## V. HEPATITIS E (viral hepatitis E, HEV infection; historically also designated as follows: enterically transmitted non-A, non-B hepatitis [ET-NANB]; epidemic non-A, non-B hepatitis; fecal-oral non-A, non-B hepatitis)

**1. Clinical features**—HEV is generally a self-limiting disease with mortality rates of less than 2% in immunocompetent patients; the ratio of symptomatic to asymptomatic infection ranges from 1:2–1:13. The clinical course is similar to that of HAV, with a short prodromal phase and a period of symptoms or jaundice lasting days to several weeks. Clinical and epidemiologic characteristics differ according to genotype.

Infection with HEV genotype 1 or 2 is common in developing countries within Asia, Africa, and Central America, and is associated with fecal-water-borne transmission, high rates of icteric disease, and a higher attack rate among adolescents and young adults. Massive outbreaks have occurred in conflict zones during humanitarian emergencies involving refugees and internally displaced populations (IDP) mainly in Africa. Mortality is high among pregnant women (about 20%). Development of chronic disease has not been reported.

By contrast, infection with HEV genotypes 3 or 4 is endemic in developed countries, with genotype 4 mainly found in Taiwan, China, and Japan; a single case caused by camelid HEV genotype 7 was diagnosed in a liver-transplant recipient who reported regular consumption of camel meat and milk. HEV caused by HEV genotype 3 is often associated with consumption of uncooked food products from pigs that harbor genotype 3. Infection with HEV genotype 3 has a low rate of icteric disease, and high rates of illness and greater mortality among older adults. Chronic infection among immunocompromised persons has been reported, and neurologic complications have occurred in some patients infected with HEV genotype

**2. Causative agents**—HEV is a spherical, nonenveloped, positive-stranded RNA virus approximately 32–34 nm in diameter classified in the *Hepeviridae* family. There are 8 genotypes, of which 1–4 and 7 belong to genus *Orthohepevirus* and infect humans.

**3. Laboratory diagnosis**—Mild infections may be detectable only through laboratory tests of liver function. HEV cannot be distinguished from other types of viral hepatitis on the basis of clinical features alone; diagnosis is established based on detection of IgM anti-HEV and IgG anti-HEV in the serum of acutely ill patients.

A majority of the commercially available tests can detect IgM anti-HEV in up to 90% of patients during the first 4 weeks of disease onset. HEV RNA is detectable in serum and fecal samples collected from patients within the first 4 weeks of disease onset. Viral genome sequencing can be used to determine the HEV genotype, which may suggest the source of infection and determine links of transmission.

Recovery is marked by viral clearance, seroconversion to IgG anti-HEV (which may persist for years), and disappearance of IgM anti-HEV (detectable up to 6 months).

Providers with questions about molecular virology methods should consult with their state health department (https://www.cdc.gov/mmwr/international/relres.html) or the CDC Division of Viral Hepatitis (https://www.cdc.gov/hepatitis/hev/labtestingrequests.htm).

**4. Laboratory capability**—Clinical specimens from unknown patients suspected of having viral hepatitis infection should always be collected and handled according to standard safety precautions. Equipment and SOPs should be in place before initiating any routine preanalytic, analytic, and postanalytic diagnostic activities, including processing and aliquoting of clinical specimens. Testing of human samples for diagnostic purposes should occur in an ISO-accredited or CLIA-regulated laboratory that routinely performs PT and CA of laboratory personnel in the established techniques.

There are no FDA-approved tests for HEV infection. All non–FDA-approved assays, including commercial and LDTs, must be validated to establish performance characteristics; SOPs must be approved by authorized qualified personnel and the laboratory quality manager. Facilities should be equipped with a validated method for decontaminating all laboratory waste (e.g., through autoclaving or chemical disinfection).

**5. Safety requirements**—HEV is a BSL-2 agent. Any material of human origin should always be considered potentially infectious and treated as such. Standard safety precautions are recommended during preanalytic, analytic, and postanalytic processing of clinical specimens and handling of diagnostic kits. Specimens and assay components should be handled, stored, and disposed of in accordance with the procedures defined by the appropriate national biohazard safety guideline or regulation (e.g., see *Biosafety in Microbiological and Biomedical Laboratories*, 5th Edition available at: https://www.cdc.gov/biosafety/publications/bmbl5).

Consistent adherence to universal/standard precautions is required, with special attention to procedures with potential to generate aerosols. Aliquoting of blood, plasma, serum or stool suspension samples should occur in a class II BSC. All laboratory supervisors are responsible for establishing and documenting specific entry requirements (e.g., baseline serum and immunizations) and any required PPE and medical surveillance programs in their laboratories.

Prevention of HEV relies primarily on good sanitation and the availability of clean drinking water. Travelers to developing countries can reduce their risk for infection by not drinking unpurified water. Boiling and chlorination of water inactivates HEV. Avoiding raw pork and venison, as well as camel milk, can reduce the risk for infection with HEV genotypes 3, 4, and 7.

No HEV vaccine is currently available in the USA; however, a recombinant vaccine was recently approved for use in China.

**6. Nonhuman hosts**—HEV strains have been detected in domestic and wild pigs, deer, camel, elk, sheep, cattle, rats, and rabbits. Some primates (e.g., chimpanzees, cynomolgus and rhesus macaques, pigtail monkeys, owl monkeys, tamarins, and African green monkeys) are reported as susceptible to infection with HEV.

**7. Sample/specimen requirements**—Collection of specimens is recommended from all patients with clinical features compatible with viral hepatitis. Blood and/or stool sample should be collected as soon as the disease is suspected, and serum or plasma should be separated promptly. The accuracy of any serologic or molecular virology technique is dependent upon the quality of the sample used. Therefore, blood, serum, plasma, and stool specimens should be handled aseptically to minimize the probability of contamination.

Serum, plasma, and stool are best stored frozen, and multiple freeze-thaw cycles should be avoided. Storage at 3°C–8°C is acceptable for 48 hours for serology, but not for molecular techniques. Storage above 15°C for more than a few hours should be avoided. Maintaining a storage history can provide valuable study data, particularly if samples are subjected to storage for a long period of time under suboptimal conditions. Specimens should be submitted for testing using accompanying documents. Those being sent to a reference laboratory should be packed by trained personnel with sufficient amounts of dry ice to prevent thawing en route, labeled "Clinical Specimens Category B," and shipped using overnight express.

**8. Testing requirements**—The initial laboratory evaluation for HEV includes a biochemical liver panel, CBC, and INR. However, acute hepatitis caused by any of the 5 hepatitis viruses cannot be clearly distinguished, clinically nor biochemically. Because HEV superinfection of patients with chronic HBV and HCV infections can ensue, differential diagnosis employs serologic tests for acute viral hepatitis profile (IgM anti-HAV, HBsAg, IgM anti-HBc, and anti-HCV), IgM and IgG antibodies to HEV (IgM anti-HEV and IgG anti- HEV), and molecular virology tests (e.g., NAT) to identify HEV RNA. If the HEV RNA test is positive, sequencing can determine HEV genotype.

**9. Reporting requirements**—HEV is not a reportable disease in the USA. Laboratories in other countries should determine reporting requirements within their respective jurisdictions.

**10. Referral network**—CDC's DVH serves as a WHO Collaborating Centre for Reference and Research on Viral Hepatitis. The CDC laboratory can provide technical assistance with diagnostic support and characterization of HEV isolates.

**11. Special considerations**—Information on the training in HEV serology and laboratory testing requests is available at: https://www.cdc.gov/hepatitis/hev/index.htm.

## VI. HEPATOCELLULAR CARCINOMA (HCC, primary liver cancer, primary hepatocellular carcinoma, hepatoma)

**1. Clinical features**—A small proportion of persons with chronic HBV or HCV infection may eventually develop HCC. HCC rarely occurs before age 40 years and peaks at approximately age 70 years. Cirrhosis is present in 80%–90% of HCV-associated HCC cases (70%–80% of persons with HBV-associated HCC). The progression to cirrhosis is often clinically silent, and some patients are not known to have underlying viral hepatitis until they present with HCC. Symptoms include anorexia, weight loss, right upper quadrant abdominal pain, or tenderness; ascites and jaundice commonly appear later in the course of the illness. Depending on lesion size and cancer stage at diagnosis, 5-year survival may be high (75%–90%) among persons with limited disease to very low (< 10% 1-year survival) among persons with extrahepatic spread or vascular involvement.

**2. Causative agents**—Approximately 50% of cases of HCC are attributable to chronic HBV infection, a slightly lower percentage to chronic HCV infection, and a small proportion to noninfectious causes. Aflatoxin, alcohol, and nonalcoholic fatty liver disease (with or without obesity, metabolic syndrome, and type 2 diabetes) may serve as important cofactors in the development of HCC.

**3. Laboratory diagnosis**—Diagnosis of HCC is often made using noninvasive imaging tests, particularly with cirrhotic patients with focal hepatic masses greater than 2 cm in diameter. Alpha-fetoprotein determination lacks adequate sensitivity and specificity; thus, surveillance has to be based on ultrasound examination. Image-guided biopsy is reserved for focal masses with atypical imaging features.

For information regarding the laboratory diagnosis of the etiological agents associated with HCC, see Hepatitis B and Hepatitis C sections in this chapter.

**4. Laboratory capability**—For information on the laboratory capability required to detect the etiological agents associated with HCC, see Hepatitis B and Hepatitis C in this chapter.

**5. Safety requirements**—See Hepatitis B and Hepatitis C in this chapter.

**6. Nonhuman hosts**—See Hepatitis B and Hepatitis C in this chapter.

**7. Sample/specimen requirements**—See Hepatitis B and Hepatitis C in this chapter.

**8. Testing requirements**—See Hepatitis B and Hepatitis C in this chapter.

**9. Reporting requirements**—Cases of HCC should be reported to a tumor registry according to standard US cancer registration procedures. Cancer reports to local health authorities is required in some other countries.

**10. Referral network**—CDC's DVH conducts epidemiologic studies of advanced liver diseases including HCC and serves as a WHO Collaborating Centre for Reference and Research on Viral Hepatitis. For information regarding DVH Laboratory diagnostic support, see Hepatitis B and Hepatitis C in this chapter.

For further information on CDC's National Program of Cancer Registries or to contact a local cancer registry, see: https://www.cdc.gov/cancer/npcr.

**11. Special considerations**—None.

[J. Drobeniuc, S. Kamili]

# HERPESVIRUS DISEASE

(varicella/herpes zoster, Epstein-Barr virus infections, cytomegalovirus disease)

| DISEASE | ICD-10 CODE |
|---|---|
| HERPESVIRAL INFECTIONS | ICD-10 A60 (anogenital herpes viral infection), B00 (herpes viral infection), P35.2 (congenital herpes viral infection) |
| HERPESVIRAL ENCEPHALITIS, SIMIAN B | ICD-10 B00.4 |
| KAPOSI'S SARCOMA | ICD-10 C46.0–C46.9 |

Although herpesvirus infections are often asymptomatic or cause only mild symptoms, these viruses cause a remarkable range of disease conditions, including but not limited to mild transient skin lesions, lymphadenopathy, encephalitis, meningitis, pneumonia, neuropathies, hepatitis, vasculopathies, neoplastic disease, stroke, retinitis, and death.

**1. Clinical features—**

1) Herpes simplex virus disease (HSV): one of the most common infections in humans. HSV infections range from asymptomatic or mild disease (typical) to severe and occasionally life-threatening conditions in all age groups. HSV-1 and HSV-2 are typically transmitted via different routes, but the epidemiology and clinical presentations caused by these viruses overlap substantially. The majority of primary infections by both viruses are asymptomatic. HSV-2 infections are usually acquired after people become sexually active. HSV-1 typically infects the oropharynx and establishes latency in the trigeminal ganglia, and HSV-2 infects the genitalia and establishes latency in the sacral ganglia. However, both viruses can infect either site, and in the USA currently over 50% of genital HSV infections are attributed to HSV-1. Antibodies to HSV-1 and HSV-2 are broadly cross-reactive, and antibody produced against HSV-1 or HSV-2 often moderates the severity of infection by the other type.

   - Skin lesions: primary HSV-1 infections most often lead to well-circumscribed, painful oropharyngeal lesions. Additional symptoms may include fever, sore throat, edema, lymphadenopathy, anorexia, and malaise. Symptomatic primary infections may require several weeks to resolve. Recurrent lesions generally progress from prodromal sensation to vesicular lesions to crusts over several days, without sequelae. Primary genital herpes, when symptomatic, can be severe with painful vesicular lesions requiring several weeks to resolve. Primary infections may also cause fever, dysuria, local lymphadenopathy, and malaise. Lesions from recurrent disease are usually less severe and heal more rapidly. The majority of both HSV-1 and HSV-2 primary infections are asymptomatic. Less common presentations in the skin include herpetic whitlow, with vesicular lesions on a finger or thumb caused by oral exposures usually in children; and herpes gladiatorum, with characteristic herpetic lesions occurring anywhere on the body subsequent to exposure to saliva containing HSV, most often seen in wrestlers.

- Encephalitis: herpes simplex encephalitis is 1 of the most serious diseases caused by HSV. In the USA, it is the most common cause of diagnosable sporadic encephalitis, with roughly 1,250 deaths annually. Untreated, the disease is fatal in about 70% of cases; among patients who receive antiviral therapy, about one-third will die and at least half of those who survive suffer long-term neurologic dysfunction. Symptoms may include fever, altered consciousness, strange behavior, disordered thought, and localized neurologic findings including seizures. The infection tends to localize to the temporal lobes.
- Herpes keratitis: herpes simplex keratitis is usually caused by HSV-1 and is often accompanied by conjunctivitis. It is regarded among the most common infectious causes of blindness in the USA. Symptoms include keratoconjunctivitis, preauricular adenopathy, photophobia, tearing, eyelid edema, and chemosis. Recurrent disease is common and can occur in 1 or both eyes and may lead to corneal scarring. Progressive disease results in loss of vision.
- Disease in immunocompromised patients: both solid organ transplant patients and bone marrow transplant patients are at increased risk of developing disease caused by HSV. Disease can result from new HSV acquisition from a HSV-positive donor organ or HSV reactivation (typical) in the recipient during therapeutic immunosuppression. Patients most often have severe oral or genital recurrences but may also develop progressive disease of the respiratory tract, esophagus, or gastrointestinal tract. Patients with human immunodeficiency virus (HIV) infection who are not virally immunosuppressed may also develop opportunistic HSV infection. Multiple recurrences of HSV reactivation during therapy can also lead to antiviral resistance. HSV-2-infected patients with symptomatic genital ulcerative disease are at increased risk of acquiring HIV

infection, and HIV-infected patients with HSV are more likely to transmit HSV.

2) Neonatal HSV: estimated to occur in 1 in 2,500 to 1 in 5,000 deliveries in the USA every year. Roughly 70% of cases are caused by HSV-2 and usually result from fetal contact with infected maternal genital secretions during delivery. The disease manifests in 3 categories: (a) skin, eye, and mouth disease; (b) encephalitis; and (c) disseminated infection. The mortality rate for each category varies from zero for skin, eye, and mouth disease, to 15% for encephalitis, and to 60% for infants with disseminated infection. Morbidity is also substantial, as children with encephalitis or disseminated infection develop normally only about 40% of the time, even with antiviral therapy. Transmission risk at delivery can be reduced through Caesarian delivery if performed shortly after labor commences. In this setting prophylactic antiviral therapy may be administered until the risk to the infant is determined. Avoidance of fetal scalp monitors in mothers with a history of HSV-2 infection is reasonable, and antiviral treatment during final weeks of pregnancy may help reduce transmission risk.
3) Other HSV-related conditions: HSV can cause aseptic meningitis, recurrent meningitis (Mollaret's meningitis), and Bell's palsy. Additional diseases associated with HSV include lower respiratory infections, acute onset bronchospasm, chronic periodontitis, pneumonitis, hepatitis, ganglionitis, and acute retinal necrosis. Some of these complications are largely confined to immunocompromised persons.
4) Varicella-zoster virus (VZV) disease: a nearly ubiquitous infection in humans, particularly in countries with a temperate climate, where more than 90%–95% of people are infected by the age of 30. The introduction of universal varicella vaccination policies in countries such as the USA has reduced the incidence of varicella by more than 90%.

   Varicella occurs following primary infection with VZV. It is a febrile, pruritic rash illness that usually resolves without complications or minor secondary bacterial skin infections and scarring. The appearance of the rash in typical varicella is distinctive, usually distributed on the trunk and face with vesicular lesions that are superficial and frequently described as dew drops on a rose petal. Primary infection during pregnancy in rare instances can lead to congenital transmission to the fetus causing congenital VZV disease, which may cause severe abnormalities in limb growth, eye, and brain development. Prior to the introduction of routine varicella vaccination in 1995, there were approximately 10,000 hospitalizations and 150 deaths annually in the USA due to varicella, most due to bacterial superinfection of skin lesions.

VZV can reactivate from latency at any age to cause herpes zoster (HZ), but the risk increases dramatically with advancing age, correlating with measurable declines in immunocompetence. It is characterized by a painful vesicular exanthema that is most often restricted to a single dermatome, reflecting the location of the dorsal root ganglion in which reactivation occurs. Rash and pain generally occur in close temporal proximity. In immunocompromised patients, potentially fatal disseminated disease targeting multiple organs can occur. HZ pain can occur in the absence of a history of rash illness, a condition known as zoster sine herpete. Approximately 10% of HZ patients continue to suffer from intense pain for months to years after the rash illness resolves, termed postherpetic neuralgia. The likelihood of this increases with advancing age.

Two vaccines to prevent HZ have been licensed and recommended in the USA. Both vaccines prevent or reduce the severity of HZ in persons over 60 years of age, although the Shingrix vaccine received preferred status by ACIP in 2017. During acute infection (i.e., varicella or chickenpox), VZV establishes latency in the dorsal root and cranial nerve ganglia, where it can reactivate to cause HZ (aka shingles). The vaccine is capable of establishing latency; early studies suggest that latent infections by varicella vaccine virus are less likely to cause HZ.

5) Other VZV-related conditions: VZV reactivation can also cause meningitis or meningoencephalitis, meningoradiculitis, acute cerebellar ataxia, and various neuropathies, such as local loss of sensation or partial paralysis. VZV vasculopathy can lead to ischemic and hemorrhagic stroke.

   Ocular disorders attributed to VZV infection include acute or chronic corneal disease, acute retinal necrosis, progressive outer retinal necrosis, optic neuritis, papillitis, and ophthalmoplegia.

   Additional complications of VZV infection include pneumonia, bacterial superinfections, hepatitis, and thrombocytopenia. Most of these conditions are associated with immune compromise.

6) Epstein-Barr virus (EBV) infections: nearly everyone will be infected with EBV at some point in their lives; 90% of adults are EBV antibody-positive by the age of 30. With infectious mononucleosis (IM), nearly all primary infections in children are asymptomatic; by contrast, about three-fourths of EBV infections from adolescence into adulthood lead to symptomatic IM. The disease is characterized by sore throat, cervical lymph node enlargement,

fatigue, hepatitis, and fever; splenomegaly is also often present. IM is clinically significant primarily because of the duration of debilitating acute illness and because symptomatic IM appears to confer an elevated risk for EBV-associated neoplastic later in life and autoimmune diseases.

7) Cancer and EBV:

- Burkitt's lymphoma (BL) is an aggressive form of non-Hodgkin lymphoma. It is the most prevalent pediatric malignancy in sub-Saharan Africa. The disease usually presents in the jaw and rapidly progresses. BL is fatal if untreated, but the majority of patients can survive with chemotherapy. Nearly 100% of BL tumors in sub-Saharan Africa are EBV positive and are most common among patients with both EBV and malaria. The immunosuppressive effects of malaria are hypothesized to curtail immune surveillance against EBV-transformed B lymphocytes. BL is uncommon outside of Africa. Approximately 1,200 people develop BL in the USA annually, and in contrast to African BL occurs mostly among patients older than 40 years. HIV-infected persons are at greatest risk for BL. Only 20% of BL tumors evaluated in the USA are EBV positive.
- Nasopharyngeal carcinoma (NPC) is a malignancy that begins in the epithelial cells that line the nasopharynx. There are 3 types: anaplastic (63%), keratinizing (25%), and differentiated (12%). Essentially all anaplastic NPC is associated with EBV infection, but EBV is found, albeit less consistently, in the other types. The disease is most common in Asia and is 3–4-fold more common in men than in women. Cofactors for developing NPC include both genetic and dietary factors. Five-year survival rates for NPC vary with the stage at diagnosis. Nearly three-fourths of NPC patients diagnosed at stage 1 will survive but only about 38% of those diagnosed at stage 4. The disease is uncommon in the USA, with only about 3,200 cases diagnosed annually.
- Hodgkin's lymphoma (HL) is a malignancy of lymphocytes, usually presenting with enlarged, painless lymph nodes in the neck, groin, or armpit. Other nonspecific symptoms include fever, itchy skin, night sweats, splenomegaly, and hepatomegaly. These symptoms are shared with non-Hodgkin lymphomas such as Burkitt's. About half of HL tumors are associated with EBV. Prognosis varies by a number of factors including age of diagnosis and stage, but 5-year survival rates are greater than 80% for patients with only a single risk factor.

- EBV-positive gastric carcinoma accounts for about 10% of all gastric carcinomas (GC) and is probably the most common EBV-associated malignancy worldwide, with an estimated 95,000 cases annually. While the role of EBV in GC is not well characterized, distinct differences in the presentation of EBV-GC have been observed, and there is also evidence that EBV-GC is more successfully treatable than other forms of GC. Rarely, EBV has been associated with leiomyosarcomas, which are soft tissue neoplasms that develop in immunocompromised patients.

8) Autoimmunity and EBV: a number of studies have sought to associate EBV infection with various autoimmune diseases. Most of these efforts lack persuasive evidence, but studies of 2 disorders, multiple sclerosis (MS) and systemic lupus erythematosus (SLE) have accumulated sufficient observations to support a possible association. The foundation for a causal link between MS and EBV infection comes from a variety of studies that show MS almost never develops until after EBV infection occurs. This included a large longitudinal study that linked development of MS to seroconversion to EBV. For SLE, the discovery that EBV nuclear antigen-1 may mimic several markers targeted by SLE, inducing an autoreactive immune response is suggestive of a role for EBV in at least some cases of SLE.
9) Other EBV-related conditions: as with all human herpesviruses (HHV), EBV can cause many disease conditions with varying frequency, including the following:

   - Neurologic: viral meningitis, encephalitis, optic neuritis, transverse myelitis, Guillain-Barré syndrome, acute cerebellar ataxia, sleep disorders, and psychoses.
   - Hematologic: neutropenia, hemolytic anemia, hemophagocytic syndrome, and x-linked lymphoproliferative disease.
   - Miscellaneous: pneumonia, interstitial lung disease, pancreatitis, and myocarditis.

10) Cytomegalovirus (CMV) disease: CMV infections are common globally and sometimes cause severe disease in immunocompetent adults and children. CMV is responsible for approximately 10% of infectious mononucleosis cases.

    - Congenital CMV disease: if actively replicating CMV from primary infection, reactivation, or reinfection occurs during pregnancy, vertical transmission to the fetus is possible. In developed countries, congenital CMV infection is a leading cause of sensorineural hearing loss and other neurological impairments such as intellectual disability, blindness, seizures, and loss of motor control. The highest risk for fetal injury occurs from primary maternal infection, which can result in severe or fatal disease.

- CMV in immunocompromised patients: CMV disease is a common, potentially serious problem among immunocompromised patients. Solid organ transplant recipients are at substantially elevated risk of CMV diseases such as pneumonitis, gastrointestinal lesions, hepatitis, retinitis, pancreatitis, and myocarditis. Stem cell recipients are also at elevated risk of CMV disease, most commonly pneumonitis. In both instances, CMV-naïve recipients receiving allografts from CMV-positive donors are at the greatest risk. Finally, HIV-positive patients who are either untreated or ineffectively treated with antiretroviral therapy are at substantially elevated risk of CMV disease, primarily from reactivated infections. Retinitis, esophagitis, and colitis are common CMV complications associated with HIV.

11) Human herpesvirus 6A, 6B and human herpesvirus 7: HHV-6A, HHV-6B, and HHV-7 are all members of the *Betaherpesvirinae* subfamily. Initially, HHV-6A and -6B were regarded as variants of the same species; however, as knowledge about their clinical associations, genomic variation, growth, and other properties expanded, the 2 viruses were reclassified in 2013 as distinct viral species. These 3 viruses compose the genus *Roseolovirus*, and all 3 viruses have been associated with exanthem subitum. HHV-6A and -6B are unique among human herpesviruses for their capacity to integrate into the telomeres of human chromosomes. These integrated genomes can be inherited, and the virus is fully capable of reactivating and causing a productive infection. An estimated 1% of persons in the USA carry a copy of the HHV-6A or -6B genome in every nucleated cell in their body. HHV-6B infection is nearly ubiquitous in the USA; 99% of persons have evidence of infection by the age of 2.

12) HHV-6A and HHV-6B: exanthem subitum, also known as roseola, is a febrile rash illness common among children between the ages of 6 months and 12 months. It typically runs a mild course, but 10%–15% of children may experience seizures due to high fever. The disease is contagious but only during the febrile phase. The virus is not spread after the onset of rash. Both HHV-6A and HHV-6B have been detected in the plasma of bone marrow patients.

HHV-6B, but not HHV-6A, has been found in the gastrointestinal tract of solid organ transplant recipients, in endodontic abscesses, and in the tonsils and adenoids. Both viruses have been observed in vitreous fluid and are implicated in inflammatory eye diseases. Both viruses are neurotropic, but some evidence suggests that HHV-6A may be associated with increased severity in cases of HHV-6 neurologic disease. HHV-6A deoxyribonucleic acid (DNA) is more frequently found than HHV-6B among MS and rhomboencephalitis patients. HHV-6A may be present in the central nervous system of MS patients and in the blood of patients with relapsing/remitting disease. There is also some evidence of an association between HHV-6A and glial tumors. HHV-6B, but not HHV-6A, has also been linked with mesial temporal lobe epilepsy and status epilepticus. HHV-6A, but not HHV-6B, may also be associated with Hashimoto's thyroiditis and with syncytial giant cell hepatitis among recipients of liver transplants. For further information, see "Exanthema Subitum."

13) HHV-7 infection: beyond its association with exanthem subitum there are no definitive disease associations with HHV-7 infection. There is a tentative association with pityriasis rosea.
14) Human herpesvirus 8 disease HHV-8, also known as Kaposi's sarcoma-associated herpesvirus, a member of the *gammaherpesvirus* subfamily. Like EBV, HHV-8 has been linked to several neoplastic diseases including Kaposi's sarcoma (KS), multifocal Castleman's disease (MCD), and primary effusion lymphoma (PEL). HHV-8 may be transmitted through several routes, notably saliva, sexual transmission, breast milk, and, more rarely, transfusion.

Four distinct forms of KS are recognized, all of which are associated with HHV-8 infection. Classic KS usually manifests as lesions on the toes and soles of the feet. It occurs primarily in elderly men of Mediterranean, Arabian, or eastern European ancestry. Classic KS is normally slow growing and chronic and is treated by removing the lesions surgically. Endemic KS occurs primarily in young people in sub-Saharan Africa. It can present as an aggressive form in children under 10, with lymph node involvement; lesions may be present or absent. In older persons (usually between ages 20–50), the disease presents with nodular, invasive masses on the extremities. The increased use of calcineurin T cell inhibitors in transplant patients led to an increase in KS incidence. Tumors develop either when an HHV-8-infected organ is transplanted into a naïve recipient or through reactivation of a latent HHV-8 infection in the recipient. Acquired immunodeficiency syndrome–associated KS usually presents with the appearance of 1 to several red to purple macules. These progress rapidly to papules, nodules, and plaques, most frequently on the head, back, trunk, and mucous membranes. As the disease progresses, involvement of the stomach and intestines, lymph nodes, and lungs is common. For the more aggressive forms, untreated disease is commonly fatal.

MCD is a lymphoproliferative disease that presents in 2 histologic forms, the hyaline vascular type and the plasma cell type. The disease may be localized or may affect multiple lymph nodes, which is why it is termed multicentric. Symptoms include fever, malaise, wasting, hypoalbuminemia, cytopenias, and hyponatremia. Among immunocompetent patients, only about half of MCD cases have detectable HHV-8; by contrast, virtually all MCD in HIV-positive patients is associated with HHV-8 infection. Long-term prognosis is poor, but new treatment regimens are promising. PEL is a disease characterized by lymphomatous effusions in any of the body cavities. PEL is uniformly associated with HHV-8 infection. The prognosis for PEL patients is poor; the disease is on average fatal within 6 months of diagnosis.

15) Herpes B virus disease: herpes B virus infection in humans is caused by the zoonotic *Macacine herpesvirus 1* (MHV-1). The virus is usually referred to as B virus but may also be called herpes B, simian B, monkey B virus, and herpesvirus simiae. The natural host for B virus are species of the Old World primate genus *Macaca*, which include multiple species of macaque monkeys. These include the rhesus and cynomolgus monkeys frequently used in primate research. B virus in macaques is analogous to typical HSV-1 infection in humans, with usually circumscribed vesicular lesions. Of all alpha herpesviruses identified in nonhuman primates, only B virus is known to be pathogenic for humans. Herpes B infection in humans usually first presents with flu-like symptoms and often with vesicular lesions at the site of exposure. Neurologic symptoms such as dizziness, weakness, neuralgia, parasthesias, and severe persistent headache foreshadow the onset of encephalomyelitis or severe neurologic impairment that is fatal if not treated with antivirals. The virus is typically transmitted through macaque bites or scratches, urine splashes, or contact with tissues or body fluids from an infected monkey. Human B virus infection is rare, and only about 50 confirmed cases have been reported since the virus was first discovered in 1932. Twenty-one of those cases have resulted in fatality. Better familiarity with the disease, monitoring of research animals for B virus history, and implementation of safe animal handling practices have reduced the risk of B virus infection in animal care facilities. However, temple parks primarily located in Asia include

populations of free-roaming macaques, many of which are B virus-positive. Tourists are encouraged to feed these animals and pose with them for professional photographers, and a number of potential exposures occur annually in that setting.

**2. Causative agents**—There are 10 currently recognized herpesvirus species that are known to cause disease in humans, 9 of which have humans as their natural host. All are capable of establishing lifelong latent infection following primary exposure. These viruses belong to 3 different subfamilies: *Alphaherpesvirinae* (herpes simplex virus, HSV-1, HSV-2; varicella-zoster virus, VZV; zoonotic herpes B virus, MHV-1); *Betaherpesvirinae* (cytomegalovirus, CMV; human herpesvirus 6, HHV-6A, HHV-6B; human herpesvirus 7, HHV7), and *Gammaherpesvirinae* (Epstein-Barr virus, EBV; human herpesvirus 8, HHV-8).

**3. Laboratory diagnosis**—The gold standard for laboratory confirmation of human herpesvirus diseases, with the exception of EBV for infectious mononucleosis, is agent-specific polymerase chain reaction (PCR). Active EBV, HHV-8, VZV, and CMV infections are generally suitable for agent-specific PCR. The alphaherpesviruses are mostly characterized by rapid growth, and in the past, virus isolation by cell culture was widely used to confirm infection. However, herpesviruses are relatively fragile, and the sensitivity of culture is limited and highly dependent on the inoculation of tissue culture immediately after sample collection from fresh lesions. PCR is much more sensitive and is the only option for herpesviruses that grow poorly in culture, such as HHV-8. Quantitative PCR is required to confirm HHV-6 disease in order to rule out chromosomal integration of HHV-6 as a consequence of inherited infection.

Serology can be useful for the agent-specific diagnosis of herpesvirus infections in several contexts. Quantitative measurement of immunoglobulin class G (IgG) from acute and convalescent sera can be used to confirm infection if either seroconversion or a 4-fold rise in titer can be observed. The chief limitation of this approach is the delay of final results due to the need to collect 2 serum specimens spaced 2 weeks apart. For EBV, detection of heterophile antibodies (monospot) or evaluation of an EBV-specific serology panel can be used to diagnose acute infectious mononucleosis. The former does not specifically identify EBV and may produce both false-positive and false-negative results. Infectious mononucleosis caused by CMV is not accompanied by the production of heterophile antibodies. Evaluation of IgG avidity for any of the herpesviruses can be used to distinguish between a recent primary infection and a remote infection. Detection of agent-specific IgM can document recent infection, reinfection, or reactivation but cannot distinguish between them. In general, IgM methods are prone to be relatively nonspecific. For VZV, measurement of intrathecal VZV IgG (compared with specific IgG in serum) has been used successfully to provide supporting evidence for active central nervous system VZV infection in cases where viral DNA is undetectable by PCR.

**4. Laboratory capability**—Serology for HSV and EBV and PCR for HSV should routinely be available from local clinical diagnostic laboratories. PCR for HHV-6, HHV-7, and HHV-8 should be available in larger specialist laboratories. Specialized PCR testing for the discrimination of vaccine VZV from wild-type virus is available in selective laboratories in the USA, Japan, the UK, Canada, and Australia. PCR and serologic testing for herpes B virus may be available from specialized reference centers (in the USA, through the National B Virus Resource Center; see: http://www2.gsu.edu/~wwwvir).

**5. Safety requirements**—Universal/standard precautions should be used whenever handling all blood and body fluids and tissues potentially containing blood. All human herpesviruses can be handled using biosafety level 2 (BSL-2) practices, and facilities including a properly maintained class II biosafety cabinet additional containment should be considered when performing certain activities such as production, purification, or concentration of virus. All herpesvirus isolation work should be performed in a biosafety cabinet after preparation of workplace and tools. Personnel responsible for diagnostic testing with infectious agents should receive regular safety training and undergo regular proficiency training for all protocols they perform. All work involving the handling of B virus-positive materials must be conducted using BSL-3 containment and practice; propagation of herpes B virus from diagnostic samples and experimental animal infections should be performed at the BSL-4 containment and practice level. Specialized training for personnel performing laboratory work in a BSL-4 facility is mandatory.

**6. Nonhuman hosts**—Humans are the natural host for all of the herpesviruses discussed in this chapter except B virus. The natural host for B virus is macaques. Like many transmissions of herpesviruses from the natural host to a closely related species, untreated herpes B disease in humans is generally devastating.

**7. Sample/specimen requirements**—

1) HSV: for vesicular skin lesions suspected to be HSV, swabs of vesicular fluid in viral transport medium are the sample of choice. It should be noted that a negative HSV PCR performed in the first 72 hours postonset does not exclude HSV encephalitis. Viral culture can be performed if samples can be immediately inoculated into culture but is substantially less sensitive than PCR. Serology with acute and convalescent sera can be used to confirm HSV infection if seroconversion or a 4-fold rise in titer is observed, but this has limited clinical value due to time considerations. For diseases

affecting specific organs, biopsy samples are the preferred PCR sample. There are also circumstances where plasma (or whole blood) is the appropriate sample for quantitative PCR (e.g., suspected fulminant HSV hepatitis).

2) VZV: for vesicular skin lesions suspected to be VZV, swabs of vesicular fluid, either dry or in viral transport medium, are the sample of choice. Scabs from crusted lesions are also excellent samples. Saliva samples collected during acute disease are also suitable. For disease affecting specific organs, biopsy samples are the preferred PCR sample. In general, IgG serologic assays have limited value, except as specified for HSV. VZV IgG avidity can be used to discriminate primary infection from remote infection. VZV-specific IgM detection indicates recent active VZV infection but does not discriminate among primary infection, reinfection, or reactivation. If cerebrospinal fluid (CSF) is collected more than a week after the onset of suspected VZV meningitis/encephalitis, VZV DNA may be undetectable. Measurements of VZV-specific intrathecal antibody synthesis may be positive for considerably longer. Assessment of VZV-specific antibody levels in CSF and serum and comparing total IgG, albumin, and antibody levels for other common infectious agents makes it possible to determine whether there is specific intrathecal synthesis of anti-VZV IgG, or alternatively there is compromise of the blood brain barrier (i.e., passive leakage of IgG from serum into the CSF or blood contamination of the sample). Careful selection of specificity controls can also rule in other possible herpesvirus etiologies (HSV, HHV-6). There are some circumstances (e.g., disseminated VZV) where whole blood may be the appropriate sample.
3) EBV: diagnosis of infectious mononucleosis is best accomplished using a panel of enzyme-linked immunosorbent assay serology methods (viral capsid antigen, early antigen, EBV nuclear antigen) which, in combination, can discriminate between active primary infection and remote infection. The monospot method, which detects the presence of heterophile antibodies, is still in common use but is not specific to EBV and can generate both false-negative and false-positive results. EBV involvement in carcinomas may be evaluated in tumor biopsies by in situ hybridization or PCR. There are some circumstances where plasma (or whole blood) may be the appropriate sample for quantitative PCR.
4) CMV: samples useful for the confirmation of congenital CMV infection include saliva, urine, and whole blood dried blood spots collected from the newborn; the former 2 samples generally have much higher viral loads. To confirm congenital CMV infection, samples must be collected within 3 weeks of delivery to distinguish

congenital infection from perinatally or postnatally acquired infection. CMV culture is generally impractical as a clinical diagnostic test due to the extended incubation times required. Amniotic fluid can be collected for antigenemia or DNAemia testing to diagnose congenital CMV infection prenatally. Quantification of CMV in whole blood or plasma may serve as a useful prognostic indicator for CMV disease onset in solid organ and hematopoetic stem cell transplant patient.

5) HHV-6/7: laboratory testing is not required for the diagnosis of exanthema subitum in infants. In cases of suspected HHV-6 neurologic disease, the appropriate sample is CSF for PCR testing. It is critical to perform quantitative HHV-6 PCR to exclude chromosomally integrated HHV6 as a cause of an encephalitis; it would be necessary to measure viral load on blood as well as CSF. There are no specific recommended laboratory diagnostic tests for additional conditions with a putative HHV-6 etiology.
6) HHV-8: tissue culture for HHV-8 is not currently feasible. HHV-8 PCR on biopsy samples from various HHV-8 associated neoplastic diseases are the appropriate specimens.
7) Herpes B: swabs of vesicular lesions are the sample of choice for the PCR confirmation of herpes B infection, although the appearance of symptoms consistent with herpes B infection in the context of known high-risk exposure warrants immediate treatment in advance of diagnostic results. Herpes B virus-specific serology can document infection but must be interpreted with the understanding that there is considerable cross-reactivity between herpes B virus and HSV. CSF samples may be collected for PCR testing if neurologic symptoms are present.

In general, for viral culture, swabs of skin lesions, saliva samples, CSF, biopsy, or other samples should be inoculated into culture as quickly as feasible after they are collected. Serum can be stored for several weeks at refrigerator temperatures or frozen indefinitely. Serum can be shipped overnight on cold packs or frozen on dry ice. Samples for PCR, such as skin lesion swabs and scabs, are stable and can be shipped dry at ambient temperature. If samples are placed in transport medium, they should be shipped on cold packs or frozen and tested as soon as possible. Saliva, CSF, urine, and tissue samples should be frozen or shipped overnight on cold packs, particularly when they will not be tested on the day of collection. Samples other than those strongly suspected to contain herpes B virus can be shipped as category B substances.

**8. Reporting requirements**—Only varicella is a nationally notifiable condition in the USA. Laboratories in other settings should determine what diseases caused by members of the *Herpesviridae* family are reportable within their respective jurisdictions.

**9. Testing requirements**—Validated and controlled methods are recommended for clinical diagnostics. All testing personnel should be regularly evaluated on accurate test performance and adherence to safety procedures. The laboratory should participate in regular external quality assessment program. Herpesvirus (HSV, VZV) culture may be performed where necessary or appropriate at 35°C–37°C in a humidified incubator containing 5% $CO_2$. PCR testing requires facilities that support unidirectional workflow, well-maintained and validated equipment, and high-quality reagents.

**10. Referral network**—Referrals for testing are generally made on the basis of clinical suspicion of infection by specific herpesvirus species. Clinical laboratories must determine if they have the requisite capability and request a confirmation of their results from accredited reference laboratories when they are available.

**11. Special considerations**—None.

Note: for further information on herpesvirus clinical features and diagnosis, see "Herpesvirus Disease" in *CCDM20*; for further information on varicella/herpes zoster, Epstein-Barr virus infections, and cytomegalovirus disease, including ICD codes, see the respective disease chapters in *CCDM20*.

[D. S. Schmid, F. P. Downes]

# HISTOPLASMOSIS

| DISEASE | ICD-10 CODE |
|---|---|
| HISTOPLASMOSIS CAPSULATI | ICD-10 B39.4 |
| HISTOPLASMOSIS DUBOISII | ICD-10 B39.5 |

Two clinically different mycoses are designated as histoplasmosis; the pathogens that cause them cannot be distinguished morphologically when grown on culture media as molds. Detailed information is given for the infection caused by *Histoplasma capsulatum* var. *capsulatum*, and a brief summary is given for that caused by *H. capsulatum* var. *duboisii*.

**1. Clinical features**—

1) Histoplasmosis capsulati (histoplasmosis due to *H. capsulatum* var. *capsulatum*, American histoplasmosis): a systemic mycosis of varying severity ranging from symptom-free, or minor self-limited, to

life-threatening illnesses. The primary lesion is usually in the lungs. While infection is common, overt clinical disease is not. Four clinical forms are recognized:

- Acute respiratory: varies from a mild respiratory illness to temporary incapacity with general malaise, fever, chills, headache, myalgia, chest pains, and nonproductive cough; occasional erythema multiforme; and erythema nodosum. Multiple, small scattered calcifications in the lung, hilar lymph nodes, spleen, and liver may be late findings.
- Acute disseminated histoplasmosis: with debilitating fever, gastrointestinal (GI) symptoms, evidence of bone marrow suppression, hepatosplenomegaly, lymphadenopathy, and a rapid course; most frequent in infants, young children, and immunocompromised patients, including those with human immunodeficiency virus infection.[1] Usually fatal unless treated.
- Chronic disseminated disease: with low-grade intermittent fever, weight loss, weakness, hepatosplenomegaly, mild hematological abnormalities, and focal manifestations of disease (e.g., endocarditis; meningitis; mucosal ulcers of mouth, larynx, stomach, or bowel; Addison disease). Subacute course progressing over the course of 10–11 months and usually fatal unless treated.
- Chronic pulmonary form: clinically and radiologically resembling chronic pulmonary tuberculosis with cavitation; occurs most often in middle-aged and elderly men with underlying emphysema. Progresses over months or years, with periods of quiescence and sometimes spontaneous cure.

2) Histoplasmosis duboisii (histoplasmosis due to *H. capsulatum* var. *duboisii*, African histoplasmosis): this usually presents as a subacute granuloma of skin or bone. Thus far, the disease has been recognized only in Africa and Madagascar. Infection, though usually localized, may be disseminated in the skin, subcutaneous tissue, lymph nodes, bones, joints, lungs, and abdominal viscera. Disease is more common in males and may occur at any age but especially in the second decade of life. Diagnosis is made through culture or demonstration of yeast cells of *H. capsulatum* var. *duboisii* in tissue by smear or biopsy. These cells are much larger than the yeast cells of *H. capsulatum* var. *capsulatum*. The true prevalence of *H. duboisii*, its reservoir, mode of transmission, and incubation period are unknown. It is not communicable from

person to person. Treatment is the same as for histoplasmosis due to *H. capsulatum*.

**2. Causative agents**—The causative agent of histoplasmosis is *H. capsulatum*. The organism grows in most soils within the endemic areas but proliferates in great concentrations in soil contaminated with bird or bat droppings due to increased nitrogen content. Thus, persons frequenting bird roosting areas or bat caves are at higher risk of contracting disease. It is a dimorphic fungus in that it exists as the mold or mycelial phase when found in the soil at ambient temperature and in the yeast phase at 37°C in the infected human or animal host. There are 2 varieties of *Histoplasma*, *H. capsulatum var capsulatum* (American histoplasmosis), which has been found worldwide but primarily in the central and eastern USA; and *H. capsulatum var duboisii* (African Histoplasmosis), which occurs in the tropical areas of Africa.[2] Both organisms cause similar diseases with *H. capsulatum var duboisii* causing mainly skin and subcutaneous infections.

**3. Laboratory diagnosis**—The diagnosis of histoplasmosis requires laboratory testing. Clinical symptoms alone are insufficient for definitive diagnosis since there is significant overlap with other diseases.

1) Skin test: in this test, an antigen prepared from the mycelial phase of *H. capsulatum* is injected just below the surface of the skin. Detection of asymptomatic cases is often by skin test screening as part of an epidemiologic investigation. The histoplasmin skin test has been a useful epidemiologic tool for surveillance purposes but does not differentiate those with disease from those exposed. In endemic areas of the USA such as the Ohio and Mississippi River valleys, estimates are that 60% of individuals react positively to histoplasmin skin testing.
2) Serology: antibody detection is a major tool to diagnose histoplasmosis. From histoplasmin, extracted from *H. capsulatum* mycelial culture, H antigens and M antigens are obtained. The H antigen is a beta-glucosidase, and the M antigen is a catalase. These antigens drive the production of 2 antibodies commonly produced by individuals with histoplasmosis, anti-H and anti-M. The 2 serologic methods frequently used by laboratories to detect anti-H and anti-M antibodies are immunodiffusion (ID) and complement fixation (CF). ID qualitatively measures precipitating antibodies to *H. capsulatum* antigen. In ID, when the antibodies in the patient serum bind with *H. capsulatum* antigen a band or line forms. There are 2 bands formed, known as the H and M precipitin bands. The CF test quantitatively measures antibodies to 2 antigens: intact yeast form and mycelial antigen.

3) Direct examination: direct wet mount, potassium hydroxide smear, or calcofluor stain are used to detect the presence of *H. capsulatum* yeast cells in sputum, urine, cerebral spinal fluid, or blood. Histopathologic staining of infected tissue or bone marrow, with methenamine silver or periodic acid-Schiff stains, is a rapid means to diagnose histoplasmosis.
4) Culture: culture is the gold standard for detection of *H. capsulatum*. Once the organism is isolated in culture, identification can be made by microscopic appearance of the hyphae, macroconidia, and microconidia, and by converting from the mold phase at 25°C to the yeast phase at 37°C. There are commercially available nucleic acid probes for rapid identification of the mold from culture. The mold phase of *H. capsulatum* produces a white to buff-brown colony at ambient temperature. Microscopically, tuberculated macroconidia and microconidia are produced. At 37°C, the yeast of *H. capsulatum* are ovoid and measure 3–5 μm in diameter, which is smaller than most other yeast. The attachment of the bud to the mother cell has a narrow base. The yeast cells of *H. capsulatum var duboisii* can be 15 μm in diameter and have a thicker wall. The mycelial forms of both varieties are identical.
5) PCR: there are several real time PCR protocols for the detection of *H. capsulatum* deoxyribonucleic acid directly from patient specimens in development.[3] There are no commercially available or FDA-approved tests yet available; however, these test products may be available in the future.
6) Antigen test: in patients with disseminated infections, *H. capsulatum* antigens are released into the tissues and enter the blood, alveolar lavage fluid, cerebrospinal fluid, and urine (antigenuria). There are commercial tests available for the detection of antigen in serum, plasma, urine, and other body fluids.

**4. Laboratory capability**—Testing for the detection of *Histoplasma capsulatum*, is designated as high-complexity testing by the Clinical Laboratory Improvement Act (CLIA) in the USA, and only laboratories certified by CLIA to perform high-complexity testing can offer this service. Similar standards may exist in other countries. Laboratory capability varies widely for clinical laboratories and public health laboratories. While most major teaching hospitals and commercial reference laboratories offer an extensive test menu for serology, direct examination, culture, PCR, and antigen testing, the specific services vary from laboratory to laboratory. Laboratories who do not offer this testing on their test menu should refer specimens to a qualified reference laboratory.

**5. Safety requirements**—Laboratory acquired histoplasmosis is a safety risk. Therefore, all work handling of cultures with mold should be performed in a biosafety level 2 laboratory in a class II biosafety cabinet. Aerosolization of microconidia when lifting the lid from a petri dish can easily occur. Pulmonary infection from handling the cultures is the major risk factor. There are also reports of infections from skin puncture and droplets into the eye. The infectious form, the microconidia, are resistant to drying and may remain viable for long periods. The small size of the microconidia makes dispersal of spores a high risk when working with cultures.

**6. Nonhuman hosts**—Since *H. capsulatum* is commonly found in the soil, many animals have a risk of exposure and acquiring the disease. Dogs and cats are most commonly infected. Most infections involve the respiratory tract, lungs, and thoracic lymph nodes. Also common are infections in the GI tract, especially in dogs. The disease can then spread via the bloodstream to other areas of the body as in humans. The infection in animals is non-contagious. Symptoms can include mild fever, weight loss, loss of appetite, labored breathing, or a chronic cough.

**7. Sample/specimen requirements**—The most common specimen type is determined by the testing used for detection.

1) Serologic detection of antibody: requires a blood (serum) specimen collected between 2–6 weeks after infection during the acute phase of infection. A convalescent serum specimen, best paired with an acute phase specimen for testing, is collected 14–21 days after the acute specimen. The convalescent phase specimen is most useful for the CF assay.
2) Direct examination: specimen types for direct examination include sputum, urine, cerebral spinal fluid, or blood.
3) Culture and PCR: specimen types for culture and PCR include sputum, urine, wound, vitreous fluid, cerebral spinal fluid, paracentesis fluid, or blood.
4) Antigen test: generally blood, alveolar lavage fluid, cerebrospinal fluid, and urine (antigenuria) are acceptable specimens.

**8. Testing requirements**—Before offering any of these tests, the laboratory must validate the test performance in their hands and enroll the laboratory in the appropriate proficiency test program. Staff who have demonstrated competency can perform testing. Performance of testing for *H. capsulatum* is within the parameters of the laboratory's quality assurance program.

1) Skin test: the histoplasmin skin test is limited to epidemiological studies and not used for diagnostic testing. A positive skin test is common in those infected and in the exposed asymptomatic patient. Cross-reactivity with other dimorphic systemic fungi (*Blastomyces dermatitidis* and *Coccidiodes immitis*) occurs

with the histoplasmin skin test. The use of the skin test can also cause a false-positive serological test.

2) Serology: diagnosis of histoplasmosis by serologic detection of antibody is common practice. Serology is not a rapid detection method since antibodies typically appear between 2–6 weeks after exposure. With ID, the H band appears first and is usually present for only 4–6 weeks after exposure. The M band appears soon after and may persist for 3 years after a patient recovers. ID has a sensitivity of 70%–100% and a specificity of 100%.[4] Consequently, ID is not useful for screening. CF is more sensitive than ID with the yeast phase antigen sensitivity of 94.3% and mycelial phase antigen sensitivity of 72.8%.[4] CF is less specific (70%–80%). CF antibodies may appear in 3–6 weeks following infection. CF will give positive results for months. A high titer ($\geq$ 1:32) or a 4-fold increase in titer indicates active histoplasmosis. Low titers ($\leq$ 1:16) can provide presumptive evidence of infection or the low titer could represent previous infection. Individuals who live in endemic regions may also have low antibody titers. Antibody titers will eventually decline and even disappear months to years after a patient recovers. Also problematic is that patients with weakened immune systems may not produce detectable antibodies and produce a false-negative serology result. Another problem with serologic testing is that cross-reactions occur in up to 40% of patients with *B. dematitidis*, *C. immitis*, and *Aspergillus fumigatus*.[5]

3) Direct examination: staining is not a sensitive method and has the risk for misdiagnosis since artifacts and other organisms may impede the correct observation. Rarely seen are mycelial forms in tissue sections in patients with histoplasmosis.

4) Culture: culture is time-consuming since *H. capsulatum* is a slow-growing organism. The time to detection often exceeds 2 weeks or longer, and culture lacks sensitivity. Estimates are that cultures can be falsely negative in about 20% of disseminated cases and 50% of chronic pulmonary diseases.[6,7] Typically, laboratories incubate the cultures for a minimum of 6 weeks.

5) PCR: when compared with direct examination and culture the PCR method demonstrates improved sensitivity of 95.4% with a specificity of 96%. Most importantly, PCR generates results much faster than culture.[8]

6) Antigen test: antigen detection can be an effective and rapid method to diagnose systemic histoplasmosis. The sensitivity of antigen detection is 91.8% in urine specimens for patients with acute primary histoplasmosis.[9] Antigen detection is particularly useful in patients with weakened immune systems. In a study of patients with

acquired immunodeficiency syndrome and disseminated histoplasmosis, 97% had a positive antigen test.[5] Typically, antigen detection occurs earlier than antibody detection. Antigen detection is also useful to evaluate treatment and detect relapse. However, false negative antigen detection tests do occur, especially if the patient is not severely ill, indicating a low burden of infection. False positives can occur with cross-reaction to blastomycosis, paracoccidioidomycosis, coccidioidomycosis, and possibly other fungal infections. Another valuable use of the antigen test is to monitor the effect of treatment since antigen concentrations decline with treatment and eventually reach undetectable levels.

**9. Reporting requirements**—Laboratories must follow the reporting requirements of their jurisdictional health department. Most health departments require reporting of histoplasmosis. If required by the health department, the laboratory must provide the organism in pure culture to the jurisdictional public health laboratory for further testing.

**10. Referral network**—There are no referral networks for *H. capsulatum*.

**11. Special considerations**—The most common laboratory tests specimen type are blood and urine for the diagnosis of histoplasmosis. Respiratory specimens and tissue biopsy may be useful depending on signs and symptoms. Other tests such as chest X-rays or computed tomography scans of the lungs may also be required. Public health prevention activities include surveillance for infections, the development of better diagnostic tools, and building laboratory capacity.

## References

1. Wheat LJ, Connolly-Stringfield PA, Baker RL, et al. Disseminated histoplasmosis in the acquired immune deficiency syndrome: clinical findings, diagnosis and treatment, and review of the literature. *Medicine (Baltimore)*. 1989;69(6):361–374.
2. Deepe GS Jr. *Histoplasma capsulatum (Histoplasmosis)*. In: Bennett JE, Dolin R, Blaser MJ, eds. *Principles and Practice of Infectious Diseases*. 8th ed. Philadelphia, PA: Elsevier; 2015:2949–2962.
3. Marwan M, Hage CA. Laboratory diagnostics for histoplasmosis. *J Clin Microbiol*. 2017;55:1612–1620.
4. Guimarães AJ, Nosanchuk JD, Zancope-Oliveira AJ. Diagnosis of histoplasmosis. *Braz J Microbiol*. 2006;37(1):1–13.
5. Wheat J, French ML, Kamel S, Tewari RP. Evaluation of cross-reaction in *Histoplasma capsulatum* serologic tests. *J Clin Microbiol*. 1986;23(3):493–499.
6. Sathapatayavongs B, Batteiger BE, Wheat J, Slama TG, Wass JL. Clinical and laboratory features of disseminated histoplasmosis during two large urban outbreaks. *Medicine (Baltimore)*. 1983;62(5):263–270.
7. Wheat LJ, Wass J, Norton J, Kohler RB, Morris ML. Cavitary histoplasmosis occurring during two large urban outbreaks: analysis of clinical, epidemiologic, roentgenographic, and laboratory features. *Medicine (Baltimore)*. 1984;63(4):201–209.

8. Simone S, Veron V, Boukhari R, Blanchet D, Aznar C. Detection of *Histoplasma capsulatum* DNA in human samples by real-time polymerase chain reaction. *Diagn Microbiol Infect Dis*. 2010;66(3):268–273.
9. Hage CA, Ribes JA, Wengenack NL, et al. A multicenter evaluation of tests for diagnosis of histoplasmosis. *Clin Infect Dis*. 2011;53(5):448–454.

[M. A. Pentella]

# HIV INFECTION AND AIDS

| DISEASE | ICD-10 CODE |
|---|---|
| HIV INFECTION AND AIDS | ICD-10 B20–B24 |

**1. Clinical features**—Acquired immune deficiency syndrome, or AIDS, is the late clinical stage of infection with the human immunodeficiency virus (HIV). Within several weeks after infection with HIV, many individuals develop an acute self-limited mononucleosis-like illness lasting for 1–2 weeks. They may then be free of clinical signs or symptoms for years before other clinical manifestations develop, the result of HIV related opportunistic infections or cancers. The frequency and severity of HIV-related opportunistic infections or cancers is, in general, directly correlated with the degree of immune system dysfunction.

**2. Causative agents**—There are 2 distinct species of HIV. These are designated as HIV-1 and HIV-2. Both are members of the genus Lentivirus within the family *Retroviridae*. HIV-1 was identified first, is the more virulent of the 2, and is responsible for the majority of AIDS cases worldwide. The subsequent material presented is for HIV-1 unless otherwise specified. The clinical manifestations of HIV infection (AIDS) were first described in 1981, and the virus (HIV-1) was first identified in 1983. Four groups of HIV-1 have been identified based on genetic relatedness: M, O, N, and P. Group M, which causes most infections, is further divided into subtypes A, B, C, D, F, G, H, J, K, and circulating recombinant forms.

**3. Laboratory diagnosis**—Various analytes are used for the laboratory identification of HIV infection. The most common is detection of antibodies to HIV-1 and HIV-2. Detection of HIV-1 p24 antigen, and viral ribonucleic acid (RNA) are also increasingly being used to test for acute infection, since these are the first measurable analytes. Molecular methods are also used to diagnose infants born to HIV infected mothers because of the passive transfer of maternal antibodies, which makes testing for antibodies in newborns unreliable. Currently multiple tests are used in a diagnostic algorithm to reach a final conclusion regarding infection status.

AIDS diagnoses are based on the presence of opportunistic infections and by measuring cluster of differentiation 4 (CD4) t-lymphocytes. When the number of CD4 cells falls below 200 cells/mm$^3$, a person is considered to have progressed to AIDS. Regardless of CD4 count, a person can be diagnosed with AIDS if they are infected with HIV and have 1 or more opportunistic infections. A list of HIV-related, common opportunistic infections can be found at: https://www.HIV.gov.

4. **Laboratory capability**—Facility requirements vary drastically depending on the format of test being used. Commercial HIV tests range from very simple, rapid, single-use device tests (antibody and antigen tests) that require no or minimal equipment or preanalytic sample preparation and minimal staff training, to very complicated tests that require substantial pre-analytical sample preparation, specialized staff training, and dedicated instruments (i.e., antigen, antibody, and nucleic acid tests). The types of tests used and laboratory capabilities often vary depending on geographic location and economic conditions. Specimen type also influences the tests and algorithms used. In the USA, simple, rapid diagnostic tests are often used in outreach settings (e.g., bars, college campuses, community-based organizations) and small clinics to screen for HIV infection for the purpose of determining a preliminary result and improving linkage to care. However, definitive diagnoses are confirmed in laboratories that are capable of conducting moderate or high complexity tests as defined under Clinical Laboratory Improvement Amendments regulations (see: https://www.cms.gov/Regulations-and-Guidance/Legislation/CLIA/index.html?redirect=/clia). These laboratories have equipment for sample preparation (e.g., centrifuges for processing serum and plasma, and nucleic acid extraction equipment), equipment for performing serologic assays (e.g., enzyme-linked immunosorbent assay plate washers and readers or dedicated random access platforms), equipment for performing molecular testing (e.g., polymerase chain reaction or transcription-mediated amplification platforms), and cold storage (4°C and -20°C) to support the complex test requirements.

By contrast, many developing countries have limited laboratory infrastructure and rely extensively on the rapid, single-use test devices that do not require cold chain storage, have minimal or no sample preparation, require minimal staff training, and have minimal equipment to perform multitest algorithms.

5. **Safety requirements**—Biosafety level 2 (BSL-2) safety practices, equipment, and facilities are used when working with clinical specimens to protect against exposure to skin and mucous membranes. Blood and blood products are the most common type of clinical specimen that is capable of causing a laboratory-acquired infection; however, other specimen types such as semen, vaginal secretions, breast milk, cerebral spinal fluid, feces, saliva, urine, tears, sweat, vomitus, and unfixed tissues can potentially contain infectious virus and thus should also be handled with the same techniques as blood. In the USA, staff should be trained and abide by the Occupational Safety and Health Administration

Bloodborne Pathogens Standard and be cognizant that bodily fluid samples often contain other bloodborne pathogens such as hepatitis B and C.

Activities such as producing research laboratory-scale quantities of HIV, manipulating concentrated virus preparations, and conducting procedures that may produce droplets or aerosols should be performed in a BSL-2 facility, using BSL-3 practices.

It is now known that postexposure prophylaxis (PEP) can be effective in preventing occupational health care/laboratory associated infection. Specific guidance on the use of PEP can be found at: https://www.cdc.gov/hiv/basics/pep.html. Facilities where occupational exposure can occur are encouraged to educate employees on the use of PEP and have systems in place to ensure employees have access to PEP

**6. Nonhuman hosts**—There are no known natural nonhuman hosts for HIV. However, HIV can infect chimpanzees in research settings, and hybrid simian immunodeficiency virus (SIV)/HIV chimeras (SHIVs) that are used in primate models of HIV infection can infect various nonhuman primates including macaques and chimpanzees. Furthermore, it has been shown that SIV (a primate virus thought to be the ancestor of HIV) can infect humans and thus work with primate samples containing HIV, SIV, or SHIV should be handled with the same precautions as human specimens.

**7. Sample/specimen requirements**—Various sample types can be used for HIV testing that is conducted using commercially available assays. These include fresh oral fluid and fresh fingerstick whole blood for rapid, single-use, point-of-care devices, dried blood spots (DBS) for laboratory-based antibody and nucleic acid tests, and serum/plasma for laboratory tests that detect antigens antibodies and nucleic acid (RNA/deoxyribonucleic acid [DNA]). Dried blood spot storage and transport can occur at room temperature if DBS are properly prepared (i.e., completely dried and stored with dessicants). Recommended specimen handling requirements are specified in commercial tests, and the test specific guidance should be followed to ensure regulatory compliance when testing in the USA and proper test performance in all locations. In general, whole blood collected for serum and plasma testing is stored at room temperature or 2°C–8°C prior to being processed to serum or plasma. Processing of whole blood should occur in the range of 12–72 hours after the blood draw for most tests, and in rare cases, unprocessed blood storage can extend up to 7 days at 2°C–8°C. Once blood has been processed to serum and plasma, storage at 2°C–8°C is common for up to a week, with extended storage at –20°C.

HIV nucleic acids can be detected in other body tissues and fluids such as breast milk, cerebrospinal fluid, semen, and vaginal secretions, but there are no commercially available tests, and exact handling requirements are defined by the test that is being performed. Testing facilities should be contacted prior to collection, storage, and shipment of such specimens to determine specific specimen handling requirements.

**8. Testing requirements**—HIV testing is generally performed by using an algorithm that consists of a series of tests to reach a definitive diagnosis. The algorithm used is generally defined by the geographic location of the testing. Most developed countries have defined algorithms. In the USA, algorithms are recommended by CDC. Currently, the recommended algorithm consists of screening with a combination antigen/antibody test, followed by an HIV-1/HIV-2 antibody differentiation assay to confirm reactive antibody results. In situations where the differentiation test result is discordant with the antigen/antibody result, a HIV-1 RNA nucleic acid test is recommended to confirm acute infection. Detailed information can be found at: https://stacks.cdc.gov/view/cdc/23447. For other countries, and specifically for developing countries, WHO provides recommendations for testing approaches and algorithms. The algorithm recommendations are linked to the prevalence of HIV in the given population. Currently, WHO recommends that any reactive HIV test result be confirmed with a second assay (in settings where prevalence is ≥5%) or with both a second and third assay (in settings where prevalence is <5%). The following link contains detailed information from WHO, http://apps.who.int/iris/bitstream/10665/179870/1/9789241508926_eng.pdf?ua=1&ua=1.

Sensitivity and specificity for HIV tests are very high. For example, in the USA, all HIV diagnostic tests approved by the FDA, except the over the counter home test, have point estimates for sensitivity in established infections (post-acute phase) that range from 99.3%–100%. Specificity point estimates range from 99.3%–100%. In general, commercial tests outside the USA have comparable reported sensitivities and specificities, but in some countries, there is less regulatory oversight to confirm the reported values.

**9. Reporting requirements**—HIV/AIDS is a reportable condition under the International Health Regulations. In most jurisdictions globally, laboratories, as well as health care providers are required to report positive HIV findings to the public health authorities. See Special Considerations section in this chapter for further information related to regulatory reporting and HIV surveillance.

For clinical reporting, all results from a single test (rapid or laboratory-based) are considered preliminary. With the exception of the rapid, single-use, point-of-care tests, preliminary results are generally not reported to individuals. In most cases, the final conclusion from the testing algorithm is reported. The most common reports are HIV positive (multiple reactive results were obtained in the algorithm), HIV indeterminate (generally corresponds to detection of some antibody reactivity, but could not be definitively confirmed by the algorithm that was used) and HIV negative (corresponds to no detection of HIV antigen or antibody, and in cases where nucleic acid testing was performed, no evidence of viral nucleic acid).

**10. Referral network**—There is no one specific referral network for HIV testing. However, in the USA, many state and local health departments can provide testing or refer individuals to clinics that conduct testing within their jurisdiction. Other countries have similar systems in place to refer individuals for HIV testing. Laboratories that require additional HIV testing support should utilize the normal process which is in place for their respective jurisdictions.

**11. Special considerations**—The surveillance criteria is as follows:

1) In the USA, HIV infection is a nationally notifiable disease and must be reported to state health departments. CDC provides the definition for a case. The CDC criteria for a confirmed case can be met by either laboratory evidence or clinical evidence, as described later. Laboratory evidence is preferred over clinical evidence. For persons aged 18 months and older and for children younger than 18 months whose mothers were not infected, laboratory criteria require reporting of the date of the specimen collection for positive test results in multitest algorithms or stand-alone virologic tests and enough information about the tests to determine that they meet any of the following criteria: a positive (reactive) result from an initial HIV antibody or combination antigen/antibody test, and an accompanying or subsequent positive result from a supplemental HIV test different from the initial test. A case can also be defined by a documented positive result or report of a detectable quantity from any of the following HIV virologic (i.e., nonantibody) tests: qualitative HIV nucleic acid amplification test (NAT; DNA or RNA), quantitative HIV NAT (i.e., viral load assay), HIV-1 p24 antigen test, HIV isolation (i.e., viral culture), or HIV nucleotide sequence (i.e., genotype). For children younger than 18 months born to mothers who have an unknown infection status or were known to be infected, a case is defined by a documented positive result or report of a detectable quantity from any of the following HIV virologic (i.e., nonantibody) tests: qualitative HIV NAT (DNA or RNA), quantitative HIV NAT (i.e., viral load assay), HIV-1 p24 antigen test, HIV isolation (i.e, viral culture), or HIV nucleotide sequence (i.e., genotype). Clinical criteria for defining a case are met by the combination of a note in a medical record by a physician or other qualified medical care provider that states that the patient has HIV infection and presumptive evidence of HIV infection (e.g., receipt of HIV antiretroviral therapy or prophylaxis for an opportunistic infection), an otherwise unexplained low CD4+ T-lymphocyte count, or an otherwise unexplained diagnosis of an opportunistic illness. More detailed information about HIV cases definitions can be found at: https://www.cdc.gov/mmwr/preview/mmwrhtml/rr6303a1.htm.
2) Outside the USA, multiple countries monitor HIV infections and associated deaths. WHO and UNAIDS work with national AIDS

programs to generate and publish country and global surveillance reports. WHO recommends the following for defining a case: "A case of HIV infection is defined as an individual with HIV infection irrespective of clinical stage (including severe or stage 4 clinical disease, also known as AIDS) confirmed by laboratory criteria according to country definitions and requirements."[1] Further information regarding WHO HIV surveillance procedures and reports can be found at: http://www.who.int/hiv/topics/me/en.

## References

1. World Health Organization. WHO case definitions of HIV for surveillance and revised clinical staging and immunological classification of HIV-related disease in adults and children. 2007. Available at: https://www.who.int/hiv/pub/guidelines/HIVstaging150307.pdf. Accessed March 25, 2019.

[S. M. Owen]

# HOOKWORM

| DISEASE | ICD-10 CODE |
|---|---|
| HOOKWORM | ICD-10 B76 |
| Cutaneous larva migrans (See "Larva Migrans") | |

**1. Clinical features**—A common chronic helminth infection of the intestine that causes anemia with a variety of symptoms, usually in proportion to the degree of iron deficiency. In heavy infections, the bloodletting activity of the nematode leads to iron deficiency and hypochromic, microcytic anemia, the major cause of disability. Children with heavy long-term infection may have hypoproteinemia and may have retarded mental and physical development. Occasionally, severe acute pulmonary and gastrointestinal reactions follow exposure to infective larvae. Light hookworm infections generally produce few or no clinical effects. Some species of the causative helminth are unable to survive in the skin and do not cause intestinal infection.

**2. Causative agents**—Patent hookworm infection: *Ancylostoma duodenale*, *Ancylostoma ceylanicum*, and *Necator americanus*. Eosinophilic enteritis: *Ancylostoma caninum*. Cutaneous larva migrans: *Ancylostoma braziliense* and *Uncinaria stenocephala*, possibly *Ancylostoma tubaeforme*, *Bunostomum phlebotomum*, and other zoonotic hookworm species.

**3. Laboratory diagnosis**—The standard method for diagnosing hookworm infection is by identifying hookworm eggs and larvae in a stool sample using microscopic techniques. The eggs of all hookworm species are ovoid or ellipsoidal, thin-shelled, colorless, 55–75 μm in length, and contain a central morula that will develop into a motile larva over 24 hours in unrefrigerated or preserved stool. The eggs of *Ancylostoma* and *Necator* cannot be reliably differentiated microscopically. In fecal samples that have not been preserved, rhabditiform (L1) larvae of hookworm may be seen. These may be differentiated from rhabditiform larvae of *Strongyloides* spp. by the presence of a long buccal cavity and absence of a prominent rhomboid genital primordium. Adult worms are rarely seen except via endoscopy, surgery, or autopsy but, if found, allow for definitive species identification based upon the morphology of the buccal cavity and male bursa. Molecular assays for identification of hookworm deoxyribonucleic acid in stool have been described. Cutaneous larva migrans is diagnosed by clinical observation alone. Eosinophilic enteritis may be diagnosed by the recovery of immature *A. caninum* on endoscopy. *A. caninum* serology has been used in diagnosis of eosinophilic enteritis for research purposes. There are no FDA-approved molecular tests for the diagnosis of hookworm disease.

**4. Laboratory capability**—Clinical diagnostic laboratory with trained fecal parasitic microscopists for microscopy. Species identification based on larval and adult worms requires advanced microscopist level skills.

**5. Safety requirements**—Infective larva in old stool samples are capable of transdermal migration and universal/standard precautions should be followed at all times. Formalin used for fixation should only be used in a well-ventilated area, preferably in a chemical fume hood. Unpreserved and preserved stools and sera should be disposed of as infectious waste.

**6. Nonhuman hosts**—Zoonotic species causing human intestinal disease are *A. ceylanicum* (humans, dogs and cats) and *A. caninum*. Zoonotic species causing cutaneous larva migrans are *A. braziliense* and *U. stenocephala* (dogs and cats), *A. tubaeforme* (cats only), and *B. phlebotomum* (cattle, sheep, and goats).

**7. Sample/specimen requirements**—For microscopic detection, use fresh (within 24 hours of passage) feces or feces preserved in 10% formalin, sodium acetate formalin, polyvinyl alcohol, or other commercial fixatives. Up to 3 fecal samples collected on separate days should be analyzed to exclude infection.

**8. Testing requirements**—Identification of eggs in feces is both diagnostic and confirmatory. Concentration procedures and subsequent microscopy are more sensitive than direct smear examinations. Individual providers will include hookworm eggs in external quality assurance programs for the morphological identification of intestinal parasites.

**9. Reporting requirements**—Report eggs of hookworm, but do not report species from egg identification alone. Report larva of hookworm, but species may be confused unless reviewed by a highly experienced morphologist. Report exact species based only upon adult worm morphology or molecular identification. Reporting of hookworm infections by laboratories to public health authorities is not normally required.

**10. Referral network**—Networks vary among countries. First line laboratories may identify eggs or larva in culture. Reference laboratories may perform molecular analysis or, based on morphology, species identification of adult worms. CDC DPDx service in the USA will identify adult worms to species level and assist with identification of eggs.

**11. Special considerations**—Exposure of humans to larva of some animal hookworms may lead to self-limited subcutaneous migration of infective larvae (cutaneous larva migrans) with associated pruritis and erythema which may persist for several months. Humans may also be aberrant hosts for the canine hookworm, *A. caninum*. This species does not reach maturity in the human gut, but it may cause eosinophilic enteritis; characterized by severe abdominal pain, diarrhea, weight loss, and melena. Peripheral eosinophilia is a common finding in all types of human hookworm infections.

Infective (L3) larvae will take from 5–20 minutes to penetrate the skin after exposure. Effective larvicidal agents for the killing of L3 larvae (≥ 90% mortality) are water at 70°C (5 minutes) or 70% ethanol (5 minutes). Exposure to 10% formalin takes 20 minutes; 1% bleach and 2% glutaraldehyde are ineffective.

[R. S. Bradbury]

# HUMAN PAPILLOMAVIRUS

| DISEASE | ICD-10 CODE |
|---|---|
| WARTS | ICD-10 B07 |
| GENITAL WARTS | ICD 10 A63 |
| CERVICAL CANCER | ICD-10 C53 |
| VULVAR CANCER | ICD-10 C51 |
| VAGINAL CANCER | ICD-10 C52 |
| PENILE CANCER | ICD-10 C60 |
| ANAL CANCER | ICD-10 C21 |
| OROPHARYNGEAL CANCER | ICD-10 C10 |

Clinical manifestations of infection with human papillomavirus (HPV) include warts (verruca) and cancers, including cervical, vulvar, vaginal, penile, anal, and oropharyngeal. There are more than 100 HPV types, and more than 40 types can infect the anogenital tract in both males and females.

Most HPV infections are asymptomatic, subclinical, or unrecognized. With respect to warts, laboratory testing is rarely indicated; when it is indicated, the biopsied samples are examined histologically.

**1. Clinical features**—In most of these cancers, invasive cancer is preceded by a preinvasive phase recognized histologically as intraepithelial neoplasia. Clinically, intraepithelial neoplasia can present as atypical lesions or skin changes, with pigmentation, erythema, very large size, or lesions that are fixed to or show induration of the underlying skin or mucosa. On the cervix, there are characteristic changes that are detected by Papanicolau (Pap) smear or by HPV deoxyribonucleic acid (DNA), which may lead to colposcopic evaluation and biopsy. In the past, clinical forms of mucocutaneous intraepithelial neoplasia have been called Bowen's disease, bowenoid papillomatosis, or erythroplasia of Queyrat; these terms have been recently replaced with the term vaginal intraepithelial neoplasia. Although the majority of cutaneous HPV cause warts, epidermodysplasia verruciformis is a rare condition caused by cutaneous HPV (usually HPV 5), which may progress to cutaneous carcinoma.

**2. Causative agents**—Cervical cancer is caused by several genotypes of HPV, with HPV genotypes 16 and 18 accounting for more than 70%. Preliminary studies have shown evidence of vaccine protection against HPV-related cancers.[1]

**3. Laboratory diagnosis**—Pap smear is a cytology test used to screen for premalignant and malignant changes in epithelial cells. Pap smears require further follow-up tests such as colposcopy, biopsy, and HPV DNA.

HPV can be detected by DNA testing. There are several molecular assays available for HPV DNA testing. The *digene* HC2 High-Risk HPV DNA Test (QIAGEN, Gaithersburg, MD) has traditionally been used for HPV DNA detection in diagnostic laboratories. However, newer, more advanced DNA detection assays have shown superior performance and higher analytical sensitivity.[2]

Routine Pap testing is being replaced with HPV nucleic acid amplification-based primary screening. This approach to HPV DNA for primary screening is being considered by many countries with the Netherlands having implemented it in early 2017 and Australia in late 2017.[3,4]

**4. Laboratory capability**—Laboratory staff must be competently trained and experienced in the detection of HPV. Pap test involves examining and differentiating cells in smear preparations using a cytological staining technique. Pap smear testing requires proficiently trained cytopathologists and cytotechnologists to perform cytological staining and differentiation and interpretation of the stained smear.

DNA testing requires trained, competent molecular microbiologists to perform polymerase chain reaction (PCR) testing and result analysis and interpretation. DNA testing involves extracting nucleic acid from a patient sample to be used in a PCR assay that targets specific genes known to be present in the virus.

Ongoing proficiency is performed through sufficient training, education, audits, and quality assurance. Laboratories must enroll in quality assurance programs and meet all regulated quality requirements in accordance with their government.

Laboratory accreditation is performed by approved accrediting organizations.

Quality assurance (QA) and quality control is an ongoing comprehensive approach to monitor and ensure true results are obtained. It is a way to ensure each platform is used in accordance with guidelines only by properly qualified and appropriately trained laboratory staff.

**5. Safety requirements**—Biosafety level 2 practices, personal protective equipment, and containment equipment and facilities are recommended for laboratory staff working with clinical specimens or materials known to contain or that may contain HPV.

Risk assessments for processes and substances relating to HPV assays should be performed before implementing an assay and when a deviation from the normal method is implemented. The goal of performing risk assessments is to consider all hazards and risks associated with processing and testing and to reduce the risk. Risks for HPV testing include cross-contamination and carry-over contamination, specimen mix-up, and use of dangerous chemicals and reagents for testing.

Contamination and specimen mix-up could occur at the specimen collection preanalytical stage, during testing at the analytical stage, or at the post-analytical stage during analysis, interpretation, and reporting. The most critical steps of testing require risk assessments to determine ways of reducing and eliminating contamination.

Good management and use of adequate personal protective equipment at all stages of HPV testing is required to minimize risk.

**6. Nonhuman hosts**—Human papillomaviruses only infect humans.

**7. Sample/specimen requirements**—Liquid-based cytology sample is the most common sample type. Samples can be transported at 2°C–30°C and stored at 2°C–8°C for up to 6 months. Liquid-based cytology samples are used to prepare smears but can also be used for HPV DNA testing.

Swab or brush sample can be collected for HPV DNA testing. Samples can be transported at 2°C–30°C depending on the transport and storage media.

**8. Testing requirements**—The assays currently approved by FDA for the detection of 13–14 high-risk HPV types include the following: Aptima HPV Assay (Hologic, San Diego, CA) and BD Onclarity HPV Assay (Becton, Dickinson and Company, Sparks, MD), Cervista HPV HR Assay and Cervista HPV 16/18 Test (Hologic), Cobas HPV Test (Roche Molecular Diagnostics, Pleasanton, CA), and *digene* HC2 High-Risk HPV DNA Test (Qiagen, Germantown, MD).

BD Onclarity HPV Assay, Cervista HPV 16/18 Test, and Cobas HPV Test provide HPV 16 and 18 genotyping results. Aptima HPV Assay, Cervista HPV HR Assay, and *digene* HC2 High-Risk HPV DNA Test detect the presence of 1 or more high-risk HPV genotypes without differentiation. No HPV tests are currently approved for use in males or for other mucosal and cutaneous genotypes.

**9. Reporting requirements**—CDC's National Program of Cancer Registries and the National Cancer Institute's Surveillance, Epidemiology, and End Results Program both have registries that measure disease burden from cervical and other HPV-related cancers. The requirements for reporting cases of cervical cancer in other countries may vary.

**10. Referral network**—WHO HPV Laboratory Network (LabNet) was established to support effective HPV surveillance and vaccination impact monitoring and improve the quality of laboratory testing through training and QA.

LabNet established the first WHO international standards for HPV genotypes 6, 11, 16, 18, 31, 33, 45, 52, and 58 DNA. LabNet developed an international HPV genotyping panel for QA and proficiency testing and distributed the panel to laboratories globally for evaluation and assessment of different HPV genotyping assays. WHO HPV LabNet information can be found at: http://www.who.int/biologicals/vaccines/hpv/en.

**11. Special considerations**—None.

For further information on warts, see "Human Papillomavirus Infection" in *CCDM20*. For further HPV information, see:

- http://www.cdc.gov/std/treatment
- http://www.who.int/topics/sexually_transmitted_infections/en
- http://www.who.int/biologicals/vaccines/hpv/en

## References

1. Luostarinen T, Apter D, Dillner J, et al. Vaccination protects against invasive HPV-associated cancers. *Int J Cancer*. 2018;(10):2186–2187.

2. Phillips S, Garland SM, Tan JH, Quinn MA, Tabrizi SN. Comparison of the Roche® 4800 HPV assay to Digene Hybrid Capture 2, Roche Linear Array and Roche Amplicor for detection of high-risk papillomavirus genotypes in women undergoing treatment for cervical dysplasia. *J Clin Virol.* 2015;62:63-65.
3. van der Veen N. Framework for the execution of cervical cancer population screening. 2017. Available at: https://www.rivm.nl/documenten/framework-for-execution-of-cervical-cancer-population-screening. Accessed March 6, 2019.
4. Cancer Australia. Changes to the National Cervical Screening Program. 2017. Available at: https://canceraustralia.gov.au/about-us/news/changes-national-cervical-screening-program. Accessed March 6, 2019.

[A. G. Costa]

# HUMAN T-LYMPHOTROPIC VIRUS TYPE-1 INFECTION

| DISEASE | ICD-10 CODE |
|---|---|
| HUMAN T-LYMPHOTROPIC VIRUS TYPE-1 INFECTION (asymptomatic, carrier) | ICD-10 Z22.6 |
| ADULT T-CELL LYMPHOMA/LEUKEMIA (acute, chronic, lymphomatoid, smoldering) | ICD-10 C91.5 |
| HUMAN T-LYMPHOTROPIC VIRUS TYPE-1 INFECTION ASSOCIATED MYELOPATHY/TROPICAL SPASTIC PARAPARESIS | ICD-10 G04.1 |
| POLYMYOSITIS | ICD-10 B97.3 |
| UVEITIS | ICD-10 B97.3 |
| INFECTIVE DERMATITIS | ICD-10 B97.3 |
| BRONCHIECTASIS | ICD-10 B97.3 |

**1. Clinical features**—Human T-lymphotropic virus type-1 (HTLV-1) causes a lifelong infection that chiefly persists by clonal proliferation of infected CD4+ T-lymphocytes. HTLV-1 causes a number of clinical manifestations in less than 5% of HTLV-1 infected individuals while about 95% remain lifelong healthy asymptomatic carriers. The 2 most common diseases are an aggressive T-cell malignancy known as adult T-cell leukemia/lymphoma (ATL) and HTLV-1 associated myelopathy (formerly known as tropical spastic paraparesis), which clinically resembles primary progressive multiple sclerosis. In addition, HTLV-1 may cause inflammatory diseases such as polymyositis, uveitis, and infective dermatitis. It is recognized that there is a high incidence of bronchiectasis among HTLV-1 carriers. The mechanisms by which HTLV-1 causes diverse manifestations are unknown, but since no viral genotype is associated with clinical disease and there is a strong antiviral immune response, the currently accepted hypothesis is that the efficiency of the host immune response is the main determinant of disease.

**2. Causative agents**—There are at least 7 genotypes of HTLV-1 mostly based on geography (e.g., Australo-Melanesian, Central African, Central African/Pygmy, Cosmopolitan, and rare Central African types), but there is no clear association between viral genotype and disease. HTLV-2, related but distinct from HTLV-1, consists of 3 genotypes that target CD8 + T-lymphocytes; these cause little clinical disease but may cause chronic low-level inflammation. HTLV-3 and HTLV-4 are related, newly identified deltaretroviruses, but little is known about their pathogenicity.

**3. Laboratory diagnosis**—HTLV-1 antibody detection by enzyme immunoassay (EIA), with confirmation and differentiation of HTLV-1 and HTLV-2 by Western Blot (WB) or line immunoassays (LIAs). Polymerase chain reaction (PCR) can be used to resolve untypable or indeterminate WB or LIA results. Quantitative real-time PCR (qPCR) to quantify the HTLV-1 proviral load—the proportion of HTLV-1 infected mononuclear cells, which is important for determining risk of clinical disease (disease risk highest with proviral load > 4% in Japan and >10% in the Caribbean). In ATL tumor cells, demonstration of monoclonal integration of HTLV-1 provirus by Southern blot, or inverse/linker mediated PCR, or whole genome sequencing techniques (to distinguish ATL from other incidental T-cell malignancies in asymptomatic HTLV-1 carriers). While HTLV-3 and HTLV-4 were detected using HTLV-1/2 screening assays and generic HTLV PCR assays, the sensitivity and specificity for their detection with these assays is currently unknown.

**4. Laboratory capability**—Institutions should have practices, equipment, facility design, and construction that meet biosafety level 2 (BSL-2) facility requirements, and preferably BSL-3 when working with concentrated virus stocks. Clinical laboratories testing biomaterials should use universal/standard precautions with all potentially infectious specimens. Training in standard microbiological procedures and practices, working with blood-borne pathogens, and using biosafety equipment are common. In Clinical Laboratory Improvements Amendments (CLIA)-certified laboratories specialized training is also required specific to the test performed. Personnel are supervised by scientists, clinicians, and others who are competent in handling infectious agents and in performing associated procedures.

**5. Safety requirements**—*Biosafety in Microbiological and Biomedical Laboratories*, 5th Edition (*BMBL*) describes retroviruses, including

HTLV, as BSL-2 pathogens, but suggests using BSL-3 procedures when working with concentrated virus stocks (see: https://www.cdc.gov/biosafety/publications/bmbl5). *BMBL* procedures also recommend limiting the use of needles, syringes, and other sharp objects; working with biomaterials in biological safety cabinets if aerosol can be produced; use of personal protective equipment and splash guards; and use of disinfectants such as 10% bleach, 70% ethanol, or 3% Lysol for decontamination of surfaces, equipment, and spills, when appropriate. Hepatitis vaccination is required for persons working with human blood and other body fluids. Specimen shipping should follow the rules of the US Department of Transportation or the International Air Transport Association.

**6. Nonhuman hosts**—Nonhuman primates (NHPs) are natural hosts for simian T-cell lymphotropic viruses (STLV) that are closely related to HTLV. These include STLV-1, STLV-2, STLV-3, and STLV-4. T-cell lymphoma and leukemia have been observed in STLV-1-infected NHPs. STLVs are believed to be the original source of HTLV in humans with both ancient and contemporary zoonotic infection occurring in persons exposed to infected material from NHPs. Persons exposed to NHPs in the wild or in captivity, including hunters and workers at zoos and research institutions, may be at risk for infection with STLV and their associated diseases.[1]

**7. Sample/specimen requirements**—Serum or plasma is suitable for use in serologic assays for HTLV antibody detection. Serum/plasma specimens can be stored at 4°C or frozen for later use. PCR can also be used to detect HTLV sequences but requires deoxyribonucleic acid (DNA) from peripheral blood mononuclear cells (PBMCs). HTLV is not shed in plasma or serum and is not detectable in these specimens by PCR. PBMCs are typically isolated from fresh ethylenediaminetetraacetic acid (EDTA)- or anticoagulant citrate dextrose solution (ACD)-treated whole blood on a Ficoll-Hypaque gradient. Whole blood should be shipped within 24 hours on cold packs using a next-morning delivery service. Heparin as a blood anticoagulant is not recommended for PCR testing because it can inhibit the amplification reaction. PBMC DNA is prepared using standard methods and can be stored at -20°C or lower until needed. PBMCs can also be used for virus isolation by cell culture, which is used in research studies.

**8. Testing requirements**—All testing should be performed following the 1988 CLIA laboratory standards and certification or similar international quality management regulations to ensure the quality of the reported test results.

The serologic testing algorithm consists of a primary screening assay followed by additional testing for confirmation and identification of HTLV type. Screening assays detect antibodies to HTLV in serum or plasma. The immunodominant regions of structural and regulatory proteins are well characterized and are used in diagnostic assays that detect and differentiate HTLV-1 and HTLV-2. Some commercial tests still use the old Roman numeral nomenclature (I or II) for HTLV-1 and -2, respectively. HTLV-3 and -4 have only been identified in small numbers of persons in Africa. Commercial serologic and PCR assays for the specific detection and discrimination of HTLV-3 and -4 are not currently available.

Primary screening assays include EIA, chemiluminescent immunoassays (ChLIA), particle agglutination (Fujirebio America, Fairfield, NJ), and immunofluorescence assays (IFAs). EIAs are sensitive and simple colorimetric tests that use purified HTLV-1 and -2-infected cell lysates and/or recombinant antigens or synthetic peptides. ChLIA is similar to EIA but uses chemiluminescence for the detection step. EIA and ChLIA can be automated and performed on a large scale. However, neither EIAs nor ChLIAs can differentiate between HTLV-1 and HTLV-2 infection because of significant antigenic similarity of the structural proteins in both viruses; therefore, these screening assays are referred to as tests for HTLV-1/2.

Comparison of various commercial screening assays containing both HTLV-1 and HTLV-2 antigens indicates that sensitivity ranges from 98.9%–100% for HTLV-1 and 91.5% –100% for HTLV-2.[2] Specificity ranged from 90.2%–100%. Currently, one HTLV-1/2 EIA (Avioq HTLV-I/II Microelisa System, Avioq, Research Triangle Park, NC) and one HTLV-1/2 ChLIA (Abbott PRISM HTLV-I/HTLV-II, Abbott Laboratories, Chicago, IL) are licensed by FDA and are available for use in the USA.[2] Both assays have reported overall sensitivity point estimates of 100% (95% confidence interval [CI] of 99.97%–100% for Avioq; 99.89%–99.96% for Abbott). Specificity of 99.93% (95% CI of 99.89%–99.96%) for Abbott and 99.95% for Avioq (95% CI of 99.89%–99.98%) were reported from clinical trial data that supported the licensure of these tests.[2] Both assays can be used for blood donor screening and as an aid in clinical diagnosis of HTLV-1 and HTLV-2 infection. The Avioq test can also be used with serum and plasma for deceased organ and tissue donors, while the Abbott test can be used to screen organ donors if specimens are obtained while the donor's heart is still beating. Further attempts have been made to develop a dual EIA algorithm to increase the predictive values of HTLV testing.[2] Pooling of samples for seroepidemiologic studies has been proposed but is not recommended for blood donor testing

Supplemental confirmatory or differentiation tests for HTLV-1 and HTLV-2 infection include Western blots (WB) containing viral lysates supplemented with recombinant proteins, and LIAs and IFAs.[2] An FDA-approved second-generation supplemental confirmatory WB assay contains type-specific gp46 envelope (Env) recombinant proteins from HTLV-1 and -2 and a truncated form of recombinant p21 Env (r21e) that reduces nonspecific reactivity, improves performance (specificity and sensitivity), and allows differentiation between HTLV-1 and HTLV-2 (MP Diagnostics WB 2.4, MP Biomedicals, Santa Ana, CA). The HTLV WB 2.4 assay is approved for using human serum and plasma specimens. The reported sensitivity and specificity of the HTLV WB 2.4 was 97.50% (95% CI of 94.26%–99.18%) and 100% (95% CI of 98.17%–100%), respectively.[2]

The LIA test consists of recombinant and synthetic HTLV-1 and HTLV-2–specific antigens printed onto strips (INNO-LIA HTLV I/II Score, Fujirebio US, Malvern, PA); this assay can differentiate between HTLV-1 and HTLV-2 infection. The LIA test does not have FDA approval but is certified for use in Europe and other areas of endemicity to confirm any repeatedly EIA-reactive sample. However, some commercial and clinical labs offer INNO-LIA as a confirmatory assay with the disclaimer that the test has not been cleared or approved by FDA, and it should not be used for diagnosis without confirmation by other medically established means. IFAs are research assays that detect binding of antibodies from a specimen to HTLV-1- or HTLV-2-infected cells and can also be used to discriminate HTLV-1/2 infections and to determine antibody titer.

Fresh whole blood specimens are used for qualitative nucleic acid testing in PBMC DNA. HTLV-1 or HTLV-2 specific PCR amplification can be used to confirm and type infection. While FDA-approved PCR kits are not available some PCR assays are commercially available using in-house tests.

**9. Reporting requirements—**HTLV is not a reportable infectious disease in the USA. Blood donations are screened for HTLV-1/2. Blood donors whose serum/plasma are confirmed as seropositive for HTLV-1/2 are notified and permanently deferred from donating blood. Blood donors repeatedly reactive on screening tests but not confirmed HTLV-1/2–seropositive on 2 separate donations are also notified and deferred. Recipients of organs and tissues from confirmed HTLV-1–positive donors as well as the transplant programs receiving organs from the donor should be informed of the HTLV results. All recipients found to be HTLV-1–positive posttransplant due to possible donor-derived infection must be reported to the Organ Procurement and Transplantation Network (OPTN) Improving Patient Safety Portal (https://portal.unos.org) as a potential donor-derived disease transmission.[3]

**10. Referral network—**

- International Retrovirology Association: https://htlv.net.
- HTLVaware: http://www.htlvaware.com/further-info.html.
- Recommendations for counseling persons infected with HTLV-1/2: https://www.cdc.gov/mmwr/preview/mmwrhtml/00021234.htm.

**11. Special considerations—**None.

## References

1. Enose-Akahata Y, Caruso B, Haner B, et al. Development of HTLV-1 associated myelopathy/tropical spastic paraparesis in a patient with simian T-lymphotropic virus type 1-like infection. *Retrovirology*. 2015;12(suppl 1):030.

2. Switzer WM, Heneine W, Owen SM. Human T-Cell Lymphotropic Viruses. In: Jorgensen JH, Pfaller M, eds. *Manual of Clinical Microbiology*. Washington, DC: ASM Press; 2015.
3. Organ Procurement and Transplantation Network. Policies. 15.4. 2019. Available at: https://optn.transplant.hrsa.gov/media/1200/optn_policies.pdf. Accessed March 6, 2019.

[W. Heneine, W. M. Switzer]

# INFLUENZA

| DISEASE | ICD-10 CODE |
|---|---|
| SEASONAL INFLUENZA | ICD-10 J10, J11 |
| OTHER INFLUENZA | ICD-10 J09 |

**1. Clinical features—**

1) Seasonal influenza: an acute viral disease of the respiratory tract characterized by fever, cough (usually dry), headache, myalgia, prostration, coryza, and sore throat. Cough is often severe and can last 2 or more weeks; fever and other symptoms generally resolve in 5–7 days. Syndromes consistent with influenza include acute upper respiratory illness, croup, bronchiolitis, febrile seizures, and pneumonia. In children, gastrointestinal (GI) tract manifestations (nausea, vomiting, diarrhea) may accompany the respiratory phase and have been reported in up to 25% of children in school outbreaks of influenza A and B. Gastrointestinal manifestations are uncommon in adults. Infants may present with atypical symptoms or a sepsis-like syndrome. Geriatric patients may not present with typical influenza-like symptoms but can present with exacerbation of underlying conditions such as congestive heart failure and may not have an elevated temperature.

   Complications of influenza include lower respiratory tract involvement such as bronchitis and pneumonitis; bacterial pneumonia caused by common community-acquired pneumonia pathogens such as *Streptococcus pneumoniae* and *Staphylococcus aureus* (associated with higher mortality and significant proportion being methicillin-resistant *S. aureus* [MRSA]); viral pneumonia; exacerbation of underlying chronic conditions; sinusitis; otitis media; febrile seizures; encephalitis/encephalopathy;

rhabdomyolysis; myocarditis; myositis; and Reye syndrome in association with use of salicylates (aspirin). Although seasonal influenza deaths can occur in any age group, more than 90% of influenza deaths occur among those aged 65 years and older. Annual epidemics of influenza can be explosive and overwhelm health care services.

2) Other influenza: humans can also be infected with influenza viruses that are circulating in animals, such as avian influenza virus subtypes A (H5N1), A (H7N9), and A (H9N2), and swine influenza virus subtypes A (H1N1) and (H3N2). Other species including horses and dogs also have their own varieties of influenza viruses. Even though these viruses may be named as the same subtype as viruses found in humans, all of these animal viruses are distinct from human influenza viruses and do not easily transmit between humans. However, some may occasionally infect humans, and may cause disease ranging from mild upper respiratory infection or conjunctivitis to severe pneumonia and even death. Usually these human infections of zoonotic influenza are acquired through direct contact with infected animals or contaminated environments and do not spread very far among humans. If such a virus acquired the capacity to spread easily among people either through adaptation or acquisition of certain genes from human viruses, it could start an epidemic or a pandemic. Pandemic viruses in the past have spread globally within weeks of detection. Modern air travel has facilitated the spread of a new pandemic virus leaving little time for vaccine development, manufacturing, or administration to the world's population. Planning for responses to pandemics ahead of actual pandemics is therefore critical for preparedness. Of the animal influenza virus infections of humans, avian influenza A (H5N1) has been the most studied.

Suspicion of a human infection with a zoonotic influenza A infection is heightened if illness has occurred after exposure to birds, pigs, or other animals that may be infected with influenza or exposure to their environments.

Human H5N1 illness, usually occurring after exposure to infected chickens or their environments, typically manifests as severe pneumonia. Common initial symptoms are fever (usually 38°C) and cough, plus signs and symptoms of lower respiratory tract involvement including dyspnea. Upper respiratory tract symptoms such as sore throat and coryza are present only sometimes. Gastrointestinal symptoms were frequently reported in cases in Thailand and Vietnam in 2004, but less frequently since

2005. Severe lower respiratory tract manifestations often develop early in the course of illness, and clinically apparent pneumonia with radiological changes has usually been found at presentation. The disease progresses rapidly, and often to an acute respiratory distress syndrome. Median times of 4 days from the onset of illness to hospitalization and 9–10 days from onset until death in fatal cases have been reported. Atypical presentations have included fever and diarrhea without pneumonia as well as fever with diarrhea and seizures progressing to coma. Common laboratory findings include leukopenia, lymphopenia, mild to moderate thrombocytopenia, and elevated levels of aminotransferases. Lymphopenia and increased levels of lactate dehydrogenase at presentation have been associated with a poor prognosis. Other reported abnormalities include elevated levels of creatine phosphokinase, hypoalbuminemia, and increased D-dimer levels and changes indicative of disseminated intravascular coagulopathy. Mild illnesses such as upper respiratory illnesses without clinical or radiological signs of pneumonia have been reported more frequently in children. Seroepidemiologic studies conducted since 2004 suggest that subclinical infection is uncommon.

The mortality among reported cases of zoonotic infection has been high (60% for A [H5N1]), but with differences between countries and over time. Potential explanation for the differences in mortality rates could be the differences in patient behaviors, types of exposure, time before case recognition, access to health care and/or clinical management, or differences in surveillance. The median age of patients with influenza A (H5N1) infection is approximately 18 years with 90% of patients aged 40 years or younger.

In most zoonotic influenza infections, with exception of A (H5N1), symptoms presented are similar to those for seasonal influenza infections. Until 2013, reported human infections with avian H7 influenza virus have mostly been subclinical, or with conjunctivitis, and mild respiratory tract symptoms with one fatal exception in the Netherlands. However, recent human infections with H7 influenza virus— influenza A (H7N9) virus in China—have caused severe disease and deaths.

**2. Causative agents**—Three types of seasonal influenza virus are recognized: A, B and C. Influenza A viruses are further divided into subtypes based on 2 viral surface glycoproteins: the hemagglutination and the neuraminidase. There are 18 different haemagglutinin subtypes and 11 different neuraminidase subtypes. The current subtypes of influenza A viruses circulating widely among humans are subtypes A (H1N1) and A (H3N2). Influenza B viruses are not divided into subtypes, but 2 antigenically and genetically distinct lineages of B viruses currently circulate among humans. Both influenza A and B viruses can cause seasonal epidemics and sporadic outbreaks. Influenza viruses are named based on their type, geographic site of detection, laboratory number, year of isolation, and subtype (e.g., A/New Caledonia/20/99 [H1N1], A/Brisbane/10/2007 [H3N2], B/Malaysia/2506/2004). Type C influenza is considered associated with sporadic cases of milder infection and minor localized outbreaks. Type C influenza imposes much less of a disease burden than influenza A and B. Levels of antibody against the haemagglutinin correlate reasonably well with protection against infection by human influenza viruses. The detailed role of antibody against the neuraminidase has been under study but is believed to contribute to the protection. Genes encoding these viral surface glycoproteins are continuously changing through mutations, a process termed "drift" that occurs during virus replication. The constant emergence of new influenza viruses through drift results in the need for the biannual review and, when needed, replacement of A (H1N1), A (H3N2), and B viruses that are contained in vaccines to be used in the northern and southern hemisphere influenza season. The constant emergence of drifted viruses is the main reason for yearly epidemics of seasonal influenza and why an individual can catch influenza illness multiple times over their lifetime.

In addition to antigenic drift, type A influenza viruses can also undergo dramatic change called antigenic shift, which often refers to a subtype influenza A virus bearing either a hemagglutination protein or a combination of hemagglutination and neuraminidase proteins that have not been in circulation among humans in recent years. The majority of the world's population will have no immunity against the new virus. If and when the new virus is capable of sustained human-to-human transmission, it means the start of a potential pandemic.

**3. Laboratory diagnosis**—Influenza may be clinically indistinguishable from disease caused by other respiratory viruses, such as rhinovirus, respiratory syncytial virus, parainfluenza, adenovirus, and other pathogens. In temperate climates, recognition of potential influenza is commonly based on clinical presentation during winter months with a syndrome consistent with influenza-like illness. Clinical diagnosis improves when influenza surveillance information is available to indicate influenza viruses are in circulation.

Laboratory confirmation of influenza infection can be done by a number of methods. Currently the primary test for the rapid detection of influenza viruses is reverse transcription polymerase chain reaction (RT-PCR) assay for the detection of virus-specific ribonucleic acid sequences from throat, nasal, and nasopharyngeal secretions or tracheal aspirate or washings. Other procedures include isolation of viruses from these specimens using cell culture or embryonated eggs and identification of viral antigens in nasopharyngeal cells and fluids (fluorescent antibody [FA] test or enzyme-linked immunosorbent assay [ELISA]). Demonstration of a 4-fold or greater rise in specific antibody titer between acute and convalescent sera using hemagglutination-inhibition or neutralization assays can also be used to confirm acute infection. A single serum specimen is not ideal for diagnosis of an acute infection. Ideally, respiratory specimens should be collected as early in the illness as possible. Virus shedding starts to wane by the third day of onset of symptoms, and, in most cases, virus is not detected after 5 days in adults, though virus shedding can occur longer in children and immunocompromised individuals.

Commercially available point-of-care tests have variable sensitivity (50%–70%) but good specificity (90%–95%). Thus, in the setting of a known influenza epidemic, negative results from patients with symptoms consistent with influenza must be interpreted cautiously. If excluding a false-negative result is important, then more sensitive testing should be considered (e.g., RT-PCR or viral culture).

4. **Laboratory capability**—The ability to test for the detection of influenza viruses varies depending on the test method employed. Testing methods range from simple to perform to highly complex, or those that require beyond normal expertise to perform. Most clinical and reference laboratories, including jurisdictional public health laboratories, have the capability to perform moderate to high complexity testing as designated by the Clinical Laboratory Improvement Amendments (CLIA), and staff must meet the appropriate qualifications and training necessary to perform these types of testing. CLIA-waived testing is performed in point-of-care facilities where testing may be performed at the bedside by staff with minimal training.

5. **Safety requirements**—Laboratory-acquired infection by influenza viruses is a safety risk, especially when new strains emerge. Biosafety level 2 laboratory practices and a class II biosafety cabinet should be used while handling and manipulating specimens that may potentially contain currently circulating human influenza strains (e.g., H1/H3/B), low pathogenic avian influenza (LPAI) strains (e.g., H1–4, H6, H8-10), or equine and swine influenza viruses. For handling these influenza types in infected animals, an animal biosafety level 2 facility is suitable. Any non-currently circulating, wild type human influenza (e.g., H2N2) strains or highly pathogenic avian influenza (HPAI) strains should be processed under biosafety level 3 or animal biosafety level 3 laboratory practices with a focus on the use of negative pressure, high-efficiency particulate air-filtered respirators, or positive air-purifying respirators while also following clothing change protocols.

The principal laboratory threats associated with influenza viruses are the inhalation of virus from aerosol generating tasks or by direct inoculation of mucous membranes from contact with virus-contaminated gloves after handling tissues or secretions from infected animals. Aerosolization of the influenza virus by infecting animals or by aspirating, dispensing, mixing, centrifuging, or otherwise manipulating virus-infected specimens is a major risk factor.

**6. Nonhuman hosts**—Infections caused by influenza viruses occur naturally in a wide range of animals, but mostly swine, horses, mink, wild aquatic mammals such as seals and whales, and the virus affects both domestic and wild avian species. The principle reservoir for most of the influenza A viruses are aquatic birds, and since the disease causes mostly asymptomatic or mild infection in the birds, it is relatively impossible to eliminate from nature. The different properties of the influenza A virus determine the severity of symptoms that birds express. Low pathogenic avian influenza viruses commonly cause outbreaks in poultry flocks and do not normally cause severe disease. On the other hand, HPAI viruses exhibit severe disease in birds, with the consequence resulting in high death rates among the aquatic bird population.

Animal influenza viruses, through direct or indirect contact, are capable of infecting humans and causing symptoms ranging from a mild infection to death.

**7. Sample/specimen requirements**—Specimens from the respiratory tract should be collected as close to illness onset as possible and preferably within 5 days of illness onset. Specimen types vary by the influenza detection method used. Typically, the preferred respiratory specimens for influenza testing include nasopharyngeal or nasal swab, and nasal wash or aspirate. A nasopharyngeal swab is collected by having the patient tip his or her head back, a swab is gently inserted into one of the nostrils until resistance is met, then the swab is rotated several times and withdrawn. Throat, sputum and other oropharyngeal specimens are less likely to contain the virus.

1) Rapid influenza diagnostic tests (RIDT): specimen types for RIDTs include nasopharyngeal swab, nasal swab, aspirate or wash, and throat swab.
2) Immunofluorescence assays (indirect or direct): specimen types for immunofluorescence assays include nasopharyngeal swab or wash, bronchial wash, and nasal or endotracheal aspirate.
3) RT-PCR: specimen types for RT-PCR include nasopharyngeal swab, throat swab, nasopharyngeal or bronchial wash, and nasal or endotracheal aspirate, and sputum.

4) Molecular assays: specimen types for rapid molecular assays include nasopharyngeal and nasal swabs.
5) Viral culture: specimen types for viral culture include nasopharyngeal swab, throat swab, nasopharyngeal or bronchial wash, nasal or endotracheal aspirate, and sputum. Specimens must be placed in Viral Transport Media.
6) Serology: the specimen type for influenza antibody detection is blood (serum).

**8. Testing requirements**—Some of the RIDT and rapid molecular assays are simple to perform, which results in their classification as waived testing by the FDA. These tests have no educational requirements or proficiency test requirements associated with them, though laboratories performing waived testing must ensure that they are complying with manufacturer's test requirements. FDA classifies many influenza tests as moderate or high complexity. These tests require an adequate facility with appropriate equipment and instruments to perform testing and a quality management system that includes requirements such as the verification of test performance and enrollment in an approved proficiency test program.

1) Viral culture: this is a high complexity laboratory assay according to FDA and requires tissue culture cells in which influenza virus will grow.
2) Serology: generally, not recommended is the diagnosis of influenza by serologic detection of antibody. Testing requires paired acute and convalescent serum samples to determine antibody titers, collected at least 10 days apart, to detect a 4-fold or greater increase in serum antibody levels. The time frame of this test makes this an impractical method for timely clinical decision-making.
3) Real-time PCR and rapid molecular assays/multiplex PCR assays: currently, these are the most sensitive and specific tests available for the detection of influenza virus. Depending on method used, results can be available within 1 hour to up to 6 hours after receipt of the specimen in the laboratory. These tests require specialized instrumentation and expertise in result interpretation.
4) Rapid influenza diagnostic tests: some of these tests only detect influenza type A; others can detect both type A and type B but not distinguish between the 2. Still others can detect and distinguish between influenza type A and type B.
5) Immunofluorescence assays: these assays require a fluorescent microscope and rely on the quality of the specimen collected since the identification of viruses found on or within the epithelial

cells from respiratory secretions is needed. Laboratory expertise in result interpretation is essential.

**9. Reporting requirements**—Laboratories must follow the reporting requirements of their jurisdictional health department. Most health departments require reporting of influenza-associated pediatric deaths, novel or variant influenza cases, and suspect or confirmed institutional outbreaks.

Public health laboratories and health departments in all 50 states, Puerto Rico, and the District of Columbia, as well as many clinical laboratories, health care providers, and emergency departments, participate in influenza surveillance throughout the USA. Several networks exist that collect vital data needed for CDC to determine where influenza activity is occurring in the USA, including WHO Collaborating Laboratories System and the National Respiratory and Enteric Virus Surveillance System.

WHO's Global Influenza Surveillance and Response System (GISRS) conducts international influenza surveillance from information provided by global National Influenza Centers (NICs), such as CDC, and the data is distributed via the global Web-based network, FluNet.

**10. Referring network**—Sentinel providers throughout each state and many clinical laboratories, health care providers, and emergency departments may forward specimens to their jurisdictional public health laboratory for virus screening or confirmatory testing. National Influenza Centers are sent a subset of these clinical specimens and perform preliminary analysis, generally viral propagation and antiviral susceptibility testing. National Influenza Centers then ship these representative specimens and isolated viruses to WHO Collaborating Centers for advanced antigenic and genetic analysis. The results form the basis for WHO recommendations on the configuration of each year's influenza vaccine, as well as to assess any potential for the virus to cause international disease distribution. National Influenza Centers form the backbone of WHO's GISRS.

The H5 Reference Laboratory is an additional component of the WHO GISRS. The H5 Reference Laboratory provides surveillance, preparedness, and response to avian influenza viruses. Any specimen from a patient suspected of being infected with an avian influenza should immediately be tested and forwarded to a WHO Collaborating Center for confirmatory testing.

**11. Special considerations**—

1) Reporting: weekly reporting from influenza sentinel surveillance sites is necessary to monitor disease activity (i.e., influenza-like illness and severe respiratory disease). Severe respiratory infection, especially when involving health care workers, should be

immediately reported and investigated. Unsubtypable or novel subtypes (including H5N1) of influenza infections should be forwarded to a qualified laboratory (jurisdictional public health laboratory) or a WHO Collaborating Center of the WHO GISRS for confirmation. Immediate notification of public health authorities and WHO is mandatory under the International Health Regulations.

2) Case definitions: the case definition for an influenza-like illness is an acute respiratory infection with a fever greater than or equal to 38°C; a cough; and onset within the last 10 days. The case definition for a severe acute respiratory infection is a history of fever or fever greater than or equal to 38°C, a cough, onset within the last 10 days; and patient requires hospitalization.

3) Epidemic measures: the severe and often disruptive effects of epidemic seasonal influenza on community activities may be reduced in part by effective health planning and education, particularly locally organized immunization programs for high-risk patients, their close contacts, and health care providers. Community surveillance for influenza illness, use of outbreak control measures, adherence to infection control recommendations, and reporting of surveillance and outbreak findings to the community are all important. Closure of individual schools can be a useful intervention during influenza outbreaks, with the greatest benefits occurring among school-age children when applied early in the course of the outbreak. The benefit has to be weighed against the cost of disruption. Hospital administrators should anticipate increased demand for medical care during epidemic periods and possible absenteeism of health care personnel as a result of influenza. Health care personnel should be immunized annually to minimize absenteeism and transmission of seasonal influenza from health care personnel to patients. In the same regard, laboratories should anticipate and plan for the increased demand for testing and for the possible absenteeism of laboratory staff who perform testing. Laboratories should maintain adequate test and ancillary supplies to ensure uninterrupted testing.

4) International measures: influenza is a disease under global surveillance coordinated by WHO. The following are recommended:

- Report regularly epidemiological and virological information to WHO electronic platforms (http://www.who.int/influenza/surveillance_monitoring/fluid/en; http://www.who.int/influenza/gisrs_laboratory/flunet/en).

- Respiratory specimens, throat and nasal swabs, nasopharyngeal swabs or aspirates, and paired blood samples may be sent to any WHO-recognized NIC (http://www.who.int/influenza/gisrs_laboratory/national_influenza_centres/list/en).
- Identify the causative virus in reports, and submit prototype virus to one of the WHO Centers for Reference and Research on Influenza in Atlanta, Beijing, London, Melbourne, or Tokyo (http://www.who.int/influenza/gisrs_laboratory/collaborating_centres/list/en).
- Conduct epidemiological studies; promptly identify and report viruses to national and international health agencies.
- Ensure sufficient commercial and/or governmental facilities provide rapid production of adequate quantities of vaccine, antiviral drugs and testing supplies, and maintain programs for vaccine and antiviral drug administration to high-risk persons and essential personnel.

## Bibliography

Atmar RL, Lindstrom SE. Influenza Viruses. In: Versalovic J, Carroll KC, Funke G, Jorgensen JH, Landry ML, Warnock DW, eds. *Manual of Clinical Microbiology*. 10th ed. Washington, DC: American Society for Microbiology Press; 2011:1333–1346.

Centers for Disease Control and Prevention. Information for clinicians on influenza virus testing. Available at: https://www.cdc.gov/flu/professionals/diagnosis. Accessed March 13, 2019.

Centers for Medicare & Medicaid Services. State operations manual. Appendix C: survey procedures and interpretive guidelines for laboratories and laboratory services. Rev. 166. 2017. Available at: https://www.cms.gov/Regulations-and-Guidance/Guidance/Manuals/Downloads/som107ap_c_lab.pdf. Accessed March 6, 2019.

Harper SA, Bradley JS, Englund JA, et al. Seasonal influenza in adults and children—diagnosis, treatment, chemoprophylaxis, and institutional outbreak management: clinical practice guidelines of the Infectious Diseases Society of America. *Clin Infect Dis*. 2009;48(8):1003–1032.

US Department of Health and Human Services, Centers for Disease Control and Prevention; National Institutes of Health. *Biosafety in Microbiological and Biomedical Laboratories*. 5th ed. 2009. Available at: https://www.cdc.gov/labs/pdf/CDC-BiosafetyMicrobiologicalBiomedicalLaboratories-2009-P.PDF. Accessed March 6, 2019.

World Health Organization. Influenza. Available at: https://www.who.int/influenza/en. Accessed March 13, 2019.

[B. Cote, M. A. Pentella]

# JAPANESE ENCEPHALITIS

| DISEASE | ICD-10 CODE |
|---|---|
| JAPANESE ENCEPHALITIS | ICD-10 A83.0 |

**1. Clinical features**—The majority of human infections with Japanese encephalitis (JE) virus are asymptomatic; fewer than 1% of people infected develop clinical disease. Acute encephalitis is the most commonly recognized clinical presentation. Milder forms of disease such as aseptic meningitis or undifferentiated febrile illness also occur.

Among persons who develop clinical disease, initial symptoms are usually nonspecific and may include fever, diarrhea, headache, and vomiting. Subsequently, mental status changes, generalized weakness, focal neurologic deficits (e.g., paresis and cranial nerve palsies), and/or movement disorders might occur. Seizures are very common, especially among children, sometimes manifesting as subtle clinical findings (e.g., twitching of a digit, eye deviation, or irregular breathing).

A distinctive clinical presentation is a Parkinsonian syndrome resulting from extrapyramidal system involvement; findings include a flat, mask-like face with wide unblinking eyes, tremor, cogwheel rigidity, and choreoathetoid movements. In some patients, JE virus infection may result in a poliomyelitis-like acute flaccid paralysis due to anterior horn cell damage, without any alteration in consciousness. After a brief febrile illness, flaccid paralysis occurs in one or more limbs, usually asymmetric, and more common in the lower than upper limbs. About 30% of these patients subsequently develop encephalitis. Abnormal behavior or acute psychosis may also be the initial clinical presentation in some patients. JE has a case-fatality ratio of approximately 20%–30%. About 30%–50% of survivors have long-term neurologic or psychiatric sequelae. JE virus infection should be considered in the differential diagnosis of acute neurologic or febrile illnesses in persons who have been in areas where JE virus transmission occurs. The differential diagnosis is broad and includes many infectious and noninfectious causes.

**2. Causative agents**—Japanese encephalitis virus, of the family *Flaviviridae* and genus *Flavivirus*.

**3. Laboratory diagnosis**—Confirmed most frequently by detection of virus-specific antibody in cerebrospinal fluid (CSF) or serum. Acute-phase specimens should be tested for JE virus-specific immunoglobulin class M (IgM) antibodies using an enzyme-linked immunosorbent assay (ELISA) or an immunofluorescence assay. JE IgM antibodies can be measured in CSF of most patients by 4 days after onset of symptoms and in serum by 7 days after onset. If JE is suspected and acute specimens collected within 10 days of illness onset lack detectable IgM, a convalescent specimen should be collected and tested. Detection of JE IgM in CSF is diagnostic of neuroinvasive disease and can help distinguish clinical disease attributable to JE virus infection from recent vaccination.

Plaque reduction neutralization tests can be performed to measure virus-specific neutralizing antibodies and to discriminate between cross-reacting antibodies in primary flavivirus infections. A 4-fold or greater rise in virus-specific neutralizing antibodies between acute- and convalescent-phase serum specimens collected 2–3 weeks apart may be used to confirm evidence of recent infection. Vaccination history, date of symptom onset, and information regarding other flaviviruses known to circulate in the geographic area that might cross-react in serologic assays should be considered when interpreting results. In patients who have been immunized against or infected with another flavivirus in the past (i.e., who have secondary flavivirus infections), cross-reactive antibodies in both ELISA and neutralization assays may make it difficult to identify which flavivirus is causing the patient's illness. Detection of viral ribonucleic acid (RNA) in CSF may be positive if collected early in illness, especially before the appearance of antibodies, while virus isolation is less sensitive and usually unhelpful. Detection of virus in blood by either of these methods is rarely positive, as humans usually have low or undetectable levels of viremia by the time distinctive clinical symptoms are recognized. Therefore, these tests are insensitive and are not routinely recommended for diagnosis of JE virus infection.

**4. Laboratory capability**—The standard commercially available assays for detection of IgG and IgM can be used in routine diagnostic laboratories if they follow the manufacturer's instructions. Where the diagnosis is uncertain and/or there is concern about the presence of cross-reacting antibodies, then further testing should be conducted in a reference laboratory that can test for other flaviviruses and carry out specific assays. Isolation of the virus, testing for JEV-RNA, and testing of tissue samples are generally conducted in reference laboratories.

**5. Safety requirements**—Clinical samples may be handled under routine physical containment 2 (PC-2)/biosafety level 2 (BSL-2) containment. JE virus is classified as a BSL-3 agent, therefore live viruses must be handled in a PC-3/BSL-3 facility. Staff working with live virus should be experienced in working safely within a PC-3/BSL-3 facility and should be vaccinated against JE virus. Inactivated virus (e.g., following nucleic acid extraction) is safe and can be handled in PC-2/BSL-2 facilities.

**6. Nonhuman hosts**—JE virus is maintained in an animal-mosquito cycle, particularly pigs and ardeid birds. Infected birds are asymptomatic and are the main mechanism of spread of the virus. Pigs also are usually asymptomatic, though JE virus may cause abortions or intrauterine deaths in pregnant sows, and encephalitis in young pigs. Other animals can be infected by the virus, including horses, donkeys, cattle, sheep, goats, dogs, cats, several wild mammals, chickens, ducks, reptiles, and amphibians.

Animals other than pigs are dead end hosts, and only horses are known to develop clinical disease which is usually severe or fatal encephalitis. Infected animals can be tested using an approach similar to that for humans, though tissue samples are more likely to be available for virus detection. Testing for virus by culture, polymerase chain reaction (PCR), or antigen detection methods can be undertaken but requires a specialist accredited veterinary laboratory. The primary vectors are *Culex* spp. mosquitoes, especially *Culex tritaeniorhynchus*. Virus can be detected in trapped mosquitoes using cell culture or PCR-based techniques, again within a specialized laboratory accredited to handle BSL-3 organisms.

**7. Sample/specimen requirements**—Serum should be collected for antibody testing, including acute and convalescent samples, 10–14 days apart. Cerebrospinal fluid should also be collected for IgM testing and nucleic acid amplification of RNA. Samples should be stored and transported at 4°C–8°C. If testing is delayed by more than 3–4 days, samples should be maintained frozen at or below −20°C. Tissue samples should be placed in virus transport medium (VTM) or kept moist in saline if VTM is not available or if the sample has to be divided for other tests such as histopathology or immunochemistry. Do not place samples for culture or RNA detection in fixatives such as formalin or alcohol. All primary containers should be shatter-proof and leak-proof and placed in a leak-proof external container. All samples must be clearly labeled with unique identifiers and accompanied by a matching request form. Staff should have undertaken formal training in packaging of dangerous goods according to regulatory requirements. Transport by air should comply with International Air Transport Association requirements.

**8. Testing requirements**—Detection of JE virus, RNA, or antigen is regarded as definitive evidence of infection, provided the tests have been conducted properly. Nucleic acid amplification tests such as PCR are particularly at risk of false-positive results if the laboratory does not have strict measures for preventing cross-contamination. If a positive PCR result is not supported by other test results (e.g., serology), then confirmation of the identity of the product by sequencing is recommended. If there is insufficient product for sequencing, then use of an alternate PCR is recommended to confirm the result. Antigen detection tests on tissues such as brain are carried out by some reference laboratories. They are less sensitive than RNA detection, though they do provide information about the location of the virus within tissues. IgM may not be detectable in serum for up to 10 days after onset. This is accompanied by a rise in IgG antibodies to JE virus. As for all flaviviruses, IgG and, to a lesser extent, IgM will cross-react with other flavivirus antigens. In areas where there are other potential infecting flaviviruses, such as West Nile virus or dengue, cross-reacting IgM can occur, and testing for IgM to these other viruses should be undertaken to exclude them. Detection of JE virus-IgM in CSF is strong evidence of encephalitis, appearing in 60% of patients within 4 days of onset of illness and in nearly all patients by

2 weeks after onset. The specificity of IgG is determined by neutralization assays, requiring the JE virus titer to be at least 4-fold higher than it is for other flaviviruses that may have infected the person. Antibody formed within the early convalescent period may not be specific, as the antibody response may not have matured sufficiently. Repeat testing at least a month after onset may be needed. Patients who have had previous flavivirus infections or vaccination may have attenuated IgM responses in both serum and CSF and a rapid rise in IgG, with the initial response being to the previously infecting virus, the so-called original antigenic sin. Convalescent serum should show a rise in specific antibody to the recently infecting virus. JE virus vaccination will produce detectable IgG, and if within the preceding 4 weeks, will also produce detectable IgM in serum. IgM is not produced in CSF postvaccination and is indicative of natural infection.

All results should be interpreted in the context of the clinical findings and the history of exposure, as well as the findings of other investigations such as cerebral scans. Reports for serological testing should include comments that indicate the possibility of cross-reacting antibodies due to current or prior infection, and recommendations for further testing. For example, if CSF and acute serum have been received, then the reports on these should recommend further serum samples in 10–14 days. Laboratories should participate in quality assurance activities for any testing they undertake. Preferably this should be part of a recognized external quality assurance program, such as the EVD-LabNet and the Royal College of Pathologists of Australasia Quality Assurance Program. Both are distributed internationally. Other programs may be available locally or supplied by reference laboratories. Where there is no external quality assurance program available, then alternatives such as specimen exchanges should be undertaken.

**9. Reporting requirements**—JE virus infection is a notifiable disease in most countries. It is of particular concern where the person has entered an area with potential vector mosquito species but which has no established activity. In that case public health authorities should be notified immediately.

**10. Referral network**—Samples for testing and/or confirmation can be sent to state or national reference laboratories, or to a WHO Regional Reference Laboratory.

**11. Special considerations**—JEV infections require reporting to local public health authorities. As JE virus may infect animals, notification to the agricultural/animal health authorities is recommended.

[D. W. Smith, J. S. Mackenzie]

# KAWASAKI SYNDROME

(Kawasaki disease, mucocutaneous lymph node syndrome, acute febrile mucocutaneous lymph node syndrome)

| DISEASE | ICD-10 CODE |
|---|---|
| KAWASAKI SYNDROME | ICD-10 M30.3 |

**1. Clinical features**—An acute febrile, mostly self-limited, systemic vasculitis of early childhood, presumably of infectious origin. Clinically characterized by a high, spiking fever, unresponsive to antibiotics, associated with pronounced irritability and mood change; usually solitary and frequently unilateral nonsuppurative cervical lymphadenopathy; bilateral nonexudative bulbar conjunctival injection; and an enanthem consisting of a strawberry tongue, injected oropharynx, or dry fissured or erythematous lips. Also present are limb changes consisting of edema, erythema, or periungual/generalized desquamation and a generalized polymorphous erythematous exanthem that can be truncal or perineal and that ranges from morbilliform maculopapular rash to urticarial rash or vasculitic exanthem. Typically there are 3 phases:

1) Acute febrile phase of about 10 days, characterized by high, spiking fever, rash, adenopathy, peripheral erythema or edema, conjunctival injection, and enanthem.
2) Subacute phase lasting about 2 weeks, with thrombocytosis, desquamation, and resolution of fever.
3) Lengthy convalescent phase, during which clinical signs fade.

The case-fatality rate is approximately 0.1%; half the deaths occur within 2 months of illness. Coronary artery vasculitis leading to lumen dilatation and aneurysm are serious complications.

**2. Causative agents**—Unknown. Postulated to be a virus or a superantigen bacterial toxin secreted by *Staphylococcus aureus* or group A streptococci. A possible association with *Pseudomonas* sepsis has also been suggested.

**3. Laboratory diagnosis**—Given that there is no known causative agent for Kawasaki syndrome (KS), there is no pathognomonic test for KS. The following laboratory tests and expected results may be seen as an adjunct to the normally observed clinical signs for KS.

1) Complete blood count: elevated white blood cell (WBC) count
2) Erythrocyte sedimentation rate: elevated
3) Platelet count: high
4) Hemoglobin/hematocrit: low
5) Urinalysis: presence of protein and/or evidence of WBCs
6) C-reactive protein: positive

The case definition for KS may vary by country or region but is based on 6 clinical signs: fever, conjunctivitis, strawberry tongue, exanthema, reddening of palms and soles, and cervical lymphadenopathy.

**4. Laboratory capability**—Most clinical laboratories are capable of performing the routine laboratory tests that may be carried out to help diagnose KS and rule out other conditions.

**5. Safety requirements**—No special safety considerations beyond standard precautions for handling blood specimens are required.

**6. Nonhuman hosts**—Some animal models (e.g., mice and guinea pigs) have been utilized for studying KS, but there are currently no known animals that naturally demonstrate KS.

**7. Sample/specimen requirements**—Blood or urine samples are normally taken for a battery of routine laboratory tests. No special handling is required.

**8. Testing requirements**—Routine blood and urine tests are performed using standard protocols for quality assurance and safety.

**9. Reporting requirements**—KS is not known to be a reportable condition for laboratory-based reporting.

**10. Referral network**—Not applicable to KS.

**11. Special considerations**—Laboratories may be asked to assist in the investigation of clusters or outbreaks of KS; therefore, laboratories may want to ascertain if the holding of specimens from KS patients is warranted for investigatory purposes.

[B. W. Wilcke]

# LARVA MIGRANS

| DISEASE | ICD-10 CODE |
|---|---|
| VISCERAL LARVA MIGRANS | ICD-10 B83.0 |
| GNATHOSTOMIASIS | ICD-10 B83.1 |
| CREEPING ERUPTION | ICD-10 B76.9 |
| CUTANEOUS LARVA MIGRANS | ICD-10 B76.9 |
| OCULAR LARVA MIGRANS | ICD-10 B83.8 |
| NEURAL LARVA MIGRANS | ICD-10 B83.8 |

# I. VISCERAL LARVA MIGRANS (larva migrans visceralis, visceral larva migrans, *Toxocara* [*canis*] [*cati*] infection)

**1. Clinical features**—Usually a chronic infection and mild disease, predominantly of young children but increasingly recognized in adults, caused by migration of larval forms of nematodes in several organs and tissues, including the eye (in this case the term ocular larva migrans [OLM] is used). *Toxocara* spp. (*Toxocara canis* and *Toxocara cati*) are the most common causes of visceral larva migrans (VLM) and OLM. While infection with few larvae is usually asymptomatic, both VLM and OLM result from high-intensity infections.

VLM is characterized by hypereosinophilia of variable duration, hepatomegaly, hyperglobulinemia, pulmonary symptoms, and fever. With an acute and heavy infection, the white blood cell count may reach 100,000/mm$^3$ or more (SI units >100 $\times$ 10$^9$/L), with 50%–90% eosinophils. Symptoms may persist for a year or longer; symptomatology is related to total parasite load. Pneumonitis, chronic abdominal pain, a generalized rash, and focal neurological disturbances may occur.

Larvae may also enter the eye, thus causing an endophthalmitis that can result in loss of vision in the affected eye (OLM). This usually occurs in older children.

VLM is rarely fatal; differential diagnosis includes larval ascariasis (which has a shorter duration) and strongyloidiasis (longer duration). OLM should be distinguished from retinoblastoma and toxoplasmosis.

**2. Causative agents**—Larvae of the zoonotic nematodes *Toxocara canis* and *Toxocara cati*, predominantly the former. *Baylisascaris procyonis* (of raccoons) is a rarer cause of VLM and OLM; VLM and OLM might also be caused by animal ascarids such as *Ascaris suum*, *Parascaris equorum*, *Toxascaris leonina*, *Toxocara* (=*Neoascaris*) *vitulorum*, and other zoonotic nematodes, although information is limited regarding the ability of these species to induce VLM in human hosts.

**3. Laboratory diagnosis**—Although biopsy has yielded positive results for *Toxocara* larvae in a small number of cases, this approach is invasive and has poor sensitivity. Diagnosis of VLM requires consideration of clinical manifestations in conjunction with serological results. The standard method for serological diagnosis is by indirect *Toxocara* excretory-secretory antigen (TES) enzyme-linked immunosorbent assay (ELISA); any specimen with a positive result should be tested by Western blot (to improve specificity). Currently, recombinant TES antigen immunoglobulin class G (IgG) ELISA kits are available from several commercial manufacturers and detect antibodies to *Toxocara* spp. larvae in humans with similar sensitivities and specificities, estimated to be 86% and 91%, respectively, though the absence of a gold standard makes definitive determination difficult. Cross-reactions can occur with sera from strongyloidiasis, trichinellosis, and ascariasis cases; these nonspecific reactions can be avoided by using TES Western blot to detect *Toxocara* low molecular weight antigenic fractions (24, 28, 30, and 35 kDa). Note that a detectable antibody response may be absent in OLM cases: because OLM typically results after a light infection (vs. a heavy infection for VLM), negative serologic results should not be the sole reason for excluding the diagnosis.

**4. Laboratory capability**—Serological reference laboratory capable of ELISA testing is required. Laboratorians should be trained in the usage and interpretation of the specific ELISA methods and should undergo regular proficiency testing.

**5. Safety requirements**—Human serum samples present a risk for laboratory-acquired infection with bloodborne pathogens. All such specimens should be collected and handled using universal/standard precautions. Laboratories performing testing should be performed at a minimum of biosafety level 2 (BSL-2) or protective containment level 2 (PC-2).

**6. Nonhuman hosts**—Larva migrans is a zoonotic disease in which the reservoir of the infective agent is the nonhuman definitive host. Humans are infected as accidental hosts only via ingestion of larvated eggs in the environment. *T. canis* is a parasite of dogs and other canids, and *T. cati* is a parasite of cats. For *B. procyonis*, the definitive hosts are raccoons, rarely dogs or exotic pets; the intermediate hosts include a wide range of birds and mammals. These animal definitive hosts shed parasite eggs in feces, which are infectious to humans after a period of about 2–3 weeks in the environment. Less common causes of VLM include *A. suum* (pigs), *P. equorum* (horses), *T. leonina* (canids and felids), and *T. vitulorum* (cattle).

**7. Sample/specimen requirements**—Blood without anticoagulant should be collected and the serum separated for serological testing. Test sera should be transported and stored at 4°C. If testing cannot be performed within 48 hours, serum should be stored frozen at -80°C.

**8. Testing requirements**—Laboratory capacity to perform ELISA testing. Laboratories performing serology should participate in regular external quality assessment. Collection of serum at least 2 weeks postinfection is advised; in *Toxocara* serology studies on rabbits, complete seroconversion had occurred in 16 of 17 (94%) subjects at that time.[1] Antibody levels in humans remain elevated for at least 5 years postinfection.[2] Serologic testing of vitreous humor for OLM has been performed in some laboratories, but the significance of *Toxocara* antibodies in these fluids has not been clinically validated; thus interpretation of results is problematic. Details for seroconversion time for *Baylisacaris* antibodies are not available, though antibody persistence has been documented in subclinically infected individuals.[3]

**9. Reporting requirements**—There are no specific reporting requirements for toxocariosis; however, laboratories should always be aware of any special reporting requirements that may exist within their jurisdiction

**10. Referral network**—Networks vary among countries. Several laboratories worldwide offer serological testing. CDC offers serological diagnosis via a *Toxocara* TES antigen ELISA testing and a *B. procyonis* immunoblot test. The DPDx service at CDC provides morphological identification of larvae recovered from human samples or found in histological sections via images submitted online through a secure file-sharing system or actual specimens; contact dpdx@cdc.gov.

**11. Special considerations**—None.

## II. GNATHOSTOMIASIS (larva migrans profundus)

**1. Clinical features**—Transient inflammatory lesions or abscesses in various parts of the body, including the subcutaneous tissue, with a typical painless, migrating, intermittent edema. Larvae may also invade the brain, producing focal cerebral lesions associated with eosinophilic pleocytosis.

**2. Causative agents**—*Gnathostoma spinigerum*, the causative agent in the vast majority of cases, has been reported from Southeast Asia and tropical Australia, as well as southern and eastern Africa and elsewhere. Other species that infect humans include *Gnathostoma hispidum* (Southeast Asia, India), *Gnathostoma binucleatum* (Central and South America), and *Gnathostoma nipponicum* and *Gnathostoma doloresi* (Japan). Two cases of possible (not confirmed) *Gnathostoma malaysiae* infection acquired in Myanmar have been reported. The geographic distribution of these species in animal hosts is wider than their reported recovery in human infections, but most human infections are not identified to the species level.

**3. Laboratory diagnosis**—Disease may be diagnosed on clinical grounds, with laboratory testing used to confirm this diagnosis. Serologic testing remains the mainstay of laboratory diagnosis. Several ELISA and immunoblot methods have been published for the detection of antibodies to *G. spinigerum* in humans, with variable sensitivities and specificities. An immunoblot that detects IgG antibodies to the 24 kDa band of a crude antigen extract of *G. spinigerum* L3 larvae has been shown to have the greatest sensitivity (91.6%) and specificity (87.8%) when validated using suspected cases of gnathostomiasis in Thailand, where *G. spinigerum* is the most common infecting species. The sensitivity and specificity of this immunoblot for human infection caused by other *Gnathostoma* spp. is unknown. An immunoblot that uses a crude antigen preparation from *G. binucleatum* larvae and that is interpreted on the basis of reactivity to the 24 kDa diagnostic band has been developed, but its sensitivity and specificity for infections with this species have not yet been determined. Seroconversion takes several weeks to occur; therefore, serologic testing typically is not useful early on in the infection.

Biopsy of migrating subcutaneous larvae may rarely yield positive results, allowing species-specific identification; but this is an invasive procedure with low sensitivity. L3 larvae of *Gnathostoma* have distinctive morphologic features in tissue transverse sections; the species may often be identified based on the shape and number of nuclei within the cells of the digestive tract. Polymerase chain reaction (PCR) and sequencing analysis of the ITS2 and COI genes of larvae may also allow species identification. *Gnathostoma* ocular larva migrans may be diagnosed by visualization of the morphologically distinct larvae in slit-lamp examination of the eye.

4. **Laboratory capability**—Serological reference laboratory capable of ELISA testing is required. For morphological diagnosis, advanced reference laboratory skills are required. Laboratories performing microscopy and/or serology should participate in regular external quality assessment.

5. **Safety requirements**—Human serum and tissue samples present a risk for laboratory-acquired infection with bloodborne pathogens. All such specimens should be collected and handled using universal/standard precautions. Laboratories performing testing should be a minimum biosafety level of PC-2 or BSL-2. Formalin used in tissue preservation requires a well-ventilated space or preferably a chemical fume hood. Formalin containing waste should be disposed of as chemical waste following local regulations.

6. **Nonhuman hosts**—Gnathostomiasis is a zoonotic disease in which the reservoir of the infective agent are the nonhuman definitive hosts. Humans only infected as accidental hosts through ingestion of infected intermediate or paratenic hosts. The definitive hosts are cats (including big cats) and dogs for *G. spinigerum*; pigs for *G. hispidum* and *G. doloresi*; Japanese minks and weasels for *G. nipponicum*; and dogs, raccoons, or opossums for *G. hispidum*. L1 and L2 larvae are found in freshwater copepods (*Cyclops*); advanced L3 larvae are found in many intermediate or paratenic hosts, such as frogs and other amphibians, fish, snakes, turtles, and birds, including domestic poultry.

7. **Sample/specimen requirements**—Blood without anticoagulant should be collected and the serum separated for serological testing. Test sera should be transported and stored at 4°C. If testing cannot be performed within 48 hours, serum should be stored frozen at -80°C. Larvae sometimes can be detected by histological examination of biopsy specimens from the advancing margin of the cutaneous lesion.

8. **Testing requirements**—Laboratory capacity to perform ELISA testing. For morphological diagnosis, advanced reference laboratory skills are required. There is no data on time to seroconversion following infection, or

antibody persistence. Some case reports described clinical disease without detectable antibody early in infection, with later seroconversion. Therefore, repeat serological testing is advised where clinical suspicion exists, and serology results are negative. Morphological identification of *Gnathostoma* spp. larvae in biopsy is both diagnostic and confirmatory. Laboratories performing microscopy serology should participate in regular external quality assessment.

**9. Reporting requirements**—There are no specific reporting requirements for gnathostomiasis; however, laboratories should always be aware of any special reporting requirements that may exist within their jurisdiction.

**10. Referral network**—*Gnathostoma* immunoblot testing directed toward the 24 kDa antigen of *G. spinigerum* is available at the Department of Helminthology, Mahidol University, Bangkok, Thailand. The Swiss Tropical and Public Health Institute, Basel, Switzerland, performs immunoblot testing directed toward the 24 kDa antigen of both *G. spinigerum* and *G. binucleatum*. The DPDx service at CDC provides morphological identification of larvae recovered from human samples or found in histological sections via images submitted online through a secure file-sharing system or actual specimens; contact dpdx@cdc.gov.

**11. Special considerations**—None.

## III. CUTANEOUS LARVA MIGRANS/CREEPING ERUPTION/LARVA CURRENS

**1. Clinical features**—A dermatitis in which each larva causes a serpiginous, reddish track, advancing several millimeters to a few centimeters a day, with intense itching, especially at night. Most common locations include feet and buttocks. The disease is self-limited, with spontaneous cure after weeks or months. *Ancylostoma caninum* larvae may migrate to the small intestine where they cause eosinophilic enteritis.

**2. Causative agents**—Cutaneous larva migrans: *Ancylostoma braziliense*, *A. caninum*, *Ancylostoma tubaeforme*, *Uncinaria stenocephala*, *Bunostomum phlebotomum*, and possibly other zoonotic hookworm species. *Strongyloides* cutaneous larva migrans (called larva currens) is most commonly caused by skin migration of *S. stercoralis* infesting the human intestinal tract. However, *Strongyloides* spp. of animals may also cause this disease (e.g., *S. procyonis*, *S. myopotami*, *S. ransomi*, *S. westeri*, and *S. papillosus*). A free-living saprophytic nematode found in decaying organic matter, *Pelodera strongyloides*, may also cause a larva currens-like infection. Eosinophilic enteritis is associated with infection with immature stages of *A. caninum*.

**3. Laboratory diagnosis**—Laboratory testing is not used in the diagnosis of Cutaneous Larva migrans. Subadult *A. caninum* recovered on colonoscopy may be identified morphologically. The laboratory confirmation of *S. stercoralis* larva currens is discussed in the chapter of this manual on strongyloidiasis (see "Strongyloidiasis").

**4. Laboratory capability**—Morphological identification of immature *A. caninum* requires advanced reference laboratory-level skills. Laboratory capability required for the diagnosis of larva currens caused by *S. stercoralis* is discussed in the strongyloidiasis chapter in this book (see "Strongyloidiasis").

**5. Safety requirements**—Cutaneous larva migrans is not a laboratory diagnosis. Safety requirements for the diagnosis of larva currens caused by *S. stercoralis* are discussed in the strongyloidiasis chapter in this manual (see "Strongyloidiasis").

**6. Nonhuman hosts**—Zoonotic hookworm species that have been implicated as causing cutaneous larva migrans include *A. braziliense*, *A. caninum* (dogs), *A. tubaeforme* (cats), *U. stenocephala* (dogs and cats), and *B. phlebotomum* (cattle, sheep, and goats). Humans and other primates are the principal reservoir of *S. stercoralis*, though transmission of dog and cat strains to humans may occur. The hosts of animal *Strongyloides* spp. causing larva currens are *S. procyonis* (raccoon), *S. myopatami* (nutria), *S. ransomi* (pigs), *S. westeri* (horses), and S. *papillosus* (sheep and goats).

**7. Sample/specimen requirements**—Cutaneous larva migrans is a clinical diagnosis. Specimen requirements for the diagnosis of larva currens caused by *S. stercoralis* are discussed in the "Strongyloidiasis" chapter in this book. Serology has been used for research-based diagnosis of *A. caninum* eosinophilic enteritis, but no diagnostic laboratories offer this testing routinely. In some cases, immature adults of *A. caninum* may be seen and recovered from the ileum or other portions of the bowel on endoscopy.

**8. Testing requirements**—Testing requirements for the diagnosis of *S. stercoralis* infection are discussed in the strongyloidiasis chapter in this manual (see "Stongyloidiasis"). The DPDx service at CDC provides morphological, species-level identification of any adult or immature hookworms recovered from the human gut via images submitted online through a secure file-sharing system or actual specimens; contact dpdx@cdc.gov.

**9. Reporting requirements**—There are no specific reporting requirements for cutaneous larva migrans.

**10. Referral network**—Networks vary between countries. Referral networks for the diagnosis of *S. stercoralis* infection are discussed in the strongyloidiasis chapter in this book (see "Strongyloidiasis").

**11. Special considerations**—None.

## IV. OCULAR LARVA MIGRANS

**1. Clinical features**—Ocular larva migrans (OLM) refers to intraocular invasion and migration within the eye by larval stages of various nematode species. For the purposes of this section, OLM should be distinguished from other ocular nematodiases in which (a) adult worms (not larvae) are implicated, (b) intraocular invasion and/or migration does not occur (e.g., conjunctival or orbital localization), or (c) ocular invasion is solely a result of broadly disseminated infection.

Clinical manifestations of OLM and the severity of visual impairment vary depending on the etiologic agent and localization within the eye. The cornea, aqueous humor, vitreous humor, anterior and posterior chamber, and the retina all are potential areas of localization. OLM is typically unilateral and commonly presents with signs such as strabismus, optic nerve atrophy, uveitis, endopthalmitis, and chorioretinitis. In severe cases, these complications can lead to permanent vision loss. Patients may report interference with vision if larvae are of a large species and/or highly motile.

*Toxocara* and *Baylisascaris* OLM typically presents with visual impairment associated with diffuse unilateral subacute retinitis and other inflammatory and degenerative lesions of the retinal and optic nerve. Occasionally, granuloma formation is observed within the anterior or posterior chamber of the eye. In ocular baylisascariasis, ocular signs are typically, but not always, present without concomitant neurologic disease. *Gnathostoma* OLM commonly presents with glaucoma, corneal ulceration, and vitreal hemorrhage. Retinoblastoma and toxoplasmosis should be included in the differential diagnosis in suspected OLM cases.

**2. Causative agents**—Most commonly, *T. canis* and *T. cati*, but also *B. procyonis*, *Onchocerca volvulus* and zoonotic *Onchocerca* spp., *Acanthocheilonema* spp., *Gnathostoma* spp., *Angiostrongylus cantonensis*, and rarely hookworms (*Ancylostoma* spp., *Necator americanus*) have been implicated.

**3. Laboratory diagnosis**—Ocular examination with visualization of the larvae with a slit-lamp is usually required. Diagnosis of OLM is often presumptive based on larval size (e.g., 200–500 μm for *Toxocara* spp. vs. ~1,000–1,800 μm for *B. procyonis*) and gross morphology, case/exposure history, clinical signs, and species specific serological results. Note that a detectable antibody response may be absent in OLM cases. Because OLM typically results after a light infection (vs. a heavy infection for VLM), negative serologic results should not be the sole reason for excluding the diagnosis.

**4. Laboratory capability**—Ability to perform ophthalmic examination and where applicable, ability to perform serological assays. However, identification of larvae based on morphology or molecular methods requires a reference diagnostic laboratory. CDC offers a telediagnostic service—DPDx—for morphological identifications.

**5. Safety requirements**—PC2 or BSL-2 practices apply when handling serum samples.

**6. Nonhuman hosts**—Refer to the chapters in this book that focus on particular nematode species.

**7. Sample/specimen requirements**—Serum/plasma for serologic diagnosis of infection with particular species. If specimens with or photographs of larvae are submitted to a reference laboratory for confirmatory diagnosis, include morphometric data.

**8. Testing requirements**—The DPDx service at CDC provides consultation on suspected ocular cases and morphological identification of migrating larvae. Serologic testing for evidence of infection with applicable species, including *Toxocara* and *Baylisascaris,* also is available through CDC.

**9. Reporting requirements**—None.

**10. Referral network**—CDC offers serological diagnosis on serum or paired specimens of serum and vitreous humor via a *Toxocara* TES antigen ELISA testing and a *Baylisascaris* immunoblot test. The DPDx service at CDC provides morphological identification of larvae recovered from human samples or found in histological sections via images submitted online through a secure file-sharing system or actual specimens; contact dpdx@cdc.gov.

**11. Special considerations**—The use of diagnostic serology on paired specimens of vitreous humor and serum for the diagnosis of OLM is controversial. Although an increased intraocular titer of antibodies compared with serum titer has been indicated by some reports as suggestive of OLM disease, limited data is available in validation of this assumption. Clinicians are required to consult with staff at CDC prior to collecting any ocular fluid specimens for testing.

## V. NEURAL LARVA MIGRANS (*Angiostrongylus cantonensis* or *Baylisascaris procyonis* infection)

Neural larva migrans (NLM) refers to the invasion of the central nervous system (CNS) by migrating larval stages of nematodes, classically *A. cantonensis* or *B. procyonis*. Clinical features of *A. cantonensis* NLM are addressed in the angiostrongyliasis (ICD-10 B83.2) chapter in this manual (see "Angiostrongyliasis").

**1. Clinical features**—The clinical manifestations of *Baylisascaris* NLM (e.g., behavioral changes, lethargy, confusion, ataxia, visual impairment, weakness/paralysis, seizures, coma) may initially be subtle but may rapidly increase in severity because of larval growth during migration, although slower progression, with a more chronic course, may be observed. Eosinophilic meningoencephalitis and peripheral eosinophilia often are present. Survivors often develop permanent neurologic sequelae, but full recovery may occur in patients with early diagnosis and treatment. Human baylisascariasis is rare, with approximately 50 cases of ocular and cerebral baylisascariasis having been reported worldwide since 1980. The actual number of cases may be greater, in part because of lack of awareness and diagnostic difficulties. *B. procyonis* and *A. cantonensis* share clinical similarities, notably eosinophilic meningitis; however, peripheral eosinophilia is moderate to high in baylisascariasis and rarely so in angiostrongyliasis. In *A. cantonensis* NLM, meningitis is a more common manifestation than meningioencaphalitis and is rarely fatal unlike *B. procyonis* NLM. Additionally, foreign travel history to Southeast Asia or the Caribbean is commonly implicated angiostrongyliasis, whereas all baylisascariasis cases thus far have been acquired in the USA or Canada.

**2. Causative agents**—Larvae of *B. procyonis* (after ingestion of infectious eggs) or *A. cantonensis* (after ingestion of infected intermediate/paratenic hosts or contaminated food items). *B. procyonis* is widely distributed in North America, with the highest prevalence in raccoons in the upper Midwest, Northeast, Mid-Atlantic, and West Coast. *B. procyonis* has also been introduced with raccoons to Europe, Japan, and China. *A. cantonensis* is endemic in parts of Asia and the Pacific Islands (including Hawaii), as well as in other regions (e.g., parts of Africa and the Caribbean). Rare human cases of *A. cantonensis* infection have been reported in the continental USA. Other parasites occasionally cause NLM (e.g., *Gnathostoma* spp., *Toxocara* spp., *Strongyloides stercoralis*).

**3. Laboratory diagnosis**—Antemortem diagnosis of baylisascariasis NLM typically is based on clinical presentation and detection of antibodies to *Baylisascaris* in serum and/or cerebrospinal fluid (CSF). An immunoblot based on a recombinant antigen has a sensitivity of 88% and a specificity of 98%. The patient's exposure history, including possible contact with raccoons and/or raccoon feces may aid in diagnosis. Larvae recovered on biopsy (e.g., brain) can be identified morphologically; however, obtaining biopsy specimens constitutes a highly invasive, low-sensitivity approach for detecting *Baylisascaris* larvae. The diagnosis of neural angiostrongyliasis (ICD-10 B83.2) is discussed in "Angiostrongyliasis."

**4. Laboratory capability**—Parasitological serological reference laboratory capability, with training in and the capacity to perform ELISA and immunoblotting. Training in and capacity to perform PCR for *A. cantonensis* is also necessary. Capability to preform morphological diagnosis from histological sections, if available.

**5. Safety requirements**—PC2 or BSL-2 practices are required for handling serum and CSF samples to avoid infection with bloodborne viruses.

Infectious stages are not encountered in human tissue for either of the parasites causing NLM.

**6. Nonhuman hosts**—For *B. procyonis*, the definitive hosts are raccoons, rarely dogs or exotic pets; the paratenic hosts include a wide range of birds and mammals. Human infections occur following ingestion of embryonated eggs shed by infected definitive hosts, after the eggs are exposed to the environment for 10–14 days. For *A. cantonensis*, the definitive hosts are rats; the intermediate hosts include several genera of mollusks. Various other animals (e.g., frogs, freshwater shrimp, land crabs, planarians) may serve as paratenic (transport) hosts for *A. cantonensis.* Ingestion of third-stage larvae from these intermediate and paratenic hosts is the primary method by which humans are infected.

**7. Sample/specimen requirements**—Serum, plasma, or CSF for serologic testing. The timing of antibody development in human baylisascariasis is not well understood, although antibodies are typically detectable at the onset of neurologic symptoms based on animal studies and past cases. Ideally, serum should be taken prior to anthelmintic treatment. Specific *A. cantonensis* IgG may not be detectable by immunoblot until more than 3 weeks after symptom onset. Tests for the presence of *A. cantonensis* antigens or deoxyribonucleic acid (DNA) in CSF may prove more useful in early diagnosis, after which serum can be collected and tested for antibodies in the convalescent phase. Serum and CSF should be stored at 4°C if testing is performed in 24 hours, or frozen and stored at -20°C if not processed within a 24-hour time frame.

**8. Testing requirements**—Laboratory capacity to perform immunoblot testing. The diagnostic immunoblot maintained by CDC has a sensitivity of 89% and a specificity of 98% based on validation using existing, biopsy-confirmed clinical samples. The PCR assay for *A. cantonensis* DNA in CSF is 100% (61 of 61 samples used in validation) when tested alongside CSF samples from patients with other CNS conditions. The sensitivity of the test is 81% (30 of 37 samples) when tested with CSF samples from patients with CNS angiostrongyliasis, as compared with immunodiagnosis. The diagnostic sensitivity for individual patients may be improved by submitting several CSF samples collected on different days. The 31 kDa *A. cantonensis* immunoblot has not been extensively validated for sensitivity and specificity values but shows little to no cross-reactivity to sera from other parasitic diseases or from healthy patients.

**9. Reporting requirements**—There are no specific reporting requirements for baylisascariasis or angiostrongyliasis; however, laboratories should always be aware of any special reporting requirements that may exist within their jurisdiction.

**10. Referral network**—The Parasitic Diseases Reference Diagnostic Laboratory, the Division of Parasitic Diseases and Malaria, CDC, offers immunoblot testing for antibodies to *B. procyonis*, as well as PCR analysis of CSF for

*A. cantonensis*. Serologic testing for *A. cantonensis* is available through Mahidol University in Thailand and ICPMR at Westmead Hospital in Sydney, Australia. The DPDx service at CDC provides morphological identification of larvae recovered from human samples or found in histological sections via images submitted online through a secure file-sharing system or actual specimens; contact dpdx@cdc.gov.

**11. Special considerations**—None.

## References

1. Fenoy S, Cuellar C, Aguila C, Guillen JL. Persistence of immune response in human toxocariasis as measured by ELISA. 1992. Available at: https://www.sciencedirect.com/science/article/pii/002075199290067U. Accessed August 25, 2018.
2. Bin LL, Santarém VA, Laposy CB, Rubinsky-Elefant G, Roldán WH, Giuffrida R. Kinetics and avidity of anti-*Toxocara* antibodies (IgG) in rabbits experimentally infected with *Toxocara canis*. 2016. Available at: http://www.scielo.br/scielo.php?pid=S1984-29612016000100099&script=sci_arttext. Accessed August 25, 2018.
3. Sapp SG, Rascoe LN, Wilkins PP, et al. *Baylisascaris procyonis* roundworm seroprevalence among wildlife rehabilitators, United States and Canada, 2012–2015. 2016. Available at: https://wwwnc.cdc.gov/eid/article/22/12/16-0467_article. Accessed August 25, 2018.

[S. G. H. Sapp, S. Handali, R. S. Bradbury]

# LEGIONELLOSIS

| DISEASE | ICD-10 CODE |
|---|---|
| LEGIONNAIRES' DISEASE | ICD-10 A48.1 |
| PONTIAC FEVER | ICD-10 A48.2 |

**1. Clinical features**—Two distinct clinical manifestations: Legionnaires' disease and Pontiac fever. Both conditions present with anorexia, malaise, myalgia, headache, and fever. Abdominal pain and diarrhea are also common.

1) Legionnaires' disease: characterized by pneumonia and a nonproductive cough. Chest imaging findings are variable and may show patchy or focal areas of consolidation or bilateral involvement. The illness can be quite severe and may ultimately progress to respiratory failure. Despite improvements in diagnostics and treatment, case-fatality rates remain at approximately 15%.

2) Pontiac fever: a self-limited, febrile illness, usually accompanied by cough, which does not progress to pneumonia or death. Patients recover spontaneously in 2–5 days without treatment. This clinical syndrome may represent reaction to inhaled *Legionella* antigen rather than bacterial invasion.

**2. Causative agents**—*Legionella,* Gram-negative bacilli. Of the multiple serogroups of *Legionellae pneumophila* currently recognized, *L. pneumophila* serogroup 1 is most commonly associated with disease. Other species including *Legionella micdadei, Legionella bozemanii, Legionella longbeachae*, and *Legionella dumoffii* have been isolated from patients including those who are immunocompromised. Currently, 65 different species are included in the *Legionella* genus (for a list, see: http://www.bacterio.net/legionella.html), and at least 70 distinct serogroups are recognized. *L. pneumophila* can be further discriminated using monoclonal antibody typing, multilocus sequence-based typing, and, increasingly, genomic phylogenic analysis. The disease caused by *L. pneumophila* has been identified worldwide with cases occurring throughout the year. Both sporadic cases and outbreaks are recognized. Outbreaks can be international in nature infecting travelers. Outbreaks can occur in the community, among travelers, and in patients within health care facilities. Person-to-person transmission has been documented only once.

**3. Laboratory diagnosis**—Legionnaires' disease: isolate the causative organism from a lower respiratory specimen using selective media (buffered charcoal yeast extract); detect *Legionella* nucleic acid in lower respiratory specimens. Detect *L. pneumophila* serogroup 1 antigens in urine. Note some urine antigen and serologic tests only detect *L. pneumophila* serogroup 1, so disease due to other serogroups or species will be missed, emphasizing the importance of polymerase chain reaction (PCR) and culture. Direct immunofluorescent antibody stain of involved tissue or respiratory secretions may be used, but sensitivity and specificity are highly variable and dependent upon the experience of laboratory personnel. The disease may be detected by demonstration of a 4-fold rise in immunofluorescent antibody titer to *L. pneumophila* serogroup 1 between acute phase serum and serum drawn 3–6 weeks later or a significant rise in specific antibody level to *L. pneumophila* serogroup 1 in paired serum samples.

Pontiac fever: this poorly defined infection is occasionally diagnosed by identifying symptoms consistent with the disease in the appropriate epidemiologic setting without demonstration of active *Legionella* infection. If disease is due to *L. pneumophila* serogroup 1, urine antigen testing may be used to confirm the diagnosis, with presumed lower sensitivity than for Legionnaires' disease.

**4. Laboratory capability**—Several rapid urine antigen tests are available for testing of infection without requirement for complex laboratory equipment. Skilled laboratory personnel should be maintained for detecting and monitoring infection in environmental sources and patients; laboratory personnel should have experience in environmental specimen processing, clinical specimen processing, *Legionella* culture, and isolation. Maintaining molecular discrimination testing in referral or specialized centers requires significant scientific and epidemiological expertise essential to identify linked cases and outbreaks and facilitate public health interventions.

**5. Safety requirements**—The UK Health and Safety Executive Approved list of Biological Agents Advisory Committee on Dangerous Pathogens lists *L. pneumophila* as a hazard group 2 organism. Biosafety level 2 laboratory practices are sufficient for handling the agent. Handling of clinical specimens of unknown respiratory infection etiology should be in accordance with local risk assessment for other potential agents.

**6. Nonhuman hosts**—Legionellosis is not known to be zoonotic.

**7. Sample/specimen requirements**—Urine and lower respiratory specimens (e.g., sputum, bronchoalveolar lavage, lung tissue) are the most appropriate specimens for detection of infection in humans, and water or swabbing of water surfaces if predrained can be used for detection in the environment. Specimens should be taken as close to onset of infection as possible or as soon after death as feasible and should be transported according to local shipping guidelines for potentially infectious specimens. Follow country-specific standard guidance for *Legionella* sampling procedures and practice (e.g., CDC [USA] and Health and Safety Executive [UK] websites) detail comprehensive sampling procedures. In practice, culture, PCR, and sequence-based typing on clinical specimens are more likely to yield a positive result if taken with 48 hours of presentation.

**8. Testing requirements**—The mainstay of diagnostics remains urine antigen testing with rapid lateral flow or enzyme-linked immunosorbent assay-based methods. Urine antigen tests designed to detect serogroup 1 have varying capacity to detect *Legionella* infections with other serogroups potentially. Urine antigen testing is increasingly complemented with detection of DNA using molecular-based methods such as PCR, which, depending on design, can detect multiple serogroups or species. Culture remains important for detection of Legionnaires' disease by the isolation of the causative organism from a lower respiratory specimen using selective media (buffered charcoal yeast extract); however, successful isolation is highly variable and dependent upon the experience of laboratory personnel. Not all patients are able to provide a lower respiratory tract specimen. These specimens are essential to enable discrimination of the type of *L. pneumophila* using sequence based typing ideally on an isolate. If an isolate is not possible, typing can be performed directly on the specimen. This is essential to enable case linkage and outbreak source identification and exclusion. Serological detection by measuring a 4-fold rise in immunofluorescent antibody titer to

*L. pneumophila* serogroup 1 between acute phase serum and serum drawn 3–6 weeks later is regarded as too slow to be of public health value in outbreak recognition and of little clinical value, although identification of cases with serology alone may be useful in outbreak review scenarios for the identification of patients past the initial event. External quality assessment schemes for urine antigen and molecular testing are available.

**9. Reporting requirements**—*Legionella* is a notifiable/reportable infection in several countries including the USA, England, and Wales. Local laboratories and regional network laboratories should provide urine antigen testing at a minimum and preferably molecular detection of infection. Reference network centers should provide culture, monoclonal antibody typing, and sequence-based typing. Submission of isolates and lower respiratory clinical specimens is recommended. Reporting of sequence-based typing to local, national, and international public health teams is commonly required and necessary to detect and control sources of infection.

**10. Referral network**—A number of *Legionella* reference laboratories exist globally and may be approached for assistance during outbreaks of infection. Some countries do not have routine testing or reference facilities. The European Centre for Disease Prevention and Control coordinates *Legionella* cases occurring in Europe and European travelers. Laboratories performing *Legionella* testing in other countries and regions should consult with their local and national reference laboratories within the public health system for guidance.

**11. Special considerations**—Legionellosis is a waterborne disease. Acquisition of infection is from contaminated water sources such as domestic water systems, spa pools, birthing pools, cooling towers, and humidifiers. Conditions that are conducive to *Legionella* growth include warm water temperatures (25°C–42°C); stagnation; scale and sediment; and low biocide levels. Infection may be acquired by inhalation, aspiration, or submersion. Risk factors for infection include increasing age (most cases are in persons >50 years), smoking, diabetes mellitus, chronic lung disease, renal disease, malignancy, and compromised immunity, particularly in organ transplant recipients and patients receiving corticosteroids. More cases are documented in males.

WHO and CDC case definitions are available on relevant websites. Epidemiological analysis is imperative to link cases and identify clusters and outbreaks. Consideration should be given to additional case finding to identify if there are other cases with the same exposures as the index case. Two or more cases of legionellosis occurring among travellers to the same destination during a 1-year period or a single case of laboratory-confirmed health care–associated Legionnaires' disease should trigger additional case finding measures and an environmental assessment. During large outbreaks meteorological factors may be considered to assist in source location. If feasible, sequence-based typing should be undertaken on isolates from patients and suspected sources. The threshold for initiating environmental sampling and remediation varies among published guidelines. During an outbreak, identify common exposures and review maintenance logs for water systems and sample potential sources where required. *Legionella* culture of water and biofilm swabs collected from the potential source(s) may be necessary to determine the cause for the outbreak and should be considered for any cluster of health care-associated legionellosis.

[V. Chalker]

# LEISHMANIASIS

| DISEASE | ICD-10 CODES |
|---|---|
| CUTANEOUS LEISHMANIASIS | ICD-10 B55.1 |
| MUCOSAL LEISHMANIASIS | ICD-10 B55.2 |
| VISCERAL LEISHMANIASIS | ICD-10 B55.0 |

**1. Clinical features—**

1) Cutaneous and mucosal leishmaniasis (Aleppo evil, Baghdad boil, Delhi boil, chiclero ulcer, oriental sore, espundia): a polymorphic disease of skin and mucous membranes that starts with a macule, then a papular or nodular lesion that enlarges and typically becomes an indolent ulcer in the absence of bacterial infection. The lesions can develop on any part of the body where the inoculation of the parasite has occurred. However, lesions usually appear on exposed surfaces of the body such as the face, arms, and legs. Lesions may be single or multiple, occasionally nonulcerative and diffuse. Lesions may heal spontaneously within weeks to months or last for a year or more. Recurrence of cutaneous lesions after apparent cure may occur as ulcers, papules, or nodules at or near the healed original ulcer.

   In some individuals, certain strains (mainly from the western hemisphere) can disseminate to cause mucosal lesions (espundia), even years after the primary cutaneous lesion has healed. In the eastern hemisphere, a chronic granulomatous lesion occurs, following anthroponotic cutaneous leishmaniasis due to *Leishmania (Leishmania) tropica* called the recidivans form. These sequelae, which involve nasopharyngeal tissues, are characterized by progressive tissue destruction and often scanty presence of parasites and can be severely disfiguring if left untreated.

Eventual spontaneous healing occurs in most cases, but the rate of healing varies by species. A small proportion of patients infected with *Leishmania (Leishmania) amazonensis* or *Leishmania (Leishmania) aethiopica* may develop diffuse parasite-rich cutaneous lesions that do not heal without treatment. Metastatic mucosal lesions may develop months or years later in a small proportion of infections with parasites of the *Leishmania (Viannia) braziliensis* complex.

2) Visceral leishmaniasis (Kala-azar): a systemic disease caused by intracellular protozoa of the subgenus *Leishmania*. The disease is characterized by fever, hepatosplenomegaly, lymphadenopathy, anemia, leukopenia, thrombocytopenia, and progressive emaciation and weakness. Untreated clinically evident disease is usually fatal. Evidence indicates that asymptomatic and subclinical infections are common. Only very few progress to develop full-blown disease. However, the role of asymptomatic infections in transmission is yet to be elucidated. Fever may have gradual or sudden onset, is persistent and irregular, and may alternate with periods of apyrexia or low-grade fever. Post–Kala-azar dermal leishmaniasis consists of macular, papular, and/or nodular skin lesions that occur weeks to years after apparent cure of systemic disease. Post–Kala-azar dermal leishmaniasis occurs in up to 50% of visceral leishmaniasis cases in Sudan and 10%–20% of cases in the Indian subcontinent. *Leishmania*/HIV coinfection is a serious form of the disease in southern Europe, eastern Africa, and southeast Asia.

**2. Causative agents**—Species in *Leishmania* and *Viannia* subgenera are obligate intracellular parasites associated with leishmaniasis. These parasites can infect humans and others mammals that serve as a source of human infection. They are transmitted by different genera and subgenera of phlebotomine sand flies such as *Lutzomyia* in the Americas and *Phlebotomus* in Europe, Africa, and Asia.

1) Cutaneous and mucosal leishmaniasis: in the eastern hemisphere (Old World), cutaneous lesions may be caused by *L. (L.) tropica* and *Leishmania (Leishmania) major* (Central Asia, Middle East, North Africa, West Africa and Sudan), *Leishmania (Leishmania) killicki* (North Africa), *L. (L.) aethiopica* (Ethiopia, Kenya and Uganda), and *Leishmania (Leishmania) arabica* (Saudi Arabia). A species belonging to the subgenus *Leishmania (Mundinia)* and *L. (L.) tropica*-like has been described in Gahna and Namibia, respectively, as causing cutaneous leishmaniasis.

There is greater diversity of *Leishmania* spp. in the Western hemisphere (Americas/New World). Leishmaniasis is endemic in many countries in South and Central America, although the distribution of species is not well defined. In South America, within the *Viannia* subgenus (*L. [V.] braziliensis, Leishmania* [*Viannia*] *panamensis, Leishmania* [*Viannia*] *guyanensis, Leishmania [Viannia] peruviana, Leishmania [Viannia] lainsoni, Leishmania [Viannia] shawi* and *Leishmania* [*Viannia*] *naiffi*), *L.* (*V.*) *braziliensis* is the primary etiological agent of mucosal leishmaniasis. More rarely *L.* (*V.*) *panamensis* and *L.* (*V.*) *guyanensis* are associated with the mucosal form of the disease. Members of the *Leishmania* (*Leishmania*) *mexicana* complex (*L.* [*L.*] *mexicana, L.* [*L.*] *amazonensis, Leishmania* [*Leishmania*] *venezuelensis, Leishmania* [*Leishmania*] *garnhami, Leishmania* [*Leishmania*] *pifanoi,* and *Leishmania* [*Leishmania*] *waltoni*) cause the cutaneous disease. Recently, within the USA, the transmission of *L.* (*L.*) *mexicana* was identified in Texas and Oklahoma. *Leishmania* (*Mundinia*) *martiniquensis* is associated with cutaneous leishmaniasis of humans in Martinique and domestic animals in Florida and Europe. *Endotrypanum colombiensis,* previously classified as *Leishmania (Viannia) colombiensis*, has been associated with cutaneous and visceral leishmaniasis in Venezuela.

2) Visceral leishmaniasis: *Leishmania* (*Leishmania*) *infantum* is found in North Africa, Southern Europe, and Central and South America, while *Leishmania* (*Leishmania*) *donovani* in India, Bangladesh, Sudan, South Sudan, and Ethiopia. *L.* (*L.*) *amazonensis* has been linked to visceral infections in Brazil and *L.* (*M.*) *martiniquensis* together with another unnamed *Leishmania* (*Mundinia*) spp. with visceral infections in Thailand.

**3. Laboratory diagnosis**—Leishmaniasis may be diagnosed by microscopy, culture, polymerase chain reaction (PCR), or serological tests. Species identification requires either culture followed by multilocus enzyme electrophoresis (MLEE), PCR with subsequent restriction fragment length polymorphism (RFLP) analysis or sequencing. Serological tests are usually unspecific and can not distinguish between active and inactive infection.

The sensitivity of microscopy is low, and the test efficiency depends on the type of specimens and experience of the operator for identification of the parasites. Multilocus enzyme electrophoresis is a technique used for parasites identification at the species level and is still considered the gold standard for differentiation of *Leishmania* spp. It is a timing consuming and laborious procedure typically requiring 4–8 weeks as it depends on parasite culture and the analysis of several isoenzymes using electrophoresis. Deoxyribonucleic acid (DNA)-based techniques typically are more sensitive, less labor intensive, and result in a more rapid specific identification of *Leishmania* parasites. DNA amplification by PCR using genus- or species-specific primers followed by postamplification analysis (e.g., PCR-RFLP or

DNA sequencing) are used for parasite species and strain identification. In PCR-RFLP, species can be identified using fragmented amplicons separated by electrophoresis, whereas DNA sequencing determines the specific sequence of DNA amplified. PCR–RFLP is an alternative for species identification at laboratories with limited technological capacity, but it is not efficient as DNA sequencing analysis for specific-species/strains identification. Real-time PCR formats usually provide fast and specific results with very low risk of laboratory environmental contamination. Multilocus sequence typing (MLST) has also been applied to the identification of *Leishmania* spp. with considerable success. Currently, there are no FDA-approved molecular tests for the diagnosis of leishmaniasis.

**4. Laboratory capability**—Laboratory capacity must include trained staff (i.e., qualified personal for culture preparation and microscopists for morphological detection). Minimal laboratory capacity includes a biosafety cabinet for specimen preparation, an incubator for parasites culture, and microscopy for morphological analysis. Ideally, laboratories must have capacity for molecular techniques and serological analysis.

**5. Safety requirements**—Clinical specimens should always be handled with universal/standard precautions including the use of proper personal protective equipment (gloves, laboratory coat, and safety glasses). Although *Leishmania* spp. are classified as biosafety level 2 organisms, and contamination via laboratory accidents have been rarely reported, the organism present in clinical specimens in most of the cases is alive and can potentially infect laboratorians.

**6. Nonhuman hosts**—Important reservoir hosts are *L. (L.) donovani*: dogs and rodents in Africa; *L. (L.) infantum*: dogs, foxes, rodents, and opossums; *L. (L.) major*: rodents; *L. (L.) aethiopica*: hyraxes and possibly rodents; *L. (L.) arabica*: rodents and feral dogs; *L. (V.) braziliensis*: rodents, dogs, and equines; *L. (V.) guyanensis*: sloths and opossums; *L. (V.) lainsoni*: pacas; *L. (V.) naiffi*: armadillos; *L. (V.) panamensis*: sloths; *L. (V.) peruviana*: dogs; *L. (V.) shawi*: sloths, monkeys, and coatimundis; *L. (L.) mexicana*: rodents; *L. (L.) amazonensis*: rodents. *L. (L.) tropica* is a predominantly anthroponotic disease, though it has been occasionally reported in hyraxes and dogs. The reservoirs of *L. (L.) killicki* and *L. (L.) waltoni* remain unknown.

**7. Sample/specimen requirements**—Specimens for visceral leishmaniasis detection can be splenic aspirates, Ethylenediaminetetraacetic acid anticoagulated peripheral blood, and lymph node or bone marrow aspirates. Specimens for the detection of cutaneous leishmaniasis include tissue biopsies (obtained from the edge of the lesions), scrapings, and aspirates. Specimens for culture must be kept in a tube/vial that contains a sterile buffered medium (e.g., buffered saline, Roswell Park Memorial Institute, Eagle's growth, Schneider's, Tobie's), with a neutral pH (~7–7.4) and should be shipped to the laboratory at room temperature as soon as possible after collection. Formalin-fixed paraffin-embedding specimens are also acceptable for identification of *Leishmania* spp. by immunohistochemistry and PCR procedures.

**8. Testing requirements**—Laboratories must have capacity to perform morphologic, culture, molecular, and serologic analysis. Ideally molecular and serological protocols must be chosen to specifically separate several species or at least species present in a focal area. To assure the quality of the results, culture and molecular tests must to be verified by using positive and negative controls. For each test run, these controls must to be tested as a real clinical specimen (i.e., control must be tested using the same protocol and equipment).

**9. Reporting requirements**—Amastigotes detected by microscopy should be reported as *Leishmania* spp. Negative microscopy results should be reported as "no parasites seen" as the limit of detection of morphology means that a true negative result cannot be reported from this test. Results can be reported as *Leishmania* spp. when culture is positive or, if available, the species identified by MLEE or molecular tests. Reporting of cases of leishmaniasis may be required within certain endemic regions of the world. Laboratories should determine if leishmaniasis is a reportable disease within their respective jurisdictions.

**10. Referral network**—First line laboratories may identify amastigotes by direct microscopy. Reference laboratories may perform molecular detection to genus or species level, though many PCR-based assays only allow identification within groups of species. CDC DPDx in the USA offers reference diagnostic services for microscopy and identification to species level by PCR and culture.

**11. Special considerations**—Correct *Leishmania* spp. identification has significant impact on patient clinical management and outcomes. Therefore, it is highly recommended that an experienced laboratorian be responsible for reviewing and interpreting the final tests results as identification has an important impact on the treatment recommendation.

[M. de Almeida, R. S. Bradbury]

# LEPROSY
(Hansen's disease)

| DISEASE | ICD-10 CODE |
|---|---|
| LEPROSY | ICD-10 A30 |

**1. Clinical features**—A chronic infectious disease of the skin and peripheral nerves whose clinical manifestations reflect a continuum between 2 forms of disease: tuberculoid and lepromatous. Under WHO classification, tuberculoid leprosy is termed paucibacillary and exhibits 1–5 hypopigmented or reddish anesthetic lesions, generally characterized as large, flat plaques with irregular borders and asymmetric distribution. Lepromatous leprosy is termed multibacillary under WHO classification, and the lesions are more numerous, typically symmetric, and consist of small, smooth hyperpigmented papules and plaques that may or may not exhibit loss of sensation. In addition, enlargement of superficial nerves (e.g., auricular, ulnar, median, radial, superficial peroneal, posterior tibial nerves) may be seen. Nerve involvement may occur together or separately as sensory, motor, and/or autonomic neuropathies.

Clinical manifestations can include 2 acute adverse events: reversal reactions and erythema nodosum leprosum (ENL). The former is characterized by edema and erythema of existing skin lesions, formation of new skin lesions, neuritis, additional sensory and motor loss, and/or edema of hands, feet, and face. ENL is characterized by appearance of tender, erythematous subcutaneous nodules on apparently normal skin and is often accompanied by systemic symptoms such as fever, malaise, anorexia, arthralgia, and edema. Both are considered medical emergencies. Differential diagnosis of leprosy includes psoriasis, vitiligo, tinea versicolor, pityriasis alba, sarcoidosis, syphilis, mycosis fungoides, miliaria profunda, and streptocerciasis, as well as other mycobacterial infections and infiltrative skin diseases.

**2. Causative agents**—*Mycobacterium leprae*. This bacterium cannot be grown in bacteriological media or cell cultures.

**3. Laboratory diagnosis**—Leprosy is usually diagnosed clinically. Clinical diagnosis is based on skin and neurologic examination.

1) Identify 1 or more chronic skin lesions that have not responded to treatment for other diagnoses, often with reduction or loss of sensation within the lesion.
2) Search for signs of peripheral nerve involvement (hypoesthesia, anesthesia, paralysis, muscle wasting, and/or trophic ulcers).
3) Conduct bilateral palpation of peripheral nerves (great auricular nerve, ulnar nerve at the elbow, radial cutaneous nerve and median nerve at wrist, peroneal nerve at the head of the fibula, and the posterior tibial nerve at the medial malleolus), examining for enlargement and/or tenderness.
4) Test skin lesions for sensation (light touch, pinprick, and temperature discrimination).
5) Check for inability to close the eyelids completely (lagopthalmos) by requesting patient to close both eyes.
6) Test for motor weakness and sensory loss (for a description of WHO disability grading, see: https://www.lepra.org.uk/platforms/lepra/files/lr/Dec03/10-366.pdf)

Laboratory diagnosis is through identification of the presence of alcohol-acid-fast bacilli in slit skin smears (incision-scrape method) or by full thickness skin biopsy (preferable). In practice, laboratory studies are not essential for the diagnosis of leprosy; however, confirmation by skin biopsy is recommended if at all possible. Polymerase chain reaction (PCR) may be used for detection of *M. leprae* deoxyribonucleic acid (DNA) in tissues. The immunological lepromin test, used in the past to classify patients, is not diagnostic and should be reserved only for research activities. No reliable blood or skin tests currently exist for the diagnosis of leprosy.

4. **Laboratory capability**—Specially equipped laboratories are not required. With proper mycobacteriology training and availability of appropriate bacterial stains (Fite-Faraco stain) and a microscope, slit skin smears may be obtained and examined in a minimally equipped clinic or hospital setting. Examination of skin biopsy by experienced laboratory scientists requires access to a histopathology laboratory and evaluation of the slides by a pathologist.

5. **Safety requirements**—*M. leprae* is not readily transmissible in a laboratory environment. Biosafety level 2 is appropriate for handling tissue samples being examined for presence of *M. leprae*. Given that *M. leprae* cannot be cultured on artificial media, generation of infectious aerosols or splashes is not a concern, and use of a biosafety cabinet is not necessary.

6. **Nonhuman hosts**—The 9-banded armadillo has been identified as a nonhuman host and is able to harbor the agent and contract disease. Evidence of transmission from the armadillo to humans (and vice versa) has been supported through genotyping studies, although routes of transmission have not been identified. *M. leprae* and *Mycobacterium lepromatosis* have also recently been identified in red squirrels in the UK; the significance of this and role in transmission is currently unknown.

7. **Sample/specimen requirements**—

1) Slit skin smears: a slit skin smear is collected by means of creating a shallow incision in the skin followed by scraping of the inner wound surface with a razor blade or scalpel blade held at a right angle to the incision. The fluid and tissue from the scraping are then transferred to a clean microscope slide by means of creating a thin smear on the slide. Six specimens are generally collected from a patient: 1 from each earlobe, 1 from each elbow, and 1 from each knee; sometimes an additional specimen is taken from a skin lesion. These are air-dried and can be transported at ambient temperature. Slides are stained using the Fite or Kinyoun methods and examined for the presence of acid-fast bacilli on a semiquantitative scale of 0–6+. Of note, slit skin smears may fail to demonstrate acid fast bacilli in tuberculoid leprosy patients due to relatively low bacterial load.

2) Skin biopsy: a full thickness skin biopsy is taken from within a skin lesion, ideally at the most active edge of the most active lesion. The biopsy is then placed in 10% neutral buffered formalin and submitted to a trained pathologist for examination. Specimens should never be stored in saline in a refrigerator, as the tissue will be macerated and lose cellular definition after such treatment, and nucleic acids will be destroyed. Specimens in formalin can be shipped at ambient temperature and pose no biosafety, infectious, or sample degradation risk. Standard 4-micron sections stained with hematoxylin and eosin are assessed for granulomatous inflammation with particular attention to perineural inflammation. Fite-stained sections are examined for acid-fast bacilli with a 100× objective (oil immersion). Demonstration of acid-fast bacilli within cutaneous nerves is pathognomonic of leprosy. Skin biopsy provides greater accuracy in diagnosis and allows for greater refinement of disease type (tuberculoid vs. lepromatous), which is important in determination of treatment approach as well as risk of disease complications such as reversal reactions and erythema nodosum leprosum. (For further information, see "Leprosy" in *CCDM20*.)

**8. Testing requirements**—Skin biopsies must be obtained and processed as described earlier and evaluated by a pathologist for the pattern of inflammatory response in hematoxylin and eosin-stained sections and for acid-fast bacilli in Fite-stained sections. The only required equipment for skin smears, described earlier, are sterile blades, glass microscope slides, and a microscope with a high magnification (oil immersion) lens. Experienced technicians are also required to obtain the samples from the skin and to stain them and count the bacilli. Tests for nucleic acids, such as PCR, can be done on formalin-fixed, paraffin-embedded tissues if the formalin fixation does not exceed 72 hours. Fixation in 70% ethanol provides optimal preservation of nucleic acid structure, and, if molecular testing is anticipated, it is prudent to obtain 2 specimens or divide 1 biopsy and fix 1 portion in formalin and the other portion in ethanol. Specimens in 70% ethanol can be stored and shipped at ambient temperature and still provide excellent preservation of DNA and ribonucleic acid. Mutations associated with resistance to various antimycobacterial agents can also be identified in DNA preparations. *M. leprae* cannot be grown in axenic culture medium but will proliferate within the footpads of mice. This technique is now used only for research purposes and only a few laboratories still retain this capability. Specimens to be used for footpad inoculation must be shipped immediately in transport medium on wet ice (not frozen or fixed). Arrangements should be made with the receiving laboratory before shipping such specimens.

**9. Reporting requirements**—In most countries, WHO provides medications for treatment of leprosy at no cost to patients; in the USA the

National Hansen's Disease Programs (NHDP) fulfills this role rather than WHO. Distribution of these medications is generally conducted through ministry of health leprosy control programs or their equivalent, and as such, leprosy should be considered reportable to these control programs (as well as state health departments in the USA) in order to allow patients access to treatment. Generally a clinical diagnosis is considered presumptive and is sufficient for initiating treatment; however, slit skin smear, or preferably skin biopsy, should be obtained for confirmatory diagnosis and determination of disease type. Results of this testing should be reported to the control program to ensure appropriate patient care and treatment as well as contact investigation.

**10. Referral network**—For most countries, ministries of health provide services for routine skin smear and biopsy studies. Within the USA, referral for laboratory services is primarily to NHDP through state health departments or CDC. WHO is also recommending 10% of all new cases be tested for mutations associated with drug resistance; the network of partners to perform this testing is still being developed.

**11. Special considerations**—None.

[D. D. Blaney, D. M. Scollard]

# LEPTOSPIROSIS

(Weil's disease, canicola fever, hemorrhagic jaundice, mud fever, canefield fever, swineherd disease, rat urine disease)

| DISEASE | ICD-10 CODE |
|---|---|
| LEPTOSPIROSIS | ICD-10 A27 |

**1. Clinical features**—A bacterial zoonotic disease that is self-limiting and often clinically inapparent in the majority of cases but can cause fulminant fatal disease. The disease typically presents as 1 of the following 4 clinical categories:

1) Mild, influenza-like illness
2) Weil's syndrome characterized by jaundice, renal failure, hemorrhage, and myocarditis with arrhythmias
3) Meningitis or meningoencephalitis
4) Pulmonary hemorrhage with respiratory failure (leptospirosis-associated pulmonary haemorrhage syndrome)

Clinical illness lasts from a few days to 3 weeks or longer. Generally, there are 2 phases in the illness. The acute, or leptospiremic, phase occurs during the first week of illness and is characterized by the abrupt onset of high fever, myalgias (calves and lumbar region), and headache (retro-orbital and frontal). Other acute manifestations can include nausea, vomiting, abdominal pain, diarrhea, cough, photophobia, and a truncal or pretibial rash. About 30% or more of patients also have conjunctival suffusion (redness of the conjunctiva)—a pathognomonic finding of leptospirosis when observed with scleral icterus. The second, or immune, phase occurs in conjunction with the development of the antibody response and is characterized by prolonged fever and systemic complications, such as jaundice, renal failure, bleeding, respiratory insufficiency with or without hemoptysis, hypotension, myocarditis, meningitis, mental confusion, and depression. The 2 phases can be separated by a 3- to 4-day abatement of fever. However, the distinction between the phases might not be apparent, and patients sometimes present only in the second phase. Recovery of untreated cases can take several months.

It is estimated that between 5% and 10% of clinical infections progress to severe illness. The icteric form (Weil's disease) is associated with severe hepatic dysfunction and hemorrhage; cardiac, pulmonary and neurological involvement; and high mortality. However, severe complications can also occur in patients without jaundice. Prognostic predictors for death include age older than 40 years, oliguria, respiratory insufficiency, pulmonary hemorrhage, cardiac arrhythmias, and altered mental status. Deaths are mainly due to renal failure, cardiopulmonary failure, widespread hemorrhage, and, rarely, liver failure. Case-fatality rates are estimated to be from 5%–15% in patients with severe illness to more than 50% in those with pulmonary hemorrhage syndrome, characterized by massive pulmonary bleeding and acute respiratory distress.

In countries where leptospirosis is endemic, it appears to be a significant cause of undiagnosed aseptic meningitis (between 5%–40% of cases). Late sequelae can occur including chronic fatigue, neuropsychiatric symptoms (paresis, depression), and unilateral or bilateral uveitis, characterized by iritis, iridocyclitis, and chorioretinitis, which can develop up to 18 months after acute illness and persist for years.

Cases are often under-recognized or misdiagnosed as dengue, malaria, aseptic meningitis, encephalitis, and influenza due to the nonspecific manifestations of acute leptospirosis. Severe leptospirosis must be differentiated from other causes of acute jaundice and renal failure, such as rickettsial disease, hantaviral infection, enteric fevers, viral hepatitis, and Gram-negative sepsis. During pregnancy infection can result in fetal death, abortion, stillbirth, or congenital infection.

**2. Causative agents**—Organisms from the genus *Leptospira* are classified into 20 named pathogenic and nonpathogenic genomospecies as determined by deoxyribonucleic acid (DNA)-DNA hybridization. They are subdivided into nearly 300 antigenically defined serovars, which are grouped into 26 serogroups based on serologic relatedness. Serologic classification continues to provide useful epidemiologic information, since serogroups and serovars are often associated with specific animal reservoirs. The severity of illness tends to vary with the infecting serovar.

**3. Laboratory diagnosis**—Diagnosis is by isolation of leptospires from blood or cerebrospinal fluid (CSF) during the first 7–10 days of acute illness, or from urine beginning in the second week of illness.

Immunoglobulin class G (IgG) assays, enzyme-linked immunosorbent assay (ELISA) assays, and antiwhole *Leptospira* IgM detection kits in enzyme-linked immunosorbent assay or rapid formats are used to provide presumptive confirmation for leptospirosis. However, sensitivity is low (39%–72%) during acute-phase illness (first 7 days). Immunofluorescence, immunohistochemical, and nucleic acid detection techniques are used for the demonstration of leptospires in clinical and autopsy specimens.

Polymerase chain reaction (PCR) assays for detection of leptospire DNA have been developed for use on clinical samples, such as blood or urine, and can be used for diagnostic testing on whole blood during the first 4 days of clinical illness and on urine after the first week of illness. These tests are available in reference and research laboratories. Direct examination of blood or urine using dark-field microscopy has poor sensitivity and specificity. Inoculation of experimental animals, such as golden hamsters, guinea pigs, or gerbils, can also confirm diagnosis but is rarely used. Where laboratory capacity is not well established, a positive test by 2 different rapid diagnostic tests could be considered as a laboratory confirmed case.

Diagnosis is most frequently confirmed by seroconversion, from a negative to a positive value, or is demonstrated by 4-fold or greater increase in serum agglutination titer on the microscopic agglutination test (MAT)—the confirmatory serologic test, using acute and convalescent specimens obtained at least 10 days apart. Seroconversion can occur as early as 5–7 days after disease onset but might not develop until after 10 days or longer, especially if antimicrobial therapy is initiated. Patients can develop cross-reactive antibodies to several serovars during acute infection; these gradually decrease weeks to months later. Different serovars of leptospires can occur in different regions. Therefore, the MAT preferably uses a panel of locally occurring leptospire serovars. However, antibody titer increase can be delayed or absent in some patients, and seroconversion can occur asymptomatically, especially in endemic areas. IgM-class antibodies can remain detectable for months to years at low titers.

Culture and isolation can be very difficult, requiring special media and incubation for up to 16 weeks, and the sensitivity of culture for diagnosis is low.

**4. Laboratory capability**—Most hospital and clinical laboratories that have diagnostic and research laboratory facilities for appropriate diagnostic testing (see Laboratory Diagnosis and Testing Requirements sections in this chapter) are suitably equipped to test for leptospirosis. Biosafety level 2 (BSL2) facilities are required.

**5. Safety requirements**—*Leptospira* spp. are classified as BSL-2, meaning that they can be handled in diagnostic and research laboratories on the bench with reasonable precautions to prevent infection. Local guidelines on the requirements for handling and working with BSL-2 organisms should be followed.

**6. Nonhuman hosts**—Pathogenic leptospires are maintained in the genital tract and renal tubules of wild and domestic animals, which serve as natural maintenance hosts and can remain asymptomatic shedders for years or even for life. Serovars are adapted to 1 or more reservoir animal species such as rats (*Leptospira copenhageni* and *Leptospira icterohaemorrhagiae*), dogs (*Leptospira canicola*), cattle (*Leptospira hardjo* and *Leptospira pomona*), sheep (*Leptospira harjo*), and horses (*Leptospira bratislava*). Human infection results from exposure to infected urine from carrier animals, either directly or indirectly through contaminated soil or water.

**7. Sample/specimen requirements**—For acute illness (<2 weeks post onset), ethylenediaminetetraacetic acid (EDTA) blood, serum, CSF and urine should be submitted for PCR or culture for laboratories where this is offered. To culture from urine, a fresh sample (<2 hours post-voiding) is required due to low survival of the leptospires in urine. For serology, serum is the best clinical sample, but EDTA blood (for ELISA) and plasma can also be used. Samples should be submitted for testing as soon as possible after collection. There are no special considerations for transport; however, local regulations regarding transport of clinical samples for diagnosis should be observed.

**8. Testing requirements**—The definitive diagnostic test for leptospirosis is direct detection of the leptospires in clinical samples. Culture is time-consuming, lacks sensitivity, and requires several weeks of incubation, making it unsuitable for routine primary diagnosis. Media should be inoculated within 24 hours from blood and CSF collected in heparin or sodium oxalate tubes for transport at room temperature. Citrate anticoagulation should be avoided due to inhibition. Clinical samples requiring culture should not be frozen. Microscopy: leptospires can be detected using dark-field microscopy or microscopy with silver staining on blood or urine. These methods lack sensitivity, have high false-positive and false-negative rates, and are generally not recommended as a diagnostic method. Serology: the main reference serology test is the MAT, which detects agglutinating antibodies in serum and is considered to be the gold standard serology test for leptospirosis. The test generally has high sensitivity and specificity; however, it requires highly experienced users to operate the test, due to the difficulties in test interpretation and requires specialist laboratory facilities to maintain the live cultures required for the test. Acute and convalescent samples are usually required. Generally, a positive MAT is demonstrated by a 4-fold increase in antibody titer or a conversion from seronegativity to a titer of 1:100 or greater using paired sera. Commercial ELISAs exist for the detection of IgM and IgG antibodies with reported high sensitivity and specificity. Commercial IgM ELISAs have been reported to be more sensitive than MAT for the diagnosis of acute-phase leptospirosis. Rapid immunochromatography tests, such as Leptocheck WB (Zephyr Biomedicals, Salcete, India), are considered to be as sensitive and specific as IgM ELISA for acute phase diagnostics and are suitable for use in resource-poor settings. Other serology assays include complement fixation, slide agglutination, indirect hemagglutination, and microcapsule agglutination tests. Antibody tests may be negative in early disease when PCR may be the preferred diagnostic method.Molecular methods: many PCR assays have been reported for direct detection of leptospires. The assays are of most use during acute illness, preferably in the first week of illness. Reported assays include those that detect genes that are widely available in bacteria, such as 16S RNA, and those that are specific for pathogenic *Leptospira*, such as LipL32. PCR assays for pathogenic leptospires, such as LipL32, can lack sensitivity compared with more generic assays targeting the 16S RNA. Real-time PCR assays based on either SYBR Green or Taqman have been described, and the assays have been shown to be sensitive, specific, and able to distinguish between pathogenic and environmental strains. Studies comparing PCR, Leptocheck WB, IgM ELISA, and MAT have shown that PCR can detect 50% of acute cases that are negative by other tests.

**9. Reporting requirements**—Leptospirosis is a notifiable disease in the USA, and many countries have surveillance systems for leptospirosis based on the number of confirmed cases. Local guidelines on reporting should be followed.

**10. Referral network**—The main WHO collaborating center is the Instituto Oswaldo Cruz (FIOCRUZ), Rio de Janeiro, Brazil. A network of 8 WHO collaborating centers and national referral centers exists (see: https://www.who.org/). Local guidelines on referral of samples for confirmation or notification of positive cases should be followed.

**11. Special considerations**—In developed countries, leptospirosis is considered to be an occupational disease, through activities such as mining, sewer maintenance and water work, livestock farming, pest control activities, abattoir working, and veterinary medicine. It is also associated with slum living and certain leisure activities, particularly water sports and caving. In tropical environments, agriculture poses a significant risk of infection, but so do general activities during high seasonal rainfall even in urban areas.

[J. Duggan]

# LISTERIOSIS

| DISEASE | ICD-10 CODE |
|---|---|
| LISTERIOSIS | ICD-10 A32 |

**1. Clinical features**—A bacterial infection that typically causes invasive disease. In older adults and persons with certain immunocompromising conditions, invasive disease usually presents as septicemia or meningitis. The onset of meningitis can be sudden—with fever, intense headache, nausea, vomiting, and signs of meningeal irritation—or subacute meningoencephalitis or rhomboencephalitis can occur. Delirium and coma may appear early; occasionally there is collapse and shock. Endocarditis, granulomatous lesions in the liver and other organs, localized internal or external abscesses, septic arthritis or osteomyelitis, and pustular or papular cutaneous lesions may occur on rare occasions. Surveillance data from the USA indicate that the case-fatality rate among nonpregnant adults with invasive listeriosis is 18%. In otherwise healthy people, *Listeria* infection is often asymptomatic but may cause an acute febrile gastroenteritis.

In pregnant women, symptoms may be mild and nonspecific—fever, headache, myalgia, or gastrointestinal symptoms—or absent. However, placental invasion can lead to fetal infection resulting in stillbirth, preterm delivery, or neonatal infection. Neonatal infection typically presents as septicemia or meningitis; meningitis is more common with late onset of symptoms (>1 week of age). *Listeria* can also cause spontaneous abortions, although the incidence is difficult to estimate since bacterial cultures are not routinely obtained. Listeriosis has not been associated with recurrent pregnancy loss. The case-fatality rate is 20%–30% in infected newborns and approaches 50% when onset occurs in the first 4 days after birth.

**2. Causative agents**—*Listeria monocytogenes*, a Gram-positive rod-shaped bacterium. Occasional cases due to other species, particularly *Listeria ivanovii,* occur.

**3. Laboratory diagnosis**—Since the clinical symptoms of human listeriosis are not sufficiently characteristic to establish a diagnosis, it is necessary to isolate and identify *L. monocytogenes* from normally sterile body sites such as blood, cerebrospinal fluid, amniotic fluid, or placenta. *L. monocytogenes* is sometimes seen in stained cerebrospinal fluid smears collected from patients with meningitis together with a moderate leucocyte reaction (usually lymphocytic), elevated protein levels and depressed sugar concentrations. Despite the species name "*monocytogenes*," monocytosis during septicemia or meningitis is rarely observed.

During pregnancy, *L. monocytogenes* can be cultured from maternal blood, especially when collected during febrile episodes. During labor, meconium-stained amniotic fluid is an indication of fetal distress and often occurs in perinatal listeriosis. At birth, *L. monocytogenes* can be readily cultured from the following: the placenta and lochia; the infant's blood, cerebrospinal fluid, respiratory and gastric tract, skin and other surface sites; and the maternal high vagina. Amniotic fluid and meconium should be cultured when available. The bacterium is present in sufficient numbers to be readily visualised in stained smears from any of the sites mentioned.

Following intrauterine death and expulsion of the fetus, necropsy should be carried out. Material taken from the infant's liver, spleen, brain, and other internal organs should be cultured for *L. monocytogenes*. Culturing maternal high-vaginal swabs may also be useful in retrospective diagnosis of intrauterine infection within several weeks after delivery.

**4. Laboratory capability**—For clinical diagnosis by conventional culture, general pathology laboratories performing standard microbiological testing should be capable of providing routine diagnostic procedures for human listeriosis.

The bacterium grows on standard blood containing nonselective media commonly used in clinical laboratories: external quality assessment is recommended. Specialized laboratories may be needed for polymerase chain reaction (PCR)-based diagnosis, although this is becoming a standard requirement within the repertoire of such laboratories and the limiting factor is likely to be the rare request for testing and not equipment and training staff to perform the test.

As listeriosis is predominantly foodborne, more specialized staff and facilities are required for its isolation from food. Since *L. monocytogenes* is a major public health problem and is included within microbiological criteria for food across many different countries, the detection of this bacterium in food, as well as the environment where food is manufactured, has become a routine capability in many food microbiology laboratories both in the public and private sector. Sold and liquid media that are used for the selective isolation of this genus of bacteria from food and the environment are widely commercially available.

**5. Safety requirements**—*L. monocytogenes* requires biosafety level 2 (BSL 2) laboratories. Some countries have recommended restrictions on pregnant laboratory workers handling live cultures of the bacterium. Laboratory-acquired infection has been described.

**6. Nonhuman hosts**—The majority of cases of human listeriosis are acquired by consumption of contaminated food. *L. monocytogenes* is widely distributed in the environment, and has been isolated from numerous sites including soil, sewage, water and decaying plant material (especially poorly fermented silage): its viability is remarkable with survival in soil or silage for more than 2 years. It is found in excreta from apparently healthy animals (including humans) although carriage in the gut is likely to be transitory. Contamination of food occurs either from the raw ingredients, or from post-process contamination in the food production environment (plant, equipment, drains, etc.). Unlike most other foodborne pathogens, *L. monocytogenes* can multiply in refrigerated foods and food types most often associated with transmission are ready-to-eat, capable of supporting the growth of the bacterium and often with extended refrigerated shelf lives.

Listeriosis has been recognized in a very wide range of mammalian and bird species as well as insects and fish. Among domestic animals, sheep and goats are most susceptible, although infection takes place in cattle. Listeriosis presents with a wide range of disorders that parallel much of that for humans (i.e., abortion, septicemia, encephalitis, diarrhea, mastitis, and ocular infections). Human listeriosis can be a zoonosis and occurs, although this probably accounts for the minority of cases. Zoonotic transmission occurs by consumption of milk contaminated from an animal with mastitis. Although this does occur, the most common route of contamination of milk is likely to be via faecal contamination or from plant and machinery within the dairy. The second mode of zoonotic transmission is by direct contact with infected animals or animal material and again this is relatively rare and accounts for a small proportion of all cases. This form of the disease principally occurs as either papular or pustular cutaneous lesions usually on the upper arms or wrists of farmers or veterinarians 1-4 days after attending bovine abortions.

**7. Sample/specimen requirements**—For diagnoses in humans, blood or cerebrospinal fluid (CSF) are the most common specimens examined. For the newly delivered infant, in addition to blood and CSF, swabs from the placenta and maternal lochia, as well as the infant's respiratory and gastric tract, skin, and other surface sites, and the maternal high vagina can be tested. Amniotic fluid and meconium should be cultured when available. Where specific anatomical sites are infected, samples directly from there should be collected (e.g., peritoneal fluid, heart valves, skin, or eyes).

For investigating foodborne infection, samples of suspected food should be tested, as well as plant, machinery, drains and environmental swabs from the food manufacturing environment.

**8. Testing requirements**—The current laboratory procedures for diagnosis require culture of *L. monocytogenes* from the patient's specimens. Special culture media and procedures are not usually required when examining samples from normally sterile sites. The bacterium generally grows within 1–2 days and produces characteristic colonies 1–2 mm in diameter. Care must be taken to distinguish this organism from other Gram-positive rods, particularly diphtheroids, although identification to the genus level of isolates from clinical cases should be straightforward using limited standard phenotypic tests.

Methods to detect specific nucleic acid sequences by PCR have been described, and these have been applied to a variety of patient's body fluids. Procedures to detect specific antibody have also been described; however, interpretation is problematic and these have not led to useful diagnostic tests. Stool samples are of limited use and are not recommended.

Selective enrichment media are readily available for isolation from food and the environment.

**9. Reporting requirements**—Reporting of cases is mandatory in some countries, and national statistics are available including mandatory consolidation of data within the EU. Pure cultures from cases, foods, and related sites such as food production environments should be referred for reference purposes (see Referral Network section in this chapter).

**10. Referral network**—Listeriosis is a rare disease (usually 1–10 cases per million of the general population). Patients can have long incubation periods (≤91 days between consumption of contaminated foods and clinical recognition of disease), and food production environments acting as reservoirs for contamination of food can be colonized by an individual strain of *L. monocytogenes* for years, even decades. Consequently, patients within an outbreak related by exposure to a common food can be very widely distributed both temporally and geographically. Prompt and thorough investigation of all cases together with national reporting and surveillance are essential for control.

Since the disease is rare and outbreaks are sometimes only detected by national or even international surveillance, the submission of isolates to reference laboratories for secondary and specialized reference testing, including application of discriminatory typing, is an essential requirement for public health control. Most human infections (95%) are caused by serovars 1/2a, 1/2b, and 4b; hence, this method provides insufficient discrimination for the purpose of epidemiological typing. Networks of laboratories using pulsed-field gel electrophoresis, as well as a range of other methods, have been highly successful for this purpose, but this has been superseded by the use of whole genome sequencing with its high resolution discrimination and phylogenetic analysis in different countries including those in North America and in Europe.

**11. Special considerations**—Preventing listeriosis requires action from the food industry to reduce, as much as possible, exposure of the public to *L. monocytogenes* in the food chain. Additional actions to ensure food safety, including avoidance of certain foods and proper preparation and storage, are especially important for groups at higher risk for invasive listeriosis (pregnant women, older adults, and immunocompromised individuals).

Human listeriosis most often affects the bloodstream, the central nervous system (CNS), or the uterus during pregnancy. In nonpregnant individuals, listeriosis most frequently presents as meningitis (with or without septicemia), or septicemia without involvement of the CNS. Septicemia is generally confined to immunocompromised individuals and rarely has identifiable foci of infection. Meningitis is the most common CNS infection: meningoencephalitis and encephalitis occur but less commonly. Focal infections caused by *L. monocytogenes* are relatively rare and are primarily confined to immunocompromised individuals. Deep-seated infections with or without abscess formation occur in a wide variety of sites. Listeria endocarditis also occurs and is usually confined to patients with underlying cardiac lesions or with prosthetic heart valves. Long-term sequalae occur following systemic infection.

Less severe forms of the disease occur in adults: cutaneous and ocular listeriosis resulting from contact with infected animals or animal material have been described. Superficial lesions may develop to serious systemic infection. Listeriosis in immunocompetent individuals may present as febrile gastroenteritis, and outbreaks of diarrhea with fever and other gastrointestinal symptoms have been described and in which a proportion of individuals go on to develop severe systemic infection. Some but not all patients with severe systemic infection have diarrhea.

In the pregnant woman, listeriosis is most often recognized as 1 or more self-limiting influenza-like episodes during or after the latter half of the second trimester, although infection can occur throughout gestation. Maternal listeriosis usually presents with pyrexia and other nonspecific symptoms, although some individuals may be asymptomatic. Maternal listeric meningitis during pregnancy is very rare.

During pregnancy infection spreads from the maternal circulatory system to the fetus via the placenta, although this is not inevitable. Fetal infection developing before the third trimester usually results in intrauterine death. The fetus has severe and overwhelming multisystem infection involving internal organs, with the widespread formation of granulomatous lesions, especially in the liver and placenta; this is named *granulomatosis infantiseptica*. Infection of the infant during the third trimester results in either intrauterine death, or the delivery of a severely ill neonate (early onset infection). Early onset sepsis is characterised by nonspecific signs of infection and prematurity. Cutaneous lesions may be present (sometimes with granulomas) and the neonate may be convulsive. Most early onset cases are septicemic, some with meningitis; however, some infants appear infected only at superficial sites. The degree of severity may be partially dependant on the gestational age at infection. Surviving infants can exhibit long-term sequelae, especially those delivered prematurely or with involvement of the CNS.

Late-onset neonatal sepsis typically occurs after uncomplicated full-term pregnancies and usually presents as meningitis about 10 days after delivery. *L. monocytogenes* is acquired either from maternal sites during or shortly after delivery (possibly during passage through the birth canal) or from the postnatal environment as a result of contact with an early onset listeriosis case.

Listeriosis has a high fatality rate at 20%–30%, which increases with age, site of infection, and underlying disease severity. The most common presentation of the disease is as septicemia in those older than 60 years.

[J. McLauchlin, K. A. Grant]

# LIVER FLUKE DISEASE

| DISEASE | ICD-10 CODE |
|---|---|
| CLONORCHIASIS | ICD-10 B66.1 |
| OPISTHORCHIASIS | ICD-10 B66.0 |
| CHOLANGIOCARCINOMA | ICD-10 C22.1 |

**1. Clinical features**—A trematode disease of the bile ducts. Clinical complaints may be slight or absent in light infections; in heavy infections (>10,000 eggs/g of stool) abdominal symptoms occur in about 10% of patients. These result from local irritation of bile ducts by the flukes. Loss of appetite, diarrhea, and a sensation of abdominal pressure are common early symptoms. Rarely, bile duct obstruction producing jaundice may be followed by cirrhosis, enlargement, and tenderness of the liver, with progressive ascites and edema. Eggs in the gall bladder increase risk of gallstones. Liver fluke disease can become chronic, sometimes lasting 30 years or longer but is rarely a direct or contributing cause of death, and it is often completely asymptomatic. However, it is a significant risk factor (≤ 15-fold increase) for the development of cholangiocarcinoma.

**2. Causative agents**—*Clonorchis sinensis* for clonorchiasis; *Opisthorchis felineus* and *Opisthorchis viverrini* for opisthorchiasis. *C. sinensis* and *O. viverrini* occur in southeast Asia; *O. felineus* occurs in Europe and Palearctic Asia.

**3. Laboratory diagnosis**—Demonstration of the characteristic eggs in concentrated feces or duodenal/bile drainage fluid. Eggs cannot be easily differentiated among these worms. Serological diagnosis by enzyme-linked immunosorbent assay can be performed but is not always specific. Immunoblot assays based on antigens have variable sensitivities. Polymerase chain reaction for detection of eggs in stools has been reported to be sensitive for heavier infections and less so in light infections; however, these laboratory-developed tests are not widely used outside of specialized reference labs. Imaging such as ultrasound, computerized tomography, and magnetic resonance imaging scans may be used as adjunct diagnostic tools.

Eggs of *C. sinensis* are oval, narrowing toward the operculum, and measure 27–35 μm long by 12–19 μm wide; the eggs have prominent opercular shoulders, a relatively thick shell, and a small abopercular knob. Eggs are embryonated when shed in feces and contain a fully developed miracidium. Eggs of *Opisthorchis* spp. are similar in morphology but are slightly smaller, measuring 19–29 μm long by 12–17 μm wide. While eggs of *Clonorchis* and *Opisthorchis* cannot be reliably separated morphologically, the eggs should be separated from the heterophyid intestinal trematodes such as *Metagonimus yokogawai* and *Heterophyes heterophyes*. Eggs of these latter 2 species are more broadly oval, lack well-defined opercular shoulders and abopercular knobs, and measure 20–30 μm long by 15–17 μm wide.

**4. Laboratory capability**—Microscopy and stool concentration/centrifugation capabilities should be available. Laboratorians should be trained in the microscopic/morphologic detection of parasites and undergo regular proficiency testing.

**5. Safety requirements**—Clinical specimens should always be collected and handled with standard precautions. Opisthorchid trematodes are biosafety level 2 organisms. Eggs are not infectious to the human host. Formalin should only be used in a well-ventilated area, preferably in a chemical fume hood. Unpreserved and preserved stools should be disposed of as infectious waste.

**6. Nonhuman hosts**—Like all trematodes that infect humans, the first intermediate host is a freshwater snail in which the miracidium develops into cercariae. Cercariae infect the second intermediate host, freshwater fish, and develop into metacercariae. Humans become infected after eating raw or undercooked fish containing metacercariae. Several other mammals (e.g., cats, dogs, rats, pigs) may act as definitive hosts and serve as potential reservoirs for human infection.

**7. Sample/specimen requirements**—Stool should be promptly preserved in an appropriate liquid medium such as 10% buffered formalin or sodium acetate-acetic acid-formalin. Single vial systems for ova and parasite (O&P) collection are also adequate. Specimens in the appropriate preservatives should remain intact indefinitely. To maximize O&P sensitivity, at least 3 stool specimens should be collected on separate days.

**8. Testing requirements**—Routine concentration procedures for stool. A calibrated ocular micrometer should be used to measure egg size. Diagnosis is confirmatory in specimens meeting morphologic criteria.

**9. Reporting requirements**—Positive stool specimens from humans may be reported as *C. sinensis/Opisthorchis* spp. Clonorchiasis and opisthorchiasis are not nationally reportable in the USA. Report to local health authority; official report not ordinarily required.

**10. Referral network**—None.

**11. Special considerations**—None.

[B. Mathison]

# LOIASIS

(*Loa loa* infection, eyeworm disease of Africa, Calabar swelling)

| DISEASE | ICD-10 CODE |
|---|---|
| LOIASIS | ICD-10 B74.3 |

**1. Clinical features**—A chronic filarial disease characterized by migration of the adult worm through subcutaneous or deeper tissues of the body, causing transient swellings several centimeters in diameter, which can be located on any body part. These swellings may be preceded by localized pain with pruritus. A major symptom is pruritus localized on arms, thorax, face, and shoulders. Migration of the adult worm under the bulbar conjunctivae may be accompanied by pain and edema. Allergic reactions with giant urticaria (large urticaria with severe edema of the skin) and fever may occur occasionally.

**2. Causative agents**—*Loa loa*, a filarial nematode.

**3. Laboratory diagnosis**—Microfilariae are present in peripheral blood during the daytime (diurnal periodicity) and can be demonstrated in stained thick blood smears, stained sediment of blood where erythrocytes and hemoglobin have been separated (laking), or through membrane filtration or concentration (Knott's). Adult worms may be extracted from the eye or subcutaneous tissue. *L. loa*-specific deoxyribonucleic acid can be detected in blood from asymptomatic infected individuals. A travel history is essential for diagnosis in non-Africans.

Microfilariae of *L. loa* are 231–250 μm long in stained blood films. The sheath, when present, does not stain with Giemsa. The microfilariae have a relatively short head space and the tail is nucleate, with the nuclei irregularly arranged to the tapered tip.

Adult female *L. loa* are 50–70 mm long; the males are smaller at 30–35 mm long. Adults of both sexes have randomly arranged cuticular nodules called bosses.

4. **Laboratory capability**—Microscopy should be available. Laboratorians should be trained in the microscopic/morphologic detection of parasites and undergo regular proficiency testing. Polymerase chain reaction capabilities recommended for labs that have proficiency in utilizing this methodology.

5. **Safety requirements**—Clinical specimens should always be collected and handled with standard precautions. Filarial nematodes are biosafety level 2 organisms. Blood and sera should be disposed of as infectious waste.

6. **Nonhuman hosts**—*L. loa* infection is transmitted by deer flies in the genus *Chrysops*. Primate infection with *L. loa* occurs, but the 2 have different transmission complexes, and therefore the infection is not zoonotic.

7. **Sample/specimen requirements**—The ideal blood specimen for morphology is a finger prick; however, blood collected in ethylenediaminetetraacetic acid is sufficient. For maximum sensitivity, blood should be collected between 12 PM and 6 PM when the microfilariae are likely to be circulating in peripheral blood.

8. **Testing requirements**—Routine staining procedures for blood parasitology (e.g., Giemsa, Wright-Giemsa, hematoxylin) and concentration procedures (e.g., Knott's). A calibrated ocular micrometer should be used to measure microfilariae. Diagnosis is confirmatory in specimens meeting morphologic criteria.

9. **Reporting requirements**—Positive cases from humans may be reported at the species level based on the morphology of the microfilariae. Loiasis is not nationally reportable in the USA. Report to local health authority; official report not ordinarily justifiable.

10. **Referral network**—None.

11. **Special considerations**—None.

[B. Mathison]

# LYME DISEASE

(Lyme borreliosis, tickborne meningopolyneuritis)

| DISEASE | ICD-10 CODE |
|---|---|
| LYME DISEASE | ICD-10 A69.2, L90.4 |

**1. Clinical features**—A tickborne, spirochetal, zoonotic disease. It is characterized by a distinctive skin lesion, systemic flu-like symptoms, and neurologic, rheumatologic, and cardiac involvement, occurring in varying combinations over months to years.

Early symptoms can vary. The first manifestation in 70%–80% of patients is a red macule or papule that expands slowly in an annular manner, often with central clearing. This lesion is called erythema migrans (formerly, erythema chronicum migrans). Erythema migrans may be single or multiple. To be considered significant for case surveillance purposes, the erythema migrans lesion must reach at least 5 cm in diameter. With or without erythema migrans, early systemic manifestations may include malaise, fatigue, fever, headache, stiff neck, myalgia, migratory arthralgias, or lymphadenopathy, all of which may last several weeks in untreated patients.

Within weeks to months following infection, patients may develop neurological abnormalities, such as aseptic meningitis and cranial neuritis—including facial palsy, chorea, cerebellar ataxia, motor or sensory radiculoneuritis, myelitis, or encephalitis. Cardiac abnormalities, including atrioventricular block, may present within weeks following infection with rare occurrence of acute myopericarditis or cardiomegaly.

Weeks to years after onset (mean 6 months), patients may develop intermittent episodes of swelling and pain in large joints (especially the knees), leading to chronic arthritis; this may recur for several years. Antibiotic-refractory Lyme arthritis is a rare complication that was previously hypothesized to be linked to cross-reactivity between the borrelial outer surface protein A and the human leukocyte function associated antigen-1. This hypothesis is now considered unlikely. Chronic neurologic manifestations may rarely occur and include encephalopathy, polyneuropathy, or leukoencephalitis; in these patients the cerebrospinal fluid often shows lymphocytic pleocytosis and elevated protein levels. In 1 published case series from Europe, which included patients of all infection stages, 89% had erythema migrans alone, 5% presented with arthritis, 3% with early neurologic manifestations, 2% with lymphocytoma, 1% with acrodermatitis chronica atrophicans, and less than 1% with cardiac manifestations. For clinical presentations that occur in the USA, similar observations have been reported.

**2. Causative agents**—The spirochete that causes Lyme disease in North America is *Borrelia burgdorferi* sensu stricto, which was identified in 1982, and *Borrelia mayonii*. Five other Lyme borrelia have been associated with human disease in Europe or Asia. These include *Borrelia afzelii*, *Borrelia bavariensis*, *B. burgdorferi*, *Borrelia garinii*, and *Borrelia spielmanii*. Three additional species, *Borrelia bissettii*, *Borrelia lusitaniae*, and *Borrelia valaisiana*, have been detected in patients, but their importance as human pathogens is not clear.

**3. Laboratory diagnosis**—In a Lyme disease endemic region, diagnosis can be made in patients presenting with an erythema migrans rash, with or without the knowledge of a tick bite, based on clinical features. Clinical findings alone are not sufficient for diagnosis of extracutaneous manifestations of Lyme disease. In later stages of illness, however, diagnosis should be supported by 2-tiered serologic testing, typically an enzyme immunoassay (EIA), followed by Western immunoblotting in patients with a positive or equivocal EIA. Serological tests in the early stages of illness should be interpreted with caution because they are insensitive during the first weeks of infection and may remain negative in people treated early with antibiotics. In patients who have been symptomatic for less than 30 days, an immunoglobulin class M (IgM)Western blot may be helpful for diagnosis. VlsE (Vls locus expression site), or C6 recombinant antigens, increase the sensitivity of IgG immunoblot. Test sensitivity increases in patients who have progressed to later stages of illness. Cross-reacting immunofluorescence assay (IFA) and enzyme-linked immunosorbent assay (ELISA) antibodies may cause false-positive reactions in patients with syphilis, relapsing fever, leptospirosis, HIV infection, Rocky Mountain spotted fever, infectious mononucleosis, lupus, or rheumatoid arthritis. Diagnosis of neuroborreliosis in Europe is typically accomplished through serologic testing for borrelial antibodies in cerebrospinal fluid.

**4. Laboratory capability**—Most clinical and public health laboratories should be capable of testing for Lyme disease. Lyme disease-causing *Borrelia* spp. may be detected in clinical specimens (humans and animals) and in arthropod (tick) vectors by direct and indirect methods. Direct methods for detecting *Borrelia* include culturing and molecular methods such as polymerase chain reaction (PCR). *Borrelia* is a fastidious organism and requires specialized media, Barbour-Stoenner-Kelly medium or its derivatives, for replication and maintenance. Verification of growing spirochetes within media is often accomplished using microscopy. A wet mount can be easily prepared and examined under dark-field microscopy to check for contaminants and proper growth. It should be noted that culture is rarely used in clinical practice, largely due to the time it takes to yield results. Indirect methods are the most common approach used for Lyme disease diagnosis, and the detection of antibody responses to infection are routinely used globally for laboratory confirmation of Lyme borreliosis. A 2-tiered testing algorithm is universal although the guidelines for performing the testing and the interpretation criteria used differ among countries.[1,2] Individuals performing these tests should be properly trained to execute the tests and interpret the results accurately and should follow the regulations for diagnostic testing set forth by each country. Laboratory support of suspect veterinary cases is also most commonly based on detection of specific antibody responses.

**5. Safety requirements**—*Borrelia* spp. are safely handled under biosafety level 2 (BSL-2) practices.[3] Laboratorians working with these agents should be properly trained to handle infectious agents and to perform associated protocols appropriately. Personnel of laboratories offering diagnostic services should undergo competency training and participate in proficiency testing programs as required by their country's regulations. When handling samples suspected to contain this agent, or the agent itself, personnel should wear personal protective equipment that includes a laboratory coat/gown, eye and face protection (e.g., goggles, face mask), and gloves. Additional requirements and guidelines for working in a BSL-2 may vary by institution and should be followed accordingly. The use of a properly functioning and certified biological safety cabinet is recommended when working with this agent. *Borrelia* are susceptible to desiccation and have not demonstrated the capacity to develop resistance to recommended treatment antibiotics. A commercial vaccine for Lyme disease was removed from the market in 2001, and there is currently no licensed vaccine available for humans.[4] Several veterinary vaccines are available, but these are not approved for human use.

**6. Nonhuman hosts**—Lyme borreliosis is a zoonotic disease caused by a number of spirochete genospecies within the *B. burgdorferi* sensu lato complex. The natural cycle of *B. burgdorferi* primarily includes small vertebrates and ixodid ticks, with humans as incidental and dead-end hosts. The species of *Ixodes* ticks that act as the main vector for Lyme disease varies among geographic regions. Casual human contact with infected mammals is not a direct risk factor for disease transfer although exposure to ticks through such contact should be considered in minimizing risk. Testing of suspect animal cases is offered by many veterinary care providers.

**7. Sample/specimen requirements**—Although the appropriate type of sample may vary depending on stage of illness and tests available in a given area, serum analysis of antibody responses to infection are widely recommended and most often available and practiced for laboratory confirmation of infection. In early infection, and some rare cases of later infection, PCR and/or culture may be of diagnostic value. The latter diagnostic services are considered specialized, and providers should be consulted prior to sample collection for specific instructions on proper sample handling and transfer.

Clinical specimens should be collected carefully to avoid contamination with other organisms (particularly important for culturing) and ideally should be processed shortly after collection. Serum for serologic testing should be kept cold (4°C) if it will be tested soon after collection or should be frozen for future use.

**8. Testing requirements**—With the exception of recently described *B. mayonii* cases of Lyme disease,[5] spirochete abundance in any clinical sample is below the limits of most direct detection methods, and amplification of targets or markers (i.e., culture, PCR) is required for useful diagnostic sensitivity. The medium used to grow *Borrelia* is a rich culture medium, and therefore, the use of a biosafety cabinet is advised to minimize the potential for contamination. Cultures of clinical samples are incubated at 33°C (91.4°C) without agitation. It is most successful (>50%) with biopsies of erythema migrans skin lesions and/or blood samples from disseminated early Lyme disease cases.[6] These include patients with multiple erythema migrans, carditis, and/or neurological symptoms. Recovery of spirochetes from any tissue or fluid in disseminated manifestations of this disease is extremely low, and culture attempts are most typically limited to research settings. Detection of the humoral response to *B. burgdorferi* is the most common means of laboratory confirmation. Current serology recommendations are for a 2-tier strategy in which the first test is an EIA or IFA, followed by second-tier Western immunoblots of all equivocal or positive first-tier samples.[2] Negative first-tier samples should not be tested further, and samples should not be tested by Western immunoblotting in the absence of an antecedent and reactive first-tier finding. A sample must have a positive or equivocal first-tier result followed by a positive Western immunoblot to be interpreted as positive by 2-tier recommendations. IgM and IgG Western immunoblots are recommended in the first weeks of illness. After 4 weeks of illness, a robust IgG response is expected, and a positive IgG Western immunoblot is required for laboratory support of infection at this time point. Technical performance of the second-tier Western immunoblot is considered highly complex. Recommended criteria for scoring of Western immunoblots differ among countries. Additionally, because *B. garinii* and *B. afzelii* are much more common in Europe than *B. burgdorferi* sensu stricto, European immunoblots are designed to detect all 3 genospecies. Some immunoblots marketed in the USA do not always detect infections from Europe. Antibody responses may require 1 to several weeks of infection before they are detectable by current tests.

Two-tier serology sensitivity for cases without prior effective antibiotic treatment correlates positively with the duration of infection, dissemination of the infecting spirochetes, and the manifestation of disease. Early Lyme disease of 2 weeks duration or less will have a 2-tier serology sensitivity of 29%–40%.[7] This sensitivity increases to 29%–78% for early Lyme disease with illness of greater than 2 weeks duration. Two-tier serology is 42%–87% sensitive for early disseminated illness and 97%–100% for late Lyme disease, which includes Lyme arthritis. Specificity of 2-tier testing ranges from 95% to more than 99%; higher specificity is observed with the use of positive IgG

Western immunoblots as opposed to IgM Western immunoblot. Antibody responses yielding positive serology test results may persist for months after treatment and clinical cure; there is no current laboratory measure of cure.

PCR is offered by some laboratories and is useful for diagnosing *B. mayonii* infections with the specimen of choice being blood.[5] When *B. burgdorferi* infections are tested by PCR, the greatest sensitivity (60%–70%) is with skin biopsies or synovial fluid from patients with early erythema migrans skin lesions and late Lyme arthritis, respectively. PCR testing is not standardized; most laboratories offering PCR have developed their own assays with variable bacterial targets and performance measures. Other nonvalidated and noncleared tests are offered by some laboratories in the USA, Europe, and Asia; caution should be exercised in utilizing these tests and interpreting their results.[8]

**9. Reporting requirements**—Lyme disease is a notifiable condition in both the USA and Canada and among some countries in Europe and Asia. Lyme disease case reports are collected and verified in accordance with each country's legal mandate and surveillance practices. Reported cases include confirmed and probable cases. The case definitions used for reporting are set forth by each country and these vary among countries.

**10. Referral network**—A formal laboratory referral network for Lyme disease testing is not established. However, the capabilities for Lyme disease testing vary among diagnostic testing laboratories. Therefore, certain laboratories may only perform first-tier testing (EIA or IFA) and subsequently send the sample to a separate laboratory for second-tier testing (Western blotting).

**11. Special considerations**—None.

## References

1. Aguero-Rosenfeld ME, Wang G, Schwartz I, Wormser GP. Diagnosis of lyme borreliosis. *Clin Microbiol Rev*. 2005;18(3):484–509.
2. Centers for Disease Control and Prevention. Recommendations for test performance and interpretation from the Second National Conference on Serologic Diagnosis of Lyme Disease. *MMWR Morb Mortal Wkly Rep*. 1995;44(31): 590–591.
3. US Department of Health and Human Services, Centers for Disease Control and Prevention, National Institutes of Health. *Biosafety in Microbiological and Biomedical Laboratories*, 5th ed. 2009. Available at: https://www.cdc.gov/labs/pdf/CDC-BiosafetyMicrobiologicalBiomedicalLaboratories-2009-P.PDF. Accessed March 7, 2019.
4. Shen AK, Mead PS, Beard CB. The Lyme disease vaccine—a public health perspective. *Clin Infect Dis*. 2011;52 Suppl 3:s247–s252.
5. Pritt BS, Mead PS, Johnson DKH, et al. Identification of a novel pathogenic *Borrelia* species causing Lyme borreliosis with unusually high spirochaetaemia: a descriptive study. *Lancet Infect Dis*. 2016;16(5):556–564.

6. Dionysios L, Schwartz I, McKenna D, et al. Comparison of five diagnostic modalities for direct detection of *Borrelia burgdorferi* in patients with early Lyme disease. *Diagn Microbiol Infect Dis*. 2012;73(3):243–245.
7. Moore A, Nelson CA, Molins C, Mead PS, Schriefer M. Current guidelines, common clinical pitfalls, and future directions for laboratory diagnosis of lyme disease, United States. *Emerg Infect Dis*. 2016;22(7):1169–1177.
8. Nelson C, Hojvat S, Johnson B, et al. Concerns regarding a new culture method for *Borrelia burgdorferi* not approved for the diagnosis of Lyme disease. *MMWR Morb Mortal Wkly Rep*. 2014;63(15):333.

[C. Molins, M. Schriefer]

# LYMPHOCYTIC CHORIOMENINGITIS

(LCM, benign [or serous] lymphocytic meningitis)

| DISEASE | ICD-10 CODE |
|---|---|
| LYMPHOCYTIC CHORIOMENINGITIS | ICD-10 A87.2 |

**1. Clinical features**—A viral infection of rodents—especially mice—transmissible to humans, in whom it produces diverse clinical manifestations. There may be influenza-like symptoms, with myalgia, retro-orbital headache, leukopenia, and thrombocytopenia, followed by complete recovery. In some cases, the illness may begin with meningeal or meningoencephalomyelitic symptoms, or these symptoms may appear after a brief remission. Orchitis, parotitis, arthritis, myocarditis, and rash occur occasionally. The acute course is usually short and very rarely fatal; even with severe manifestations (e.g., coma with meningoencephalitis), prognosis for recovery without sequelae is usually good, although convalescence with fatigue and vasomotor instability may be prolonged. The cerebrospinal fluid (CSF) in cases with neurological involvement typically shows a lymphocytic pleocytosis and, at times, a low glucose level. The primary pathological finding in the rare human fatality is diffuse meningoencephalitis. Fatal cases of hemorrhagic fever-like disease have been reported in immunosuppressed patients after organ transplantation from lymphocytic choriomeningitis virus-infected donor. Transplacental infection of the fetus leading to hydrocephalus and chorioretinitis occurs and should be tested for lymphocytic choriomeningitis virus in such cases.

**2. Causative agents**—LCM virus is an enveloped ambisense ribonucleic acid (RNA) virus in the genus *Arenavirus*, family *Arenaviridae*. Among viruses in the *Arenavirus* genus, LCM virus is the prototype of the Old World arenaviruses, which include Lassa and Lujo viruses.

**3. Laboratory diagnosis**—Laboratory methods include detection of the virus RNA by conventional or real-time polymerase chain reaction (PCR) or isolation of the virus by inoculation of cell cultures with CSF collected early in the course of illness. Specific immunoglobulin class M (IgM) in serum or CSF, as evidenced by IgM capture enzyme-linked immunosorbent assay (ELISA) or rising antibody titers by immunofluorescence assay in paired sera, are considered diagnostic. LCM requires differentiation from other aseptic meningitides and viral encephalitides in young adults or differentiation from other TORCH (toxoplasmosis, rubella cytomegalovirus, herpes simplex virus) etiologies in neonatal hydrocephalus and chorioretinitis.

**4. Laboratory capability**—Most clinical and public health laboratories that perform viral diagnostic testing should be able to provide LCM testing; however, the lack of experience with LCM or lack of reagents may require referral to regional reference laboratories. LCM is rare, and diagnostic reagents are available only in a few laboratories. Molecular, serological, and classical virology capabilities are necessary.

**5. Safety requirements**—LCM viruses are classified as biosafety level 2 (some laboratory strains are biosafety level 3). Clinical specimens should always be collected and handled with universal/standard precautions. Collection and handling of infectious or suspected infectious clinical specimens should be performed by trained personnel with proper personal protective equipment. No human vaccines are currently available.

**6. Nonhuman hosts**—The infected house mouse *Mus musculus* is the natural reservoir. Infected females transmit infection to their offspring, which become asymptomatic persistent viral shedders. Infection also occurs in mouse and hamster colonies. Virological surveillance of commercial rodent breeding establishments, especially those producing hamsters and mice, is recommended.

**7. Sample/specimen requirements**—During acute febrile stages of disease, virus or viral RNA can be detected in CSF (rarely in serum, heparinized plasma, or whole blood except in immunosuppressed patients), and serologic techniques in serum or CSF can be performed on late acute or convalescent samples of the same type. Virus may also be detected or isolated in biopsy or in autopsy specimens in the rare fatal cases. Diagnostic samples should be stored and shipped frozen, if possible, on dry ice or liquid nitrogen vapor. Formaldehyde-fixed tissues collected during autopsies and paraffin-embedded blocks should be stored and shipped at room temperature. During investigation of human disease, rodent blood could be screened by serology and tissues from positive animals tested by PCR and confirmatory sequencing to confirm the source of infection.

**8. Testing requirements**—As for other infectious diseases, the diagnosis should always be based on the results of a combination of clinical and laboratory data. During acute febrile stages of disease, virus can be detected by conventional or real-time PCR using primers and probes targeting the L gene, or by virus isolation, followed by confirmatory sequencing from CSF. In late acute and convalescent stages, IgM or IgG antibodies can be detected by ELISA from blood or CSF. Viral antigens can be detected by immunohistochemistry in tissue samples collected post-mortem. Direct detection of virus, viral genome, IgM, or rising IgG antibodies titer in an individual with a clinically compatible illness or an individual with a known high-risk exposure to the virus constitutes a confirmed case of infection.

**9. Reporting requirements**—LCM infections in the USA are only reportable in a few states. LCM virus is not a select agent and does not need to be reported to the Federal Select Agent Program.

**10. Referral network**—Testing can only be performed in a few laboratories. For shipping potentially infectious material, samples should be packaged and shipped by trained personnel in accordance with current International Airline Transportation Association recommendations and forwarded, after consultation, to one of the laboratories with diagnostic capability for these agents.

**11. Special considerations**—Occurrence of LCM infection does not constitute an International Health Regulations reportable event to WHO. If LCM infection is suspected in the USA, contact the Viral Special Pathogens Branch at CDC by phone (470-312-0094 or 404-639-1115) or e-mail (spather@cdc.gov).

[P. E. Rollin]

# LYMPHOGRANULOMA VENEREUM

(lymphogranuloma inguinale, climatic or tropical bubo, LGV)

| DISEASE | ICD-10 CODE |
|---|---|
| LYMPHOGRANULOMA VENEREUM | ICD-10 A55 |

**1. Clinical features**—A sexually acquired chlamydial infection, which, in its classic form, consists of 3 stages. The first stage is characterized by a small, painless, self-limited papule at the site of inoculation (e.g., on the penis or within the urethra in men; on the vulva, vaginal wall, or cervix in women), which has often resolved by the time the patient seeks care. The second stage involves extension to the regional lymph nodes draining the area of the primary lesion, where suppuration may occur. In men, inguinal and/or femoral buboes are seen, which may become adherent to the skin, fluctuate, and result in sinus formation. In women, these external nodes are less frequently affected and involvement is mainly of the pelvic nodes with extension to the rectum and rectovaginal septum. This stage can be associated with fever and other systemic symptoms. If untreated, some patients progress to a chronic inflammatory stage that can be prolonged and debilitating, with fibrosis and lymphatic obstruction that can lead to formation of colorectal strictures, fistulas, lymphedema, and genital elephantiasis. Rectal exposure in women and men who have sex with men can result in proctocolitis, with mucoid and/or hemorrhagic rectal discharge, anal pain, constipation, fever, and/or tenesmus. This syndrome may be difficult to distinguish clinically or histologically from other conditions such as inflammatory bowel disease, colorectal cancer, and lymphoma; if untreated, it can lead to chronic fistulas and strictures.

**2. Causative agents(s)**—The invasive *Chlamydia trachomatis*, genotypes L-1, L-2, and L-3. These are related to, but distinct from, those genotypes that cause ocular (trachoma) and nonlymphogranuloma venereum (non-LGV or genital) infections.

**3. Laboratory diagnosis**—Direct detection of chlamydial organisms in swabs from lesions or bubo aspirates by direct immunofluorescence, nucleic acid detection, or culture is suggestive of lymphogranuloma venereum (LGV), since non-LGV chlamydial infections rarely result in lesion formation or lymphadenopathy. However, most tests are not specific for LGV and specimens may need additional testing to differentiate LGV from non-LGV chlamydia infections. LGV specific tests include serotyping, genotyping, or LGV-specific polymerase chain reaction (PCR). Serological tests, such as complement fixation (CF) and microimmunofluorescence (MIF), can be used in conjunction with the clinical presentation to support the diagnosis (a single titer of ≥ 1:64 and 1:256 in the CF and MIF tests respectively). However, these tests have not been validated for proctitis presentation.

**4. Laboratory capability**—Most hospital and clinical laboratories should be capable of testing for chlamydial infections including LGV. Genital and lymph node specimens (i.e., lesion swab or bubo aspirate) can be tested for *C. trachomatis* by culture, direct immunofluorescence, or nucleic acid detection. Commercially available nucleic acid amplification tests (NAATs) for *C. trachomatis* detect both LGV and non-LGV *C. trachomatis* but cannot distinguish between them. Additional molecular procedures (e.g., PCR-based genotyping) can be used to differentiate LGV from non-LGV *C. trachomatis*, but these are not widely available. The same laboratory procedures detailed in "Chlamydial Infections" apply to LGV.

**5. Safety requirements**—Biosafety level 2 level facilities are required. All specimens, microbial cultures, and inoculated products should be considered infectious and handled appropriately. Aseptic technique and usual precautions for handling the bacterial group studied should be observed throughout this procedure.

6. **Nonhuman hosts**—Humans are the only known reservoir for *C. trachomatis* LGV genotypes. Primate animal models have been used to investigate pathogenesis but are limited by the inability to establish chronic infections similar to those observed in humans.

7. **Sample/specimen requirements**—Specimen types for *C. trachomatis* LGV culture and NAATs are the same as outline under "Chlamydial Infections." Direct lesion swabs can be taken if the primary lesion is present. There is little diagnostic utility in aspirates from fluctuating regional lymph nodes. Serum samples should be stored at 4°C or frozen until testing.

8. **Testing requirements**—Commercially available NAATs detect *C. trachomatis* LGV genotypes with the same level of confidence as non-LGV *C. trachomatis* (see "Chlamydial Infections"). However, differentiation requires a second amplification test that targets nucleic acid sequences unique to LGV. These reflex tests are not commercially available and are only offered by specialized laboratories. Though the major outer membrane protein can be sequenced to distinguish LGV and non-LGV genotypes, most tests target the polymorphic membrane protein H gene (*pmpH*), since LGV genotypes have a unique 36-base pair (bp) deletion. PCR tests can be further refined by targeting a second 9-bp insertion within the *pmpH* gene, which is specific for the L2b variant of LGV that has been frequently reported in rectal infections.

Serologic testing for LGV is not widely available. The chlamydial CF test, which measures antibody against group-specific lipopolysaccharide antigen, has been used as an aid in the diagnosis of LGV. A CF test titer greater than or equal to 1:64 can typically be measured in the serum of patients with bubonic LGV. The MIF test can be used detect type-specific antibody and different immunoglobulin classes. The MIF test is more sensitive than the CF test with a larger proportion of patients developing an antibody response and at a higher titer. Patients with LGV tend to have broadly cross-reactive MIF titers that are often greater than 1:256. Microtiter plate format enzyme immunoassays have been developed but comparative performance data are lacking. Serologic test interpretation for LGV is not standardized; tests have not been validated for clinical proctitis presentations, and *C. trachomatis* serovar-specific serologic tests are not widely available. If culture is performed (see "Chlamydial Infections"), LGV specific antibodies must be used to identify *C. trachomatis* LGV.

9. **Reporting requirements**—Results should be reported based on differential testing between LGV and non-LGV *C. trachomatis*. In the absence of specific LGV tests, the results should be reported as LGV or

non-LGV *C. trachomatis*. LGV may be a reportable disease in some settings. Laboratories should check with the state or provincial public health authorities.

**10. Referral network**—No specific referral networks exist.

**11. Special considerations**—LGV infections are classified under but not distinct from *C. trachomatis* as a notifiable disease in several countries.

[J. R. Papp]

# MALARIA

| DISEASE | ICD-10 CODE |
|---|---|
| MALARIA | ICD-10 B50–B54 |

**1. Clinical features**—Malaria is an acute febrile illness. The clinical syndrome initially resembles that in early stages of many other febrile illnesses due to bacterial, viral, or parasitic causes and is similar enough among *Plasmodium* spp. to make differentiation impossible without laboratory studies. Malaria should be part of the differential diagnosis in all cases of fever starting at any time between 7 days after the first possible exposure to malaria and 3 months (or, rarely, later) after the last possible exposure. It is imperative to ask for a travel history. The diagnosis must be considered in all febrile patients who have traveled to or live(d) in malaria-endemic areas during the preceding 12 months or who have received blood products, tissues, or organs from persons who have been to such areas.

Persons infected with *Plasmodium falciparum* may present with variable clinical features including fever, chills, headache, muscular aching and weakness, vomiting, cough, diarrhea, and abdominal pain. In a young child there may be irritability, refusal to eat, and vomiting. If treatment is delayed after the onset of clinical symptoms, severe malaria may develop and death may result. This is especially so for malaria due to *P. falciparum*. Clinical features of severe falciparum malaria include impaired consciousness (including coma), prostration (inability to walk or sit without assistance), multiple convulsions (>2/24 hours), deep breathing and respiratory distress (acidotic breathing), acute pulmonary edema and respiratory distress syndrome, circulatory collapse and shock, acute kidney failure, clinical jaundice plus evidence of other vital organ dysfunction, and coagulation defects. Severe falciparum malaria should be considered as a possible cause of coma and/or other central nervous system symptoms in any person living in or recently returned from an endemic area. Case-fatality rates of children and nonimmunes with uncomplicated falciparum malaria are about 0.3%. This increases to 15%–20% once complications appear. Untreated severe falciparum malaria is almost always fatal.

The other human malarias (vivax, ovale, and malariae) are not usually considered life-threatening, although there are increasing reports of severe vivax malaria. Illness generally begins with malaise and fever for several days, followed by shaking chills and rapidly rising temperature, accompanied by headache and nausea, followed by profuse sweating with defervescence. After a fever-free interval, the cycle of chills, fever, and sweating recurs daily, every other day, or every third day. An untreated primary infection may last from a week to a month or longer and be accompanied by prostration, anemia, and splenomegaly. True relapses following periods with no parasitemia can occur in vivax and ovale infections at irregular intervals for up to 4 years due to a relapsing parasite stage sequestered in the liver (hypnozoites).

Persons who have grown up in endemic areas and acquired partial immunity, or nonimmune persons who have been taking prophylactic antimalarial drugs, may show an atypical clinical picture of malaria and a prolonged incubation period.

**2. Causative agents**—Human malaria is caused by the protozoan parasites *P. falciparum*, *Plasmodium vivax*, *Plasmodium ovale*, and *Plasmodium malariae*. Zoonotic infection with *Plasmodium knowlesi* also occurs. *P. falciparum* is common in all malaria-endemic areas of the world but has particularly high prevalence in sub-Saharan Africa. *P. vivax* is very common in endemic areas of Asia and the Americas; it is rare in sub-Saharan Africa south of 5°N but, contrary to some references, human malaria due to *P. vivax* may occur in this region. *P. malariae* is rare but found in all malaria endemic areas of the world. *P. ovale* is rare but has been found in all malaria endemic areas except the Americas to date. The prevalence of *P. ovale* infections is higher in West Africa than in other regions. Mixed species infections are frequent in endemic areas. Humans occasionally become infected with *Plasmodium* spp. that normally only infect nonhuman primates, such as *P. knowlesi, P. cynomolgi*, and *P. simium. P. knowlesi* is found only in Southeast Asia and is common in forest-dwelling people living in association with macaques, particularly in parts of Malaysian Borneo. Several cases of confirmed human *P. simium* infection have occurred in humans in Rio de Janeiro, Brazil, and 1 naturally acquired human infection with *P. cynomolgi* has been reported from Peninsular Malaysia.

**3. Laboratory diagnosis**—WHO recommends that every suspected case of malaria receive a diagnostic test. Several diagnostic methods exist, including microscopy, lateral flow immunochromatographic antigen detection assays (widely known as rapid diagnostic tests, or RDTs), polymerase chain reaction (PCR)–based assays, and serological tests. Direct microscopic examination of intracellular parasites on stained blood films allows identification of species, quantification of parasite density and detection of gametocytes which is important for transmission intervention programs. High-quality RDTs that detect malaria parasite antigens (histidine-rich protein 2 [HRP2], parasite lactate dehydrogenase [pLDH], and aldolase) have comparable sensitivity and specificity to quality-assured microscopy and are useful for the initial diagnosis of malaria when quality microscopy is not available. RDTs may target 1 or more *Plasmodium* spp. Combination RDTs can distinguish between *P. falciparum* and non-*P. falciparum* infections, and some are specific for both *P. falciparum* and *P. vivax*. HRP2-detecting RDTs may remain positive for a few weeks after parasite clearance. The sensitivity of RDTs decreases with lower parasitemia, particularly for pLDH-based assays. Lower quality RDTs may also have poor sensitivity. Furthermore, HRP2-negative strains of *P. falciparum* have been reported to be circulating in Latin America (Peruvian and Colombian regions) and most recently in part of Africa (Eritrea). This has directly resulted in a risk of false-negative HRP2-RDT results in these regions.

Microscopy remains the gold standard method for the detection of malaria when carried out by an expert microscopist. A minimum of 3 specimens, collected 12–24 hours apart, is recommended for the detection of malaria. Both thin films and thick films should be prepared and examined before a microscopic screen is declared negative. Discrimination of species by morphology relies on several specific factors, including the size and any distortion of infected red cells, the observation of red cell inclusion bodies such as Maurer's clefts and Shüffner's dots, the size and shape of different life stages of the parasites, and the relative abundance of those life stages. Staining with fresh Giemsa stain at pH 7.2 produces ideal morphological discrimination of species, including subtle morphological features such as Shüffner's dots.

Serological tests may not detect current infection. They generally determine past exposure and are therefore not useful in the acute management of individual patients. Species-specific serologic tests using recombinant antigen in multiplex serology platforms have been applied with good success for the retrospective diagnosis of infecting species.

PCR and loop-mediated isothermal amplification (LAMP) methods for malaria diagnosis have been published. All methods show high sensitivity, though this varies depending on the primers employed. Care should be taken when applying some multiplex PCR approaches to potential mixed infections as competitive primer inhibition in the PCR reaction may result in only the predominant species being detected. Some laboratories employ nested PCR to avoid this issue.

Diagnosis of resistance in malaria may be undertaken by specialized reference laboratories through PCR amplification, Pyrosequencing and Sanger sequencing of a genomic region containing 1 or more resistance mutations. Due to the limitation of these conventional genotyping methods in the detection of minor allele frequencies, recent work has focused on utilizing next generation sequencing methods to detect all malaria drug resistant alleles in an infecting population of parasites within the host.

**4. Laboratory capability**—Regional or district level clinical diagnostic laboratories with trained microscopists should be capable of performing morphological detection and determination of species. Tertiary level laboratories with PCR facilities are required for molecular techniques. Serological detection requires reference laboratory level skills.

**5. Safety requirements**—Clinical specimens should always be collected and handled with standard precautions. *Plasmodium* spp. are biosafety level 2 organisms. Blood specimens should be disposed of as infectious waste.

**6. Nonhuman hosts**—Chimpanzees have been found to be capable of naturally harboring all 4 species of human malaria. *Macaques* (*Macaca* spp.) are considered to be the reservoir of *P. knowlesi* and can carry *P. cynomolgi*, although other monkeys may also be infected with both of these species.

**7. Sample/specimen requirements**—Ethylenediaminetetraacetic acid (EDTA) anticoagulated blood or fresh blood from a fingerstick is acceptable for microscopy and RDT analysis. EDTA anticoagulated blood is recommended for molecular diagnosis, while serum or EDTA plasma is best for serology. Thin and thick blood smears for morphologic identification should ideally be prepared within 1–2 hours and no later than 6 hours after collection. Serum or plasma are required for serology.

**8. Testing requirements**—Morphological diagnosis should be carried out on thick and thin blood smears. Smears should be stained with a Giemsa, Fields, Wright-Giemsa, or Wright's stain or and examined thoroughly by light microscopy. Use of Giemsa at pH 7.2 is recommended as staining at this pH highlights morphological features such as Schüffner's dots and haemozoin (malaria pigment).

The sensitivity of microscopy varies based upon the experience and skill of the microscopist. Quality assurance of microscopic analysis is recommended to maintain and monitor these skills. Reported sensitivities of microscopy, RDT, and LAMP compared with PCR varies. Comparisons of microscopy and PCR have reported sensitivities of between 68%–95.7%. Microscopy sensitivity is also adversely affected by low parasitemias and the level of experience of the microscopists performing the test. RDT sensitivity varies greatly by the brand of RDT employed and the species of *Plasmodium* prevalent in the study. RDT sensitivity is lower for non-*P. falciparum* infections and low parasitemia infections. The Binax-NOW Malaria RDT, combining the *P. falciparum* HRP-2 and panmalaria aldolase antigen RDT, is the only malaria RDT that is FDA approved for use in the USA. In 1 study comparing the sensitivity of this RDT with PCR in febrile returned travelers, the Binax-NOW Malaria RDT showed 94% sensitivity for the detection of *P. falciparum*, 87% sensitivity for *P. vivax* infections, and 62% for *P. ovale* and *P. malariae* infections. Sensitivity is lowest for detecting *P. ovale* infections.

LAMP methods have reported sensitivity of between 95%–100% compared with PCR. Multiplex real-time PCR is often used in diagnosis and has a sensitivity approaching 100%, but for the detection of mixed infection, nested PCR may be advisable, due to competitive priming of different species in multiplex real-time PCR.

**9. Reporting requirements**—Reporting requirements/criteria may vary by country and local jurisdiction but cases of malaria are routinely reportable under the IHR. Malarias is currently reportable in all US states and territories.

**10. Referral network**—Networks vary among countries. First-line laboratories may perform RDTs, LAMP, and/or microscopy. Reference laboratories may perform PCR and confirm microscopic findings. The Parasitic Diseases Diagnostic Reference Laboratory at CDC offers morphological, PCR, and serological diagnosis of malaria infections and diagnosis to species level based on submission of images through the DPDx website. The Malaria Branch of CDC offers antimalarial resistance screening by genomic methods for epidemiological purposes.

**11. Special considerations**—Due to the evolutionary plasticity of *Plasmodium* parasites, drug resistance has evolved and spread rapidly, leading to the failure of many previous first-line antimalarial drugs such as chloroquine (CQ) and sulfadoxine-pyrimethamine (SP) in *P. falciparum*. Resistance emerged in Southeast Asia, where originally both CQ and SP resistant parasites evolved and spread to Africa and other parts of Asia. Notwithstanding that artemisinin-based combination therapy was introduced relatively recently (after 2000) in most parts of the world, numerous reports have already provided compelling evidence for the emergence of artemisinin resistance.

[R. S. Bradbury, H. S. Bishop, E. Talundzic]

# MEASLES

(rubeola, hard measles, red measles, morbilli)

| DISEASE | ICD-10 CODE |
|---|---|
| MEASLES | ICD-10 B05 |

**1. Clinical features**—An acute, highly communicable viral disease with prodromal fever, conjunctivitis, coryza, cough, and small spots with white or bluish-white centers on an erythematous base on the buccal mucosa (Koplik spots). A characteristic red blotchy rash appears on the face on the third to seventh day, becomes generalized, lasts 4–7 days, and sometimes ends in brawny desquamation. Leukopenia is common and serum vitamin A levels are often decreased. Complications, resulting from direct viral replication or bacterial superinfection, may occur up to 4 weeks after rash and include otitis media, pneumonia, laryngotracheobronchitis (croup), diarrhea, febrile seizures, and encephalitis. In malnourished children, measles may be associated with hemorrhagic rash, protein-losing enteropathy, otitis media, oral sores, dehydration, diarrhea, blindness, and severe skin infections. Persons with deficiencies of cell-mediated immunity may lack the characteristic rash and may have progressive measles inclusion-body encephalitis.

Very rarely (in 4–11/100,000 cases), subacute sclerosing panencephalitis develops several years after infection; more than 50% of subacute sclerosing panencephalitis cases had measles diagnosed in the first 2 years of life. In adults, hepatitis, hypocalcemia, and elevated creatinine phosphokinase levels are also seen.

The case-fatality rate is estimated to be less than 1% in developed countries but can be 3%–5% in developing countries, reaching 10%–30% in some localities. Both acute and delayed mortality in infants and children have been documented.

**2. Causative agents**—Measles virus, a member of the genus *Morbillivirus* of the family *Paramyxoviridae*.

**3. Laboratory diagnosis**— Fever, maculopapular rash, and cough/coryza/conjunctivitis. Diagnosis is usually made on clinical and epidemiological grounds, although laboratory confirmation is preferred. The detection of measles-specific immunoglobulin class M (IgM) antibodies, which present 4 days after rash onset, remains the most common method of laboratory confirmation, but reverse transcription polymerase chain reaction (RT-PCR) is gaining utility in many laboratories. Time and labor intensive methods are less effective for early diagnosis (e.g., those requiring the collection of 2 serum specimens and testing for a 4-fold rise in IgG antibody concentrations between acute and convalescent sera as measured by semiquantitative or quantitative assays [plaque-reduction neutralization]). Less commonly used techniques include the identification of viral antigen in nasopharyngeal mucosal swabs by fluorescent antibody techniques, or virus isolation in cell culture from blood or nasopharyngeal swabs collected before day 4 of rash, or from urine specimens before day 8 of rash. Virus isolation, however, is now vastly improved due the availability of cell lines bearing the human receptors for measles. RT-PCR can be used to identify measles ribonucleic acid (RNA) in urine, blood, and nasopharyngeal mucus.

**4. Laboratory capability**—A measles laboratory should be appropriately resourced in terms of space, equipment, and support to permit the simultaneous operation of serology, virology, and molecular biological methods. Likewise, staffing levels should be adequate to enable each of the expected functions. Methods such as cell culture, RT-PCR, sequencing, and nucleotide sequence analysis and genotyping require experienced and highly trained personnel. Thus, both technical and scientific staff would likely have to be identified and, if not already appropriately trained, afforded access to training courses and workshops to acquire the knowledge and skills. In this regard, WHO organizes training workshops to members of the WHO Measles/ Rubella Laboratory Network (LabNet). As mentioned later (see Referral Network section in this chapter), this multitiered network consists of national (and subnational), regional reference, and global specialized laboratories. Each laboratory has prescribed functions in terms of providing laboratory testing, training, test protocol development, as well as quality assurance and quality control standardization and panel distribution. The performance of all LabNet member laboratories is reviewed annually using a standard list of accreditation criteria.[1]

**5. Safety requirements**—The recommended biosafety level (BSL) for measles is BSL-2. BSL-2 conditions and guidelines should be used for handling any samples that are known or suspected to contain measles virus. These guidelines are published in *Biosafety in Microbiological and Biomedical Laboratories*.[2] Moreover, WHO has made available *Laboratory Biosafety Manual*.[3] Personnel who handle measles virus containing samples should be trained in BSL-2 methods pertaining to specimen handling and storage, sterile technique, decontamination, and sharps and biohazardous waste disposal.

Personal protective equipment should include a laboratory coat, gloves, and eye protection. The most common risk to staff in the measles laboratory is in handling serum samples. Serum should always be considered as a potentially infectious material, and personnel should wear gloves when opening packages containing serum, aliquoting samples, transferring samples, and when performing assays. A class II biological safety cabinet should be used for handling samples that contain a high concentration of virus or when performing tasks that have a potential for creating infectious aerosols. Disinfectants should be available in case of spills.

A safe and effective live attenuated vaccine has been available for measles for almost 50 years.[4] Vaccination with measles containing vaccine is recommended for all laboratory staff, especially in laboratories that are attempting to culture measles virus from clinical samples. Presumptive evidence of immunity may be accepted in lieu of vaccination in many facilities. Acceptable presumptive evidence of measles immunity for laboratory workers includes laboratory evidence of immunity or laboratory confirmation of disease. Women of child bearing age working in the measles laboratory should have demonstrable immunity to rubella, since the clinical diagnosis of rubella is often confused with that of measles, and specimens containing rubella virus are often referred to the measles laboratory for testing.

**6. Nonhuman hosts**—Measles is considered a uniquely human disease although many species of nonhuman primates can be infected by the virus.[5]

**7. Sample/specimen requirements**—For laboratory confirmation of measles infection, clinical samples should be taken for both serologic testing and virologic detection. Specimens for RT-PCR and virus isolation should be collected at the same time as samples taken for serologic testing, which is usually at first contact with the suspected case. In some cases, a second serum sample may be requested.

The preferred specimens for virus isolation or RT-PCR are throat or nasopharyngeal swabs, but urine may also contain virus. Oral fluid is also a good sample for detection of viral RNA by RT-PCR but not for virus isolation. Virus isolation and RNA detection are more likely to be successful when the specimens are collected within 3 days of rash onset, but samples collected up to 10 days post rash may give positive results.

Measles virus is sensitive to heat and desiccation and viability decreases markedly when samples are not kept cold. It is important to transport samples from the point of collection to the laboratory with cold packs as soon as possible following sample collection. Samples should be kept at 4°C and processed within 48 hours before being stored at −70°C. Samples are stable at −70°C for several months and, once frozen, will need to be transported on dry ice. For throat, nasopharyngeal or nasal swabs, and oral fluid samples that have low volumes (1–4 mL), the entire sample can be processed and frozen at −70°C. For detection of virus from urine, the sediment from 10–50 mL of urine should be resuspended in 2–3 mL of sterile transport medium, tissue culture medium, or physiological buffered saline. The sample can be stored at −70°C. There is no minimum volume for samples for virologic detection, though at least 0.5 mL is preferred.

Blood samples are typically collected by venipuncture, but capillary tubes from heel or finger sticks are sometimes used to collect blood from infants. In all cases, serum should be separated from the blood as soon as possible and stored at 4°C until it can be shipped to the laboratory on cold packs. It is best to avoid repeated freezing and thawing, as this may affect the stability of IgM. Serum can be stored for longer periods at −20°C or −70°C. The minimal volume for a serum sample is approximately 0.1 mL.

Though tissue samples are not used for routine surveillance, they may be tested for presence of measles RNA or antigen. Paraffin fixed tissues should be shipped at room temperature, and fresh tissue must be shipped on dry ice.

All samples should be shipped in appropriate packaging so as to conform to requirements for UN 3373 (category B). Viral isolates and clinical specimens arriving from outside the USA will require a CDC Import Permit. A copy of the import permit must accompany the shipping documents.

**8. Testing requirements**—A suspected measles case is considered laboratory confirmed by isolation of measles virus from a clinical specimen, detection of measles-virus specific nucleic acid from a clinical specimen by using PCR, IgG seroconversion or a 4-fold rise in measles IgG antibody by using any validated method, or by detection of measles-specific IgM antibody. The gold standard for confirmation of infection is isolation of measles virus in cell culture; however, this method is time consuming and few laboratories have access to the cell line required for isolation of measles, Vero/hSLAM.[6] Detection of measles-specific IgM antibody and detection of measles RNA by real-time RT-PCR are the most common methods for confirmation of measles infection.

The most widely used serologic method is IgM detection by enzyme immunoassay (EIA), though several laboratories use immunofluorescence. Commercial EIA tests are available with excellent sensitivity and specificity. IgM EIAs can be performed relatively quickly, and results are generally available in 1 day. A drawback to IgM detection is that up to 23% of samples taken with 3 days of rash onset may give false-negative results.[7] If a negative result is obtained from serum collected within 72 hours after rash onset, a second serum should be collected 72 hours or longer after rash onset. Measles IgM is detectable for at least 30 days after rash onset and frequently longer. IgM responses are often not detectable in cases of secondary vaccine failure.[8,9]

Isolation of measles virus in culture or detection of measles RNA by conventional RT-PCR or real-time RT-PCR in clinical specimens confirms the diagnosis of measles. Successful virus isolation or detection of RNA by RT-PCR is helpful when serologic results are inconclusive, so laboratories are encouraged to request samples for viral detection in addition to serum samples. The availability of the Vero/hSLAM cell line, a cell line expressing with a receptor for wild type measles viruses, has greatly improved the ability to isolate measles virus in cell culture.[6] However, negative cell culture or negative conventional or real time RT-PCR results do not rule out measles, because both methods are affected by the timing of specimen collection and the quality and handling of the clinical specimens. Because virus isolation is time consuming and requires cell culture facilities, conventional RT-PCR or real time RT-PCR are the preferred virus detection assays because they offer rapid testing and flexible platforms. There are no commercial RT-PCR assays available for measles, though protocols have been published and are available online.[10,11] To avoid contamination of RT-PCR assays, laboratories should establish strict unidirectional workflow. Sequencing the amplicon from conventional RT-PCR reaction can help confirm the result.

Conventional or real time RT-PCR can also be used to detect measles RNA in nucleic acid extracts from either fixed or frozen tissue samples. In addition, there are commercially available monoclonal antibodies that can be used to detect measles antigens in fixed tissue samples by immunohistochemistry.

Tests for IgG rise or seroconversion, plaque reduction neutralization[12] and avidity testing[13] may be helpful in certain situations. In immunologically naïve persons, the measles IgG response starts slowly and, depending on the assay, can be detected by day 3–7 after rash onset (range: 1–10 days) but typically persists for a lifetime. IgG antibody seroconversion or demonstration of a rise in titer using IgG EIA can be determined by testing a convalescent serum sample collected 10–30 days after the acute serum. IgG testing of paired serum samples requires the demonstration of a significant (usually 4-fold) rise in the titer of antibody against measles using an assay that has been validated for this use. The test for IgG antibody should be conducted with acute and convalescent serum samples at the same time using the same test. IgG avidity assessments would also be informative on such specimens since low avidity results would rule in a case of measles in this instance.[13–15]

If measles RNA is detected in clinical samples, a standard region of the genome should be sequenced to determine the viral genotype.[11,16–19] Determination of the measles genotype provides the only means to distinguish between wild type virus infection and a rash caused from a recent measles vaccination. In addition, molecular epidemiologic data are used to track transmission pathways of measles and to suggest possible sources of imported cases. Genetic characterization of circulating measles strains has been used to help document the absence of endemic circulation of measles in the USA.[20] Genotyping of measles virus is conducted at the CDC measles laboratory and in regional reference laboratories that are part of the WHO Global Measles and Rubella Laboratory Network.[1]

The routine serologic and molecular diagnostic tests for measles can be performed by individuals with a bachelor of science level education in biology, chemistry, or microbiology, or medical technology and some specialized training. In the USA, diagnostic testing is regulated by the Clinical Laboratory Improvement Amendments, which requires regular competency assessments and proficiency testing. Quality control measures for serologic and molecular tests are well established. Genetic analysis of measles virus requires additional specialized training in sequencing and sequence analysis. The minimal testing algorithm would be to conduct testing to detect measles IgM in acute phase serum samples, with samples for virus detection referred to another, specialized laboratory. In many areas where measles is well controlled, the number of suspected cases may be quite low, and the minimal testing strategy with appropriate referral options will be adequate. The optimal testing scheme would be for a laboratory to perform both serologic and molecular diagnostic testing.

**9. Reporting requirements**—Measles is a reportable disease in the USA and in many countries. In the USA, uniform case definitions are established by the Council of State and Territorial Epidemiologists. Most countries in the world are currently performing case-based surveillance for measles with data complied nationally on at least a monthly basis and regularly reported to WHO.

**10. Referral network**—In the USA, most of the serologic testing is performed in private, commercial laboratories. Most state public health laboratories are capable of IgM detection and many are currently initiating molecular diagnostic methods. The Measles, Mumps, Rubella and Herpes Viruses Laboratory Branch at the CDC is the national reference laboratory for measles. CDC also performs genetic characterization of wild type measles viruses for molecular epidemiologic studies. On the global level, WHO supports LabNet, consisting of 690 laboratories providing services to 183 countries. LabNet is a 3-tiered laboratory system composed of national laboratories, regional reference laboratories, and global specialized laboratories. Large countries support subnational laboratory networks.[1]

**11. Special considerations**—Measles is not covered by the International Health Regulations.

## References


1. Featherstone DA, Rota PA, Icenogle J, et al. Expansion of the global measles and rubella laboratory network 2005-09. *J Infect Dis*. 2011; 204(suppl 1):S491–498.
2. US Department of Health and Human Services, Centers for Disease Control and Prevention; National Institutes of Health. *Biosafety in Microbiological and Biomedical Laboratories*. 5th ed. 2009. Available at: https://www.cdc.gov/labs/pdf/CDC-BiosafetyMicrobiologicalBiomedicalLaboratories-2009-P.PDF. Accessed March 7, 2019.
3. World Health Organization. *Laboratory Biosafety Manual*. 2004. Available at: https://www.who.int/csr/resources/publications/biosafety/WHO_CDS_CSR_-LYO_2004_11/en. Accessed March 7, 2019.
4. Sanders R, Dabbagh A, Featherstone D. Risk analysis for measles reintroduction after global certification of eradication. *J Infect Dis*. 2011;204(suppl 1):S71–7.
5. Ono N, Tatsuo H, Hidaka Y, Aoki T, Minagawa H, Yanagi Y. Measles viruses on throat swabs from measles patients use signaling lymphocytic activation molecule (CDw150) but not CD46 as a cellular receptor. *J Virol*. 2001;75(9):4399–4401.
6. Helfand RF, Heath JL, Anderson LJ, Maes EF, Guris D, Bellini WJ. Diagnosis of measles with an IgM capture EIA: the optimal timing of specimen collection after rash onset. *J Infect Dis*. 1997;175(1):195–199.
7. Hickman C, Hyde T, Sowers S, et al. Laboratory characterization of measles virus infection in previously vaccinated and unvaccinated individuals. *J Infect Dis*. 2011;204(suppl 1):S549–S558.
8. Rota JS, Hickman CJ, Sowers SB, Rota PA, Mercader S, Bellini WJ. Two case studies of modified measles in vaccinated physicians exposed to primary measles cases: high risk of infection but low risk of transmission. *J Infect Dis*. 2011;204(suppl 1):S559–63.
9. Hummel KB, Lowe L, Bellini WJ, Rota PA. Development of quantitative gene-specific real-time RT-PCR assays for the detection of measles virus in clinical specimens. *J Virol Methods*. 2006;132(1–2):166–73.
10. Rota PA, Brown KE, Hubschen JM, et al. Improving global virologic surveillance for measles and rubella. *J Infect Dis*. 2011;204(suppl 1):S506–513.
11. Cohen BJ, Audet S, Andrews N, Beeler J; WHO working group on measles plaque reduction neutralization test. Plaque reduction neutralization test for measles antibodies: description of a standardised laboratory method for use in immunogenicity studies of aerosol vaccination. *Vaccine*. 2007; 26(1):59–66.
12. Mercader S, Garcia P, Bellini WJ. Measles virus IgG avidity assay for use in classification of measles vaccine failure in measles elimination settings. *Clin Vaccine immunol*: 2012;19(11):1810–1817.
13. Pannuti CS, Morello RJ, Moraes JC, et al. Identification of primary and secondary measles vaccine failures by measurement of immunoglobulin G avidity in measles

cases during the 1997 Sao Paulo epidemic. *Clin Diagn Lab Immunol.* 2004;11(1): 119–122.
14. Paunio M, Hedman K, Davidkin I, Peltola H. IgG avidity to distinguish secondary from primary measles vaccination failures: prospects for a more effective global measles elimination strategy. *Expert Opin Pharmacother.* 2003;4(8):1215–1225.
15. Rota PA, Bellini WJ. Update on the global distribution of genotypes of wild type measles viruses. *J Infect Dis.* 2003;187(suppl 1):S270–276.
16. Rota PA, Brown K, Mankertz A, et al. Global distribution of measles genotypes and measles molecular epidemiology. *J Infect Dis.* 2011;204(suppl 1):S514–S523.
17. Rota PA, Featherstone DA, Bellini WJ. Molecular epidemiology of measles virus. *Curr Top Microbiol Immunol.* 2009;330:129–150.
18. Measles virus nomenclature update: 2012. *Wkly Epidemiol Rec.* 2012;87(9):73–81.
19. Rota PA, Liffick SL, Rota JS, et al. Molecular epidemiology of measles viruses in the United States, 1997–2001. *Emerg Infect Dis.* 2002;8(9):902–908.
20. Hilleman MR, Buynak EB, Weibel RE, Stokes J, Whitman JE, Leagus MB. Development and evaluation of the Moraten measles virus vaccine. *JAMA.* 1968;206(3): 587–590.

[W. J. Bellini, P. A. Rota]

# MELIOIDOSIS
(Whitmore's disease)

| DISEASE | ICD-10 CODE |
|---|---|
| MELIOIDOSIS | ICD-10 A24.1–A24.4 |
| GLANDERS | ICD-10 A24.0 |

**1. Clinical features**—Clinical manifestations range from subclinical infection to localized acute or chronic cutaneous or visceral abscesses, necrotizing pneumonia, and/or a rapidly fatal septicaemia. Melioidosis may simulate typhoid fever or tuberculosis, with pulmonary cavitation, emphysema, chronic abscesses, and osteomyelitis. Overwhelming infection can occur, resulting in death from septic shock within 48 hours of generalized symptoms. Infection can become persistent and result in latent, recurrent, and recrudescing infections. A specific syndrome of meningoencephalitis with flaccid paraparesis or peripheral motor weakness occurs in 5% of cases in northern Australia. Cerebral abscess is occasionally reported. Mortality rates range from 15%–40% despite use of appropriate antimicrobial therapy.

In humans, signs and symptoms of glanders—a highly communicable disease of horses, mules, and donkeys—are similar to melioidosis. Human glanders is associated with contact with sick animals, contaminated fomites, tissues, or bacterial cultures, and it no longer occurs in the Western Hemisphere.

**2. Causative agents**—*Burkholderia pseudomallei* is the causative agent for melioidosis; *Burkholderia mallei* for glanders. *B. pseudomallei* is a saprophytic, Gram-negative, motile rod; *B. mallei* is a Gram-negative, non-motile rod and is an obligate, mammalian, zoonotic pathogen, which can survive for only a short period in the environment.

**3. Laboratory diagnosis**—Depends on isolation of the causative agent from clinical specimens (e.g., blood, urine, sputum, skin lesions, and throat swabs); a rising antibody titer in serological tests in conjunction with clinical signs and symptoms is suggestive. In some highly endemic areas, more than 50% of individuals have demonstrable antibodies but no history of overt disease. Direct immunofluorescent microscopy is 98% specific but only about 70% sensitive compared with culture. The possibility of melioidosis must be kept in mind in any unexplained suppurative disease and sepsis, especially cavitating pulmonary disease, in patients living in or returning from endemic areas; disease has become manifest after exposure.

Infection with *B. pseudomallei* cannot be differentiated serologically from infection with *B. mallei*; characterization of the isolated organism alone can lead to specific diagnosis.

**4. Laboratory capability**—Biosafety level 3 (BSL-3) laboratories are required for culture and isolation of *B. pseudomallei* in developed countries (when there is strong clinical suspicion). BSL-2 laboratories can be used for primary sample processing when the clinical index of suspicion is not high, and for techniques such as polymerase chain reaction (PCR) and serology directly from clinical samples. Manipulation of cultures should be performed inside a microbiological safety cabinet.

**5. Safety requirements**—See Laboratory Capability section in this chapter. *B. pseudomallei* is infectious by the aerosol route, and cases of laboratory-acquired infection have been recorded, so extreme caution is required when handling this organism. Human-to-human transmission is extremely rare, however.

**6. Nonhuman hosts**—While *B. pseudomallei* can infect other animal species such as goats, pigs and cattle, the main route of transmission is environmental exposure to infected soil and water. Melioidosis is not considered to be a zoonotic infection.

**7. Sample/specimen requirements**—Organisms can be isolated by culture from various sample types such as blood, sputum, urine, throat swab, and pus. A complete screen is recommended for culture in any patients with suspected melioidosis. Plasma and serum are required for serology

**8. Testing requirements**—The gold standard for diagnosis of melioidosis remains culture and identification of the organism. Due to very close genetic relationships, it can be difficult to distinguish between *B. pseudomallei*, *B. mallei*, and other closely related species such as *Burkholderia*

*thailandensis*; therefore, diagnosis by molecular methods is difficult. Serology can be used in addition to culture/molecular methods, although serological assays tend to lack sensitivity and specificity. Numerous serology tests such as enzyme-linked immunosorbent assay (ELISA), lateral flow assays (LFA), and immunochomatographic assays have been developed, although very few are commercially available.

1) Culture and identification: *B. pseudomallei* can be cultured from blood, sputum, abscess aspirates, cerebrospinal fluid, skin lesions, and other clinical specimens. *B. pseudomallei* can grow on blood agar and MacConkey's agar, but the best medium for the isolation of *B. pseudomallei* from nonsterile sites is Ashdown's medium. Ashdown's medium contains crystal violet and gentamicin, and colonies appear as purple, dry, and wrinkled. A long incubation (i.e., 96 hours) is required, although colonies may appear at 24 hours. The sensitivity of culture from sites with abnormal flora such as throat swabs can be enhanced by culturing in an enrichment broth based on Ashdown's medium with colistin, followed by plating on Ashdown's medium. Identification of *B. pseudomallei* from culture is dependent on biochemical analysis and commercial bacterial identification kits can be used, although misidentification can occur. *B. pseudomallei* is included in the databases of API 20NE (bioMérieux, Durham, NC) and VITEK 1 and 2 systems (bioMérieux). More recently, methods such as matrix-assisted laser desorption/ionization time-of-flight (MALDI-TOF) analysis and 16S ribosomal ribonucleic acid (rRNA) sequencing have been used to identify *B. pseudomallei.* These methods are becoming increasingly reliable and available in routine microbiology laboratories, although care must be taken to ensure that the organism is included in the database. Care must also be taken when analyzing the results of 16S rRNA sequencing, as the sequence difference of the 16S gene between *B. pseudomallei* and *B. thailandensis* is about 1%, and *B. pseudomallei* and *B. mallei* differ by a single nucleotide. Recently, a 3-disc method of antibiotic susceptibility testing has been shown to be predictive of melioidosis. Suspected *B. pseudomallei* colonies have been defined as being oxidase positive, Gram-negative bacilli with resistance to gentamycin and colistin but sensitive to amoxicillin/clavulonic acid (zone diameter 21–26 mm). A number of latex agglutination assays are described using monoclonal antibodies against O polysaccharide (OPS) and C polysaccharide (CPS) whole extracts or antigen derivatives. The assays have a high reported sensitivity (>95%) and specificity (100%) and can distinguish between *B. pseudomallei* and *B. thailandensis.* These assays are mostly in-house assays; further information

and a standard operating procedure for producing latex agglutination assays can be found at: http://www.melioidosis.info.

2) Molecular methods: diagnosis by PCR can be problematic due to the genetic relatedness of *B. pseudomallei* and other species of the *Burkholderia* genus, particularly *B. mallei* and *B. thailandensis*. PCR assays that have been developed tend to rely on interspecies multilocus differences and need extensive validation. Many PCR assays have been described targeting various genes and gene clusters such as 16S rRNA, type 3 secretion system, flagellin, and serine metalloprotease (*mprA*), as well as assays that target particular gene loci. Reported sensitivity and specificity of these assays vary greatly. Multispecies differentiation assays have also been developed that can detect 2 or more *Burkholderia* spp., usually *B. pseudomallei* and *B. mallei*. For direct detection from clinical samples, detection in sputum gives the best results due to the high bacterial load of *B. pseudomallei* in sputum, although high background contamination can lead to false-positive results. PCR should not be used alone, as in their current state, they cannot be used with 100% confidence. Rather, they should be used alongside culture or other tests to ensure greater confidence in the diagnostic result. PCR may be used as an alternative to serological or conventional methods for identification of the organisms.

3) Serology: given the low sensitivity and time consuming nature of culture, serologic assays are used to give a preliminary diagnosis in endemic areas. However, the results are often misleading due to the high rates of seroprevalence that exist. These assays have low sensitivity and specificity in these settings but may be useful in non-endemic areas. Indirect hemagglutination assays are commonly used in endemic regions. The assay can be variable depending on the antigens used and interpretation can be difficult in areas with high antibody prevalence. A number of immunoglobulin class M (IgM) and IgG ELISAs have been developed. Bacterial lipopolysaccharide (LPS) is a common antigen for these assays although whole cells and exopolysaccharide have been used. There is little reported difference in the assays based on sensitivity, although LPS-based assays may provide better specificity. Other assays include indirect immunofluorescence, lateral flow immunoassays and complement fixation, but these are not commercially available. The reported sensitivity of these assays is low. As with PCR, serologic methods should be used in combination with other methods such as culture due to a lack of sensitivity and specificity.

**9. Reporting requirements** Melioidosis is a reportable disease in some countries and should be reported according to local regulations and guidelines.

**10. Referral network**—There is as yet no WHO collaborating center for melioidosis. The International Melioidosis Society hosts a website (http://www.melioidosis.info) that raises awareness of melioidosis through research networks and provides an online platform to report cases and for disseminating information on melioidosis.

**11. Special considerations**—A number of underlying conditions have been found to be associated with increased risk of contracting melioidosis. The most significant underlying condition is diabetes mellitus. Other conditions include renal disease, thalassemia, immunosuppression, primary tuberculosis, hematologic malignancy or solid tumor, or history of previous trauma or surgery. In endemic areas, occupational exposure is also a risk factor.

*B. pseudomallei* is tier 1 biothreat agent and is listed in the Select Agents and Toxins, 7 CFR Part 331, 9 CFR Part 121, and 42 CFR Part 73 (http://www.selectagents.gov). In the USA, confirmed isolates of select agents identified in a clinical or diagnostic laboratory must be reported. Each country may have specific registration requirements for laboratories working with *B. pseudomallei*, and these should be checked.

[J. Duggan]

# MENINGITIS

| DISEASE | ICD-10 CODE |
|---|---|
| VIRAL MENINGITIS | ICD-10 A87 |
| NONPYOGENIC MENINGITIS | ICD-10 G03.0 |
| BACTERIAL MENINGITIS | ICD-10 G00 |
| MENINGOCOCCAL MENINGITIS | ICD-10 A39.0 |
| HAEMOPHILUS MENINGITIS | ICD-10 G00.0 |
| PNEUMOCOCCAL MENINGITIS | ICD-10 G00.1 |
| NEONATAL MENINGITIS ICD-10 | P37.8, P35–P37, G00, G03 |

## I. VIRAL MENINGITIS (aseptic meningitis, nonbacterial meningitis)

**1. Clinical features**—A relatively common but rarely serious clinical syndrome with multiple viral etiologies, characterized by sudden onset of febrile illness with signs and symptoms of headache with meningeal involvement. Cerebrospinal fluid (CSF) findings are pleocytosis (usually mononuclear, occasionally polymorphonuclear in early stages), increased protein, normal sugar, and absence of bacteria. A rubella-like rash characterizes certain types caused by enteroviruses, including coxsackieviruses, echoviruses, and the more recently identified numbered enteroviruses (e.g., EV68-EV115), and excluding the rhinoviruses. Vesicular and petechial rashes may also occur. Active illness seldom exceeds 10 days. Transient paresis and encephalitic manifestations may occur; paralysis is unusual. Residual signs lasting a year or more may include weakness, muscle spasm, insomnia, and personality changes. Recovery is usually complete. Gastrointestinal and respiratory symptoms may be associated with enterovirus infection.

Various diseases caused by nonviral infectious agents may mimic viral meningitis. These include inadequately treated pyogenic meningitis; tuberculous and cryptococcal meningitis; meningitis caused by other fungi; cerebrovascular syphilis; and lymphogranuloma venereum. Postinfectious and postvaccinal reactions require differentiation from sequelae to measles, mumps, varicella, and immunization against rabies and smallpox; these syndromes are usually encephalitic in type. Leptospirosis, listeriosis, syphilis, lymphocytic choriomeningitis, viral hepatitis, infectious mononucleosis, influenza, and other diseases may produce the same clinical syndrome.

Infection by enteroviruses (excluding rhinoviruses) transmitted from the mother is a frequent cause of neonatal fever with neurological signs. In polio-free countries, the most prevalent infectious agent causing flaccid paralysis is enterovirus 71, responsible for outbreaks of meningitis and paralysis in many countries. Children and adults with B-cell deficiencies are subject to chronic relapsing meningitis, usually caused by enteroviruses.

**2. Causative agents**—A wide variety of causative agents exist, many associated with other specific diseases. Predominant causative agents can vary by geographic location and season. Several viruses can produce meningeal features. The causative agent may not be identified in a large proportion of viral meningitis cases (e.g., 50%). In epidemic periods, mumps may be responsible for more than 25% of cases of established etiology in nonimmunized populations. In developed countries, enteroviruses (coxsackieviruses, echoviruses, and the numbered enteroviruses) cause many epidemics/outbreaks of known etiology. Arboviruses, measles, herpes simplex and varicella viruses, lymphocytic choriomeningitis virus, adenovirus, enterovirus, and others may cause sporadic cases. Incidence of specific types varies with geographic location and time. Leptospira may cause up to 20% of cases of aseptic meningitis in various areas (see "Leptospirosis"), and this bacterial infection should be included in the differential diagnosis of viral meningitis.

**3. Laboratory diagnosis**—Epidemiologic patterns, patient characteristics (e.g., age, clinical findings, vaccination history), and laboratory information should be used to make a diagnosis and identify the causative agent. Under optimal conditions, specific identification is possible in about half of all viral meningitis cases, through molecular diagnostic, serological, and isolation techniques. Molecular diagnostic methods often yield a more rapid diagnosis and are available for the detection and characterization of most viruses. Viral agents may be detected in early stages from nasopharyngeal and oropharyngeal swabs and stool, CSF, and blood/serum. Other specimens such as pathologic specimens may also be useful in some instances.

4. **Laboratory capability**—Hospital laboratories may offer a limited range of testing for detection of viral etiologies of meningitis. Commercially available molecular assays can detect enteroviruses, herpes simplex virus 1 and 2, varicella zoster virus, parechovirus, cytomegalovirus, and human herpesvirus 6. Larger laboratories including reference and public health laboratories may have the ability to perform viral culture, serologic testing, and molecular testing for other viral pathogens. Testing is generally restricted to laboratories that perform moderate- or high-complexity testing.

5. **Safety requirements**—Many of the viruses that cause meningitis can be safely handled under biosafety level 2 precautions (BSL-2). BSL-3 practices are required for certain agents, such as lymphocytic choriomeningitis virus and certain arboviruses, for activities that have a high potential for aerosol production, or when working with high concentrations of infectious materials.

6. **Nonhuman hosts**—Enteroviruses are generally spread fecal–orally or from respiratory shedding, but they have also been recovered from houseflies. The common house mouse is the main host of lymphocytic choriomeningitis virus. Arboviruses have a wide range of vectors including mosquitoes, ticks, midges, and sand flies that transmit the viruses from a variety of vertebrate reservoirs, including birds, small mammals (e.g., rodents), and large mammals (e.g., horses).

7. **Sample/specimen requirements**—Specimens usually include CSF for molecular, antibody, and viral culture assays, and serum for serodiagnosis. Specimens for antibody and molecular testing may be refrigerated or frozen. Specimens for viral culture generally should be refrigerated and not frozen. For optimal results, specimens should be sent to the laboratory as soon as possible after collection. Specimen stability varies depending on the test being performed and the laboratory performing the test; specimen stability for molecular testing may be a few days refrigerated and a few months frozen, for serologic testing a few days or weeks refrigerated and up to a year frozen, and for viral culture a few days refrigerated.

8. **Testing requirements**—Testing for viral meningitis utilizes examination of CSF for cell count, glucose, and protein levels. Depending on the suspected etiology, diagnosis is typically accomplished using a molecular method, such as for enterovirus and herpes simplex virus infections, for which molecular methods are more sensitive than viral culture, or by serology, such as for arboviruses. Standard quality control and quality assurance practices used for molecular, serologic, and viral culture testing should be followed.

**9. Reporting requirements**—Common causes of viral meningitis, such as enteroviruses and herpes simplex viruses, typically do not need to be reported to public health authorities; however, arboviruses and other less common viruses, such as lymphocytic choriomeningitis virus, mumps virus, and measles virus, may require reporting to local, state, and/or federal authorities. Requirements for reporting and specimen submission should be determined in conjunction with the relevant authorities.

**10. Referral network**—If testing cannot be performed locally, serologic, molecular, and viral culture testing can be performed at reference or public health laboratories.

**11. Special considerations**—None.

## II. BACTERIAL MENINGITIS

*Neisseria meningitidis, Streptococcus pneumoniae* and *Haemophilus influenzae* type b (Hib) are thought to cause more than 75% of all bacterial meningitis and 90% of bacterial meningitis in children. Meningitis due to Hib, previously the most common cause of bacterial meningitis, has largely been eliminated in many industrialized countries through immunization programs. Meningococcal disease is unique among the major causes of bacterial meningitis in that it causes both endemic disease and large epidemics. The less common bacterial causes of meningitis, such as staphylococci, enteric bacteria, group B streptococci and *Listeria*, occur in susceptible persons (such as neonates and patients with impaired immunity) or as the consequence of head trauma.

Infants with neonatal meningitis develop lethargy, seizures, apneic episodes, poor feeding, hypo- or hyperthermia, and sometimes respiratory distress, usually in their first week of life. The white blood cell count may be elevated or depressed. CSF culture yields group B streptococci, *Listeria monocytogenes* (see "Listeriosis"), *Escherichia coli* K-1, or other organisms acquired from the birth canal. Infants aged 2 weeks to 2 months may develop similar symptoms, with recovery from the CSF of group B streptococci or organisms of the *Klebsiella-Enterobacter-Serratia* group, acquired from the nursery environment. Meningitis in both groups is associated with septicemia. Treatment is with ampicillin, plus a third-generation cephalosporin or aminoglycoside until the causal organism has been identified and its antimicrobial susceptibilities determined.

**1. Clinical features**—

1) Meningococcal meningitis (cerebrospinal fever): an acute bacterial meningitis, characterized by sudden onset of fever, intense headache, nausea and often vomiting, stiff neck, and photophobia. A petechial rash with pink macules or occasionally vesicles may be observed in Europe and North America, but rarely in Africa. Even with antibiotics,

case-fatality remains high at 8%–15%. In addition, 10%–20% of survivors will suffer long-term sequelae, including neurologic deficits, hearing loss, and limb loss. Invasive disease is characterized by 1 or more clinical syndromes including meningitis (the most common presentation), bacteremia, and sepsis. Meningococcemia, or meningococcal sepsis, is the most severe form of infection, with petechial rash, hypotension, disseminated intravascular coagulation, and multiorgan failure. Other forms of meningococcal disease, such as pneumonia, purulent arthritis, and pericarditis, are less common.

2) *Haemophilus influenzae* meningitis (meningitis due to *Haemophilus influenzae*): in industrialized countries, before widespread use of Hib conjugate vaccines, Hib most commonly presented as meningitis. Epiglottitis and bacteremia without focus were the next most common presentations. In developing countries, the primary manifestation of Hib is lower respiratory tract infection. It may account for 5%–8% of all pneumonia in children in these areas and causes an estimated 480,000 pneumonia deaths each year among children younger than 5 years.

   Infection is usually associated with bacteremia. Onset can be subacute but is usually sudden, including fever, vomiting, lethargy, and meningeal irritation, with bulging fontanelle in infants or stiff neck and back in older children. Progressive stupor or coma is common. Occasionally, there is a low-grade fever for several days, with subtler central nervous system symptoms. Overall mortality rate for Hib meningitis is 5%; 6% of the survivors have permanent sensorineural hearing loss; 25% have significant disability of some type.

3) Pneumococcal meningitis: onset is usually sudden with high fever, lethargy or coma, and signs of meningeal irritation. It can be fulminant and occurs with bacteremia but not necessarily with any other focus, although there may be otitis media or mastoiditis. Pneumococcal meningitis has a high case-fatality rate.

**2. Causative agents—**

1) Meningococcal meningitis (cerebrospinal fever): *N. meningitidis*, also called meningococcus, is a Gram-negative, aerobic diplococcus. *Neisseria* are divided into serogroups according to the immunological reactivity of their capsular polysaccharide. Groups A, B, and C account for at least 90% of cases worldwide, although the proportion of groups W, X, and Y is increasing. In most European and many Latin American countries, serogroups B and C cause the majority of disease, while A is the main cause in Africa and Asia. Serogroup Y causes about one-third of disease in the

USA, but less in other countries. As countries introduce meningococcal conjugate vaccine programs against the most common circulating serogroups (serogroup C in Europe, serogroup A in Africa), the proportion of disease caused by serogroup B is increasing.

2) *Haemophilus influenzae* meningitis (meningitis due to *H. influenzae*): *H. influenzae* are Gram-negative coccobacilli that are divided into unencapsulated (nontypeable) and encapsulated strains. The encapsulated strains are further classified into serotypes a through f, based on the antigenic characteristics of their polysaccharide capsules. Hib is the most pathogenic.

3) Pneumococcal meningitis: *S. pneumoniae,* a Gram-positive diplococcus. Nearly all strains causing meningitis and other severe forms of pneumococcal disease are encapsulated. There are 90 known capsular serotypes. The distribution of serotypes varies regionally and with age. In North America the 13 serotypes in pneumococcal conjugate vaccine are those that cause a substantial proportion of pneumococcal meningitis in children and adults.

**3. Laboratory diagnosis—**

1) Meningococcal meningitis (cerebrospinal fever): the gold standard for diagnosis is recovery of meningococci from a sterile site, primarily CSF or blood. However, the sensitivity of culture, especially in patients who have received antibiotics, may be low. In culture-negative cases, identification of group-specific meningococcal polysaccharides in CSF by latex agglutination can help, but false-negative results are common, especially for serogroup B. Polymerase chain reaction (PCR) offers the advantage of detecting meningococcal deoxyribonucleic acid (DNA) in CSF or plasma and does not require live organisms, but it is not yet widely available in many countries. Microscopic examination of Gram-stained smears from petechiae may show Gram-negative diplococci suggestive of *Neisseria*.

2) *Haemophilus influenzae* meningitis (meningitis due to *H. influenzae*): may be made through isolation of organisms from blood or cerebrospinal fluid. Specific capsular polysaccharide may be identified by slide agglutination or latex agglutination techniques. PCR offers the advantage of detecting *H. Influenzae* DNA in CSF or plasma and does not require live organisms, but it is not yet widely available in many countries.

3) Pneumococcal meningitis: may be by isolation of organisms from blood or CSF. Pneumococcal capsular polysaccharide may be identified by the Quellung reaction or PCR.

**4. Laboratory capability**—Most bacteria that cause meningitis can be recovered by standard clinical microbiology laboratories using routine media, such as blood agar, chocolate agar, and/or enriched media containing X and V factors. Commercially available molecular assays are available and detect several bacterial agents including *E. coli*, *H. influenzae*, *L. monocytogenes*, *N. meningitidis*, *Streptococcus agalactiae*, and *S. pneumoniae*.

**5. Safety requirements**—Many bacteria that cause meningitis, including *S. pneumoniae* and *H. influenzae*, and noninvasive *N. meningitidis*, can be handled under BSL-2 precautions. *N. meningitidis* recovered from sterile sites should be handled in a biosafety cabinet, and BSL-3 practices should be applied to activities that are likely to produce aerosols or droplets or high concentrations of infectious materials. Depending on risk of exposure, laboratory personnel should be encouraged to receive vaccination against bacteria for which vaccines are available.

**6. Nonhuman hosts**—Bacterial meningitis is generally not due to zoonosis.

**7. Sample/specimen requirements**—CSF and other specimens, such as blood, are ideally collected before initiation of antimicrobial therapy when possible. For optimal results, specimens should be sent to the laboratory as soon as possible after collection for Gram stain and bacterial culture. Molecular testing may be performed on CSF that has been refrigerated for several days.

**8. Testing requirements**—The gold standard for diagnosis of bacterial meningitis is through recovery of the bacterial agent via bacterial culture of CSF. Isolation of bacteria from other specimen types, such as blood, may support the diagnosis. Greatest sensitivity is obtained when specimens are collected prior to initiation of antimicrobial therapy. Molecular assays may be useful if patients have already received antimicrobials because they do not require organism viability for detection. Gram stain and CSF examination for cell count, glucose, and protein levels are useful in the diagnosis of bacterial meningitis. The utility of performing routine bacterial antigen tests has been questioned in that they demonstrate suboptimal sensitivity and specificity. Standard quality control and quality assurance practices used for molecular testing, Gram staining, and bacterial culture should be followed.

**9. Reporting requirements**—Bacterial meningitis—including meningitis caused by *S. pneumoniae*, *H. influenzae*, and *N. meningitidis*—typically requires reporting to local, state, and/or federal authorities. Requirements for reporting and specimen submission should be determined in conjunction with the relevant authorities. Other less common causes of bacterial meningitis should also be reported, including *Leptospira*, *Listeria*, *Borrelia*, *Mycobacterium*, and *Treponema*.

**10. Referral network**—Reference and public health laboratories may provide additional testing for bacterial agents of meningitis. Additionally, public health laboratories may request submission of isolates for further testing, such as typing of *N. meningitidis*, *H. influenzae*, and *S. pneumoniae*.

**11. Special considerations**—None.

[D. Chen]

# MERS, SARS, AND OTHER HUMAN CORONAVIRUS INFECTIONS

| DISEASE | ICD-10 CODE |
|---|---|
| SEVERE ACUTE RESPIRATORY SYNDROME | B97.21 |
| MIDDLE EAST RESPIRATORY SYNDROME | B97.29 |
| OTHER HUMAN CORONAVIRUS INFECTIONS | B97.29 |
| Common cold (see "Common Cold and Other Acute Viral Respiratory Diseases") | |

**1. Clinical features**—

1) Severe acute respiratory syndrome coronavirus (SARS-CoV) infection: early signs and symptoms of SARS-CoV infection are nonspecific and consistent with influenza-like illness, with a spectrum of disease ranging from milder or atypical presentations to severe respiratory illness. SARS should be considered in the differential diagnosis in an individual presenting with fever above 38°C (100.4°F) and with symptoms of lower respiratory tract illness (e.g., cough, dyspnea, shortness of breath); with radiological evidence of lung infiltrates consistent with pneumonia or acute respiratory distress syndrome (ARDS); or with autopsy findings consistent with pneumonia or ARDS without an identifiable cause and with no alternative diagnosis that can fully explain the illness. Cases can become severe quickly, progressing to respiratory distress coinciding with peak viremia that occurs during the second week of illness (e.g., 10 days), with about 20%–30% requiring intensive care.
2) Middle East respiratory syndrome coronavirus (MERS-CoV) infection: since its emergence in 2012, signs and symptoms of MERS-CoV infections in the majority of primary human cases have been reported as severe respiratory disease as judged by admission to intensive care, mechanical ventilation, use of extra corporeal

membrane oxygenation and vasopressors, and death; however, recently milder clinical presentations and even some asymptomatic cases have been reported. Secondary human cases have had a spectrum of disease ranging from milder influenza-like illness to severe respiratory illness. There have also been cases with atypical presentation such as immunosuppressed individuals presenting with gastric involvement. Coinfections with other respiratory viruses (in particular influenza A [H1N1], herpes simplex virus, rhinovirus, parainfluenza virus, influenza B) have been reported.

3) Other human coronavirus (HCoV) infections: in contrast with SARS-CoV and MERS-CoV, infections with the 4 common seasonal HCoVs (see Causative agents) are more often associated with subclinical infections or self-limited mild upper respiratory illnesses (common colds) presenting with nasal and pharyngeal symptoms, sometimes accompanied by low-grade fever. However, these viruses can infrequently cause severe lower respiratory tract infections, especially in medically compromised persons.

**2. Causative agents**—Coronaviruses are large, enveloped, positive-sense, single-stranded ribonucleic acid (RNA) viruses with surface spike protein projections imparting a crown-like appearance to the virus particle. Coronaviruses are classified in the *Nidovirales* order, family *Coronaviridae,* and subfamily *Coronavirinae,* with 4 designated genera: *Alphacoronovirus, Betacoronavirus, Gammacoronavirus*, and *Delacoronavirus*. Coronaviruses that infect humans include the 4 common seasonal HCoVs: alphacoronaviruses 229E and NL63 and betacoronaviruses OC43 and HKU1. SARS-CoV and MERS-CoV are betacoronaviruses that recently emerged from animal reservoirs.

**3. Laboratory diagnosis**—Diagnosis of HCoV infections requires a specific laboratory test to confirm infection. Laboratory diagnosis is most often accomplished by reverse transcription polymerase chain reaction (RT-PCR) or alternative molecular assays, and less commonly by virus isolation or serology. A wide variety of laboratory-developed and commercial diagnostic molecular assays are available for HCoVs. Because there have been no documented cases of SARS-CoV infection worldwide since 2004, available diagnostic testing for this virus is limited, and testing is not recommended unless there is compelling evidence that SARS-CoV may be involved (e.g., someone engaged in SARS-CoV-related laboratory work who develops an acute respiratory illness). MERS-CoV infections continue to be reported and all cases to date have been linked back to the Middle East, so a travel history should be obtained as part of the diagnostic evaluation. Within the Middle East, surveillance of cases of severe acute respiratory illness for MERS-CoV is recommended. Diagnosis of MERS-CoV infection is usually accomplished by detection of viral RNA by RT-PCR during the early course of infection. Qualified diagnostic reagents for MERS-CoV are available from CDC to select laboratories, and FDA-cleared commercial molecular assays are now available. Confirmation of a MERS-positive case requires a positive RT-PCR test on at least 2 independent genomic targets or a single positive target with sequencing from a different genomic region. For serology, a symptomatic patient can be considered a confirmed MERS case if they have evidence of seroconversion (a minimum of a 4-fold increase in antibody titer) in at least 1 screening immunoassay (e.g., enzyme immunoassay or immunofluorescence assay) with confirmation by a neutralization assay in samples ideally taken at least 14 days apart. A symptomatic patient can be considered a probable case if they have a positive screening serologic assay with confirmation by a neutralization assay in a single serum sample. An asymptomatic contact with a positive serological test result on a single serum specimen does not currently meet the WHO definition for a confirmed or probable acute case. It is also recommended to test for other common respiratory pathogens (e.g., influenza virus), but identification of another respiratory pathogen should not preclude MERS-CoV testing.

4. **Laboratory capability**—A biosafety level 2 (BSL-2) laboratory facility with certified class II biological safety cabinets, diagnostic test equipment, and materials and personnel with specific training in diagnostic procedures for molecular detection and identification of MERS-CoV/HCoVs. Capacity to inactivate (e.g., gamma irradiate) potential infectious virus in serum/plasma specimens used for serologic assessment of SARS-CoV or MERS-CoV infection. An appropriately outfitted BSL-3 facility and trained personnel certified for handling select agents are required for primary culture isolation or propagation of SARS-CoV or MERS-CoV. US laboratories must meet Clinical Laboratory Improvement Amendments requirements for performing moderate- to high-complexity molecular tests; those requirements include proficiency testing, quality control and assessment, and personnel requirements. If testing for MERS-CoV, the laboratory would need to participate in biannual proficiency testing, which is supported by CDC.

5. **Safety requirements**—Handling of infectious or potentially infectious clinical diagnostic specimens can be performed by trained laboratory personnel using appropriate BSL-2 facilities and work practices.
Viral culture should not be performed for persons suspected of having SARS-CoV or MERS-CoV infection unless appropriate biosafety measures are instituted. Primary culture isolation or propagation of SARS-CoV or MERS-CoV must be performed in a BSL-3 facility or higher using BSL-3 work practices by trained laboratory personnel.

6. **Nonhuman hosts**—Bats are the likely natural reservoirs for the progenitor viruses of SARS-CoV and MERS-CoV. During the SARS outbreak, the

Himalayan masked palm civet (*Paguma larvata*) and other wet-market animals in Guangdong Province, China, served as intermediate hosts and the main source of animal-to-human transmission of SARS-CoV. Dromedary camels are a reservoir of MERS-CoV and are likely the major animal source of human infections. Viruses similar to MERS-CoV have also been identified in European hedgehogs. Serological surveys have shown no evidence of MERS-CoV infection in other animals found in the Arabian Peninsula, including goats, cattle, sheep, water buffalo, swine, chickens, and wild birds.

**7. Sample/specimen requirements**—The type and timing of specimens collected can greatly impact the diagnostic sensitivity for coronaviruses that infect humans. Upper and/or lower respiratory tract specimens collected within the first week of symptoms onset are optimal for RT-PCR or culture isolation of HCoVs. For SARS-CoV and MERS-CoV, multiple respiratory specimens from the upper and lower respiratory tract and serum/blood should be collected early after symptoms onset for diagnosis with lower respiratory tract specimens (e.g., sputum, bronchial/tracheal aspirates/washes) preferred for RT-PCR detection. Stool is uniquely useful for detection of SARS-CoV later in the course of illness. For serology, serum should first be separated from whole blood. A negative serologic test can help rule out SARS-CoV infection if the serum specimen is collected 28 or more days after onset of illness. For MERS-CoV, paired serum samples are required to confirm acute infection, with samples collected at least 14 days apart and the first sample ideally being taken during the first week of illness. If only a single serum sample is available for MERS-CoV antibody detection, this should be collected no earlier than 14 days after the onset of symptoms. Respiratory and other specimens can be kept at 2°C–8°C for up to 72 hours before testing. If testing is delayed more than 72 hours, specimens should be frozen at −80°C and shipped frozen on dry ice. For immunohistochemistry, formalin-fixed tissue or paraffin-embedded blocks should be stored and shipped at room temperature.

**8. Testing requirements**—HCoVs can be detected by RT-PCR or culture isolation. RT-PCR is preferred due to its greater sensitivity and lower biosafety risk. Only laboratories with adequate biosafety containment should attempt culture of SARS-CoV or MERS-CoV. During the SARS outbreak of 2002–2003, confirmation of a positive SARS case required a positive RT-PCR test on at least 2 different clinical specimens (e.g., sputum and stool), the same specimen type collected on 2 or more days during illness, repeat RT-PCR on new extract from the original clinical sample, or 2 different RT-PCR assays. Routine testing for SARS-CoV is no longer recommended except under special circumstances as there is no evidence that the virus is currently circulating within human populations. For MERS-CoV, WHO recommends screening by RT-PCR assay (validated assays targeting MERS-CoV upE, ORF1a, and nucleocapsid genome regions have been described) using appropriate assay controls. A positive screening test must be confirmed by an independent RT-PCR assay or by nucleic acid sequencing. In the USA, RT-PCR assays for MERS-CoV must be cleared for use as an in vitro diagnostic test by FDA. In addition to the test algorithm described earlier, positive RT-PCR tests performed locally are considered presumptive and must be confirmed by CDC before reporting a positive MERS case. Serology is performed by only a few experienced reference laboratories that possess qualified reagents and well validated assays. No universal standard serological assay has been established.

**9. Reporting requirements**—Both SARS-CoV and MERS-CoV infections are notifiable under the 2005 International Health Regulations (IHR). Because there have been no documented cases of SARS-CoV infection worldwide since 2004, routine surveillance for this virus is no longer performed. Testing for SARS-CoV is now limited to a few international reference laboratories, and testing should only be undertaken when there is compelling evidence that SARS-CoV may be involved (e.g., someone engaged in SARS-CoV-related laboratory work who develops an acute respiratory illness). US health care providers should report any person being evaluated for MERS-CoV infection who meets clinical and epidemiological criteria for a patient under investigation to their state or local health departments who in turn should notify CDC. A presumptive positive RT-PCR test for MERS-CoV must be confirmed by CDC before final reporting.

**10. Referral network**—RT-PCR testing for MERS-CoV is provided by many individual countries through their health ministries and an international network of referral laboratories that WHO supports for member states and is available for primary detection or confirmatory testing. In the USA, real-time RT-PCR testing for MERS-CoV is available at most state public health departments through the CDC Laboratory Response Network (https://emergency.cdc.gov/lrn/index.asp). RT-PCR, genome sequencing, virus culture, and serology services for MERS-CoV are available from CDC and other international reference laboratories.

**11. Special considerations**—

- SARS-CoV and MERS-CoV infections are notifiable under IHR.
- SARS-CoV is subject to Select Agent Regulations as designated by the Federal Select Agent Program; MERS-CoV is under consideration for a select agent designation.
- WHO MERS case definitions are available at: http://www.who.int/csr/disease/coronavirus_infections/case_definition/en.
- CDC interim patient under investigation guidance and case definitions are available at: http://www.cdc.gov/coronavirus/mers/case-def.html.

[D. Erdman]

# MOLLUSCUM CONTAGIOSUM

| DISEASE | ICD-10 CODE |
|---|---|
| MOLLUSCUM CONTAGIOSUM | ICD-10 B08.1 |

**1. Clinical features**—A viral infection of the skin resulting in smooth-surfaced, firm, and dome-shaped or hemispherical papules with central umbilication. The lesions may be flesh-colored, white, translucent, or yellow. Most papules are 2–5 mm in diameter; lesions with large size or giant mollusca' (10–30 mm) are occasionally seen. Lesions in adults are most often on the lower abdominal wall, pubis, genitalia, or inner thighs; on children, they are most often on the face, trunk, and proximal extremities. In immunocompetent hosts the course of infection is usually benign, typically resulting in the development of 15–35 lesions with no other symptoms present. Immunocompromised hosts (e.g., patients with human immunodeficiency virus infection) may develop hundreds of disseminated lesions of the body and face. Occasionally the lesions itch and show a linear orientation, which suggests autoinoculation by scratching. In some patients, 50–100 lesions may become confluent and form a single plaque. Without treatment, molluscum contagiosum can persist for 6 months to 2 years. Any one lesion has a life span of 2–3 months. Lesions may resolve spontaneously or as a result of inflammatory response following trauma or secondary bacterial infection. Treatment (including mechanical removal of the lesions) may shorten the course of infection.

**2. Causative agents**—Molluscum contagiosum virus (MCV), a member of *Poxviridae* family, genus *Molluscipoxvirus*. The genus comprises at least 4 distinct genetic types (MCV-1 to -4), differentiated by deoxyribonucleic acid (DNA) endonuclease cleavage maps. The virus has not been grown in cell culture.

**3. Laboratory diagnosis**—The diagnosis of MCV can be made clinically when multiple lesions are present. Lesions visualized by dermatoscopy, showing orifices and vessels (in crown, radial, or punctiform patterns), are suggestive of MCV. For laboratory confirmation, however, the core can be expressed onto a glass slide and examined by ordinary light microscopy for classic basophilic, Feulgen-positive, intracytoplasmic inclusions, and molluscum or Henderson-Paterson bodies. Histology or molecular analysis (polymerase chain reaction [PCR]) confirms the diagnosis.

**4. Laboratory capability**—Testing via light microscopy and histology can be performed by most clinical laboratories with qualified personnel. Confirmatory testing via electron microscopy and molecular analysis generally require reference laboratory capabilities and personnel with advanced training.

**5. Safety requirements**—Biosafety level 2 is recommended for work with MCV.

**6. Nonhuman hosts**—Transmission of MCV between humans and animals has not been documented; however, MCV lesions have been diagnosed in several animal species including donkeys, horses, and chimpanzees by histology, electron microscopy, and PCR.

**7. Sample/specimen requirements**—Molluscum lesion material expressed directly onto a glass slide or into a sterile screw-capped plastic tube with O-ring can be used for laboratory testing. Alternatively, sterile, dry polyester or Dacron swabs can be used to collect lesion material for molecular analysis. Lastly, lesion biopsy specimens can be used for evaluation by histopathology and/or molecular analysis. Viral transport medium should not be used as this can dilute the sample for molecular analysis. Specimens should be stored at 4°C until shipment.

**8. Testing requirements**—When the clinical appearance of lesions is insufficient to make the diagnosis, confirmatory laboratory testing can include light microscopy, electron microscopy, histopathology, and molecular analysis. Serologic testing is not routinely available, and the virus has not been successfully cultured using cell culture methods.

**9. Reporting requirements**—Molluscum contagiosum is not a nationally notifiable condition.

**10. Referral network**—CDC provides MCV specific molecular detection. Clinical consultation with the CDC Poxvirus Program (404-639-4129) is required prior to specimen shipment to determine testing appropriateness and urgency.

**11. Special considerations**—None.

[B. Petersen]

# MUCORMYCOSIS

(zygomycosis)

| DISEASE | ICD-10 CODE |
|---|---|
| INFECTIONS DUE TO MUCORALES | ICD-10 B46.0–B46.5 |
| INFECTIONS DUE TO ENTOMOPHTHORALES | ICD-10 B46.8 |
| BASIDIOBOLOMYCOSIS | ICD-10 B46.8 |
| CONIDIOBOLOMYCOSIS | ICD-10 B46.8 |

**1. Clinical features**—Infections caused by fungi of the order Mucorales result in disease that is typically rapidly progressive, destructive, and associated with high mortality. These fungi have an affinity for blood vessels and cause thrombosis, infarction, and tissue necrosis. The mycosis has an acute or subacute course. In debilitated persons it is the most fulminant fungal infection known.

The 4 main systemic forms of the disease are the rhinocerebral, pulmonary, gastrointestinal, and disseminated types. Cutaneous infection may also occur. The underlying disease influences the portal of entry of the fungus. Rhinocerebral disease represents one-third to one-half of all cases and usually presents as nasal or paranasal sinus infection, most often in patients with poorly controlled diabetes mellitus. Necrosis of the turbinates, perforation of the hard palate, necrosis of the cheek or orbital cellulitis, proptosis, and ophthalmoplegia may occur. Infection may penetrate to the internal carotid artery or extend directly to the brain and cause infarction.

Pulmonary mucormycosis (zygomycosis) appears to occur most commonly among hematological malignancy patients with neutropenia and recipients of hematopoietic stem cell transplants. In this form, the fungus causes thrombosis of pulmonary blood vessels and infarcts of the lung.

Gastrointestinal mucormycosis has been associated with severe malnutrition and has been reported in preterm neonates. In this form, mucosal ulcers or thrombosis and gangrene of stomach or bowel wall may occur.

Disseminated mucormycosis usually occurs in severely immunosuppressed patients, such as those with profound neutropenia and hematological malignancy. Deferoxamine therapy has been associated with disseminated mucormycosis. Nosocomial infections have been reported.

**2. Causative agents**—Those species most often implicated in human disease are members of the subphylum Mucormycotina, which encompasses the orders Mucorales and Entomophthorales. The species *Rhizopus arrhizus, Rhizopus microsporus* group, *Rhizopus rhizopodiformis, Rhizomucor pusillus, Mucor circinelloides,* and *Lichthiemia corymbifera* (previously *Absidia corymbifera*) of the order Mucorales are encountered most frequently, with other genera such as *Cunninghamella, Apophysomyces, Saksenaea*, and *Syncephalastrum* implicated on occasion. Less common, and usually associated with specific geographical locations, are infections due to the order Entomophthorales: *Conidiobolus coronatus* and *Basidiobolus ranarum* are the 2 species most frequently reported.

**3. Laboratory diagnosis**—Early detection of pulmonary or sinus lesions by computerized tomography (CT) can provide evidence of angioinvasive fungal infection although there are few signs that specifically indicate mucormycosis. One feature that has been reported is the appearance on occasion on chest CT of a lesion with a reverse halo.

Definitive diagnosis requires the visualization of broad, ribbon-like, aseptate, or pauciseptate hyphae with right-angled branching on microscopic examination of tissue or body fluids from the affected area. Useful histopathological stains include Grocott's methamine silver, which stains tissues green and fungal hyphae silver-black. With the Entomophthorales, fragments of broad mycelium may be seen surrounded by an irregular deposit of eosinophilic Splendore-Hoeppli material best demonstrated in a hematoxylin and eosin stain. Microscopy of fresh tissue is enhanced by presoftening with 10% KOH and application of optical brighteners followed by examination under an ultraviolet light. Culture onto a glucose peptone agar containing chloramphenicol to inhibit bacterial overgrowth and incubation, aerobically at 30°C and also at 37°C, may yield the infecting pathogen. It is very important not to homogenize tissues containing suspected agents of mucormycosis as this may render the pathogen nonviable. Instead, samples should be minced and portions gently pushed into the surface of the agar. Agents of mucormycosis are often fast growing, producing a luxuriant aerial growth that invades the available air space of a culture plate within 48 hours incubation. As they are also frequent environmental contaminants, culture without positive direct microscopy is not definitive, but isolation should prompt a thorough clinical assessment of a patient in one of the risk groups. Many environmental Mucorales will be unable to grow at body temperature, and this can be helpful in determining their significance. Agents from the Entomophthorales produce flat, spreading, waxy cultures with radial grooves and often produce forcibly discharged balistospores, which are propelled away from the culture and can be seen producing secondary spores on the underside of the culture plate lids. If an organism fails to grow from tissue or body fluids—which happens quite often even when hyphae have been seen in the tissues—panfungal or specific polymerase chain reaction (PCR) may be helpful either on formalin-fixed or fresh tissue; however, the deoxyribonucleic acid (DNA) yield is often better from the latter.

Isolates can usually be identified based on their phenotypic characteristics, but amplification of DNA followed by sequencing can be a useful pointer in some poorly sporing, unusual, or atypical isolates.

With the increasing choice of antifungal agents with activity against this group of opportunistic pathogens, specific antifungal susceptibility testing may be helpful in selecting therapy.

**4. Laboratory capability**—Local microbiology laboratories should be able to provide an isolation and identification service for the agents of mucormycosis, although the identification of some of the less common species may require referral to a specialist mycology laboratory. Laboratories should have the facilities and expertise for examining fungal structures seen in microscopic mounts of tissues treated with optical brighteners.

**5. Safety requirements**—In the UK, the Advisory Committee on Dangerous Pathogens lists the causative agents of mucormycosis as hazard group 2 organisms; therefore, biosafety level 2 laboratory practices are sufficient for handling the agents. In the USA, mycology work should be conducted in a certified type 2 laminar-airflow biosafety cabinet.

**6. Nonhuman hosts**—Many of the agents of mucormycosis are important saprobes on decaying plant material, thus the opportunistic pathogens are usually acquired from an environmental source. The most common presentations are rhinocerebral mucormycosis or pulmonary infection following inhalation of spores, although infection can follow ingestion or deposition of spores onto the susceptible tissue of wounds such as burns leading to a rapidly invasive infection with marked necrosis. Most often infections are sporadic occurring as isolated cases, but there have been instances where contaminated fomites such as dressings or wooden tongue depressors have caused localized outbreaks. Wooden tongue depressors used to splint lines and other medical equipment have caused outbreaks of disseminated infection on neonatal units following cutaneous infection and subsequent dissemination and have also been implicated in an outbreak of gastric mucormycosis when used to mix nasogastric feeds.

The Entomophthorales are often found in association with decaying vegetation, soil, insects, and in the gastrointestinal tracts of amphibians and reptiles. Infection arises due to inoculation of spores under the dermis or in the nasal mucosa by minor trauma, often in otherwise healthy individuals.

**7. Sample/specimen requirements**—The ideal sample is a tissue biopsy sample from the affected area taken during surgery or endoscopy, although body fluids and bronchoalveolar lavage may also be helpful. Surgical debridement is often an important part of the treatment, so portions of tissue should be reserved for mycological examination and histology. The sample for mycology should be transported to the laboratory at ambient temperature in a leak-proof, sterile container with a few drops of saline to keep tissue samples moist and processed as soon as possible to reduce the chances of bacterial overgrowth.

**8. Testing requirements**—On arrival in the laboratory, the sample should be examined microscopically and cultured on selective media incubated at 30°C and 37°C for a minimum of 2 weeks, although growth is often apparent within 24–48 hours. Biopsy samples should not be homogenized but cut into small (1 $mm^2$) pieces for microscopy and culture. Microscopic examination of the test sample following presoftening in 10% KOH is enhanced by the application of optical brighteners and examination under a fluorescence microscope. Molds causing mucormycosis can usually be recognized by their characteristic broad, ribbon-like aseptate or pauciseptate hyphae with right-angled branching. Histological stains such as Grocott's methamine silver stain may be helpful to visualize the fungal hyphae in fixed tissue samples.

Biomarkers such as beta-glucan are not usually helpful in diagnosis as these molds have little beta-glucan in the cell wall, and there are currently no serological tests available. In-house panfungal or specific PCR tests may be helpful as pointers toward identifying isolates to species level and also have great potential as diagnostic tools for use on tissue, blood, or other body fluids.

**9. Reporting requirements**—Local laboratories should provide isolation and identification services for the agents of mucormycosis; there is no national surveillance. Outbreaks are rare, but infections due to the same species in more than 1 patient, occurring simultaneously or sequentially, in a health care facility should trigger investigation by the appropriate state or local public health agency as outbreaks have been reported due to contaminated medical supplies.

**10. Referral network**—Isolates that are unusual or difficult to identify should be referred to specialist mycology reference laboratories.

**11. Special considerations**—The most common agents of mucormycosis (previously referred to as zygomycosis and more recently as mucoromycosis) are in the subphylum Mucoromycotina, order Mucorales. They typically cause life-threatening, rapidly invasive, destructive infection in which there is angioinvasion leading to spread to contiguous tissues, thrombosis, infarction, and extensive necrosis. Spores of the causative agents are often larger than those of other opportunistic pathogenic fungi and when inhaled impact on the nasal turbinates initiating localized infection of the sinus, cheek, orbit, or hard palate. However, the infection can rapidly progress to the devastating and often fatal disease rhinocerebral mucormycosis following penetration to the internal carotid artery or by contiguous extension into the brain. Due to the localized bulk of the fungal growth, proptosis and ophthalmoplegia may occur. Rhinocerebral mucormycosis, which accounts for 30%–50% of infections with this group of agents, occurs most often in individuals with defects in their cell-mediated immunity. Traditional risk factors include uncontrolled diabetes mellitus, solid organ or stem cell transplant, corticosteroid use, and increased levels of available iron due to acidosis or the administration of deferoxamine. If inhaled spores reach the alveoli, especially in neutropenic patients, then the resulting infection is clinically indistinguishable from pulmonary aspergillosis but may follow a more rapidly progressive and fulminant course with hemorrhagic infarcts of the lung and spread across adjacent tissue planes. Disseminated infection can follow hematogenous spread to other organs, especially the brain, and usually only occurs in severely immunocompromised patients.

Gastrointestinal mucormycosis may follow ingestion and traditionally was thought to predominantly affect preterm neonates in the form of a necrotizing enterocolitis and those adults with severe immunosuppression or malnutrition. However, in recent years this form seems to have become more prevalent and is also seen as a nosocomial infection in patients without the previously reported risk factors but who have suffered peptic, gastric, or colonic ulceration. The symptoms are nonspecific and mimic those of an intra-abdominal abscess, including abdominal pain, distention, nausea, and vomiting, often with accompanying fever and gastrointestinal hemorrhage.

Deposition of spores of the agents of mucormycosis onto open wounds such as those caused by burns or physical trauma may result in cutaneous infection, with associated localized necrosis. Penetrating injuries following accidents, natural disasters, or bomb blasts may introduce spores deep into wounds. Devastating limb infections have been reported in which fungal infection has progressed along blood vessels and extended well beyond the obvious area of necrosis, ultimately necessitating much more radical surgical debridement than anticipated.

Entomophthoromycosis is the term given to infection by 2 agents of the order Entomophthorales, which also merit their own disease names—conidiobolomycosis and basidiobolomycosis—but which, as members of the Mucoromycotina, also come under the collective terminology of mucormycosis, which may in time be replaced by the more encompassing mucoromyosis. They are seen most often in tropical and sub-tropical areas of Asia, Africa, and Latin America. Infection arises due to inoculation of spores under the dermis or in the nasal mucosa usually by minor trauma that may have been forgotten by the time the infection becomes apparent. Unlike the Mucorales, the agents of entomophthoromycosis are not angioinvasive and do not cause tissue infarction. Rather, infection is characterized by slow but relentlessly progressive growth within the subcutaneous and mucosal tissue eliciting a marked eosinophilic inflammatory response, usually in otherwise healthy individuals.

Conidiobolomycosis most often affects the paranasal skin or nasal mucosa of adult males leading to marked and often disfiguring swelling of contiguous areas such as the lips, cheek, palate, and nasopharynx. Basidiobolomycosis is also more common in males but affects mainly children and adolescents and most often involves cutaneous infection of the buttocks, thighs, and chest in which the area of infection is a large, firm, painless, well-circumscribed mass.

[E. M. Johnson]

# MUMPS
(infectious parotitis)

| DISEASE | ICD-10 CODE |
|---|---|
| MUMPS | ICD-10 B26 |

**1. Clinical features**—An acute viral disease characterized by fever, swelling, and tenderness of 1 or more salivary glands—usually the parotid, and sometimes the sublingual or submaxillary glands. Parotitis may be unilateral or bilateral, and typically lasts 7-10 days in unvaccinated individuals. Prodromal symptoms are nonspecific, consisting of myalgia, anorexia, malaise, headache, and low-grade fever. Not all cases of parotitis are caused by mumps infection, but other parotitis-causing agents do not produce parotitis on an epidemic scale.[1] Orchitis, most commonly unilateral, occurs in 20%-30% of affected postpubertal males, but sterility is extremely rare. Mumps orchitis has been reported to be a risk factor for testicular cancer. As many as 40%-50% of mumps infections have been associated with respiratory symptoms, particularly in children younger than 5 years. Mumps can cause sensorineural hearing loss in both children and adults. Pancreatitis, usually mild, occurs in 4% of cases.

Symptomatic aseptic meningitis occurs in up to 10% of mumps cases; patients usually recover without complications, though many require hospitalization. Mumps encephalitis is rare (1-2/100,000 cases) but can result in permanent sequelae, such as paralysis, seizures, and hydrocephalus; the case-fatality rate for mumps encephalitis is about 1%. Mumps infection during the first trimester of pregnancy has been associated with spontaneous abortion, but there is no firm evidence that mumps during pregnancy causes congenital malformations.

**2. Causative agents**—Mumps virus is a member of the family *Paramyxoviridae*, genus *Rubulavirus*.

**3. Laboratory diagnosis**—Acute mumps infection can be confirmed through the following: detection of virus by reverse transcription polymerase chain reaction (RT-PCR); or isolation of mumps virus from an appropriate clinical specimen (buccal swab or cerebrospinal fluid [CSF]); or a positive serological test for mumps-specific immunoglobulin class M (IgM) antibodies or seroconversion, or detection of a significant (at least 4-fold) rise in serum mumps IgG titer as determined by a quantitative serological assay. Collection of paired serum samples from vaccinated persons, even if appropriately timed, is not recommended since IgG begins to rise soon after exposure, making detection of a 4-fold rise difficult.

Diagnosis may be more challenging in vaccinated populations where the IgM response may be absent or short lived and the viral load may be lower.

The ability to confirm cases by ribonucleic acid (RNA) detection using real-time reverse-transcriptase polymerase chain reaction (rRT-PCR) is improved when samples are collected within 2 days after symptom onset regardless of vaccination status.[1,2] Collection of serum from 5–10 days after parotitis onset may improve the ability to detect IgM among persons who have received 1 or 2 doses of measles, mumps, rubella vaccine (MMR).[2,3] Absence of a positive PCR result or a mumps IgM response in a vaccinated or previously infected individual presenting with clinically compatible mumps does not rule out mumps as a diagnosis.

**4. Laboratory capability**—The isolation, identification, and characterization of mumps virus require specific microbiology experience and training, special specimen collection materials and techniques, as well as specialized media and equipment. Laboratories that are not experienced or equipped to perform virus culture should refer testing to a qualified reference laboratory.

**5. Safety requirements**—Virologic and serologic specimens should be shipped in containers specifically designed for the transport of clinical specimens (that retain potential fluid spills or leaks), and labeled appropriately to indicate the presence of biohazardous material and dry ice (as needed).

Biosafety level 2 (BSL-2) conditions and guidelines should be used for handling any samples that are known or suspected to contain mumps virus. These guidelines are published in *Biosafety in Microbiological and Biomedical Laboratories.*[4] Personnel who handle mumps-containing samples should be trained in BSL-2 methods pertaining to specimen storage, sterile technique, decontamination, and sharps and biohazardous waste disposal. Personal protective equipment (PPE) should include a laboratory coat, gloves, and eye protection. A biological safety cabinet should be used for handling samples that contain a high concentration of virus or when performing tasks that have a potential for creating infectious aerosols. All laboratory personnel should have documentation of 2 doses of live mumps virus containing vaccine or other acceptable presumptive evidence of immunity.

**6. Nonhuman hosts**—Humans are believed to be the only natural host of mumps virus infection, although nonhuman primates, rodents, and other species can be experimentally infected. A bat virus conspecific with the human mumps virus has been identified as a potential reservoir.[5] This virus was found to have a direct antigenic relatedness as well as a close genetic proximity to the human mumps virus. It is not yet known if this virus is transmissible to humans.

**7. Sample requirements**—Collection of specimens for both serology and molecular testing are recommended from all patients with clinical features compatible with mumps. Specimens should be collected as soon as mumps disease is suspected. Virologic specimens should be tested for the presence of virus by RT-PCR or by culture, and serum should be tested for the presence of mumps-specific antibody as described later.

Mumps virus can be detected from fluid collected from the parotid duct, other affected salivary gland ducts, the throat, from urine, and from CSF. Parotid duct swabs yield the best viral sample. Urine samples are less likely than oral specimens to contain sufficient virus copies or virus-infected cells for culture or detection by molecular methods and therefore are not recommended. Samples collected when the patient first presents with symptoms have the best chance of having a positive result by RT-PCR or virus culture since the amount of virus shed in the saliva rapidly decreases and is often undetectable by 4 days postsymptom onset.

The buccal or oral swab specimens are obtained by massaging the parotid gland area for 30 seconds prior to swabbing the area around Stensen's duct. A commercial product designed for the collection of throat specimens or a flocked polyester fiber swab can be used. Synthetic swabs are preferred over cotton swabs, which may contain substances that are inhibitory to enzymes used in RT-PCR. The swab should be immediately placed in 2 ml of standard viral transport medium at 4°C for at least 1 hour. In preparation for shipping, the swab should be reamed around the rim of the tube to retain cells and fluid in the tube. The swab can then either be left inside the collection tube or discarded.

Following collection, samples should be maintained at 4°C and shipped on cold packs (4°C) within 24 hours. If there is a delay in shipment, the sample is best preserved by freezing at –70°C. Frozen samples should be shipped on dry ice.

Serologic specimens are obtained by collecting 7–10 ml of blood in a red-top or serum-separator tube. Serum specimens should be stored at 4°C and shipped on wet ice packs.

**8. Testing requirements**—Commonly used methods for identifying mumps virus infection include both virologic and serologic assays. Early collection (prior to day 3 postparotitis onset) of a buccal or oral swab provides the best means of laboratory confirmation, particularly among suspected patients with a history of vaccination. Acute mumps infection can be confirmed by detection of virus by rRT-PCR or by positive mumps virus culture. The presence of serum mumps IgM or a significant rise in IgG antibody titer in 2 appropriately timed serum specimens using a quantitative assay or by IgG seroconversion can also be used to aid in the diagnosis of mumps. Because IgG levels may be quite elevated in acute samples from vaccinated persons, the use of diagnostic tests measuring IgG is not recommended for previously vaccinated persons. Infected individuals who have previously been exposed to mumps through vaccination may not have a detectable IgM response, and the amount and duration of virus shedding may be blunted. As a result, negative laboratory test results do not necessarily rule out mumps infection and must be considered along with clinical and epidemiologic observations.

Viral detection methods include standard methods of culturing virus in appropriate cell lines and molecular techniques, such as RT-PCR and real time RT-PCR to detect mumps viral RNA. Virus culture is the gold standard for mumps confirmation. However, sample quality must be maintained to ensure viability of the virus. Laboratories are strongly encouraged to perform cell culture isolation of mumps from buccal or oral swab specimens. Primary monkey kidney cells and Vero cells are frequently used to isolate virus. Successful virus isolation should always be confirmed by immunofluorescence with a mumps-specific monoclonal antibody or by molecular techniques such as RT-PCR. Virus can often be detected in culture or using RT-PCR when infection cannot be confirmed by serology. It may be necessary to grow the virus in culture to have adequate material for viral sequencing. Sequence analysis allows the determination of the mumps genotype (there are currently 12 recognized genotypes).[6] The sequence information can help to identify the source of the virus and can provide confirmation of suspected epidemiologic links. A positive RT-PCR result indicates the presence of mumps virus RNA in the patient sample and provides laboratory confirmation of mumps infection in persons with symptoms consistent with mumps who have not been vaccinated within the preceding 45 days.

Failure to detect mumps virus RNA by RT-PCR in samples from a person with clinically compatible mumps symptoms does not rule out mumps as a diagnosis. Successful detection of mumps virus depends primarily on the timing of collection and quality of the clinical sample. Vaccinated individuals may shed virus for a shorter period and less virus may be present.

Assays to detect mumps specific IgM and IgG are available commercially and include the indirect fluorescent antibody test, indirect enzyme immunosorbent assay (EIA), and capture EIA assay. IgM test methods and kits vary considerably in their sensitivity and specificity. While most IgM assays perform well for the diagnosis of primary mumps infection in unvaccinated persons, commercial indirect fluorescent antibody tests and indirect EIA IgM tests are less sensitive than mumps IgM capture assays when used to detect mumps specific IgM among patients with an anamnestic response.[2]

Acute-phase mumps specimens may contain significant levels of mumps-specific IgG, especially among persons with a history of 1 or 2 doses of MMR. The indirect fluorescent antibody format is particularly susceptible to interference by high levels of mumps IgG. Treatment of serum with an agent to remove human IgG antibody, such as Gullsorb or a similar IgG inactivation reagent, is necessary to avoid false-positive IgM test results. Absence of a mumps-specific IgM response in a vaccinated or previously infected individual presenting with clinically compatible mumps does not rule out mumps as a diagnosis.

If the first (acute) serum specimen is IgM negative, a second serum may be drawn and tested for mumps-specific IgM from 5–10 days later. A 4-fold increase in IgG titer between acute- and convalescent-phase samples, as measured in plaque-reduction neutralization assays or similar quantitative assays, or a seroconversion from negative to positive from acute to convalescent phase is considered a positive diagnostic result for mumps. Paired serum samples from vaccinated persons, even if appropriately timed, may not show a rise in IgG titer because the existing IgG often rises soon after infection. At the time of symptom onset and collection of the acute-phase serum sample, IgG may already be quite elevated, which would obviate the 4-fold rise in titer expected when comparing acute-and convalescent-phase titers. A second negative IgM result does not rule out mumps unless the IgG result is also negative.

A single serum sample tested for mumps-specific IgG is not useful for diagnosing acute mumps infections. There is no known correlate of protection for mumps, and the presence of mumps-specific IgG as detected using a serologic assay (EIA or indirect fluorescent antibody test) does not necessarily predict the presence of neutralizing antibodies or protection from mumps disease. A positive IgG result is expected among previously vaccinated persons. Older persons with no history of mumps illness or vaccination may have detectable mumps IgG due to a previous subclinical infection.

Parainfluenza viruses 1, 2, and 3, Epstein-Barr virus (EBV), adenovirus, and human herpesvirus 6 have all been noted to interfere with mumps serologic assays.[1] EBV can be particularly troublesome since the initial immune response to EBV produces not only a rise in IgM antibodies against EBV but also a polyclonal B cell stimulation; the antibodies are broadly reactive and can result in a positive mumps IgM result. However, the heterophile antibody test for EBV should be considered less susceptible to false-positive results with serum collected from true cases of mumps.

**9. Reporting requirements**—WHO recommends making mumps a notifiable disease in all countries. Mumps occurs worldwide with cases reported throughout the year and epidemics occurring regularly. Mumps remains endemic in many countries, and only 121 of 194 (62%) of WHO Member States included mumps vaccine in their national immunization schedules in 2016. When mumps is endemic, disease incidence and coverage should be monitored to assess progress and to identify high-risk populations and predict and prevent outbreaks. When mumps is widespread, outbreaks rather than individual cases should be investigated. By contrast, many industrialized countries have had long-standing mumps immunization programs, and mumps is a reportable disease in most countries that have achieved high routine mumps coverage and have low disease incidence. Case-based surveillance is used to detect, investigate, and confirm each suspect mumps case in the community, although in very large outbreaks this may not be possible.

Routine mumps vaccination is recommended in countries with a well-established, effective childhood vaccination program, the capability to maintain high-level vaccination coverage with measles and rubella vaccines (coverage that is >80%), and where the reduction of mumps incidence is a public health priority. In countries that decide to use mumps vaccine, the combination of mumps vaccine with measles and rubella vaccines is recommended. In this case, surveillance for mumps should progress with the level of control, and adjustments should be made to match regional and country-specific program goals and objectives. Countries with the objective of interrupting mumps transmission require thorough case-based surveillance to detect, investigate, and confirm each suspect mumps case in the community. They should include mumps in their list of notifiable diseases and routinely monitor disease incidence by age, vaccination status, and geographical distribution. As mumps incidence declines, case-based surveillance should be developed with laboratory confirmation of disease. Laboratory capacity for the diagnosis of measles and rubella should be used to develop similar capabilities for mumps. Countries using MMR vaccine should conduct surveillance for adverse events following immunization.

**10. Referral network**—There are no known referral networks specifically set up for mumps virus testing. Laboratories that are not set up for virus testing should refer all testing for mumps to their reference laboratory.

**11. Special considerations**—None.

## References


1. Barskey AE, Juieng P, Whitaker BL, et al. Viruses detected among sporadic cases of parotitis, United States, 2009–2011. 2013. Available at: https://academic.oup.com/jid/article-lookup/doi/10.1093/infdis/jit408. Accessed August 23, 2018.
2. Rota JS, Rosen JB, Doll MK, et al. Comparison of the sensitivity of laboratory diagnostic methods from a well-characterized outbreak of mumps in New York City in 2009. 2013. Available at: http://cvi.asm.org/content/20/3/391.full.pdf+html. Accessed August 23, 2018.
3. Krause CH, Molyneaux PJ, Ho-Yen DO, McIntyre P, Carman WF, Templeton KE. Comparison of mumps-IgM ELISAs in acute infection. 2007. Available at: http://www.sciencedirect.com/science/article/pii/S1386653206004069?via%3Dihub. Accessed August 23, 2018.
4. US Department of Health and Human Services, Centers for Disease Control and Prevention, National Institutes of Health. *Biosafety in Microbiological and Biomedical Laboratories*. 5th ed. 2009. Available at: https://www.cdc.gov/labs/pdf/CDC-BiosafetyMicrobiologicalBiomedicalLaboratories-2009-P.PDF. Accessed March 7, 2019.
5. Katoh H, Kubota T, Ihara T, Maeda K, Takeda M, Kidokoro M. Cross-neutralization between human and African bat mumps viruses. 2016. Available at: https://wwwnc.cdc.gov/eid/article/22/4/15-1116_article. Accessed August 23, 2018.
6. Jun L, Rima B, Brown D, et al. Proposal for genetic characterisation of wild-type mumps strains: preliminary standardisation of the nomenclature. 2005. Available at: https://link.springer.com/article/10.1007/s00705-005-0563-4. Accessed August 23, 2018.


[C. J. Hickman, D. R. Latner]

# MYCETOMA AND NOCARDIOSIS

| DISEASE | ICD-10 CODE |
|---|---|
| ACTINOMYCETOMA | ICD-10 B47.1 |
| EUMYCETOMA | ICD-10 B47.0 |
| NOCARDIOSIS | ICD-10 A43 |

Mycetoma has 2 distinct etiologies. Infections caused by fungi are termed eumycotic mycetoma or eumycetoma; those caused by aerobic actinomycetes (filamentous bacteria) are termed actinomycotic mycetoma or actinomycetoma. The latter manifest either as a mycetoma or as a pulmonary infection of varying severity (nocardiosis).

## I. EUMYCOTIC MYCETOMA (eumycetoma)

**1. Clinical features**—A clinical syndrome characterized by formation of small subcutaneous nodules that enlarge and become fixed to the underlying tissue and the skin, eventually forming sinus tracts that drain purulent material with visible granules (or grains) composed of a matrix component and masses of mycelial fungi; this is considered as pathognomonic. Eventually, the lesions result in destruction of structures, deformity, and loss of function. Pain is not a feature; bone invasion is common, but pathological fractures are rare. Mycetoma may spread directly or through the lymphatic system with secondary lesions; hematogenous spread occurs but is uncommon.

Lesions are usually on the foot or lower leg; sometimes on the hand, shoulders, and back; and rarely at other sites. Lesions on the head may invade the brain. It is unusual to have lesions on more than 1 extremity or area of the body.

Eumycetoma may be difficult to distinguish from osteosarcoma, rhabdomyosarcoma, sporotrichosis, chronic osteomyelitis, and botryomycosis (a clinically and pathologically similar entity caused by a variety of bacteria, including staphylococci and Gram-negative bacteria).

**2. Causative agents**—Eumycetoma is mainly caused by *Madurella mycetomatis*, *Trematosphaeria* (formerly *Madurella*) *grisea*, *Pseudallescheria boydii* spp. complex, *Falciformispora* (formerly *Leptosphaeria*) *senegalensis*, and *Medicopsis romeroi*, but other fungi have been implicated as well. Some species are more frequent in certain regions depending on the climate (i.e., rainfall).

**3. Laboratory diagnosis**—Specific diagnosis depends on visualizing the grains in fresh preparations; the color of the grain may indicate the organism involved. Fine needle aspiration or a true cut biopsy is often required, and identification of the causative bacteria or fungus is best made by culture. Molecular methods such as sequencing the internal transcribed spacer region may be used. The extent of the lesion is determined with ultrasound, computerized tomography (CT) scan, or magnetic resonance imaging (MRI); the latter may show the individual grain as the dot-in-circle sign.

**4. Laboratory capability**—A basic laboratory or a research laboratory with experience in the handling of fungi, stains, and simple biochemical tests and with the support of molecular diagnostic equipment such as polymerase chain reaction (PCR) instrumentation is required. Laboratory personnel who obtained at least a diploma or a degree in microbiology, biomedical science, biology, biotechnology, or similar and also underwent training in operating testing/diagnostic equipment are required.

**5. Safety requirements**—Mycetoma research and diagnostic culturing is performed under the biosafety level 2 (BSL-2) requirement. BSL-2 is suitable for work involving agents of moderate potential hazard to personnel and the environment.

**6. Nonhuman hosts**—Cats, dogs, cows, horses, goats, dolphins, parrots, and hamsters have been known to be infected. However, eumycetoma is not a zoonotic disease since there is no evidence of transmission from those animal hosts to humans. Mice, monkeys, and larvae of the greater wax moth *Galleria mellonella* have been known to be infected as models of experimental studies for eumycetoma.

**7. Sample/specimen requirements**—Grains obtained from true cut biopsy of infected patients are required for testing. Fungi in grains obtained via true cut biopsy are viable and can be used for testing while grains excreted from sinus tracts are often not viable and cannot be used for testing. Grains obtained from patients are stored in transport medium containing glycerol and should be processed as soon as possible.

**8. Testing requirements**—In most laboratories, culturing of the grains and examination of the fungi using microscopy are used as the primary method for diagnosing this disease. However, misdiagnosis often occurs because this method is not sensitive or specific enough.

Molecular diagnosis by sequence comparison of the internal transcribed spacer regions of cultured fungi has also been used to determine the causative agents of this disease. These molecular methods have been shown to be both sensitive and specific.

**9. Reporting requirements**—Mycetoma is not known to be a laboratory-based reportable disease.

**10. Referral network**—Several mycetoma laboratory referral networks exist and are as follows:

- The Mycetoma Research Centre (http://www.mycetoma.edu.sd), University of Khartoum, Sudan (WHO Collaborating Centre on Mycetoma). Contact the Centre by e-mail (info@mycetoma.edu.sd).
- Mycetoma working group, Erasmus Medical Centre, Rotterdam, The Netherlands. Contact Wendy van de Sande by e-mail (w.vandesande@erasmusmc.nl).
- Westerdijk Fungal Biodiversity Institute, Royal Netherlands Academy of Arts and Sciences, Utrecht, The Netherlands.

**11. Special considerations**—None.

## II. NOCARDIOSIS AND ACTINOMYCETOMA

**1. Clinical features**—Pulmonary infection is the most common clinical presentation of infection with *Nocardia* and can present as pneumonia, lung abscesses, or cavitary lesions. Contiguous spread within the thoracic cavity and hematogenous dissemination, particularly to the central nervous system, is common. Subcutaneous abscess or localized cellulitis also occurs following inoculation injuries with contaminated soil. Actinomycetoma is a specific chronic progressive clinical syndrome involving infection with *Nocardia* spp. (or other aerobic actinomycetes) characterized by swelling and suppuration of subcutaneous tissues and formation of sinus tracts, predominately located in the distal extremities.

**2. Causative agents**—Overall, there are now at least 94 recognized species within the aerobic actinomyces. *Nocardia farcinica*, *Nocardia nova*, *Nocardia carnea*, *Nocardia brasiliensis*, *Nocardia otitidiscavearum*, *Nocardia cyriacigeorgica*, *Nocardia abscessus*, *Actinomadura madurae*, and *Streptomyces somaliensis* are the more common species associated with disease in humans. For actinomycetoma, etiology is dependent on the country. In Mexico and South America, *Nocardia* spp. are more commonly seen, having as main etiological agent *N. brasiliensis* (70%). In Africa and India, *S. somaliensis* is also seen. *A. madurae* is seen globally and represents depending on the endemic area from 10%–50% of cases.

**3. Laboratory diagnosis**—Diagnosis of nocardiosis is difficult since clinical manifestations are nonspecific, requiring identification from clinical samples. Presumptive diagnosis may be provided from microscopic examination of stained smears of sputum, pus, cerebrospinal fluid, and bronchial washings, or tissues may reveal beaded Gram-positive branched filaments which may or may not be modified acid-fast positive in direct stains; colonies generally appear with aerial filaments and may be white or orange/yellow. Culture confirmation is desirable but often difficult, and any suspicion of nocardial infection should be passed on to the microbiology laboratory to enhance diagnosis. Biopsy or autopsy usually clearly establishes involvement, although histopathology may be nonspecific. Current serological tests are nonspecific with an exception of a serological test for detecting *N. brasiliensis.*

Diagnosis for actinomycetoma depends on visualizing the grains in fresh preparations; the color of the grain may indicate the organism involved (most are yellowish white and some red). The majority of grains are microscopic, and some such as those of *A. madurae* and *S. somaliensis* are visible to the naked eye and must be distinguished from white eumycetomas. Fine needle aspiration or a biopsy is often required, and identification of the causative bacteria is best made by culture. Identification of the agents may be difficult in most instances using biochemical tests; therefore, 16S rRNA gene amplification, gene sequencing, or use of matrix-assisted laser desorption/ionization time-of-flight mass spectrometry (MALDI-TOF MS) are now preferred methods for species identification of the *Nocardia*. The extent of the lesion is determined with ultrasound, computerized tomography scan, or magnetic resonance imaging; the latter may show the individual grain as the dot-in-circle sign (especially for cases caused by *A. madurae* and *S. somaliensis*).

**4. Laboratory capability**—A basic laboratory or a research laboratory with molecular diagnostic equipment such as PCR instrumentation is required. Laboratory personnel who obtained at least a diploma or a degree in microbiology, biomedical science, biology, biotechnology, or similar scientific discipline, and also underwent training in operating testing/diagnostic equipment are required.

**5. Safety requirements**—Norcardiosis and actinomycetoma research or diagnostic testing are both performed under the BSL-2 requirement. BSL-2 is suitable for work involving agents of moderate potential hazard to personnel and the environment.

**6. Nonhuman hosts**—Nocardiosis has been reported in cats, dogs, cattle, horses, goats, dolphins, birds (pigeons, parrots, Pesquet's parrots, warblers, royal parakeets), cetaceans (dolphins, seals, beluga whales, and killer whales), and rodents. Actinomycetoma has been reported in dogs, cats, and dolphins. However, nocardiosis and actinomycetoma are not zoonotic diseases since transmission from these animal hosts to humans has not been demonstrated. Mice, rats, and hamsters have been known to be infected as models of experimental studies for nocardiosis and actinomycetoma.

**7. Sample/specimen requirements**—In pulmonary nocardiosis, sputum or bronchoalveolar lavage are required for cutaneous cases with exudate of lesions and/or biopsies fragments. In actinomycetoma, grains obtained from true cut biopsy of infected patients are required for testing. Actinomycetes in grains obtained via true cut biopsy are viable and can be used for testing, while grains excreted from sinus tracts are often not viable and cannot be used for testing. Grains obtained from patients are stored in transport medium containing glycerol or saline isotonic solution and should be processed as soon as possible. The work with the actinomycetes causing nocardiosis and actinomycetoma is of moderate risk, and a biosafety cabinet 2 is required; personnel must be specialized in handling puncture-cutting material.

**8. Testing requirements**—In most laboratories, culturing of exudates, sputum, or the grains and examination of the fungi using microscopy are used as the primary method for diagnosing this disease. However, misdiagnosis often occurs because this method is not sensitive or specific enough. It should be noted that it is necessary to distinguish *Nocardia* spp. from *Actinomyces* spp., the first being aerobic and modified acid-fast positive, while the second is anaerobic and modified acid-fast negative. For nocardiosis, it is necessary to observe Gram-positive filaments in exudates and biopsies, while for the actinomycetomas it is necessary to see grains and to classify them. For *Nocardia* spp., the fundamental biochemical tests are hydrolysis or degradation of the following: casein, gelatin, tyrosine, xanthine, hypoxanthine, and urease. Biochemical tests only allow identification of complexes, and because these comprise several species, the best test is molecular identification by testing 16S rRNA gene amplification and whole gene sequencing. Identification by proteomics is also useful via the MALDI-TOF MS technique; however, it has a lower sensitivity and specificity than molecular identification.

Additionally, susceptibility testing of the *Nocardia* is recommended as susceptibilities to a wide variety of antimicrobial agents vary amongst the species.

**9. Reporting requirements**—Nocardiosis and actinomycetoma are not known to be laboratory-based reportable diseases.

**10. Referral network**—The following referral networks exist for these diseases and their laboratory testing requirements:

- Medical Mycology Reference Laboratory, National Centre for Microbiology, Instituto de Salud Carlos III, Majadahonda, Madrid, Spain. Contact Ana Alastruey Izquierdo by e-mail (anaalastruey@isciii.es).
- Mycology Reference Centre Manchester, Education & Research Centre, Wythenshawe Hospital, Manchester, UK. Contact Malcolm Richardson by e-mail (malcolm.Richardson@manchester.ac.uk).
- PHE Mycology Reference Laboratory, Bristol, UK. Contact Andy Borman by e-mail (Andy.Borman@uhBrisotl.nhs.uk).
- Department of Medical Mycology, Vallabhbhai Patel Chest Institute, University of Delhi, Delhi, India. Contact Anuradha Chowdhary by e-mail (dranuradha@hotmail.com).
- WHO Collaborating Center for Reference & Research of Fungi of Medical Importance, Chandigarh, India. Contact Arunaloke Chakrabarti by e-mail (arunaloke@hotmail.com).

- Mycology Branch, CDC, Atlanta, GA. Contact Tom Chiller by e-mail (tnc3@cdc.gov).
- Mexico Department of Dermatology, Hospital General de México "Dr. Eduardo Liceaga," Mexico City, México. Contact Alexandro Bonifaz by e-mail (a_bonifaz@yahoo.com.mx).

**11. Special considerations**—None.

[W. Lim, A. Bonifaz, W. van de Sande]

# NIPAH AND HENDRA VIRAL DISEASES

| DISEASE | ICD-10 CODE |
|---|---|
| NIPAH VIRUS INFECTION | ICD-10 B33.8 |
| HENDRA VIRUS INFECTION | ICD-10 B33.8 |

**1. Clinical features**—Nipah virus (NiV) manifests primarily as encephalitis. Since 1994 and as of 2013, Hendra virus (HeV) has been identified in 7 humans and appears to manifest either as a respiratory illness or as a prolonged and initially mild meningoencephalitis.

Symptoms range in severity from mild to coma and/or respiratory failure and death and include fever and headaches, sore throat, dizziness, drowsiness and disorientation, or influenza-like symptoms and atypical pneumonitis. Subclinical cases also occur.

Pneumonitis was prominent in the 2 initial HeV cases—one of which was fatal—whereas NiV cases have been largely encephalitic and were initially misdiagnosed as Japanese encephalitis. A proportion of NiV patients displayed pulmonary involvement with atypical pneumonitis, and the majority of patients who survive acute NiV encephalitis make a full recovery, but up to 20% have residual neurologic deficits. Mild late-onset disease and relapse encephalitis have been observed several months after initial infection, and the case-fatality rate varies from 40%–75%.

**2. Causative agents**—HeV and NiV are members of a new genus, *Henipaviruses*, of the *Paramyxoviridae* family. Both viruses are classified as select agents in the Federal Select Agent Program.

**3. Laboratory diagnosis**—NiV or HeV infection can be confirmed by direct detection of virus in cerebrospinal fluid (CSF), urine, oropharyngal secretions, nasal or oral swabs, and bronchial wash by virus isolation, or polymerase chain reaction (PCR) if collected at the early stage of infection. At a later stage, immunoglobulin class M (IgM) and IgG antibodies may be detectable in the serum and CSF by enzyme-linked immunosorbent assay (ELISA) or by serum neutralization assays. If death occurs rapidly and only tissues (e.g., brain, spleen) are available, diagnosis should be confirmed by PCR, virus isolation, or by immunohistochemistry (IHC) in formalin-fixed tissues and paraffin embedded blocks.

4. **Laboratory capability**—Clinical specimens from suspect patients should always be collected and handled with standard precautions within the appropriate containment facilities. Molecular and serological techniques should be available in those regions where these viruses are known to cause disease. If HeV- or NiV-infection is confirmed, potentially infectious specimens should be transferred to a national Select Agents-approved laboratory or destroyed.

5. **Safety requirements**—HeV and NiV are biosafety level 4 (BSL-4) agents, and virus isolation attempt should be performed in a BSL-4 facility. No human vaccines are currently available. Handling of infectious or suspected infectious clinical specimens should be performed by trained personnel with disposable caps, gowns, shoe covers, surgical gloves, and face masks (N99 or N100 [HEPA] filters). Procedures generating aerosols (e.g., centrifugation) should be minimized. The infectivity of samples may be greatly reduced, if not totally inactivated, by the addition of Triton X-100 and heating treatment, and the samples may be safely tested by serologic or antigen capture assays in the field. Heating to 60°C for 1 hour renders diagnostic specimens noninfectious. Ribonucleic acid extraction, using the guanidinium acid-phenol method, which also inactivates the specimen, must be conducted in a laminar-flow safety cabinet or a class III biosafety cabinet. In the absence of BSL-4, primary virus isolation from suspect samples could be conducted under strict BSL-3 conditions. Cell culture and the manipulation of potentially infectious specimens should be stopped when cytopathic effect with syncytia is observed. Fixed cells should be stained with proper reagents if available; in case of positive results, specimen should be transferred to the appropriate reference laboratory.

6. **Nonhuman hosts**—Fruit bats, particularly members of the genus *Pteropus*, are the major reservoir hosts of HeV and NiV, but the viruses do not cause overt disease in their hosts. HeV has been isolated from all 4 Australian members of the genus *Pteropus*, and NiV has been isolated from *Pteropus hypomelanus* in Malaysia. Elsewhere, NiV has also been isolated from Pteropid bats in Cambodia, and antibodies to a Nipah-like virus have been found in sera from fruit bats collected in Timor Leste, Indonesia, Thailand, India, and Madagascar. Antibodies to a Hendra-like virus have been found in sera from fruit bats collected in Papua New Guinea and Madagascar. It is therefore probable that related viruses exist throughout the

range of Pteropid bats, spanning a geographic area stretching from Oceania to the Middle East and including islands off the east coast of Africa.

The major spillover hosts are horses for HeV, and domestic swine for NiV (in Malaysia). The viruses cause an acute febrile illness in animals that may lead to severe respiratory and central nervous system involvement and death. Dogs infected with NiV show a distemper-like manifestation, but their epidemiological role has not been defined. Nipah-seropositive horses have been identified, but their role is also undetermined. Testing of other animals is underway; susceptibility testing suggests that cats and guinea pigs can be infected, sometimes with fatal outcomes. Mice, rabbits and rats appear refractory to infection.

**7. Sample/specimen requirements—**

1) Human clinical specimens: during the febrile stage of disease, virus can be detected in CSF, urine, oropharyngeal secretions, nasal or oral swabs, bronchial wash, or urine. Nasal or oral swabs, bronchial washes, and urine samples should be mixed with an equal volume buffered diluent containing serum protein. These samples should be stored and shipped frozen, if possible, on dry ice or liquid nitrogen. Serology can be performed on late acute or convalescent samples from serum, heparinized plasma, or whole blood, and samples should be stored and shipped at 4°C or frozen. For IHC, formaldehyde-fixed tissue or paraffin-embedded blocks should be stored and shipped at room temperature.
2) Nonhuman clinical specimens: secretions, serum, and tissues from livestock or other animals collected by veterinarian authorities should be processed with the same techniques.

**8. Testing requirements**—Hendra and Nipah virus infections are rare, and diagnostic reagents are available only at select reference laboratories equipped with appropriate biosafety containments. There are no commercially available assays. As for other infectious diseases, the diagnosis should always be based on the results of a combination of clinical laboratory data. During acute febrile stages of disease, virus can be detected by PCR or virus isolation, followed by sequencing. In late acute and convalescent stages, IgM or IgG antibodies can be detected by ELISA. Because of cross-reactivity, it is impossible to distinguish between ELISA antibodies against HeV or NiV, and neutralization assays are necessary to allow the proper identification of the etiologic agent. Virus antigens can be detected by IHC in tissue samples collected post-mortem. Direct detection of virus, viral antigens, or IgM or IgG antibodies in an individual with a clinically compatible illness or an individual with a known high-risk exposure to the virus constitutes a confirmed case of infection.

**9. Reporting requirements**—Suspicion of Hendra or Nipah viruses must be reported to the local health authorities. Laboratory testing could be performed at international WHO reference laboratories or nationally in select laboratories (e.g., European Network for Diagnostics of Imported Viral Diseases). If Hendra or Nipah disease are suspected in the USA, contact the Viral Special Pathogens Branch at CDC by phone (1-470-312-0094 or 1-404-639-1115; after hours, 1-770-488-7100) or by e-mail (spather@cdc.gov).

**10. Referral network**—Testing can only be performed at select reference laboratories with BSL-4 capabilities. For shipping potentially infectious material, samples should be packaged in accordance with current recommendations (International Airline Transportation Association) and forwarded, after consultation, to one of the BSL-4 facilities with diagnostic capability for these agents.

**11. Special considerations**—Occurrence of Hendra or Nipah virus infection does not constitute an International Health Regulations reportable event to WHO. Isolation of Hendra or Nipah viruses must be reported to the Federal Select Agent Program in the USA.

[P. E. Rollin, S. Nichol]

# NOMA

(cancrum oris)

| DISEASE | ICD-10 CODE |
|---|---|
| NOMA | ICD-10 A69.0 |

**1. Clinical features**—Noma is a debilitating inflammatory condition that starts as a localized gingival ulceration and spreads rapidly through the orofacial tissues, establishing itself with a fairly well-defined perimeter surrounding a blackened necrotic center. The word "noma" derives from the Greek "voun," meaning to devour, emphasizing the rapid progression of the disease. The noma lesion often disrupts anatomic barriers and spreads through muscles and bone. In general, there are 3 stages of noma development, which may overlap with one another: an acute phase, a gangrenous phase, and the final scarring phase. The acute phase is characterized by chronic malnutrition as evidenced by severe stunting and weight loss as well as hair discoloration and edema of the limbs. Other prominent symptoms include marked depletion of serum level of leptin (a polypeptide involved in the inflammatory response and immune function), halitosis, mouth soreness, excessive salivation, facial swelling, and difficulty eating. A child with noma often presents with a body temperature of 101.3°F (38.5°C) or more; enlarged submandibular lymph nodes; variable degree of loss of interdental papillae with alveolar bone exposure; and a medical history notable for antecedent illnesses such as gastroenteritis, measles, malaria, bronchopneumonia, tuberculosis, or human immunodeficiency virus (HIV) infection. The gangrenous phase coincides with the spread of the gingival inflammatory lesion to the labiogingival fold and then to the mucosal surface of the cheek and lip. Subsequently, an area of bluish-black discoloration may appear on the cheek. After this finding appears, rapid progression results in perforation of the cheek, usually in a matter of days. This phase is characterized by extensive intraoral tissue destruction. Soft tissue sloughing leaves a fairly well-demarcated deep wound with exposed bones and teeth. The disease is usually unilateral but can occur bilaterally. The scarring phase sets in following the gangrenous stage and results in trismus and facial disfigurement. Sequelae of noma depend on the sites affected and the extent of tissue destruction. The sequelae may include displacement or exfoliation of teeth, facial mutilation, bony fusion between the maxilla and mandible, trismus, poor speech, difficulty feeding, persistent leakage of saliva, and severe emotional problems. Atypical sites of noma lesions may occur (e.g., in the mastoid region, scalp, perineum) concurrently with the orofacial lesions. Noma neonatorum occurs during the first few weeks of life in premature and low birthweight babies, and resembles noma in children. Other infections with similar manifestations include ecthyma gangrenosum (associated with *Pseudomonas aeruginosa*), Buruli ulcer, leishmaniasis, niocervical necrotizing fasciitis in the elderly (associated with diabetes mellitus or other chronic condition), and necrotizing lesions associated with HIV-infection.

**2. Causative agents**—Noma is a polymicrobial infection of the oral cavity. The specific microbial etiology has not been well established. It has been difficult to establish which microorganisms contribute to the disease process versus those that are only incidentally associated. The following microbes, including some specific genera and species, have been isolated from the site of infection in patients with noma: *Actinobacillus actinomycetemcomitans, Actinomyces* spp., *Bacteroides forsythus, Campylobacter rectus, Capnocytophaga* spp., *Eikenella corrodens, Eubacterium* spp., *Flavobacterium* spp., *Fusobacterium necrophorum, Microbacterium* spp., *Peptostreptococcus micros, Porphyromonas gingivalis, Prevotella intermedia, Prevotella oralis, Prevotella melaninogenica, Pseudomonas* spp., *Streptococcus* spp., *Sphingomonas* spp., and *Treponema* spp. In addition, *Escherichia coli and Klebsiella* spp. have been isolated from noma lesions of neonates.

**3. Laboratory diagnosis**—Given that there are no definitively established causative organisms for noma, microbiological testing is not necessary to supplement the clinical diagnosis. Individuals with noma will frequently have other infectious diseases at the time of their noma diagnosis. The laboratory diagnostic procedures for these other diseases (e.g., measles, malaria, diarrhea, pneumonia, tuberculosis, and HIV-infection) are included under their respective chapters.

**4. Laboratory capability**—Most clinical laboratories can perform the laboratory tests that may be carried out to help diagnose the infectious diseases commonly associated with noma patients.

**5. Safety requirements**—Not applicable.

**6. Nonhuman hosts**—Many of the organisms found in noma lesions are also found in animals; however, there is no evidence that noma is zoonotically spread.

**7. Sample/specimen requirements**—Not applicable.

**8. Testing requirements**—Testing for noma-related infections may be required.

**9. Reporting requirements**—Noma is not known to be a reportable condition for laboratory-based reporting.

**10. Referral network**—Not applicable.

**11. Special considerations**—Laboratories may be asked to assist in the diagnosis of noma-related infections. Laboratories may also be asked to perform microbiological examination of noma lesions, but the results generated are not likely to influence treatment.

[B. W. Wilcke]

# NOROVIRUS INFECTION
(Norwalk-like virus, winter vomiting disease)

| DISEASE | ICD-10 CODE |
|---|---|
| NOROVIRUS INFECTION | ICD-10 A08.1 |

**1. Clinical features**—Usually a self-limited, mild to moderate disease that often occurs in outbreaks, with clinical symptoms of nausea, vomiting, diarrhea, abdominal pain, myalgia, headache, malaise, low-grade fever, or a combination of these symptoms. Gastrointestinal symptoms typically last 24–72 hours. Dehydration is the most common complication.

**2. Causative agents**—Noroviruses are small (27–32 nm), structured ribonucleic acid viruses classified within the family *Caliciviridae*; they are highly contagious and recognized as the most common causal agent of sporadic gastroenteritis across all age groups and of gastroenteritis outbreaks worldwide. Differential diagnoses include another member of the *Caliciviridae* family, sapovirus as well as the family *Astroviridae* (astrovirus), *Rioviridae* (rotavirus), and *Adenoviridae* (adenovirus).

**3. Laboratory diagnosis**—Reverse transcription quantitative real-time polymerase chain reaction (RT-qPCR) assays are the preferred method for norovirus detection on whole stool samples and vomitus. These assays are highly sensitive and are able to differentiate between norovirus genogroups I and II. Conventional PCR followed by sequencing of PCR products is used for genotyping. Multiplex nucleic acid-based assays for a panel of gastrointestinal pathogens and an enzyme immunoassay (EIA) for the detection of norovirus antigen have been cleared by FDA. The sensitivity of the norovirus EIA is limited, and testing with this method is indicated only during outbreaks when multiple specimens are available. EIA negative samples should be confirmed by nucleic acid amplification testing (NAAT).

**4. Laboratory capability**—In the USA, human testing for norovirus should occur in a Clinical Laboratory Improvement Amendments (CLIA)-, College of American Pathologists (CAP)-, or Clinical Laboratory Evaluation Program (CLEP)-certified laboratory capable of performing low to high complexity testing, depending on the methods used. In other countries, laboratories of similar capability are required for norovirus testing. Only properly trained personnel should handle potentially norovirus-infected specimens. Depending on the jurisdiction, clinical diagnostic testing personnel may require state licensure. Minimally, after training, testing personnel should perform an initial validation and annual competency testing on the test method(s) performed.

**5. Safety requirements**—Biosafety level 2 standards should be used at all times as recommended in the current edition of *Biosafety in Microbiology and Biomedical Laboratories*, which can be found at: https://www.cdc.gov/labs/pdf/CDC-BiosafetyMicrobiologicalBiomedicalLaboratories-2009-P.PDF. Use of a biosafety cabinet, laboratory coat, and gloves are intended to provide protection from splashes, aerosols, or direct skin contact with vomitus or stool. All procedures that may produce splashes, aerosols, or involve high concentrations of virus or large volumes should be conducted in a biosafety cabinet.

**6. Nonhuman hosts**—Norovirus genogroups GI, GII, and GIV are known as human norovirus. However, norovirus GII has been detected in swine and norovirus GIV in canine. There has been no documentation of interspecies transmission to date; however, potential for zoonotic transmission exists.

**7. Sample/specimen requirements**—Whole stool is the most common specimen type and should be stored at 4°C and tested within 72 hours for EIA or within 3 weeks by NAAT. If testing will be delayed, stool specimens should be frozen at -20°C. Repeated freeze/thaw cycles should be avoided. Some RT-qPCR and multiplex PCR syndrome panels have specimen requirements such as collecting the stool in Cary-Blair media or freezing the specimen if testing will be delayed beyond 72 hours after collection. Refer to the assay package insert for detailed instructions. Vomitus may be tested to support an outbreak investigation. Not all laboratories test vomitus; medical personnel should consult with their testing laboratory prior to collection. Vomitus specimens may be stored in the same way as stool specimens. Serum specimens for acute- and convalescent-phase IgG titers are not recommended for clinical diagnosis. Studies involving norovirus IgG titers should refer to the study protocol for specimen requirements. Food, water, and environmental sample testing are limited to public health investigations. Testing these specimen types may be indicated in support of an outbreak investigation and may assist environmental health specialists and epidemiologists during remediation and educational activities. Only specialized laboratories conduct testing on these sample types. Disease control specialists should consult with their public health laboratory and outbreak investigator to discuss the utility of this type of testing.

**8. Testing requirements**—Individual patients can be tested with RT-qPCR or laboratory developed tests. This is considered a diagnostic result when performance characteristics are determined by the testing laboratory and approved through CLIA, CAP, or CLEP. Single pathogen and multiplex PCR syndrome panels that are FDA cleared are considered a diagnostic result. Sensitivity and specificity have been documented from 84.9%–98.9% and from 89.6%–99.3%, respectively. During outbreak investigations, additional testing may be employed for further characterization. EIA is considered a presumptive result. Due to low sensitivity (65% [59%–71%]), negative results should be confirmed by RT-qPCR. Specificity has been documented at 90% (86%–93%).

RT-qPCR is considered a confirmatory result when following EIA or diagnostic when performed as the primary test. Single pathogen and multiplex PCR syndrome panels that are FDA cleared are considered a diagnostic result. Performing PCR followed by sequencing is considered a surveillance tool for determining the genotype of individual specimens and the relatedness of specimens to each other. Genotype information is uploaded to CaliciNet, the national norovirus outbreak surveillance network.

Recent advances in culturing norovirus make this a promising area for norovirus research into infectivity beyond current detection only testing. Testing by IgG titers and electron microscopy are applicable to special studies only.

**9. Reporting requirements**—Norovirus is not included in the 2019 list of Nationally Notifiable Conditions. Public health jurisdictions are at liberty to include norovirus on their own list of reportable conditions; however, it is common to request only outbreaks of norovirus as reportable. Local, state, and territorial health departments are not required to report individual cases of norovirus illness to a national surveillance system. Public health departments are encouraged to report suspected norovirus outbreaks through the National Outbreak Reporting System (NORS), and laboratories can participate in CaliciNet either directly or through their designated CaliciNet Outbreak Support Center. CDC launched both NORS and CaliciNet in 2009.

NORS collects information on outbreaks of foodborne, waterborne, and enteric diseases through a Web-based system. The information is used to determine norovirus outbreak geography, its transmission, and food or water sources involved. The data and subsequent analysis is used to improve norovirus outbreak prevention and control.

CaliciNet is a repository for both epidemiology and laboratory data from norovirus outbreaks. The laboratory sequencing data is used to identify the outbreak strain and monitor for newly emerging norovirus strains. Due to standardized laboratory protocols, strains can be compared within the national database to assist in linking outbreaks to a common source.

**10. Referral network**—Physicians' offices and hospitals may provide testing on site or send samples to a reference laboratory. Increased use of culture-independent diagnostic testing multiplex syndrome panels has led to the detection of more norovirus cases. Norovirus may be detected purely because it was on the testing panel, not because it was specifically requested.

Local, state, and territorial health departments are either certified to conduct norovirus sequencing for surveillance purposes or they are assigned to a CaliciNet Outbreak Support Center to refer their outbreak specimens for inclusion in the CaliciNet national database.

**11. Special considerations**—Prevention measures include washing hands with soap and water; hand sanitizers may not be effective against norovirus. Clean surfaces with a freshly prepared bleach solution (1 cup regular strength bleach per gallon of water). There is a potential for large-scale outbreaks where water supplies, sanitation, or food preparation do not meet accepted hygiene standards.

[A. M. Woron]

# ONCHOCERCIASIS

| DISEASE | ICD-10 CODE |
|---|---|
| ONCHOCERCIASIS | ICD-10 B73 |

**1. Clinical features**—A chronic, nonfatal filarial disease. Adult worms are found in superficial fibrous nodules in subcutaneous tissues, particularly in the head and shoulders (Americas) or pelvic girdle and lower extremities (Africa). Nodules also occur in deep-seated bundles lying against the periosteum of bones or near joints. Female worms discharge microfilariae that migrate through the skin, often causing an intense pruritic rash as the microfilaria die, with disfiguring skin lesions, including chronic papular and lichenified dermatitis, altered pigmentation, edema, and atrophy of the skin. Pigment changes result in the condition known as leopard skin, while loss of skin elasticity and lymphadenitis may result in hanging groin. Microfilariae frequently reach the eye, causing visual impairment and blindness. Symptoms are predominantly due to the inflammatory response to endosymbiotic *Wolbachia* bacteria, which are released upon the death of microfilariae. The greater the body load of microfilariae, the greater the risk of developing skin and eye disease. Microfilariae may be found in organs and tissues other than skin and eye, but the clinical significance is unclear; in heavy infections they may also be found in blood, tears, sputum, and urine. Onchocerciasis has been associated with epilepsy and nodding syndrome.

Disease manifestations vary between geographical zones, with onchocercal blindness most prevalent in the African savanna, while skin manifestations predominate in forest areas. In Yemen and central Sudan, the major disease manifestation is Sowda, a pruritic skin condition usually affecting one limb. In the Americas, the manifestations are most consistent with those in the African savanna.

**2. Causative agents**—*Onchocerca volvulus*, a filarial nematode. Humans can also serve as hosts for zoonotic *Onchocerca* spp., such as *Onchocerca lupi. O. volvulus* is native to Africa and the Middle East and has been introduced to Central and South America.

**3. Laboratory diagnosis**—Laboratory diagnosis is made through microscopic examination of fresh superficial skin snips or through the finding of adult worms in excised nodules. Different species cannot be distinguished morphologically, but species-specific deoxyribonucleic acid probes exist that are routinely used for species differentiation in control programs. Differentiation of the microfilariae from those of other filarial diseases is required where the latter are also endemic. Other diagnostic clues include evidence of ocular manifestations and slit-lamp observations of microfilariae in the cornea, anterior chamber, or vitreous body. Serum antibody testing (using recombinant antigens) may be used for diagnosis. Immunochromatographic tests utilizing the Ov16 antigen (Standard Diagnostics, Yongin-si, South Korea) have been shown to be effective for diagnosis and evaluation for elimination programs in endemic areas; however, this test is not currently approved for diagnostic testing in the USA.

Microfilariae of *O. volvulus* are unsheathed and measure 304–315 μm in length. The tail tapers to a point and is often sharply flexed; the nuclear column does not extend to the tip of the tail. Microfilariae of *O. volvulus* need to be differentiated from those of *Mansonella streptocerca*.

Adults of *Onchocerca* spp. in biopsy specimens are sexually dimorphic, with females measuring 33–50 cm long by 270–400 μm wide and males smaller at 19–42 mm long by 130–210 μm wide. The cuticle is multilayered; the middle layer is divided into striae which are best visible in lateral sections. Musculature is reduced, with only a few cells per quadrant. Lateral chords are short but conspicuous. Females have paired reproductive tubes, which often contain developing or mature microfilariae; males have a single reproductive tube, which may contain spermatozoa.

**4. Laboratory capability**—Microscopy should be available. As adult worms are usually identified by examination of biopsy specimens, diagnosis of adults is often performed by pathologists or parasitologists in specialized reference laboratories. Laboratorians should be trained in the microscopic/ morphologic detection of parasites and undergo regular proficiency testing.

**5. Safety requirements**—Clinical specimens should always be collected and handled with standard precautions. Filarial nematodes are biosafety level 2 organisms. Skin snips and biopsy specimens should be disposed of as infectious waste.

**6. Nonhuman hosts**—*Onchocerca volvulus* is transmitted by black flies in the genus *Simulium*. Nonhuman primates such as gorillas and chimpanzees may serve as reservoir hosts.

**7. Sample/specimen requirements**—For microfilariae, skin snips should be collected from selected sites on the body; common locations include the hip, scapular area, and lower calf. Surveys have demonstrated that when the microfilarial density is high, 2 snips can be adequate, but if the density is low, 4 snips at multiple sites improves the sensitivity. *Onchocerca* does not exhibit periodicity, so the time of collection during the day is not significant. Skin snips should be placed in physiological saline or water at room temperature for 30 minutes to 3 hours before microscopy; if still negative, hold overnight at 37°C. After incubation, the liquid may be placed in alcohol or formalin to preserve microfilariae. Preserved material can then be stained with Giemsa for confirmatory diagnosis.

For adult worms, biopsies should be taken from subcutaneous nodules (onchocercomata) that are soft, palpable, and may be found anywhere on the body. Biopsy specimens should be collected and processed per standard histological procedures

**8. Testing requirements**—Routine microscopy for helminth identification. A calibrated ocular micrometer should be used to measure microfilariae. Diagnosis is confirmatory in specimens meeting morphologic criteria.

**9. Reporting requirements**—Positive cases of *O. volvulus* may be reported at the species level based on the morphology of the microfilariae or adults in conjunction with epidemiologic data. Non-*volvulus* spp. are usually reported at the genus level when identified morphologically.

Onchocerciasis is not nationally reportable in the USA. Report to local health authority; official report not ordinarily required.

**10. Referral network**—None.

**11. Special considerations**—Epidemic measures: in areas of high prevalence, concerted efforts to provide community mass drug administration.

[B. Mathison]

# PARACOCCIDIOIDOMYCOSIS

(South American blastomycosis, paracoccidioidal granuloma)

| DISEASE | ICD-10 CODE |
|---|---|
| PARACOCCIDIOIDOMYCOSIS | ICD-10 B41 |

**1. Clinical features**—Paracoccidioidomycosis is a polymorphic disease, often severe and progressive, although some self-limited cases have been reported. In younger patients, the disorder is subacute and carries a severe prognosis; in adults, the course is chronic and the outcome better if appropriate therapy is given. The lungs are the site of primary infection, but the patient's symptoms may not reflect this. The acute or subacute form (less common) usually affects children, adolescents, and young adults who present clinical manifestations compatible with involvement of the reticuloendothelial system (i.e., lymph node hypertrophy, hepatomegaly, and/or splenomegaly). Cervical and submandibular chains of hypertrophic lymph nodes are the most obvious manifestation. In this clinical form, mucosal and pulmonary involvement is infrequent. In adult form, most patients present with respiratory problems and seek medical advice as a result of the following symptoms in order of decreasing frequency:

1) Mucosal ulcerations occurring in the upper respiratory and digestive tracts, mostly in the mouth and nose
2) Difficulties swallowing and changes in voice
3) Cutaneous lesions, often located on the face or limbs
4) Enlarged lymph nodes (mostly patients <30 years), especially in cervical area
5) Respiratory problems such as shortness of breath and persistent cough
6) Purulent or blood-tinged sputum and chest pain
7) Brain lesions

These symptoms are accompanied by weakness, malaise, fever, and weight loss. Hematogenous spread of *Paracoccidioides brasiliensis* can result in widespread dissemination, including lesions of the small or large intestine, adrenal gland destruction, osteomyelitis, arthritis, and meningoencephalitis or focal cerebral lesions. The disease may require differentiation from tuberculosis, Hodgkin's disease, squamous cell carcinoma, and other cutaneous systemic mycoses.

**2. Causative agents**—*P. brasiliensis*, a dimorphic fungus geographically restricted to areas of South and Central America. Three phylogenetic species have been recognized to date. *Paracoccidioides lutzii* has been named to designate Pb01-like isolates endemic to Central-West Brazil.

**3. Laboratory diagnosis**—Direct examination of histopathology or culture; both may have a low sensitivity. Serology may be useful but has a low specificity.

**4. Laboratory capability**—Laboratories with biosafety level 3 (BSL-3) mycology testing capability are the most appropriate for receipt and testing of specimens.

**5. Safety requirements**—Specimens suspected of containing *P. brasiliensis* as well as cultures of the agent should be handled in a class II biological safety cabinet under BSL-3 containment conditions.

**6. Nonhuman hosts**—The fungus is found in soils, mainly in the moist climates of the tropical and subtropical rainforests of Central and South America. Several reports have stated that armadillos may be a natural reservoir of this fungus.

**7. Sample/specimen requirements**—The most common specimen type is lower respiratory samples; however, oral and pharyngeal lesions, cutaneous lesions, lymph nodes, adrenal glands, and gastrointestinal tract materials are all acceptable.[1]

**8. Testing requirements**—A wet mount from a clinical specimen may be used to identify *P. brasiliensis* in more than 85% of patients.[1] Staining of wet preparations with lactophenol cotton blue, methylene blue, calcofluor white, or Gram stain may assist with visualizing characteristic structures. *P. brasiliensis* is a thermally dimorphic fungus. Colony characteristics are helpful for identification. Sabouraud dextrose agar or potato dextrose agar may assist in recovery of the yeast phase. At 25°C colony appearance will have a texture of glabrous to velvety with a white, pink, beige, or brown surface color and reverse color of yellowish-brown. Colonies may look very similar to *Blastomyces dermatitidis*. At 37°C there will be slow growth resulting in a creamy white colored colony. Conversion to a yeast phase is slow, and additional media may be utilized (i.e., Kelly or cysteine agar). Microscopically there are septate hyphae with some intercalary and terminal chlamydospores present at 25°C (mycelial form), while at 37°C (yeast-like form) a ship's wheel or satellite budding is present as indicated by multiple thin-necked buds developing around the parent cell. No commercial serological kits are available, although in-house serological tests may assist in more expedient diagnosis.

Real-time PCR assays generally target the gp43 gene. Antigen detection is not currently available as a routine clinical diagnostic test in the USA; however, several international studies have indicated diagnostic use from specimen such as bronchoalveolar lavage wash fluids, urine, or cerebral spinal fluid.[2,3,4] Antigenic detection assays for gp43 and gp70 are used for detection and for monitoring antigen clearance after antifungal treatments in some locations outside the USA.[4] Although most reports include the use of both the gp43 and gp70, there are some studies that suggest the use of gp43 alone being sufficient.[4,5] The definitive diagnosis requires microscopic examination and culture. The isolation and identification of the organism may take up to 30 days.

**9. Reporting requirements**—Public health authorities may require notice of cases or isolates; all laboratories should check with state/provincial public health authorities for further requirements.

**10. Referral network**—When assistance with testing is required, reference laboratories at the regional or federal level should be contacted. If shipping of specimens is required, then all applicable International Air Transport Association recommendations should be followed.

**11. Special considerations**—The AccuProbe test for *B. dermatitidis* will cross-react with *P. brasiliensis.* Research developed serological tests may cross-react with *Histoplasma capusulatum.*

## References


1. Thompson GR, Gomez BL. Histoplasma, blastomyces, coccidioides, and other dimorphic fungi causing systemic mycoses. In: Jorgensen JH, Pfaller MA, Carroll KC, et al., eds. *Manual of Clinical Microbiology*. Vol. 2. 11th ed. Washington, DC: ASM Press; 2015:2109–2127.
2. Marques-da-Silva SH, Colombo AL, Blotta MHSL, et al. Diagnosis of paracoccidioidomycosis by detection of antigen and antibody in bronchoalveolar lavage fluids. *Clin Vaccine Immunol*. 2016;13(12):1363–1366.
3. Salina MA, Shikanai-Yasuda MA, Mendes RP, Barraviera B, Giannini MJSM. Detection of circulating *Paracoccidioides brasiliensis* antigen in urine of paracoccidioidomycosis patients before and during treatment. *J Clin Microbiol*. 1998;36(6): 1723–1728.
4. Pires de Camargo Z. Serology of paracoccidioidomycosis. *Mycopathologia*. 2008; 165:289–302.
5. Oliveria dos Santos P, Rodrigues AM, Ferdeandes GF, Marques da Silva SH, Burger E, Pires de Camargo Z. Immunodiagnosis of paracoccidioidomycosis due to *Paracoccidioides brasiliensis* using a latex test: detection of specific antibody Anti-gp43 and specific antigen gp43. *PLoS Negl Trop Dis*. 2015;9(2):e0003516


[M. Soehnlen]

# PARAGONIMIASIS

(pulmonary distomiasis, lung fluke disease)

| DISEASE | ICD-10 CODE |
| --- | --- |
| PARAGONIMIASIS | ICD-10 B66.4 |

**1. Clinical features**—A trematode (flat worm) disease most frequently involving the lungs. Symptoms include cough, hemoptysis, and pleuritic chest pain. Chest X-ray findings may include diffuse and/or segmental infiltrates, nodules, cavities, ring cysts, and/or pleural effusions. Extrapulmonary disease is not uncommon; flukes may be found in organs such as the central nervous system, subcutaneous tissues, intestinal wall, peritoneal cavity, liver, lymph nodes, and genitourinary tract. Patients with cerebral infection can present with headache, mental confusion, behavioral changes, convulsion, visual impairment, and cerebral hemorrhage. Infection usually lasts for years, and the infected person may appear well. The disease may be mistaken for tuberculosis clinically and on chest X-rays.

**2. Causative agents**—In Asia (including India), infection may be caused by *Paragonimus westermani*, *Paragonimus skrjabini*, *Paragonimus heterotremus*, *Paragonimus miyazakii*, *Paragonimus hueitungensis*, and other species. Infections in West and Central Africa are caused by either *Paragonimus africanus* or *Paragonimus uterobilateralis*. Several species may cause human infection in Central and South America, including *Paragonimus mexicanus*, *Paragonimus caliensis*, and *Paragonimus ecuadoriensis*. Some of these species may be synonymous, and other poorly described species may also occur in this region. In North America, *Paragonimus kellicotti* is the only species known to infect humans. Infections with an undetermined *Paragonimus* spp., possibly *Paragonimus siamensis*, have been described from New Guinea.

**3. Laboratory diagnosis**—Sputum generally contains orange-brown flecks, sometimes diffusely distributed, in which masses of eggs are seen microscopically, and this establishes the diagnosis. However, acid-fast staining for tuberculosis destroys the eggs and precludes diagnosis. Eggs are also swallowed upon expectoration, especially by children, and may be found in feces by some concentration techniques. Eggs are unembryonated when passed in stool or respiratory secretions. Eggs are large, operculate, and ovoid to cylindrical or pyriform, sometimes tapering at the abopercular end. There are prominent opercular shoulders and an abopercular thickening in the egg wall, and eggs have a brown or golden coloration. Size and morphology vary depend on the species infecting. Eggs of species infecting humans in Asia have a size range of 80–120 μm × 45–70 μm. Smaller eggs may be seen in species from other regions, such as *P. africanus* (70–112 μm × 43-68 μm), *P. uterobilateralis* (50-95 μm × 35–55 μm), *P. kellicotti* (83–100 μm × 55-65 μm), and *P. mexicanus* (65-75 μm × 37–47 μm). In histological section, eggs have a thick shell, and the shell has a golden color and may be deformed or split. The egg shells do not retain acid-fast stains. Miracidia may or may not be seen, depending upon the age of the egg. Adult worms, when recovered, are typically reddish-brown, measuring 7–16 mm by 4–8 mm; eggs have a golden brown tinge. Microscopic detection of adult worms or eggs in sputum, feces, or biopsies is diagnostic. Deoxyribonucleic acid extraction from eggs in feces and sputum, followed by polymerase chain reaction (PCR) and sequencing of portions of the internal transcribed spacer 2 region 2 (ITS2) and cytochrome c oxidase subunit 1 gene (*cox1*) has been successfully employed on several occasions to differentiate species of *Paragonimus* from human and animal specimens.

A serological immunoblot (western blot) assay may aid the diagnosis especially when eggs are not seen in sputum or stool or in ectopic infections. The *P. westermani* immunoblot assay has a sensitivity of 96% against *P. westermani* from Southeast Asian subjects and has a specificity of 99%. The sensitivity for detection for *P. kellicotti* infection is 71%; the sensitivity for the serological detection of other species infecting humans is unknown. A soluble adult worm extract western blot of *P. kellicotti* recognized 100% of *P. kellicotti* infected subjects but is available for research purposes only (see: https://www.ncbi.nlm.nih.gov/pmc/articles/PMC3752799). There is no information on the cross-reactivity of these 2 immunoblot-based assays regarding their reaction to other species of *Paragonimus.* There are no FDA-approved molecular tests for the diagnosis of paragonimiasis.

4. **Laboratory capability**—Clinical diagnostic laboratories with trained parasitic microscopists are required. Morphological identification of larval and adult worm speciation requires reference laboratory level skills. Laboratories should be equipped to perform serologic assays, including blotting, if they wish to perform the *P. westermani* western blot assay. Laboratories should be equipped to perform conventional PCR if they wish to undertake *cox1* and ITS2 analysis. Sequencing of these PCR products may be performed at the primary testing laboratory if equipment is available, or they may be shipped to reference laboratories (commercial or public health) that perform sequencing of PCR products.

5. **Safety requirements**—Biosafety level 2 facilities are required to handle sputum and fecal samples. Formalin should only be used in a well-ventilated area, preferably in a chemical fume hood. Unpreserved and preserved stools and respiratory specimens and sera should be disposed of as infectious waste.

6. **Nonhuman hosts**—Definitive hosts are cats (including large cats such as tigers, leopards, and panthers), wolves, dogs, wolverines, gray fox, raccoons, skunks, opossums, coatis, beavers, pigs, rats, mongoose, and nutria. Intermediate hosts include several species of freshwater snails and, secondarily, several species of freshwater crabs, crayfish, and shrimp.

7. **Sample/specimen requirements**—For microscopic detection: fresh (within 48 hours) sputum; sputum preserved in 10% formalin, sodium

acetate formalin, or polyvinyl alcohol is required. Histology specimens include tissue biopsies of cystic lesions. Blood without anticoagulant should be collected and the serum separated for serological testing.

**8. Testing requirements**—Morphological identification of either eggs in sputum or eggs with or without adult trematodes in lung biopsy is diagnostic and confirmatory. *P. westermani* serology is effective for the diagnosis of *P. westermani* infections, but its sensitivity and specificity for other species of *Paragonimus* infecting humans is not well defined.

**9. Reporting requirements**—Report eggs of *Paragonimus* spp., but do not report species from egg identification alone. Exact species may be reported based upon adult worm morphological identification or upon detection of species specific sequences by molecular methods. Paragonimiasis is not known to be reportable by laboratories, but it is always recommended that laboratories contact their local and regional public health facilities to confirm which laboratory findings must be reported.

**10. Referral network**—Networks vary among countries. First-line laboratories may identify eggs or larva in culture. Reference laboratories may perform molecular analysis or morphological species identification of adult worms. The CDC DPDx service in the USA will identify adult worms to species level and assist with identification of eggs. *Paragonimus* serology is available through the CDC parasite diagnostics reference laboratory.

**11. Special considerations**—Consumption of freshwater crustaceans—raw or pickled in vinegar, brine, or wine, without cooking—is the primary risk factor acquisition of paragonimiasis. In some parts of Asia and Africa, the use of raw freshwater crabs and crayfish in traditional medicine practices may also pose a risk.

[R. S. Bradbury, I. T. McAuliffe, S. Handali]

# PEDICULOSIS AND PTHIRIASIS

| DISEASE | ICD-10 CODE |
|---|---|
| PEDICULOSIS AND PTHIRIASIS | ICD-10 B85 |

**1. Clinical features**—Infestation by head lice occurs on hair, eyebrows, and eyelashes; infestation by body lice is via clothing, especially along the seams of inner surfaces. Crab lice usually infest the pubic area, and—more rarely—facial hair (including eyelashes in heavy infestations), axillae, and body surfaces. Infestation may result in severe itching and excoriation of the scalp or body. Secondary infection may lead to regional lymphadenitis (especially cervical).

**2. Causative agents**—The ectoparasites *Pediculus humanus capitis* (head louse), *P. humanus humanus* (body louse), and *Pthirus pubis* (crab louse) are found worldwide. Adult lice, nymphs, and nits (eggs) infest people for *P. h. capitis* and *P. pubis*; nits of *P. h. humanus* are laid on fomites such as bedding and clothing. Lice are host-specific; those that infest non-human hosts do not infest humans, although they may be present transiently. Both sexes feed on blood. The body louse is the arthropod vector involved in outbreaks of epidemic typhus caused by *Rickettsia prowazekii*, trench fever caused by *Bartonella quintana*, and epidemic relapsing fever caused by *Borrelia recurrentis*.

**3. Laboratory diagnosis**—A head lice infestation is best diagnosed by finding a live nymph or adult louse in the hair or scalp. However, they are small, move quickly, and can be difficult to see. Use of a fine toothed louse comb may help in identifying live lice. If they are not found, then finding nits (eggs) on hair shafts (within one-fourth inch of the base of the shaft) suggests but does not confirm a lice infestation. If no nymphs or adults are seen and the only nits seen are more than one-fourth inch from the base of hair shafts, then the infestation is probably old, is no longer active, and does not need to be treated.

An infestation with body lice is usually diagnosed by finding nits and crawling lice in the seams of clothing. Sometimes a body louse can be seen crawling or feeding on the skin.

Pubic lice infestation is diagnosed by finding lice or nits on hair in the pubic region or, less commonly, elsewhere on the body.

Adult head and body lice are 2.0–4.0 mm long and are longer than broad; have 3 distinct body regions (head, thorax, abdomen); possess 3 pairs of legs ending in raptorial claws (i.e., adapted for grasping hair shafts), with all claws subequal in size; 1 pair of antennae; 1 pair of eyes; and lack wings. Adult pubic lice are 1.5–2.0 mm long and are nearly as broad as long; have 3 distinct body regions (head, thorax, abdomen); possess lateral protuberances on the abdominal segments; possess 3 pairs of legs ending in raptorial claws (the claws on the middle and hind legs are larger than those on the front legs); 1 pair of antennae; 1 pair of eyes; and lack wings.

Nits of head lice and pubic lice are about 1.0 mm in length. Nits of head lice have a flattened operculum while the nits of pubic lice have a conical operculum.

**4. Laboratory capability**—Microscopy/morphologic testing should be available. A dissecting/stereo microscope is preferred, but a diagnosis can be made on a standard compound (light) microscopy at low power (4x). Laboratorians should be trained in the morphologic identification of arthropod ectoparasites and undergo regular proficiency testing.

**5. Safety requirements**—Clinical specimens should always be collected and handled with universal precautions. Living lice are biosafety level 2 organisms. Lice are highly contagious; head and body lice are easily transmitted through direct person-to-person contact and contaminated fomites (e.g., hair brushes, bed linens). Pubic lice are less likely to be transmitted by contact with contaminated fomites. Because body lice may transmit the agents of some vector-borne diseases, specimens should be disposed of as infectious waste.

**6. Nonhuman hosts**—None.

**7. Sample/specimen requirements**—Whole intact adults, nymphs, and nits should be collected in a sterile container, mounted on a microscope slide, or promptly placed in a liquid preservative, such as 10% buffered formalin or 70% laboratory grade ethanol, to prevent desiccation and alteration of morphologic features. Specimens in an appropriate preservative should remain intact indefinitely.

**8. Testing requirements**—Routine examination of gross (whole) arthropods. A calibrated ocular micrometer or other measuring device should be used to measure adults and nits. Diagnosis is confirmatory in specimens meeting morphologic criteria.

**9. Reporting requirements**—Lice should be identified to the species level. Report to local health authority; official report not ordinarily justifiable. School authorities should be notified in cases involving children.

**10. Referral network**—None.

**11. Special considerations**—

1) Epidemic measures: mass treatment with the treatments recommended, using insecticides clearly known to be effective against prevalent strains of lice. In typhus epidemics, individuals may protect themselves by wearing silk or plastic clothing tightly fastened around wrists, ankles, and neck and by treating their clothes with repellents or permethrin.
2) Disaster implications: diseases for which body and head lice are vectors are particularly prone to occur at times of social upheaval (see Epidemic Louse-Borne Typhus Fever section in "Typhus").

[B. Mathison]

# PERTUSSIS
(whooping cough)

| DISEASE | ICD-10 CODE |
|---|---|
| PERTUSSIS | ICD-10 A37.0, A37.9 |
| PARAPERTUSSIS | ICD-10 A37.1 |

**1. Clinical features**—An acute bacterial infection of the respiratory tract classically characterized by paroxysmal cough and inspiratory whoop. The initial (catarrhal) stage consists of an insidious onset of upper respiratory infection with an irritating cough. Over the course of 1-2 weeks, paroxysms develop (paroxysmal phase) and increase in frequency and intensity before gradually improving after 1-2 months. Paroxysms are characterized by repeated violent coughing; each series of paroxysms has many coughs without intervening inhalation, which may be followed by a characteristic high-pitched inspiratory whoop. Paroxysms frequently end with the expulsion of clear, tenacious mucus often followed by vomiting. Between paroxysms, infected persons may appear well. Infants younger than 6 months may have cough without the typical whoop or may present with apnea.

In many industrialized countries with long-standing infant immunization and high coverage, an increasing number of cases are reported in adolescents and adults. Many such cases occur in previously immunized persons and suggest waning immunity following immunization. In those with partial immunity, symptoms vary from a mild, atypical respiratory illness to the full whooping syndrome.

Complications include pulmonary hypertension, pneumonia, atelectasis, seizures, encephalopathy, weight loss, hernias, and death. Pulmonary complications are the most common cause of death; fatal encephalopathy, probably hypoxic, and inanition from repeated vomiting occasionally occur. The number of fatalities in vaccinated populations is low. Most severe disease and deaths occur in infants younger than 6 months, often in those too young to have completed primary immunization. Case-fatality rates are less than 1 per 1,000 in industrialized countries; in developing countries they are estimated at 3.7% for children younger than 1 year and 1% for children aged 1-4 years. Pertussis remains among the most lethal diseases of unimmunized infants and young children, especially in those with underlying malnutrition and simultaneous enteric or respiratory infections.

Parapertussis is a similar but occasional and milder disease.

**2. Causative agents**—*Bordetella pertussis*, the bacillus of pertussis sensu stricto; *Bordetella parapertussis* causes parapertussis. *Bordetellae* are Gram-negative aerobic bacteria; *B. pertussis* and *B. parapertussis* are similar species, but the latter lacks the expression of the gene coding for pertussis toxin. *Bordetella holmesii* has also been reported to cause a pertussis-like syndrome.

**3. Laboratory diagnosis**—Laboratory confirmation requires demonstration of the causal organism from nasopharyngeal specimens obtained during the catarrhal and early paroxysmal stages. Culture is performed on Bordet-Gengou or Regan-Lowe culture media both supplemented with 15% defibrinated sheep or horse blood and is considered the gold standard of laboratory confirmation. While it is the most specific diagnosis, culture has limited sensitivity (60%). Polymerase chain reaction (PCR) can be highly sensitive and can be performed on the same biological samples as cultures. Direct fluorescent antibody staining of nasopharyngeal secretions is not recommended because of the occurrence of false-positive and -negative results. Indirect diagnosis is possible by determining a rise in specific immunoglobulin class G (IgG) antibodies directed against the pertussis toxin (anti–PT IgG) in an acute serum of the infected individual collected at the beginning of cough and in a convalescent serum collected 1 month later. In many developed countries, single-point anti-PT antibody tests are readily available and useful for diagnosis late in the course of illness when culture and PCR may be negative. Single-point serology results should be interpreted with caution as they do not differentiate between antibodies due to vaccination and those due to infection.

Differentiation among *B. parapertussis, B. pertussis,* and *B. holmesii* are based on phenotypic, genetic, biochemical, and immunological differences.

**4. Laboratory capability**—Most clinical and public health laboratories can perform culture, PCR testing as well as the serology testing for *B. pertussis.* Analysts should be trained on each testing methodology, and their competency should be assessed prior to their performing the tests independently.

**5. Safety requirements**—*B. pertussis* and *B. parapertussis* may be transmitted by droplets or aerosol generation during the manipulation of cultures. Contaminated clinical specimens present the greatest potential biohazard; therefore, biosafety level 2 (BSL-2) practices, containment equipment, and facilities are recommended for all activities involving the use or manipulation of known or potentially infectious clinical material and cultures. Personal protective equipment, such as laboratory coat, gloves, and goggles, should be worn when handling clinical specimens and pure cultures. Primary containment devices and equipment, including biological safety cabinets, safety centrifuge cups or safety centrifuges should be used for activities likely to generate potentially infectious aerosols. When handling serum samples, OSHA Bloodborne Pathogens Standard should be followed in addition to BSL-2 practices.[1]

Pertussis vaccines are available for adolescents and adults in addition to persons under 6 years of age. Review the current recommendations of the Advisory Committee on Immunization Practices published by CDC in the *Morbidity and Mortality Weekly Report* and on the Vaccines & Immunizations website or by another authoritative body for the latest detailed vaccination schedule.[2,3] The vaccine is available through occupational health care facilities and health care providers.

**6. Nonhuman hosts—***B. pertussis*, an exclusively human respiratory pathogen of worldwide distribution. Humans, sheep, goats, and pigs are known to be hosts for *B. parapertussis*.[4] Humans are the only known host for *B. homesii*.

**7. Sample/specimen requirements[5–7]—**

1) Culture:

- Time to collect: during the first 3 weeks of cough onset; ideally the first 2 weeks of cough onset.
- Sample type: nasopharyngeal (NP) swab, NP aspirate. The procedure of NP swab and aspirate collection are illustrated in videos by CDC and are available at: http://www.cdc.gov/pertussis/clinical/diagnostic-testing/index.html.
- Transport condition: Regan-Lowe (RL) transport medium, Amies medium with charcoal, half-strength RL charcoal-blood medium, and Casamino Acids are common transport media. Once an NP swab has been collected, it should be plated directly or placed into transport medium immediately. The transport time should not exceed 48 hours.

2) PCR:

- Time to collect: during the first 3 weeks of cough onset but may provide accurate results for up to 4 weeks in infants or unvaccinated persons. If antibiotic therapy has been initiated, it may result in false-negative results; therefore, PCR testing after 5 days of antibiotic use is not recommended.
- Sample type: NP aspirates, NP swabs with Dacron, or rayon-tipped swabs are optimal. Calcium alginate swabs and swabs with aluminum shafts should not be used for PCR.
- Transport condition: Swabs can be transported dry at ambient temperature.

3) Serology:

- Time to collect: during the first 2 to 8 weeks following cough onset optimally and may be collected up to 12 weeks following cough onset.
- Sample type: serum; the serum specimens should be collected using serum separator tubes.
- Transport condition: the specimens should be stored and shipped at refrigeration temperature.

All specimen types, NP swabs, NP aspirates, sera, and isolates should be packaged and shipped as category B biological substance according to International Air Transport Association regulation if commercial shipping services are used.

**8. Testing requirements—**

1) Direct fluorescent-antibody assay is a microscopic visualization of fluorescent antibodies directed toward *B. pertussis* cell of nasopharyngeal sample and is no longer recommended for diagnosis.[8]
2) Culture continues to be the gold standard for pertussis diagnosis because of its high specificity despite its low sensitivity compared with that of PCR. The sensitivity of culture is affected by the stage of disease in which the specimen is taken, the vaccination status of a patient, the age of a patient, antibiotic therapy, and culture methods. Various culture media, such as RL medium, Bordet-Gengou medium, and Stainer-Scholte medium, are commonly used for culturing *B. pertussis* and *B. parapertussis*. Most media are supplemented with cephalexin to suppress concomitant bacteria.[8] It should be incubated at least 1 week at 35°C–37°C or ambient atmosphere. The isolation of *B. pertussis* or *B. parapertussis* is the diagnosis of pertussis.
3) PCR assays have become an established method for detection and identification of etiology of pertussis. PCR assays are more sensitive compared with culture. The specificity and sensitivity of PCR assays may vary by the platform used, the deoxyribonucleic acid target(s) included, and the duration of disease at the time of sampling. The most used targets include IS*481*, IS*1001*, IS*1002*, h-IS*1001*, *ptxP*, and *recA*.[7] The presence and absence of different targets can be used to differentiate *B. pertussis*, *B. homesii*, *B. parapertussis*, and *B. bronchiseptica*. While PCR testing is increasingly used as the sole diagnostic test for pertussis, it is recommended that PCR be used in conjunction with culture when feasible, instead of as an alternative test.[6]

   Contamination is a significant challenge that the diagnostic application of nucleic acid amplification methods faces, which may cause false-positive results due to contaminating nucleic acids. To prevent contamination of clinical samples, these measures may be implemented: unidirectional workflow, air pressure control, and removal of amplicons. Appropriate controls, such as positive control, reagent blank control, negative control, and internal control, should be included in each PCR run to monitor the validity of the PCR mixture, carryover of amplification products or samples, cumulative effects during manipulations, and PCR inhibition of samples.

4) Serological tests, enzyme-linked immunosorbent assays, or bead-based assays to quantify anti-PT antibody levels are the recommended serodiagnostic methods and can be performed with paired (acute and convalescent phase) or single-serum samples. Paired-sample serology is an optimal method of diagnosis, while single-sample serology also provides good sensitivity and specificity to determine cases in older children, adolescents, and adults. IgG anti-PT antibodies are primarily measured and have the best sensitivity for all age groups, while IgA anti-PT may be useful to differentiate between recent vaccination and recent infection.[9] Serology is unable to detect infection with *B. parapertussis*.[8] The accuracy and sensitivity of serologic assays are affected by the time a pertussis vaccine was given, the type of vaccine (primary series or booster), the content of vaccine, and the age of patients.

   The quality of commercial assays varies and is in need of further standardization.[8] A positive serological test result meets the requirement for case confirmation in some countries but not in others.

5) Participation in an external quality control program is highly recommended to assure the quality of tests performed. Most laboratories participate in proficiency challenges or specimen exchanges at least twice per year. Review of statistics and test performance in the performance summaries can provide valuable information about the testing environment and the assay performance consistency.

**9. Reporting requirements**—Reporting of suspected and confirmed pertussis cases to local health authorities is required in most countries. The requirement of submitting *B. pertussis* isolates to reference laboratories varies by local jurisdictions.

**10. Referral network**—Testing for *B. pertussis* does not require a tiered referral laboratory testing system. Most routine clinical and public health laboratories can perform the isolation and identification of *B. pertussis*, PCR and serology testing.[10] The submission of pertussis isolates to reference laboratories for typing is required by some countries to actively monitor the possible emergence of new strains. Various typing methods such as conventional and next-generation sequencing, pulsed-field gel electrophoresis, multilocus variable-number tandem repeat analysis, and others may be employed to address different problems. Similar typing methods are also being used for *B. homesii* isolates.[0]

**11. Special considerations**—Different countries may use different criteria to define a laboratory confirmed case; however, isolation and identification of *B. pertussis* or positive PCR result are common criteria to define a laboratory confirmed case. Although WHO recommends positive paired serology results as a confirmed case,[7] some countries use single serum-positive results, while other countries do not include serology results as case definition.

As recommended by WHO, the data elements included in reporting and the frequency of reporting depend on the vaccine coverage of a region and the type of surveillance. WHO recommends immediate reporting of outbreak investigations to the WHO regional office.[11]

*B. parapertussis* causes milder disease, is not responsible for significant mortality, and is not a priority for surveillance in most countries.[7]

Detection of IgG-PT antibodies in oral fluids is used in the UK for older children suspected of having pertussis. A positive IgG-PT of oral fluid from a patient who was not vaccinated within the past year is considered to be a laboratory confirmed case.[12]

## References

1. US Department of Health and Human Services, Centers for Disease Control and Prevention, National Institutes of Health. *Biosafety in Microbiological and Biomedical Laboratories*. 5th ed. 2009. Available at: https://www.cdc.gov/labs/pdf/CDC-BiosafetyMicrobiologicalBiomedicalLaboratories-2009-P.PDF. Accessed March 8, 2019.
2. Centers for Disease Control and Prevention. Morbidity and Mortality Weekly Report (*MMWR*). Available at: https://www.cdc.gov/mmwr/index.html. Accessed March 8, 2019.
3. Centers for Disease Control and Prevention. Vaccines & immunizations. Available at: https://www.cdc.gov/vaccines/index.html. Accessed March 8, 2019.
4. Kilgore PE, Salim AM, Zervos MJ, Schmitt HJ. Pertussis: microbiology, disease, treatment, and prevention. *Clin Microbiol Rev*, 2016;29(3):449–486.
5. Centers for Disease Control and Prevention. Pertussis (whooping cough) specimen collection. Available at: https://www.cdc.gov/pertussis/clinical/diagnostic-testing/specimen-collection.html. Accessed August 24, 2018.
6. Centers for Disease Control and Prevention. Pertussis (whooping cough) diagnosis confirmation. Available at: https://www.cdc.gov/pertussis/clinical/diagnostic-testing/diagnosis-confirmation.html. Accessed August 24, 2018.
7. World Health Organization. *Laboratory Manual for the Diagnosis of Whooping Cough Caused by* Bordetella pertussis/Bordetella parapertussis. 2014. Available at: http://apps.who.int/iris/bitstream/10665/127891/1/WHO_IVB_14.03_eng.pdf. Accessed August 24, 2018.
8. Wirsing von König CH, Riffelmann M, Coenye T. *Bordetella* and related genera. In: *Manual of Clinical Microbiology*. 11th ed. Washington, DC: ASM Press; 2015.
9. van der Zee A, Schellekens JFP, Mooi FR. Reviews: laboratory diagnosis of pertussis. *Clin Microbiol Rev*. 2015;28(4):1005–1026.
10. Centers for Disease Control and Prevention. manual for the surveillance of vaccine-preventable diseases. Chapter 10: pertussis. 2017. Available at: https://www.cdc.gov/vaccines/pubs/surv-manual/chpt10-pertussis.html. Accessed August 24, 2018.
11. World Health Organization. Immunization, vaccines and biologicals: WHO-recommended surveillance standards of pertussis. 2008. Available at: http://www.

who.int/immunization/monitoring_surveillance/burden/vpd/surveillance_type/passive/pertussis_standards/en. Accessed March 7, 2019.

12. Public Health England. Guidelines for the public health management of pertussis in England. 2018. Available at: https://www.gov.uk/government/uploads/system/uploads/attachment_data/file/576061/Guidelines_for_the_Public_Health_Management_of_Pertussis_in_England.pdf. Accessed August 24, 2018.

[L. Liu]

# PINTA
(carate)

| DISEASE | ICD-10 CODE |
|---|---|
| PINTA | ICD-10 A67 |

**1. Clinical features**—Pinta is a chronic, nonvenereal, treponemal skin infection without systemic manifestations. From 1–8 weeks after exposure, a single or several scaly, pruritic, erythematous papules, or small plaques with regional lymphadenopathy appear usually on the extremities or other uncovered area. These primary lesions may resolve entirely without treatment. After 3–12 months, the initial lesions appear smaller, and scaly papules develop over a wider area of the body. These secondary lesions vary in size from less than 0.5 cm to several centimeters and also vary in color and form from macules to small plaques. Over time, these lesions evolve into tertiary patches of altered (dyschromic) skin pigmentation of variable size. These treponema-containing patches sometimes pass through stages of blue to violet to brown pigmentation, finally becoming treponema-free depigmented (achromic) areas. Lesions coexist at different stages of evolution and are most common on the face and extremities. The differential diagnosis includes syphilis, psoriasis, yaws, and fungal infections in early lesions and vitiligo, tinea versicolor, and other pigmentary disorders in late lesions.

**2. Causative agents**—*Treponema carateum*, a spirochete.

**3. Laboratory diagnosis**—Spirochetes are demonstrable in primary, secondary, and dyschromic (but not achromic) lesions through dark-field or direct fluorescent antibody microscopic examination. Other diseases in the differential might be ruled out by histological examination of the skin lesions. Serological tests for syphilis usually become reactive before or during the secondary lesions, and thereafter behave as in venereal syphilis. Point-of-care tests for syphilis, which have not been validated, may also be reactive in pinta.

**4. Laboratory capability**—Serological testing can be performed in laboratories with standard equipment and minimal scientific and technical knowledge, but the high throughput tests require automation, which are usually found in sophisticated laboratories. Point-of-care serological tests can be performed by staff with minimal laboratory training and can be used at all levels of health care facilities, even those without a laboratory. Specialized scientific and technical knowledge including sophisticated laboratory equipment is essential for performing polymerase chain reaction (PCR) testing.

**5. Safety requirements**—Biosafety level 2. Standard precautions should be taken when working with blood or clinical specimens as other infectious agents may also be present.

**6. Nonhuman hosts**—No nonhuman host for pinta has been identified.

**7. Sample/specimen requirements**—Serum is the specimen of choice for treponemal and nontreponemal serological tests, but plasma can be used for some tests. Rapid point-of-care tests use whole blood obtained through a finger stick. Serum and plasma should be stored at 4°C if testing cannot be performed within 4 hours and at −20°C or lower if testing will be done more than 5 days from collection. Serous exudate from moist lesions of primary and secondary syphilis are amenable to dark-field microscopy (DF) and PCR. Specimens for DF must be tested within 20 minutes of collection. Tissue for silver staining and immunohistochemistry (IHC) should be fixed in 10% buffered formalin as soon as possible at ambient temperature and then paraffin embedded and sectioned for staining. PCR can be performed on either fixed or unfixed tissue, although unfixed tissue is preferred. All samples for PCR should be stored at −70°C if testing cannot be performed immediately.

**8. Testing requirements**—Serology is the mainstay for diagnosis of pinta, although serological tests may be negative in early primary pinta. Treponemal antibody tests (e.g., treponema pallidum particle agglutination assay, treponema pallidum hemagglutination assay) and fluorescent treponemal antibody absorption remain positive for life. Quantitative nontreponemal tests become positive following infection, and the titer then falls following successful treatment.

Traditionally samples were screened using a nontreponemal test (e.g., rapid plasma regain or Venereal Disease Research Laboratory), and if this test was positive a confirmatory treponemal test was performed. Many laboratories have now adopted an alternative algorithm (the reverse syphilis screening algorithm). Using this approach, the initial test is a treponemal antibody test. When this test is positive, a quantitative nontreponemal test is then performed. If the nontreponemal test is negative, a second treponemal test (preferably antibodies against different *T. pallidum* antigens using a different test platform) can be performed.

Point-of-care serological tests are now available. The majority detect only treponemal antibodies (commonly referred to as rapid syphilis tests). Point-of-care tests, which detect both treponemal and nontreponemal antibodies, are now available. When using a point-of-care test, it is important to ensure the kit meets appropriate quality standards.

It should be noted that serological assays cannot distinguish pinta from other endemic treponematoses or syphilis. When both treponemal and nontreponemal tests are positive, the diagnosis is confirmed. A quantitative nontreponemal test is required for assessing response to therapy. Participation in the WHO/CDC Syphilis Serology Proficiency Programme is recommended for maintaining proficiency in treponemal and nontreponemal testing.

IHC, silver stain, or PCR is used for tissue biopsies. Use of a hematoxylin counterstain with IHC allows tissue structure to be observed with localization of treponemes. On molecular testing, many clinically suspicious lesions will not have detectable treponemal deoxyribonucleic acid present.

Lesion samples could be screened with a pantreponemal PCR (such as polA or tp47). Unlike for other treponemal infections, there is no specific PCR for pinta because type/laboratory strains of *T. carateum* do not exist.

**9. Reporting requirements**—Reactive treponemal and nontreponemal test results are consistent with current or past pinta infection but cannot distinguish from infection with an alternative treponemal infection (most importantly syphilis). If the nontreponemal titer is less than 1:4, this could be associated with a serofast state where nontreponemal titers neither increase nor decrease 4-fold after treatment. If the treponemal test is nonreactive, then there is no laboratory evidence of pinta infection. If the nontreponemal test is reactive but the treponemal test is nonreactive, then it is most likely a biological false-positive. If the first treponemal test in the reverse algorithm is reactive and the nontreponemal test is nonreactive but the second/supplemental treponemal test is reactive, then this is consistent with past or potential early infection with yaws or an alternative treponemal infection. If nonreactive, it is inconclusive for pinta infection or is false-positive.

Laboratories should determine if pinta is reportable to the public health authorities in their specific setting.

**10. Referral network**—No specific referral networks exist.

**11. Special considerations**—None.

[M. Marks, A. Pillay]

# PLAGUE

(pestis)

| DISEASE | ICD-10 CODE |
|---|---|
| PLAGUE | ICD-10 A20 |

**1. Clinical features**—Plague has 3 possible presentations: bubonic, septicemic, and pneumonic. Initial signs and symptoms for all phases may be nonspecific, with fever, chills, malaise, myalgia, nausea, prostration, sore throat, and headache. With bubonic plague, lymphadenitis often develops in those lymph nodes that drain the site of the flea bite that causes infection and are called buboes. The location of buboes can vary depending on the circumstances of exposure, with flea bites on the legs typically resulting in the appearance of buboes in the inguinal area. Axillary buboes can be associated with flea bites as well and are often seen after the handling of infected animals. Cervical buboes are rare in industrialized countries but are relatively common in many developing countries where people sleep on the dirt floors of flea-infested huts. Regardless of the location, the buboes are inflamed and tender and may suppurate. The septicemic form of plague can occur subsequent to bubonic plague (secondary septicemic plague) or without prior lymphadenopathy (primary septicemic plague) and involves bloodstream dissemination to diverse parts of the body, including in some instances the meninges. Septicemic cases also can experience endotoxic shock and disseminated intravascular coagulation, in some instances without localizing signs of infection. Secondary involvement of the lungs results in pneumonia; mediastinitis or pleural effusion may develop. Secondary pneumonic plague is of special significance since respiratory droplets may serve as the source of person-to-person transfer with resultant primary pneumonic or pharyngeal plague; this can lead to localized outbreaks or more widespread epidemics. Though naturally acquired plague usually presents as bubonic plague, purposeful aerosol dissemination as a result of deliberate use would be manifest primarily as pneumonic plague. Untreated bubonic plague has a case-fatality rate of about 50%–60%. Untreated primary septicemic plague and pneumonic plague are almost invariably fatal. Modern therapy markedly reduces fatalities from bubonic plague; pneumonic and septicemic plague also respond if recognized and treated early (within 2 days). Plague is a medical and a public health emergency. Further information on this and other plague-related topics or updates can be found at: http://www.cdc.gov/plague.

**2. Causative agents**—*Yersinia pestis*, the plague bacillus.

**3. Laboratory diagnosis**—Visualization of characteristic bipolar staining, safety-pin ovoid, Gram-negative organisms in direct microscopic examination of material aspirated from a bubo, sputum, or cerebrospinal fluid (CSF) is suggestive, but not conclusive, evidence of plague infection. Examination by fluorescent antibody test, antigen capture by enzyme-linked immunosorbent assay (ELISA) or dipstick formats, or polymerase chain reaction (PCR) are more specific and particularly useful in some instances. In the USA, cases are considered confirmed following isolation of *Y. pestis* by culture of bubo aspirates, blood, CSF, or sputum samples or by demonstration of a 4-fold or greater rise or fall in antibody titer. Slow growth of the organism at normal incubation temperatures may lead to misidentification by automated systems. The passive hemagglutination test using *Y. pestis* Fraction-1 antigen and ELISA are used for serodiagnosis. Recently, WHO and others proposed the use of dipstick (horizontal flow) assays designed to detect *Y. pestis* antigen in clinical samples as a means for rapid diagnosis of cases, but these tests are not widely available. Medical personnel should be aware of areas where the disease is endemic and should entertain the diagnosis of plague early on; unfortunately, plague is often misdiagnosed, especially in travellers who develop illness after returning from an endemic area, and delays in diagnosis can result in fatalities.

4. **Laboratory capability**—Routine diagnostic laboratories conforming to biosafety level 2 (BSL-2) standards can be used for the initial isolation and identification of *Y. pestis* in clinical settings. In many cases the disease will be part of a broader differential diagnosis in which other organisms may be the primary suspect (e.g., in primary pneumonic plague).

5. **Safety requirements**—Routine diagnostic work can be carried out at a BSL-2 facility. BSL-3 facilities should be used for work involving aerosol-generating procedures, animal inoculation, necropsy of animals, and large-scale culture.

6. **Nonhuman hosts**—Plague is a zoonotic disease present in more than 200 species of rodents and 14 species of lagomorphs in different parts of the world. Rats, gerbils, marmots, rabbits, and prairie dogs are common reservoirs and often act as the source of human infections. Classically bubonic plague is transmitted to humans through the bite of an infected flea, usually *Xeonopsylla cheopis,* which bite humans after the death of their rat hosts. Primary pneumonic plague can be transmitted to humans by domestic cats, which prey on sick rodents and transmit the organism in respiratory and oral secretions to their owners, often succumbing themselves. Domestic dogs (*Canis lupus familiaris*) may facilitate transmission of infected fleas or bring infected rodents they have caught into contact with humans. Plague is usually a mild and self limiting disease in dogs, and in endemic areas dogs frequently have antibodies to *Y. pestis* in serosurveys. Camels and goats are susceptible to plague, and humans are occasionally infected by contact with sick animals or consumption of contaminated meat. Sheep, pigs, and cattle may develop antibodies to *Y. pestis*, but consumption of their meat has not been implicated directly in human cases.

**7. Sample/specimen requirements**—The choice of sample depends on the clinical presentation of the disease.

1) Blood cultures: 1 or more sets of blood cultures should be taken in febrile patients and transported at ambient temperature to the laboratory as promptly as possible. If plague is considered likely, an additional broth bottle should be inoculated and incubated at 22°C–28°C as *Y. pestis* will grow more rapidly at this temperature.
2) Lower respiratory tract samples in pneumonic plague: a bronco-alveolar lavage (BAL, bronchial wash) or transtracheal aspirate (≥ 1 ml) should be transferred to a sterile, screw-capped container and transported at ambient temperature to the laboratory. If the sample transport is likely to be delayed for 2–24 hours, the sample should be refrigerated and transported at 2°C–8°C. Sputum can be used but is contaminated with throat flora and likely to be of limited value.
3) Biopsy of affected tissues or aspirates: biopsies of lymph nodes, liver, spleen, bone marrow, and lung should be submitted in a sterile screw capped container, adding 1–2 drops of sterile saline to small samples to prevent drying out. Formaldehyde-saline or other fixatives must not be used. Aspirates rarely yield much material, but can be flushed into a sterile container with a small amount of sterile saline. Samples should be transported at ambient temperature but refrigerated if processing is delayed.
4) Swabs: swabs have a poor diagnostic yield, but if they are the only specimen available they should be transported by replacing the swab in the original transport package, ideally one containing a bacterial transport medium.
5) Blood for PCR or antigen detection: 2–5 ml of blood should be drawn into an Ethylenediaminetetraacetic acid or sodium citrate tube for PCR, and 2–5 ml into a clotted or serum separation gel tube for serology by F1 antigen or antibody. Transport should be at ambient temperature, or specimens should be refrigerated if transport is delayed.

**8. Testing requirements**—Microscopy and culture, serology, and PCR are the principal technologies in the diagnosis of plague, supplemented by rapid antigen detection tests. Microscopy and culture can be used to give a presumptive diagnosis in an acute case, and should be confirmed by secondary methods as detailed earlier.

1) Culture: *Y. pestis* will grow on general nutrient rich media, ideally horse or sheep blood agar, brain heart infusion or base-hemin broths, as well as selective agar such as MacConkey, eosin methylene blue, or Congo red agar. The organism typically takes 48 hours to form clearly visible colonies at 37°C, but if plague is actively

suspected and the incubation options are available, it should be grown at 28°C since it grows more rapidly at that temperature. Pinpoint colonies are usually visible on blood agar at 24 hours. The organism is a nonlactose fermenter, catalase positive, and oxidase and urease positive. Colonies can be confirmed as *Y. pestis* using matrix-assisted laser desorption/ionization time-of-flight mass spectrometry, biochemical methods, or PCR. Further information can be found in the Sentinel Laboratory Guidelines at: https://www.asm.org/images/PSAB/LRN/Ypestis316.pdf.

2) Microscopy: microscopy can be performed on smears of pus or other samples or on smears made from suspect colonies. *Y. pestis* is a Gram-negative rod, typically with bipolar staining (safety-pin staining) on Gram stains, more easily seen with a Wright-Giemsa or Wayson stain. This appearance is not diagnostic as it may not occur and can be seen in other organisms. Specialist labs may use specific immunofluorescent antibodies to verify the presence of *Y. pestis* on microscopy preparations.
3) PCR: advances in molecular biology make PCR a rapid and sensitive technique for a variety of samples, including the primary diagnosis of plague from respiratory samples[1] and lymph node aspirates[2] with 100% specificity. The positivity rate in lymph node samples has been shown to be significantly higher than with culture, highlighting a problem with PCR when the traditional gold standard may be inferior to the newer technique. A quadriplex assay using multiple gene targets gave 100% specificity for Yersinia pestis against other *Yersinia* spp. with a sensitivity of 85 colony-forming units per reaction[3] and has been adopted by other laboratories as a basis for clinical assays. PCR can be applied to blood samples directly, to positive blood cultures, aspirate, and tissues, and has been used successfully on archaeological material.
4) Antigen detection and rapid diagnostic tests: a number of ELISA and lateral flow assays have been developed to detect plague antigens in blood and other samples, mostly based on the F1 surface antigen.[4] These are not commercially available at present.
5) Antibody tests in clinical cases and outbreak investigation: antibodies to *Y. pestis* F1 antigen appear around 7 days after infection and can be detected using ELISA and other standard methods. Diagnosis requires a 4-fold rise in titer and is practicable for acute cases.[5] Rapid diagnostic tests (lateral flow) have been evaluated in Madagascar to follow up on outbreaks with around 95% sensitivity and specificity.
6) Quality assurance: the standard of quality control systems for assays will vary among laboratories, but as a minimum the laboratory should be able to demonstrate that the batches of culture plates

used have the ability to grow standard controls strains of common pathogens and that microscope stains perform adequately on a range of samples. PCR assays require qualified reagents, positive and negative controls, extraction, and inhibition controls on all runs. Serology assays require positive and negative controls. The laboratory should maintain a quality management system compliant with local regulations. In some countries, this will equate to ISO15189 standards,[6] but regional schemes such as the East African networks are more suitable for many users.

**9. Reporting requirements**—Plague is a reportable disease under International Health Regulations. Laboratories suspecting plague should refer isolates or samples to a reference center for confirmation, and inform the national ministry or agency responsible for communicable disease surveillance.

**10. Referral network**—A list of referral centers in the USA can be found at: https://www.asm.org/index.php/guidelines/sentinel-guidelines. In other countries, the central public health laboratory or agency is the best source to contact for advice on referral for confirmation.

**11. Special considerations**—Plague is a notifiable disease under the 2005 International Health Regulations, and all cases of human disease must be investigated and reported to WHO.[7] CDC case definitions for plague can be found at: https://wwwn.cdc.gov/nndss/conditions/plague/case-definition/1996. WHO case definitions can be found on page 50 of the WHO manual at: https://www.who.int/csr/resources/publications/plague/WHO_CDS_CSR_EDC_99_2_EN/en.

Plague is classified as a biothreat agent and in the USA is controlled under the Select Agent Rules described in Select Agents and Toxins, 7 CFR Part 331, 9 CFR Part 121, and 42 CFR Part 73.[8] In the USA, confirmed isolates of select agents identified in a clinical or diagnostic laboratory must be reported. Each country may have specific registration requirements for laboratories working with *Y. pestis*, and these should be checked.

## References

1. Loiez C, Herwegh S, Wallet F, Armand S, Guinet F, Courcol RJ. Detection of *Yersinia pestis* in sputum by real-time PCR. *J Clin Microbiol*. 2003;41(10):4873–5.
2. Riehm JM, Rahalison L, Scholz HC, et al. Detection of *Yersinia pestis* using real-time PCR in patients with suspected bubonic plague. *Mol Cell Probes*. 2011;25(1):8–12.
3. Woron AM, Nazarian EJ, Egan C, et al. Development and evaluation of a 4-target multiplex real-time polymerase chain reaction assay for the detection and characterization of *Yersinia pestis*. *Diagn Microbiol Infect Dis*. 2006;56(3):261–8.
4. Tomaso H, Thullier P, Seibold E, et al. Comparison of hand-held test kits, immunofluorescence microscopy, enzyme-linked immunosorbent assay, and flow cytometric analysis for rapid presumptive identification of *Yersinia pestis*. *J Clin Microbiol*. 2007;45(10):3404–7.

5. Rajerison M, Dartevelle S, Ralafiarisoa LA, et al. Development and evaluation of two simple, rapid immunochromatographic tests for the detection of *Yersinia pestis* antibodies in humans and reservoirs. *PLoS Negl Trop Dis*. 2009;3(4):e421.
6. Centers for Medicare & Medicaid Services. Clinical Laboratory Improvement Amendments (CLIA). 2019. Available at: https://www.cms.gov/Regulations-and-Guidance/Legislation/CLIA/index.html. Accessed March 8, 2019.
7. World Health Organization. *Plague Manual: Epidemiology, Distribution, Surveillance and Control*. Available at: http://www.who.int/csr/resources/publications/plague/whocdscsredc992a.pdf. Accessed March 8, 2019.
8. Department of Health and Human Services, Centers for Disease Control and Prevention. Select agents and toxins. Available at: https://www.selectagents.gov/SelectAgentsandToxins.html. Accessed March 8, 2019.

[T. Brooks]

# PNEUMONIA

| DISEASE | ICD-10 CODE |
|---|---|
| PNEUMOCOCCAL PNEUMONIA | ICD-10 J13 |
| MYCOPLASMA PNEUMONIA | ICD-10 J15.7 |
| PNEUMOCYSTIS PNEUMONIA | ICD-10 B59 |
| PNEUMONIA DUE TO *CHLAMYDIA TRACHOMATIS* | ICD-10 P23.1 |
| PNEUMONIA DUE TO *CHLAMYDIA PNEUMONIAE* | ICD-10 J16.0 |
| OTHER PNEUMONIAS | ICD-10 J12, J15, J16.8, J18 |

There are a plethora of potential microbial causes of pneumonia, including viral, bacterial, fungal, and parasitic pathogens, and a wealth of diagnostic tests are available. These include molecular techniques for viral, fungal, and bacterial organisms; culture for common and fastidious bacterial, mycobacterial and fungal pathogens; selective staining and microscopy of deep clinical specimens for fungal and parasitic identification; and serological studies (with antigen and antibody detection in both serum and urine). Specimens to be collected include sterile (blood and urine) and nonsterile (upper and lower respiratory tract specimens, such as bronchoalveolar lavage fluid) specimens, some of which require trend analysis (e.g., monitoring of β-d-glucan levels in blood for fungal infection monitoring or the appropriate timing of acute and convalescent sera). There can often be coexisting pathologies, such as bacterial superinfection in patients infected with influenza or advanced immunosuppressed patients presenting with both *Pneumocystis jiroveci* pneumonia and nontuberculous mycobacterial infection. Therefore, appropriate test selection depends on the potential etiology, dependent on factors such as patient age, comorbid status, travel history, and animal contact, among others. It is therefore critical that the clinician and laboratory scientist are in close communication to determine the correct laboratory diagnostic pathway to be followed. Since the pathogen content of samples received for workup of respiratory infections is unknown, respiratory tract samples should be handled in a biosafety level 2 (BSL-2) facility according to standard microbiology procedures (unless Middle East respiratory syndrome [MERS]-coronavirus or other hazard group 3 pathogens are considered part of the differential diagnosis).

# I. PNEUMOCOCCAL PNEUMONIA

**1. Clinical features**—Clinical manifestations include sudden onset, high fevers, rigors, pleuritic chest pain, dyspnea, tachypnea, and cough productive of rusty sputum. Onset may be less abrupt, especially among the elderly; fever, shortness of breath, or altered mental status may provide the first evidence of pneumonia. In infants and young children, fever, vomiting, and convulsions may be the initial manifestations. Laboratory findings include leukocytosis (neutrophilia) and elevated C-reactive protein. Typical chest radiograph findings show lobar or segmental consolidation; consolidation may be bronchopneumonic, especially in children and the elderly. Pneumococcal pneumonia is an important cause of death in infants and the elderly.

Infection can be complicated by empyema, acute respiratory distress syndrome, septic shock, and purpura fulminans. The case-fatality rate varies widely from 5%–35%, depending on the setting (e.g., outpatients vs. inpatients) and the population (e.g., healthy adults vs. persons with alcohol dependency). In developing countries, case-fatality rates among children are often more than 10%, and as high as 60% among infants younger than 6 months. Pneumococcal pneumonia among previously healthy individuals with other respiratory infections (e.g., influenza) is well described.

**2. Causative agents**—*Streptococcus pneumoniae* (pneumococcus) is a Gram-positive, lancet-shaped, encapsulated diplococcus that often asymptomatically colonizes the human nasopharynx. Children are colonized with *S. pneumoniae* more often than adults. Current data suggest that 6 serotypes (1, 5, 6B, 14, 19F, 23F) account for the majority of invasive disease worldwide.

**3. Laboratory diagnosis**—A microbiologic diagnosis of pneumococcal pneumonia can guide antibiotic therapy. The presence in sputum of many Gram-positive diplococci together with polymorphonuclear leukocytes suggests pneumococcal pneumonia; however, Gram stain and culture of respiratory secretions are often not performed, largely due to technical aspects of obtaining good quality specimens and the difficulty of distinguishing infection from respiratory tract colonization. Definitive diagnosis of pneumococcal pneumonia is established by isolation of pneumococci from blood or, less commonly, pleural fluid. Among adults, the diagnosis can also be established by identification of pneumococcal polysaccharide in urine. For children, urine antigen testing is not useful because nasopharyngeal colonization can cause excretion of pneumococcal antigen in urine. Most pediatric cases are diagnosed by isolation of pneumococci from blood. Patients suspected of having pneumococcal pneumonia should be treated promptly, preferably after collection of appropriate diagnostic specimens according to established guidelines. If pneumococcus is isolated, susceptibility testing should be performed and antimicrobial therapy tailored to susceptibility results.

**4. Laboratory capability**—Laboratories capable of detecting pneumococcal infections should have BSL-2 facility design as well as training in standard microbiology procedures and practices.

**5. Safety requirements**—The UK Advisory Committee on Dangerous Pathogens (ACDP) lists *S. pneumoniae* as a hazard group 2 organism, and containment level 2 laboratory practices are sufficient for handling the agent (equivalent to BSL-2 conditions.) Since the content of samples received for workup of respiratory infections is unknown, they should be handled in a BSL-2 facility according to standard microbiology procedures (unless MERS-coronavirus or other hazard group 3/BSL-3 pathogens are considered part of the differential diagnosis).

**6. Nonhuman hosts**—Zoonotic reservoirs do not contribute to *S. pneumoniae* infection in humans.

**7. Sample/specimen requirements**—Lower respiratory specimens (e.g., expectorated or induced sputum, bronchoalveolar lavage fluid) should be transported to the laboratory in a sterile container at room temperature within 2 hours of collection and should be stored at refrigeration temperature (4°C) for not more than 24 hours before plating. Blood agar, chocolate blood agar, and MacConkey agar are typically used for plating of respiratory specimens. Blood cultures should also be collected if invasive pneumococcal disease is suspected. Blood culture bottles (aerobic and anaerobic) should be inoculated with 8–10 mL of blood each (for adult patients) and transported at room temperature to the laboratory within 2 hours of collection. Urine specimens for pneumococcal antigen testing should be collected in standard containers and transported to the laboratory within 24 hours of collection.

**8. Testing requirements**—Although multiplex nucleic acid testing panels have become commonplace for detecting respiratory viruses and more recently for atypical bacterial pneumonia, culture remains a mainstay of detecting most bacterial pneumonias, including those caused by *S. pneumoniae*. However, sputum cultures lack sensitivity and specificity and must be interpreted within the patient's clinical context. An important quality measure for sputum specimens submitted for culture is assessment by Gram stain. Using one of several grading systems, the quantitation of polymorphonuclear cells (neutrophils) and squamous epithelial cells allows for determination of adequacy of the sample. Specimens that contain a predominance of squamous epithelial cells should not be cultured as they represent sampling of secretions from the oral cavity. *S. pneumoniae* can colonize the tonsils and nasopharynx and can therefore be present in improperly collected sputum samples that do not truly represent the lower respiratory tract. If such specimens are not rejected based on Gram stain results, patients may be inappropriately treated. By contrast, growth of *S. pneumoniae* in a blood culture is diagnostic of invasive disease. Blood cultures are positive in 30% of cases of community-acquired pneumonia due to pneumococcus.

On Gram stain, *S. pneumoniae* often presents as Gram-positive, lancet-shaped diplococci. However, definitive distinction from *Enterococcus* and other species of *Streptococcus* is not possible based on microscopic morphology alone. Although no longer used frequently in many laboratories, performing a Quelling reaction directly on a sputum sample containing organisms morphologically consistent with pneumococcus will highlight the organism's capsule and allow for a presumptive diagnosis of *S. pneumoniae*.

Colonies of *S. pneumoniae* are alpha-hemolytic and can have 2 distinctive morphologies: both large and mucoid (if large amounts of capsular polysaccharides are produced), or with a central depression (if pneumococcal autolysin is present). Like other viridans group streptococci, *S. pneumoniae* is leucine aminopeptidase–positive and pyrrolidonyl arylamidase–negative. Biochemical reactions that distinguish pneumococcus from the other viridans group streptococci include optochin sensitivity and bile solubility. Newer technologies in the clinical microbiology laboratory such as matrix-assisted laser desorption/ionization time-of-flight mass spectrometry and 16s ribosomal nucleic acid (RNA) nucleic acid testing have difficulty distinguishing *S. pneumoniae* from other members of the *S. mitis* group.

In adults, the urine antigen test is a helpful adjunct test for pneumococcal pneumonia, especially in patients who have already received antibiotic therapy. While not as sensitive as respiratory testing (between 50%–80%), urine antigen testing has good specificity (>90%). However, the test should not be used in infants and small children because it can be positive in the setting of upper respiratory tract colonization.

Susceptibility testing on isolates causing invasive disease is important as up to 30% of these isolates are resistant to at least 1 antibiotic.

**9. Reporting requirements**—In the USA, since 2010, CDC's Notifiable Diseases Surveillance System has classified invasive *S. pneumoniae* infection as a notifiable disease whenever the organism is recovered from a sterile body site such as blood or cerebrospinal fluid (CSF). Public Health England (PHE) has similar reporting guidelines. In other settings laboratories must determine whether the isolation of *S. pneumoniae* is a finding that requires reporting to the public health authorities.

**10. Referral network**—Referral networks vary by country. In the USA, isolates causing invasive disease should be referred to CDC's StrepLab, which offers serotyping of selected isolates causing invasive disease for 92 capsular antigen serotypes as part of the national population-based Active Bacterial Core surveillance. PHE's respiratory and vaccine preventable bacteria reference unit also undertakes enhanced surveillance of invasive pneumococcal disease.

**11. Special considerations**—National diagnostic laboratories will collect information for surveillance purposes, particularly to inform national vaccination policy and review of different circulating serotypes in response to recent changes in valence. Continuous monitoring of the serotypes implicated in invasive disease is important because in the setting of vaccine-induced herd immunity nonvaccine strains become more prevalent. The pneumococcal polysaccharide vaccines recommended for people older than 65, as well as those older than 19 with certain chronic illnesses, contain 22 capsular serotypes (1, 2, 3, 4, 5, 6B, 7F, 8, 9N, 9V, 10A, 11A, 12F, 14, 15B, 17F, 18C, 19A, 19F, 20, 22F, and 33F). Starting in 2000, the pneumococcal conjugate vaccine 7 (PCV7) became available for use in infants and children, targeting the 7 serotypes that caused 80% of pneumococcal disease occurring in children younger than 5 (serotypes 4, 6B, 9V, 14, 18C, 19F, and 23F). Subsequently in 2010, a 13-valent conjugate vaccine became available that added 6 additional serotypes (1, 3, 5, 6A, 7F, and 19A) that had been found to cause 64% of cases of invasive disease in children younger than 5 in the wake of implementation of PCV7.

## II. MYCOPLASMA PNEUMONIA

**1. Clinical features**—Predominantly a febrile lower respiratory infection causing about 20% of pneumonias; less often, a pharyngitis that sometimes progresses to tracheobronchitis or pneumonia. Clinical pneumonia occurs in about 3%–30% of infections with *Mycoplasma pneumoniae*. Disease varies from mild afebrile pharyngitis to febrile illness of the upper or lower respiratory tract. Onset is gradual with headache, malaise, cough (often paroxysmal), sore throat, and sometimes chest discomfort that may be pleuritic. Sputum, scant at first, may increase later. Early patchy infiltration of the lungs is often more extensive on X-ray than clinical findings suggest. In severe cases, the pneumonia may progress from one lobe to another and become bilateral. Leukocytosis occurs after the first week in approximately one-third of cases. Duration varies from a few days to a month or more. Complications such as central nervous system involvement (e.g., encephalitis, acute disseminated encephalomyelitis) and Stevens Johnson syndrome are infrequent; fatalities are rare.

Differentiation is required from atypical pneumonia due to many other agents: other bacteria; adenoviruses; influenza; respiratory syncytial virus;

parainfluenza; measles; Q fever; psittacosis; certain mycoses; severe acute respiratory syndrome or other coronavirus infections; and tuberculosis.

**2. Causative agents**—*M. pneumoniae* belongs to the mycoplasmas (*Mollicutes*). As mycoplasmas lack cell walls, cell wall synthesis inhibitors such as the penicillins and cephalosporins are not effective in treatment. There are increasing reports globally of resistance to macrolides. Genomic data indicate 2 major genetic lineages. Along with *S. pneumoniae* and *Haemophilus influenzae*, *M. pneumoniae* is one of the most common agents of community-acquired pneumonia. *Mycoplasma amphoriforme* has to date only been found in humans, of which some have had pneumonia.

**3. Laboratory diagnosis**—Although serology-based tests are commercially available and widely used, many have proven to be unreliable due to inherent difficulties in interpretation. A 4-fold rise in antibody titers between acute and convalescent sera collected 3–6 weeks apart may provide some diagnostic utility, and serological assays may add value when used as supportive evidence of infection in concert with other testing modalities. Molecular diagnostics, most notably qualitative and quantitative real-time polymerase chain reaction (qPCR) assays, have become a more common and reliable method for rapid diagnosis of *M. pneumoniae*. Respiratory specimens such as throat swabs, nasopharyngeal, and oropharyngeal sputum are acceptable specimen types for molecular testing. These tests are commercially available in some specialty public health laboratories, but there is an absence of standardization among laboratories. Some specialized laboratories can also perform culture using special media. However, due to the low recovery rate and lengthy incubation time required, culturing is not routinely attempted or useful for rapid diagnosis.

**4. Laboratory capability**—Laboratories capable of detecting *Mycoplasma* infections should have BSL-2 facility design as well as training in standard microbiology procedures and practices. Many laboratories will have appropriate capability for serological detection of immune response. Limited facilities may have the capacity to culture *Mycoplasma* isolates. Increasingly multiplex PCRs are available for routine testing of respiratory specimens, which include *Mycoplasma* targets, and laboratories that maintain expertise in molecular testing will be able to perform this. Antigen detection tests for respiratory specimens have largely been replaced by molecular techniques.

**5. Safety requirements**—The UK ACDP lists *M. pneumoniae* as a hazard group 2 organism, and BSL-2 laboratory practices are sufficient for handling the agent. Since the content of samples received for workup of respiratory infections is unknown, they should be handled in a BSL-2 facility according to standard microbiology procedures (unless MERS-coronavirus or other hazard group 3/BSL-3 pathogens are considered part of the differential diagnosis).

**6. Nonhuman hosts**—*M. pneumoniae* is a human pathogen. Zoonotic *Mycoplasma* spp. have been found in various mammals, for example

*Mycoplasma phocicerebrale* from seals and *Mycoplasma canis and Mycoplasma edwardii* from dogs.

**7. Sample/specimen requirements**—Serum for serological diagnosis should be taken via venipuncture and transported routinely.

Lumbar punctures for extrapulmonary neurological manifestations, such as *Mycoplasma* encephalitis, should be performed using routine techniques, with CSF collected in sterile containers and transported to the laboratory as soon as possible following collection. Paired CSF and respiratory specimens should be tested. CSF samples should be tested in parallel with a respiratory specimen such as throat swab for *M. pneumoniae*. There have been instances of CSF-negative patients with detectable *M. pneumoniae* on throat swab testing with symptoms of central nervous system infection.

Acceptable specimen types for identification of *M. pneumoniae* in suspected cases of pneumonia include induced sputum, bronchoalveolar lavage (BAL) specimens, lung biopsy, pleural fluid, tracheal aspirate, and bronchial brush washings. For nonproductive patients, throat swabs may yield a positive result. Lower respiratory specimens should be collected in sterile containers and transported to the laboratory within 2 hours of collection if culture is to be attempted and should be stored at refrigeration temperature (4°C) for not more than 24 hours before plating. Centrifuging of liquid specimens should be performed to concentrate any organisms present.

**8. Testing requirements**—Serum, both acute and convalescent samples taken approximately 3–4 weeks after infection, should always be tested in parallel to look for 4-fold increase in antibody titers, either through complement fixation or microparticle agglutination assays. A single, 1-off high titer gives a less sensitive indication of acute infection, though in isolation it can be difficult to interpret. Additionally, the age of the patient must be considered because adult patients are more likely to have had previous exposure.

*Mycoplasma* culture, though thought to be the gold standard for diagnosis, is a specialized procedure that requires both selective growth media (including broad spectrum beta-lactam antibiotics and antifungal agents to prevent overgrowth) and longer-term incubation conditions to enable the significant enrichment environment required for recovering *Mycoplasma* present in samples. Fried-egg-shaped colonies are the classic morphology seen on microscopic examination.

Nucleic acid amplification techniques, including specific primer sets as part of multiplex assays (commonly also testing for *Chlamydia* respiratory pathogens), 16S ribosomal deoxyribonucleic acid (rDNA) (with detection to species level), RNA amplification, and nested PCRs with reamplification by specific *M. pneumoniae* primers, are all highly sensitive diagnostic tests. Molecular typing includes multilocus sequence typing, multiple-locus variable number tandem repeat analysis, and P1 type determinations.

**9. Reporting requirements**—In the USA, there is no national reporting for *M. pneumoniae* infections, and in the UK, *M. pneumoniae* is not a notifiable infection, though data can be extracted from routine hospital and laboratory surveillance databases. A 2012 European Centre for Disease Prevention and Control (ECDC) review of 30 countries highlighted that 13 of the 20 that responded have some degree of surveillance activities. As of 2016, CDC has been given funding to perform sentinel surveillance given increasing concerns about macrolide-resistant *M. pneumoniae.* Laboratories in other countries should determine whether mycoplasma-caused infections are reportable within their respective jurisdiction.

**10. Referral network**—There are current attempts led by WHO to standardize and harmonize real-time PCR protocols and platforms across international laboratories.

**11. Special considerations**—Antibiotic resistance is a recognized global problem for *M. pneumoniae* with resistance rates to macrolides greater than 90% in some regions of the world. Given the difficulties in culture, and increasing concerns about resistance across many *Mycoplasma* spp., increasing the national collection of antimicrobial resistance data including molecular resistance detection is imperative for the international community to monitor resistance. Mixed infections with bacterial and viral respiratory pathogens have been documented.

## III. PNEUMOCYSTIS PNEUMONIA (interstitial plasma cell pneumonia, PCP)

**1. Clinical features**—An acute to subacute, often fatal, pulmonary disease, especially in persons with immunosuppression and in malnourished, premature infants. Clinically, patients present with dyspnea on exertion, dry, nonproductive cough, and fever. Auscultatory signs are usually minimal or absent. Chest radiographs typically show bilateral diffuse interstitial infiltrates.

**2. Causative agents**—*Pneumocystis jiroveci* (previously known as *Pneumocystis carinii* and classified as a protozoa). Currently it is considered a fungus, based on nucleic acid and biochemical analysis.

**3. Laboratory diagnosis**—Established through demonstration of the causative agent in material from induced sputum, bronchoalveolar lavage, or transbronchial or open lung biopsy. Staining with methenamine silver or Giemsa can identify the organism. There is no commercially available routine culture method or serological test at present, though several exist in research laboratories.

**4. Laboratory capability**—Laboratories successfully capable of detecting *Pneumocystis* infections should have BSL-2 facility design as well as training in standard microbiology procedures and practices.

**5. Safety requirements**—Although *P. jiroveci* cannot be cultured and does not cause disease in immunocompetent people, the content of samples received for workup of respiratory infections is unknown, and therefore all such specimens should be handled in a BSL-2 facility according to standard microbiology procedures (unless MERS-coronavirus or other hazard group 3 pathogens are considered part of the differential diagnosis, in which case BSL-3 conditions are required).

**6. Nonhuman hosts**—The species *P. jiroveci* is unique to human hosts. However, other host-specific *Pneumocystis* spp. have been found in various mammals.

**7. Sample/specimen requirements**—Acceptable specimen types for identification of *Pneumocystis* in suspected cases of pneumonia include induced sputum, BAL specimens, lung biopsy, pleural fluid, tracheal aspirate, and bronchial brush washings. Lower respiratory specimens should be collected in sterile containers and transported to the laboratory within 2 hours of collection. If testing is performed by staining methods, specimens should be lysed with a mucolytic agent such as N-acetyl-L-cysteine (except for BAL specimens which do not require treatment) and then centrifuged to concentrate any organisms present. Serum can also be tested for elevated beta-D-glucan levels, although this is not specific to *Pneumocystis* infection.

**8. Testing requirements**—*P. jiroveci* is a nonculturable fungus. Currently, the most common method used to diagnose *Pneumocystis* infection is microscopic detection of the organism in an induced sputum or BAL specimen, or more rarely, a lung biopsy, pleural fluid, tracheal aspirate, or bronchial brush specimen. A variety of common stains can be used to detect the cyst (and sometimes trophozoite) forms of the organism in these sample types, some of which stain *Pneumocystis* cyst walls (methenamine silver, toluidine blue O, and calcofluor white) and some of which stain cyst contents (Giemsa, Gram, Weigert, and Papanicolau stains). Another common morphologic detection method is direct fluorescent antibody staining, which requires use of a fluorescence microscope. A positive test for the presence of *P. jiroveci* by staining methods should be communicated promptly to clinicians so that adequate therapy may be initiated.

Commercial options for nucleic acid testing are becoming more widely available and are more sensitive and specific for detection of *P. jiroveci*. However, due to high colonization rates in immunocompetent hosts, one must correlate a positive test with clinical symptoms.

**9. Reporting requirements**—In the USA, *Pneumocystis* pneumonia is reportable in 2 states (New Hampshire and Idaho). In the USA, *Pneumocystis* is considered a pathogen of public health concern (but not notifiable) and all clinically significant identifications should be reported. In the UK, any *Pneumocystis* pneumonia in human immunodeficiency virus (HIV) infected individuals is routinely reported through the HIV and AIDS Reporting System. Laboratories testing for *Pneumocystis* pneumonia in other settings must determine if it is a reportable condition within their jurisdiction.

**10. Referral network**—Although there are no known formal laboratory referral networks in place to test for *Pneumocystis*, there are several specialist laboratories located throughout the world in academic settings and elsewhere, and they could be used for reference testing.

**11. Special considerations**—None.

## IV. PNEUMONIA DUE TO CHLAMYDIA TRACHOMATIS (neonatal eosinophilic pneumonia, congenital pneumonia due to *Chlamydia*)

**1. Clinical features**—A subacute chlamydial pulmonary disease typically occurring between 4–11 weeks of age among infants whose mothers have chlamydial infection of the cervix. Clinically, the disease is characterized by insidious onset, cough (characteristically staccato), lack of fever, patchy infiltrates on chest radiograph with hyperinflation, eosinophilia, and elevated immunoglobulin class M (IgM) and IgG. About half of cases show prodromal rhinitis and conjunctivitis. Duration of illness is commonly 1–3 weeks but may extend as long as 2 months. The illness is usually moderate but can progress to severe pneumonia. One study suggests that infants with chlamydial pneumonia are at increased risk of chronic cough and abnormal lung function.

**2. Causative agents**—*Chlamydia trachomatis* of immunotypes D to K.

**3. Laboratory diagnosis**—A wide variety of diagnostic tests are available, including direct fluorescent antibody tests, enzyme immunoassays, DNA probes, and nucleic acid amplification systems. Although elevated serum IgM suggests recent infection, microimmunofluorescent assays, considered optimal for detection of antibody, are not widely available.

**4. Laboratory capability**—Laboratories capable of detecting *Chlamydia* infections should have BSL-2 facility design as well as training in standard microbiology procedures and practices and should be familiar with the running of molecular panels. Increasingly multiplex PCRs are available for routine testing of respiratory or genitourinary specimens that include *Chlamydia* targets.

**5. Safety requirements**—The UK ACDP lists *C. trachomatis* as a hazard group 2 organism, and BSL-2 laboratory practices are sufficient for handling the agent. Since the content of samples received for workup of respiratory infections is unknown, they should be handled in a BSL-2 facility according to standard microbiology procedures (unless MERS-coronavirus or other hazard group 3 pathogens are considered part of the differential diagnosis, in which case BSL-3 conditions are required).

**6. Nonhuman hosts**—Zoonotic reservoirs do not contribute to *C. trachomatis* infection in humans; however, *Chlamydia psittaci* (psittacosis), which may be found in psittacine birds, may be a cause of atypical pneumonia in humans.

**7. Sample/specimen requirements**—Serum for serological diagnosis should be taken via venipuncture and transported routinely. Upper genital tract specimens from mothers of at-risk infants should be taken for molecular testing using cotton, Dacron, or calcium alginate swabs (though not those with wooden shafts). Routine culture would not be indicated for most routine samples. Samples appropriate for antigen or nucleic acid testing include induced sputum, BAL specimens, pleural fluid, tracheal aspirate, and bronchial brush washings. These should be stored in sterile containers and transported to the laboratory in a timely manner.

**8. Testing requirements**—Many laboratories may have appropriate capability for serological detection of immune response though current commercial serological tests do not distinguish between *C. trachomatis, C. pneumoniae* and *C. psittaci*; this is not recommended for routine diagnosis. Specialist research centers can identify specific antibodies to the pgp3 specific antigen of *C. trachomatis*. Direct fluorescent antibody and enzyme immunoassay (EIA) tests for antigen/antibody detection have largely been replaced by nucleic acid amplification tests (NAAT), though these tests have lower sensitivity and specificity for nasopharyngeal specimens. Samples suspected to be due to *C. trachomatis* can be run on NAAT platforms for suspected genital ulcer disease as can maternal upper genital tract specimens though these have not been validated for use in infant nasopharyngeal specimens. Laboratories that maintain expertise in managing molecular panels for genitourinary infections will be able to perform these assays. Culture is considered the gold standard diagnostic test though it is available only in a few specialist centers. *Chlamydia* spp. are obligate intracellular bacteria; therefore, to be cultured, they require growth in tissue culture cells such as human epithelial cells.

**9. Reporting requirements**—Though there is mandatory reporting through PHE for genital *C. trachomatis* infections through the genitourinary medicine clinic activity dataset to evaluate the national screening program, *C. trachomatis* is not a notifiable disease in the UK. From 2010, CDC's National Notifiable Diseases Surveillance System has classified all *C. trachomatis* infections as a notifiable disease. Many countries, such as the USA, have national guidelines for laboratory-based detection of *C. trachomatis*. Laboratories testing for *C. trachomatis* pneumonia in other settings must determine if it is a reportable condition within their jurisdiction.

**10. Referral network**—Referral networks for *C. trachomatis* are limited.

**11. Special considerations**—None.

## V. PNEUMONIA DUE TO CHLAMYDIA PNEUMONIAE

1. **Clinical features**—An acute respiratory disease with cough, frequently a sore throat and hoarseness, and fever at the onset; sputum is scanty and chest pain is rare. Inflammatory signs are sometimes subtle. Pulmonary rales are usually present. The clinical picture is similar to pneumonia caused by *Mycoplasma*. Radiographic abnormalities include bilateral infiltrates, sometimes with pleural effusions. Illness is usually mild, but recovery is slow with cough persisting for 2–6 weeks. Death is rare in uncomplicated cases.

2. **Causative agents**—*Chlamydophila pneumoniae* is the species name for the human-specific organism with distinct morphological and serological differences from *C. psittaci* and *C. trachomatis*.

3. **Laboratory diagnosis**—Historically, laboratory diagnosis has been primarily serological. Microimmunofluorescence testing of paired sera collected 4–8 weeks apart is commercially available but requires a fluorescent microscope, and there are specificity problems due to cross-reaction with chlamydial antigens of other species. More recently, real-time PCR assays have been employed to provide rapid, specific, and sensitive antigen detection of nasopharyngeal/oropharyngeal sputum or other respiratory tract specimens. The organism can be isolated from throat swab specimens in special cell lines, but this is not routinely performed due to cost, length of time to result, and low recovery rates.

4. **Laboratory capability**—Laboratories capable of detecting *Chlamydia* infections should have BSL-2 facility design as well as training in standard microbiology procedures and practices. Many laboratories may have appropriate capability for serological detection of immune response, though current commercial serological tests do not distinguish between *C. trachomatis, C. pneumoniae,* and *C. psittaci;* this is not recommended for routine diagnosis. Increasingly multiplex PCRs are available for routine testing of respiratory or genitourinary specimens, which include *Chlamydia* targets, and laboratories that maintain expertise in managing molecular panels will be able to perform this.

5. **Safety requirements**—The UK ACDP lists *C. pneumoniae* as a hazard group 2 organism, and BSL-2 laboratory practices are sufficient for handling the agent. Since the content of samples received for workup of respiratory infections is unknown, they should be handled in a BSL-2 facility according to standard microbiology procedures (unless MERS-coronavirus or other hazard group 3 pathogens are considered part of the differential diagnosis, in which case BSL-3 conditions are required).

6. **Nonhuman hosts**—Zoonotic reservoirs do not contribute to *C. pneumoniae* infection in humans; however, *C. psittaci* (psittacosis) is a zoonotic cause of pneumonia in humans.

**7. Sample/specimen requirements**—Serum for serological diagnosis should be taken via venipuncture and transported routinely. Culture would not be indicated for most routine samples. Samples appropriate for antigen or nucleic acid testing include induced sputum, BAL specimens, pleural fluid, tracheal aspirate, and bronchial brush washings. These should be stored in sterile containers and transported to the laboratory in a timely manner.

**8. Testing requirements**—Commercial multiplex PCR testing is now the mainstay of current diagnostics, with both high sensitivity and specificity. Cell culture is difficult to perform and often does not give a timely answer, and serology has poor predictive value. Direct fluorescent antibody tests are no longer in routine use as they are prone to interference and are limited by sensitivity and the expertise of the operator. In addition, samples for respiratory EIA require mucolytic processing, with poorer specificity.

**9. Reporting requirements**—There is no national reporting or surveillance system for *C. pneumoniae* infections in the USA. In the UK, national laboratory reports of respiratory infections including those caused by *C. pneumoniae* are routinely published, extracted from routine hospital and laboratory data surveillance systems. Pneumonia caused by *C. pneumoniae* are not notifiable, whereas those caused by *C. psittaci* are reportable. Laboratories testing for *C. pneumoniae* pneumonia in other settings must determine if it is a reportable condition within their jurisdiction.

**10. Referral network**—Although there are no known formal laboratory referral networks in place to test for *C. pneumoniae,* there are several specialist laboratories located throughout the world in academic settings and elsewhere, and they could be used for reference testing.

**11. Special considerations**—*C. psittaci* is considered a hazard group 3 organism, and special considerations are required for handling and storage of the organism, specimens known to be positive, and for those specimens carrying DNA. See "Psittacosis."

## Bibliography


Brown RJ, Nguipdop-Djomo P, Zhao H, Stanford E, Spiller OB, Chalker VJ. *Mycoplasma pneumoniae* epidemiology in England and Wales: a national perspective. *Front Microbiol.* 2016;7:157.

Chemesky MA. The laboratory diagnosis of *Chlamydia trachomatis* infections. *Can J Infect Dis Med Microbiol.* 2005;16(1):39–44.

Clark AE, Kaleta EJ, Arora A, Wolk DM. Matrix-assisted laser desorption ionization-time of flight mass spectrometry: a fundamental shift in the routine practice of clinical microbiology. *Clin Microbiol Rev.* 2013;26(3):547–603.

Cunha BA. The atypical pneumonias: clinical diagnosis and importance. *Clin Microbiol Infect.* 2006;12 Suppl 3:12–24.

Dalpke AH, Hofko M, Zimmermann S. Development and evaluation of a real-time PCR assay for detection of *Pneumocystis jirovecii* on the fully automated BD MAX platform. *J Clin Microbiol.* 2013;51(7):2337–2343.

Daxboeck F, Krause R, Wenisch C. Laboratory diagnosis of *Mycoplasma pneumoniae* infection. *Clin Microbiol Infect*. 2003;9(4):263–273.

Dowell SF, Garman RL, Liu G, Levine OS, Yang YH. Evaluation of Binax NOW, an assay for the detection of pneumococcal antigen in urine samples, performed among pediatric patients. *Clin Infect Dis*. 2001;32:824–825.

Gutierrez F, Masia M, Rodriguez JC, et al. Evaluation of the immunochromatographic Binax NOW assay for detection of *Streptococcus pneumoniae* urinary antigen in a prospective study of community-acquired pneumonia in Spain. *Clin Infect Dis*. 2003;36(3):286–292.

Jorgensen JH, Pfaller MA, Carroll KC, et al, eds. *Manual of Clinical Microbiology*. 11th ed. Washington, DC: ASM Press; 2015.

Lenglet A, Herrador Z, Magiorakos AP, et al. Surveillance status and recent data for *Mycoplasma pneumoniae* infections in the European Union and European Economic Area, January 2012. *Euro Surveill*. 2012;17(5):20075.

Lentino JR, Lucks DA. Nonvalue of sputum culture in the management of lower respiratory tract infections. *J Clin Microbiol*. 1987;25(5):758–762.

Morris A, Norris KA. Colonization by *Pneumocystis jirovecii* and its role in disease. *Clin Microbiol Rev*. 2012;25:297–317.

Nuorti JP, Whitney CG; Centers for Disease Control and Prevention. Prevention of pneumococcal disease among infants and children - use of 13-valent pneumococcal conjugate vaccine and 23-valent pneumococcal polysaccharide vaccine - recommendations of the Advisory Committee on Immunization Practices (ACIP). *MMWR Recomm Rep*. 2010;59(RR-11):1–18.

Roson B, Fernandez-Sabe N, Carratala J, et al. Contribution of a urinary antigen assay (Binax NOW) to the early diagnosis of pneumococcal pneumonia. *Clin Infect Dis*. 2004;38(2):222–226.

Zbinden A, Kohler N, Bloemberg GV. recA-based PCR assay for accurate differentiation of *Streptococcus pneumoniae* from other viridans streptococci. *J Clin Microbiol*. 2011;49(2):523–527.

[I. Martin, V. Chalker, C. S. Brown]

# POLIOMYELITIS
(polioviral fever, infantile paralysis)

| DISEASE | ICD-10 CODE |
|---|---|
| POLIOMYELITIS | ICD-10 A80 |

**1. Clinical features**—A viral infection recognized by acute onset of flaccid paralysis. Infection occurs in the gastrointestinal tract with spread to regional lymph nodes and, in a minority of cases, to the central nervous system. Flaccid paralysis occurs in less than 1% of infections; the rate of paralysis among infected nonimmune adults is higher than among nonimmune infants and young children. Approximately 90% of infections are unapparent or result in nonspecific fever. Aseptic meningitis occurs in about 1% of infections. Fever, malaise, headache, nausea, and vomiting are recognized in 10% of infections. If disease progresses to major illness, severe muscle pain and stiffness of the neck and back with flaccid paralysis may occur. Paralysis is usually asymmetric with fever present at onset; maximum extent is usually reached within 3–4 days. The site of paralysis depends on the location of nerve cell destruction in the spinal cord or brain stem; legs are affected more often than arms. Paralysis of the respiration and/or swallowing muscles can be life-threatening. Some improvement in paralysis may occur during convalescence, but paralysis still present after 60 days is likely to be permanent. Infrequently, recurrence of muscle weakness following recovery may occur many years after the original infection has resolved (postpolio syndrome); this is not believed to be related to persistence of the virus itself.

With progress made towards global eradication, poliomyelitis must now be distinguished from other paralytic conditions by isolation of virus from stool. Other enteroviruses (notably enterovirus 71), echoviruses, and coxsackieviruses have been reported to cause an illness simulating paralytic poliomyelitis. The most frequent cause of acute flaccid paralysis (AFP) that must be distinguished from poliomyelitis is Guillain-Barré syndrome (GBS). Paralysis in GBS is typically symmetrical and may progress for periods as long as 10 days. Fever, headache, nausea, vomiting, and pleocytosis characteristic of poliomyelitis are usually absent in GBS; high protein and low cell counts in cerebrospinal fluid (CSF) and sensory changes are seen in the majority of GBS cases. Acute motor axonal neuropathy (China paralytic syndrome) is an important cause of AFP in northern China and is probably present elsewhere; it is seasonally epidemic and closely resembles poliomyelitis. Fever and CSF pleocytosis are usually absent, but paralysis may persist for several months. Other causes of AFP include transverse myelitis, traumatic neuritis, infectious and toxic neuropathies, tick paralysis, myasthenia gravis, porphyria, botulism, insecticide poisoning, polymyositis, trichinosis, and periodic paralysis. Differential diagnosis of acute nonparalytic poliomyelitis includes other forms of acute nonbacterial meningitis, purulent meningitis, brain abscess, tuberculous meningitis, leptospirosis, lymphocytic choriomeningitis, infectious mononucleosis, the encephalitides, neurosyphilis, and toxic encephalopathies.

**2. Causative agents**—Poliovirus (genus *Enterovirus*, family *Picornaviridae*) types 1, 2, and 3; all types cause paralysis. Circulating wild type 2 poliovirus has not been detected since October 1999 and was declared eradicated in 2015. As of the end of 2018, wild type 1 still circulates in 3 countries—Nigeria, Pakistan, and Afghanistan—but wild poliovirus (WPV) type 3 has not been detected since 2012. Paralytic polio cases have also been reported due to outbreaks caused by circulating vaccine-derived polioviruses types 1, 2, and 3. Presently most circulating vaccine-derived polioviruses are caused by type 2 viruses. Paralytic polio also occurs rarely in association with vaccination (vaccine-associated paralytic poliomyelitis) in vaccine recipients, in their healthy contacts at a rate of approximately 1 in every 2.5 million doses administered, or in 1 in 800,000 first vaccinations.

**3. Laboratory diagnosis**—Definitive laboratory diagnosis requires isolation of the poliovirus from stool samples (gold standard; highest sensitivity), CSF, or oropharyngeal secretions. Specialized laboratories can differentiate wild-type from vaccine-derived and vaccine virus strains. Rises in antibody levels (> 4-fold) are less helpful in the diagnosis of wild poliomyelitis infection; type-specific neutralizing antibodies may already be present when paralysis develops, and significant titer rises may therefore not be demonstrable in paired sera. Antibody response following immunization mimics the response after infection with wild type viruses, and the widespread use of live polio vaccines makes interpretation of antibody levels difficult, except to rule out polio in cases where no antibody has developed in immunocompetent children. Poliovirus is demonstrable in throat secretions as early as 36 hours and in feces 72 hours after exposure to infection in both clinical and unapparent cases.

**4. Laboratory capability**—The current gold standard for detection of poliovirus in cases of acute flaccid paralysis requires virus isolation in cell culture, followed by intratypic differentiation (ITD) of positive cultures using specific real-time polymerase chain reaction (PCR) reagents. Viruses of potential programmatic importance (wild, VDPV, or any type 2 after August 1, 2016) are further characterized by partial genome sequencing. In countries that conduct formal AFP surveillance, specimens should be referred to the designated national or regional reference laboratory. In the USA, some state public health laboratories are capable of isolating poliovirus in culture, but isolates should be referred to CDC for further characterization.

**5. Safety requirements**—All human enteroviruses, including polioviruses, are categorized as biosafety level 2 agents, with standard precautions recommended. Staff should have received the full childhood series of poliovirus immunizations. An adult booster dose is recommended for health care workers, including laboratorians, who may come into contact with virus or virus-infected specimens. Also see Special Considerations section in this chapter.

**6. Nonhuman hosts**—Several species of nonhuman primates, including macaques and chimpanzees can be experimentally infected with poliovirus, but they are not considered a reservoir for transmission to humans.

**7. Sample/specimen requirements**—To rule out poliovirus infection in a paralytic case, 2 stool specimens should be collected at least 24 hours apart during the first 14 days following onset of paralysis. Specimens should be sent to the laboratory at 4°C–8°C, to arrive within 3 days of collection. Specimens should be frozen if transport will take > 72 hours.

**8. Testing requirements**—Isolation in culture remains the gold standard for poliovirus detection. The standard WHO algorithm requires inoculation of a 10% stool suspension into RD cells (human rhabdomyosarcoma) and L20B cells (mouse L cells engineered to express the human poliovirus receptor, CD155). A few human enteroviruses can replicate in L cells, but an enteric virus that causes cytopathic effect in L20B cells is presumed to be poliovirus pending further characterization. Poliovirus is identified by ITD using real-time reverse transcription (RT) PCR primers and probes distributed through the WHO Global Polio Laboratory Network (GPLN), consisting of 146 laboratories. This set of assays specifically detects (a) any enterovirus, (b) each of the 3 Sabin vaccine strains (with primers that can flag potential VDPV for further investigation), (c) wild poliovirus (WPV) type 1, (d) any type 2 poliovirus, and (e) WPV type 3. Virus isolation and ITD are generally screening assays, though the Sabin RT-PCRs are considered definitive. Any type 2 virus, any WPV, and potential VDPV must be referred to a polio sequencing laboratory for confirmation by sequencing the complete VP1 region (~900 nucleotides). All polio diagnostic methods used in the GPLN are supported by a quality assurance system that includes annual accreditation and proficiency testing, administered by WHO.

**9. Reporting requirements**—Poliovirus infection (either paralytic poliomyelitis or non-paralytic infection with detection of poliovirus are the only enterovirus infections that are nationally reportable in the USA (see: https://wwwn.cdc.gov/nndss/conditions/notifiable/2018). This applies to any person "in whom a poliovirus isolate was identified in an appropriate clinical specimen, with confirmatory typing and sequencing performed by the CDC Poliovirus Laboratory, as needed."[1] Reporting of poliovirus detection is also required under the 2005 International Health Regulations.

**10. Referral network**—WHO coordinates a global network of 146 polio laboratories; the GPLN, which includes laboratories at subnational and national levels; as well as regional and global reference laboratories. Every WHO member state is served by at least 1 GPLN laboratory, though in some cases the laboratory may be located in a neighboring country. The laboratory network is organized by the type of testing available: virus isolation (from stool and/or sewage), intratypic differentiation, and sequencing.

**11. Special considerations**—In 2015, type 2 poliovirus was declared eradicated. As a result, the type 2 component was removed from the oral polio vaccine, and any work with type 2 poliovirus (wild-type, vaccine, or vaccine-derived) must be conducted under enhanced containment, as described by WHO.[2] As of August 1, 2016, all type 2 poliovirus isolates must be referred to a WHO-accredited polio sequencing laboratory for detailed characterization.

## References

1. Centers for Disease Control and Prevention, National Notifiable Diseases Surveillance System. Poliovirus infection, nonparalytic 2010 case definition. 2012. Available at:

https://wwwn.cdc.gov/nndss/conditions/poliovirus-infection-nonparalytic/case-definition/2010. Accessed April 1, 2019.

2. World Health Organization. *WHO Global Action Plan to Minimize Poliovirus Facility-Associated Risk After Type-Specific Eradication of Wild Polioviruses and Sequential Cessation of OPV Use*. 2015. Available at: https://apps.who.int/iris/handle/10665/208872. Accessed April 1, 2019.

[M. S. Oberste]

# PRION DISEASES
(transmissible spongiform encephalopathies)

| DISEASE | ICD-10 CODE |
|---|---|
| CREUTZFELDT-JAKOB DISEASE | ICD-10 A81.0 |
| GERSTMANN-STRÄUSSLER-SCHEINKER SYNDROM | ICD-10-CM A81.09 |
| VARIANT CREUTZFELDT-JAKOB DISEASE | ICD-10-CM A81.01 |
| FATAL FAMILIAL INSOMNIA | ICD-10-CM A81.09 |

A group of brain diseases characterized by a clinical and neuropathologic picture of progressive neurodegeneration resulting from tissue deposition of prions, which are believed to be an abnormally folded form of a host encoded cellular protein (the prion protein). Prions are believed to be the causative agents, and their deposition in neurons is the hallmark of prion disease pathology and pathogenesis. Human prion diseases are as follows:

- Creutzfeldt-Jakob disease (CJD), occurring in 3 different forms: sporadic CJD (~85% of cases), familial CJD (10%–15% of cases), and iatrogenic CJD (<1% of cases).
- Variant CJD (vCJD), which has been causally linked with bovine spongiform encephalopathy (BSE), a prion disease of cattle.
- Gerstmann-Sträussler-Scheinker syndrome (GSS).
- Fatal familial insomnia (FFI).

The most common prion disease in humans, sporadic CJD, is not thought to be exogenously acquired, and it occurs sporadically. Other prion diseases not thought to be exogenously acquired include familial CJD, GSS, and FFI, and they are associated with mutations of the prion protein gene and inherited within families. Still, other prion diseases in humans (Kuru, vCJD, iatrogenic CJD) are thought to be acquired exogenously, have generally long incubation periods (i.e., many years), and have no demonstrable inflammatory or immune response. Even those diseases thought not to be acquired exogenously, and some that are genetically associated, may be transmissible to others in certain settings (e.g., iatrogenic CJD, vCJD).

**1. Clinical features**—Signs and symptoms of CJD are limited to central nervous system (CNS) dysfunction. It typically presents as a subacute illness in the middle-aged and elderly (median age at death is 68 years) as a rapidly progressive encephalopathy with confusion, dementia, and other neurologic signs such as cerebellar dysfunction and myoclonus. However, clinical heterogeneity and atypical presentations have been reported. Patients have no fever, and routine blood tests and cerebrospinal fluid (CSF) cell count are normal. Typical periodic high-voltage complexes are present in the electroencephalogram (EEG) in about 70% of cases, and the CSF 14-3-3 and tau proteins are elevated in the majority of patients. Brain magnetic resonance imaging (MRI) shows signal hyperintensity in the caudate/putamen in many cases, especially on fluid attenuation inversion recovery sequences. High signal may be seen in some cerebral cortical regions.

Variant CJD, first identified in 1996, has a longer clinical course (median 14 months vs. 4 months for sporadic CJD) and usually presents with psychiatric or behavioral disturbances, followed by signs of neurologic dysfunction, usually delayed by several months after the onset of illness. The typical EEG changes of sporadic CJD are seen only rarely in vCJD. MRI scan in vCJD shows high signal in the pulvinar area of the posterior thalamus in more than 90% of cases, especially on fluid attenuation inversion recovery sequences. The CSF 14-3-3 may be elevated but in only about 45% of cases. With one exception, all tested confirmed cases of vCJD to date have been homozygous for methionine (MM) at the polymorphic codon 129 of the prion protein gene. It remains unclear whether or not vCJD will occur in non-MM individuals who may be infected at present.

The clinical picture for genetic prion diseases is highly variable, and traditionally they have been classified as familial CJD, GSS, and FFI. GSS is used to describe a heterogeneous group of inherited prion diseases that are characterized by long illness duration and the presence of amyloid plaques, primarily in the cerebellum. FFI predominantly involves the thalamus, resulting in an illness characterized by intractable insomnia and autonomic nervous system dysfunction.

CJD must be differentiated from other forms of dementia (especially Alzheimer's disease), other infections (including encephalitis and vasculitis), and toxic, endocrine, autoimmune, and metabolic encephalopathies.

**2. Causative agents**—CJD and other related diseases are caused by prions, which are abnormally folded (misfolded), self-replicating isoforms of the normal host-encoded prion protein. The normal cellular prion protein is a structural component of cell membranes of neurons and other mammalian cells. Genetic prion diseases are associated with autosomal dominant mutations in PRioN Protein (*PRNP*) gene located on chromosome 20 that encodes for the normal prion protein. The mutations are thought to predispose the individual to prion protein misfolding and subsequent prion disease. The pattern of inheritance and penetrance is variable, but up to 40% of cases may have no family history of a prion disease. Many prion diseases are transmissible in the laboratory to other species, including wild and transgenic mice and nonhuman primates.

**3. Laboratory diagnosis**—Prion diseases can be diagnosed based on clinical and laboratory findings although laboratories that provide prion disease testing are highly specialized facilities. All forms of CJD are diagnosed based on clinical features, family history, MRI, and CSF findings. The real-time quake induced conversion assay (RT-QuIC) is a recently developed diagnostic method, which directly detects prions in CSF. In vCJD, immunohistochemical or Western blot testing of tonsil biopsy can be very helpful but is probably best reserved for those cases with atypical features and/or without the MRI pulvinar sign. A definite diagnosis of all prion diseases depends on brain tissue testing and is most reliable when undertaken at postmortem examination. Genetic testing using a peripheral blood sample is of importance in the diagnosis of suspect genetic prion disease. Brain biopsy can provide antemortem diagnosis, but this is an invasive procedure and is arguably best reserved for those cases in which an alternative diagnosis is otherwise not possible.

**4. Laboratory capability**—CDC recommends that laboratories handling prions from human tissue should use biosafety level 2 (BSL-2) laboratory practices. Although prions have been identified from many sites in individuals with CJD, central nervous tissues typically contain prions at much higher titers than other tissues, blood, or CSF. CDC recommends that central nervous system tissues from autopsy specimens containing prions should be processed with extreme care in a BSL-2 facility utilizing BSL-3 practices during autopsy. In the USA, the National Prion Disease Pathology Surveillance Center, sponsored by CDC, has expertise in performing CJD autopsies and can be consulted. For those laboratories that are accredited by the College of American Pathologists (CAP), the CAP Anatomic Pathology Checklist explicitly describes special handling instructions for histology tissue specimens suspected of containing prions.

**5. Safety requirements**—Prions are not inactivated using routine decontamination methods commonly employed in the clinical microbiology laboratory. For example, prions can maintain infectivity after alcohol fixation, formalin fixation, and standard autoclaving. Although prions can maintain their infectivity after harsh treatment, no confirmed iatrogenic transmission of prions via contaminated surgical equipment has been identified since the 1970s, and human transmission of prions from potentially contaminated surfaces has never been identified.

CNS tissues are known to harbor the highest titer of transmissible prions, but detectable prions have also been identified from other body sites, even blood. Individuals with vCJD have been noted to have infectivity in reticuloendothelial tissues, albeit lower than in CNS. The current WHO guidelines published in 1999 recommend handling blood and body fluids other than CSF using routine handling precautions.

Several infection control guidelines for prion diseases are available as follows:

1) *Guidance: Minimise Transmission Risk of CJD and vCJD in Healthcare Settings*, available at: https://www.gov.uk/government/publications/guidance-from-the-acdp-tse-risk-management-subgroup-formerly-tse-working-group.
2) *WHO Infection Control Guidelines for Transmissible Spongiform Encephalopathies*, available at: http://www.who.int/csr/resources/publications/bse/WHO_CDS_CSR_APH_2000_3/en.
3) *Biosafety in Microbiological and Biomedical Laboratories,* 5th Edition (Section VIII, Part H) available at: https://www.cdc.gov/biosafety/publications/bmbl5.

Generally, if materials to be decontaminated can withstand the harsh treatment, the rule of thumb for decontamination of possible prion-contaminated material is to immerse the material or cover the contaminated surface with 1N sodium hydroxide (or 20,000 ppm of sodium hypochlorite) for 1 hour before neutralizing the chemical decontaminant and then proceed with routine disinfection procedures. Specific biosafety recommendations and protocols are available at: https://www.cdc.gov/biosafety/publications/bmbl5.

**6. Nonhuman hosts**—Humans are the only species affected by the CJD prions in nature, with the exception of vCJD, which represents zoonotic spread of BSE from its reservoir, thought to be in cattle. Subclinical infection with the BSE prion appears to be present in human populations (especially in the UK where the estimated prevalence ranges from 1 in 1,250 to 1 in 3,500). The magnitude of the risk from such infections is unknown, but it may represent a potential reservoir of infection for secondary, human-to-human spread by blood transfusion, organ transplantation, or surgery.

Another reservoir of prions with zoonotic potential is chronic wasting disease (CWD) in farmed and free-ranging cervids. The disease has been endemic for decades in areas of Colorado and Wyoming. Since 2000, the disease has been detected in 19 additional states, 2 Canadian provinces, South Korea, Norway, and Finland. Unlike the BSE outbreak in cattle, CWD prions are highly infectious among cervids, and the disease is readily transmissible animal to animal through contact and through exposure to CWD prions in the environment. No convincing evidence indicates that exposure of humans to CWD prions can cause disease in humans. The experimental evidence suggests the existence of a species barrier against CWD transmission to humans, but it is unclear how protective this is in primates. As many as 100% of intracerebrally and 92% of orally exposed squirrel monkeys developed CWD, and ongoing macaque experiments also suggest susceptibility. The potential transmission of CWD to humans directly or via an intermediate animal host warrants an ongoing surveillance focusing on populations with high level of exposure to CWD.

**7. Sample/specimen requirements**—Standard precautions are necessary when collecting and handling specimens that may contain prions. Surgical instruments used to collect specimens for prion testing should ideally be disposed of after use. Alternatively, instruments and devices should be decontaminated using methods known to inactivate prions. *Biosafety in Microbiological and Biomedical Laboratories,* 5th Edition *(BMBL)* recommends that unfixed samples of brain, spinal cord, and other tissues containing human prions should be processed with extreme care in a BSL-2 facility utilizing BSL-3 practices. Specimens such as blood for genetic testing, CSF and biopsies for diagnostic testing, and brains for autopsy should be stored and transported according to the reference laboratory's protocols. Neurologic tissue to be sectioned for histopathologic analysis should be handled and processed in accordance with CAP recommendations, which ideally involve formic acid decontamination of the tissue before paraffin embedding. Shipping of specimens should be performed by trained individuals in accordance with government regulations. The National Prion Disease Pathology Surveillance Center recommends shipping all specimens as UN3373, category B material (see: https://case.edu/medicine/pathology/divisions/prion-center).

**8. Testing requirements**—Autopsy is currently the gold standard for diagnosing and classifying prion diseases and determination of disease origin. However, antemortem studies have diagnostic value, and a confident diagnosis of CJD can often be made before death. Brain tissue studies, CSF analyses, and genetic testing can all contribute to arriving at the diagnosis of prion disease.

1) Classification of prions: human prion diseases are phenotypically heterogeneous, and premortem clinical diagnosis has poor specificity. Although RT-QuIC testing on CSF and brain MRI are helping to improve the reliability of clinical diagnosis, examination of brain tissue specimens remains the gold standard for determining disease origin. Two major determinants of prion disease phenotype and origin is the conformational structure of the pathogenic prion protein ($PrP^{Sc}$), which generates higher (type 1) or lower (type 2) molecular weight fragments after proteolysis on Western blot and the *PRNP* codon 129 polymorphism with MM or valine (V). In combination with neuropathological characteristics, these aspects are now used to classify sporadic human prion diseases and have been adopted by prion surveillance centers worldwide. This

classification scheme describes 6 subtypes of sporadic CJD (sCJD): MM1, MV1, VV1, MM2, MV2, and VV2. sCJD subtypes MM1 and MV1 are often considered a single subtype due to their similar phenotypic findings. Over half of sCJD cases can be classified as subtype MM1, but mixed subtypes can be found in one-fifth of individuals. Notably, these subtypes correlate strongly with unique histopathological findings of the brain at autopsy to the extent that neuropathological findings often are predictive of the prion subtype. Different prion subtypes are associated with different clinical courses of disease and represent different prion strains with distinctly different conformational structure of prion particles.

2) Western blot: $PrP^{Sc}$ is typically proteinase K-resistant, and brain tissue can be treated with proteinase K, which digests proteins other than $PrP^{Sc}$. Any $PrP^{Sc}$ that remains after proteinase K treatment can be detected and classified by electrophoretic migration pattern. Three bands of $PrP^{Sc}$ with increasing molecular weight are visible by Western blot: an unglycosylated band, a mono-glycoslyated band, and a di-glycoslyated band. Unglycosylated $PrP^{Sc}$, with a molecular weight of 20-21 kDa, is classified as type 1, and unglycosylated $PrP^{Sc}$, with a molecular weight of 19 kDa, is classified as type 2. Notably, variably protease-sensitive prionopathy (VPSPr) has been reported in which the $PrP^{Sc}$ can be digested with proteinase K.
3) Histopathological: brain tissue obtained by biopsy or autopsy can be used for histology studies. Classic histological findings of the brain in individuals with CJD include spongiform degeneration, neuron loss, and astrogliosis. Specific neuropathological findings can be used to predict the prion subtype. Immunohistochemical staining of PrP is used to characterize the disease (e.g., florid plaques of $PrP^{Sc}$ deposited in the cortex are a key feature of vCJD). Other histological features and the location within the brain where those features are identified can be used to suggest 1 of the 6 subtypes of sCJD. $PrP^{Sc}$ has been reliably identified in lymphoid tissues and tonsils in individuals with vCJD but is absent in individuals with sCJD.
4) CSF: several diagnostic tests can be performed on CSF, which can be helpful in diagnosing or ruling out prion disease. Two types of tests are typically performed. The first type examines the CSF for nonspecific markers of neurodegeneration. The second type examines the CSF for $PrP^{Sc}$, which is the causative agent of disease.

Multiple assays can be used to identify brain tissue breakdown products in the CSF including 14-3-3, tau, neuron-specific enolase, and α-synuclein. A 14-3-3 assay is the classic test used to detect prion disease, and it is often still used despite the availability of more sensitive and specific assays.[1] Either a Western blot or an enzyme-linked immunosorbent assay (ELISA) can be used to identify elevated 14-3-3. Another important nonspecific marker is total tau, which is commonly identified by ELISA. Because prion disease causes rapid deterioration of the brain tissue, these markers are sensitive in detecting prion disease. However, many other diagnoses can cause elevated levels, so these markers lack specificity. More slowly progressive forms of prion disease, such as some genetic prion diseases, may have levels of markers of neurodegeneration that are lower than more rapidly progressive prion diseases.

5) Real-time quake induced conversion was recently developed as a novel assay to detect $PrP^{Sc}$. This assay does not identify surrogate markers of disease, but it detects replication (i.e., seeding) activity of prions. The assay uses recombinant $PrP^{C}$ as a reagent substrate, and the assay is seeded with CSF from a patient who is suspected of having prion disease. If $PrP^{Sc}$ is present in the CSF, the $PrP^{Sc}$ template induces misfolding of the $PrP^{C}$ substrate in vitro. These misfolded proteins are detected by an increase in relative fluorescence of the reporter reagent, thioflavin T. The second generation of CSF RT-QuIC reached a sensitivity of 92%–95% and specificity of 98.5% in the detection of human prion diseases. Genetic testing of *PRNP* gene: as with any genetic testing, a genetic counselor should be consulted before a living individual is tested. *PRNP* sequence analysis can be performed to determine the codon 129 genotype and to interrogate the gene for mutations which can cause genetic prion diseases. The most common mutation associated with genetic CJD is E200K, but many other *PRNP* mutations have also been described.
6) Blood, urine, and nasal brushings: research is being done to try to detect prions in peripheral blood, urine, nasal brushings, skin, and internal organs in individuals who may have prion disease, but this testing is not currently available for routine diagnostic use.

**9. Reporting requirements**—Many countries have made CJD (including vCJD) a notifiable disease. The World Organisation for Animal Health lists BSE as a reportable disease for international trade in livestock and livestock products. International measures for the prevention of vCJD are as follows: To avoid human exposures to the BSE agent in food of bovine origin, no part or product of any animal that has shown signs of a prion disease should enter the human food chain. Countries should not permit tissues that are likely to contain the BSE agent to enter any (human or animal) food chain.

Prevention of bloodborne transmission: as a precautionary measure to reduce the risk of transmission of vCJD through blood or blood products, some countries, including Canada, the USA, and some continental European countries, have requested that blood centers exclude potential blood donors who have resided for a specified period in the UK or other European countries.

**10. Referral network**—Prion centers monitoring human prion disease were established in countries of the EU, the USA, and Canada, and the referral networks should be used as circumstances and regulations dictate.

**11. Special considerations**—Ideally, laboratories should be informed when the possibility of prion disease is being considered by the ordering provider, so appropriate laboratory precautions and subsequent decontamination can be undertaken. Laboratory evaluation of CSF or CNS tissue from individuals suspected of having prion disease should follow their institutional policies and procedures for handling, testing, and decontamination. The diagnosis or exclusion of prion disease should be based on the complete laboratory results. Autopsy remains the gold standard in definitively diagnosing and characterizing prion diseases, and autopsy plays an essential role in investigating the etiology and epidemiology of each individual's prion disease.

## References

1. Weber T, Aguzzi A. The spectrum of transmissible spongiform encephalopathies. *Intervirology* 1997;40:198–212.

[J. Safar]

# PSITTACOSIS

(*Chlamydia* [or *Chlamydophila*] *psittaci* infection, ornithosis, parrot fever, avian chlamydiosis)

| DISEASE | ICD-10 CODE |
|---|---|
| PSITTACOSIS | ICD-10 A70 |

**1. Clinical features**—An acute disease with systemic presentations and respiratory symptoms. Acute onset of fever, headache, myalgia, and dry cough are typical clinical features. Respiratory symptoms are often mild when compared with pneumonia demonstrable by chest X-ray. Cough is initially absent or nonproductive; when present, sputum is mucopurulent and scant. Pleuritic chest pain and splenomegaly occur infrequently; pulse may be slow in relation to temperature. Respiratory failure, hepatitis, endocarditis, and encephalitis are occasional complications; relapses may occur. Although usually mild or moderate, human disease can be severe, especially in untreated elderly persons.

**2. Causative agents**—The causative agent of psittacosis is *Chlamydophila psittaci*, which is a small bacterium (0.5 μm) that undergoes several transformations during its life cycle. It exists as an elementary body when the disease is quiescent. The elementary body is not biologically active but is resistant to environmental stresses and can survive outside a host. The elementary body travels from an infected bird (usually in feces or respiratory secretions) to the lungs of an uninfected bird or person in small droplets and is responsible for infection. Once in the lungs, the elementary body is phagocytized within an endosome and transforms into a reticulate body and begins to replicate within the endosome. The reticulate bodies must use some of the host's cellular machinery to complete their replication. The reticulate bodies then convert back to elementary bodies and are released back into the lung, often after causing the death of the host cell. The elementary bodies are thereafter able to infect new cells, either in the same organism or in a new host.

*C. psittaci* is currently grouped into 7 avian genotypes (A through F and a newly identified genotype, E/B) and 2 nonavian genotypes (M56 and WC). *C. psittaci* serovar A is endemic among psittacine birds and has caused sporadic zoonotic disease in humans, other mammals, and tortoises. Serovar B is endemic among pigeons, has been isolated from turkeys, and has also been identified as the cause of abortion in herds of dairy cattle. Serovars C and D are occupational hazards for slaughterhouse workers and for people in contact with birds. Serovar E isolates have been obtained from a variety of avian hosts worldwide and, although they were associated with the 1920s–1930s outbreak in humans, a specific reservoir for serovar E has not been identified.

**3. Laboratory diagnosis**—Psittacosis can be diagnosed in the laboratory by performing serological tests on clotted serum samples or by using molecular assays to detect *C. psittaci* deoxyribonucleic acid (DNA) in respiratory samples.

Serology is usually performed by means of the complement fixation (CF) test. The patient's serum is heated to inactivate complement in the sample. It is then tested in 2-fold dilution steps in a reaction mixture including complement, sheep red blood cells with antisheep red blood cell antibodies attached, and *C. psittaci* antigen. If the patient's serum contains antibodies against the *C. psittaci* antigen, they will bind to the antigen to form antigen-antibody complexes. The complement proteins will react with these complexes and be depleted. When the sheep red blood cell antibody complexes are added, there will be no complement left in the serum. However, if no antibodies against the *C. psittaci* antigen are present, the complement will not be depleted, and it will react with the sheep red blood cell antibody complexes, lysing the sheep red blood cells. Nonlysed sheep red blood cells will form a red button at the bottom of the reaction wells. If a single blood is tested for *C. psittaci* antibody, an antibody titer (the reciprocal of the serum dilution, which is positive) of 16–64 or greater is an indication of possible recent *C. psittaci* infection, depending on the sensitivity of the test. A preferred and more reliable method of diagnosis is to test paired serum samples, 1 taken in the first 7–10 days after the onset of symptoms and a second taken at least 10–14 days after the onset of symptoms. A 4-fold or greater rise in *C. psittaci* antibody titer is more indicative of recent *C. psittaci* infection. However, since the CF test is not specific for *C. psittaci*, a rise in antibody titer could be due to infection with *Chlamydia trachomatis* or *Chlamydia pneumoniae* infection, which is why CF test results need to be interpreted after consideration of the clinical symptoms and epidemiological factors (e.g., bird contact).

4. **Laboratory capability**—Complement fixation tests are only conducted in a few microbiology laboratories in the UK and in the USA. Real time polymerase chain reaction (PCR) for detecting *C. psittaci* DNA in sputum samples is only available in reference laboratories, with prior consultation on suitability of the request. Given the challenges in providing laboratory diagnostic support for suspected psittacosis cases, most clinical and public health laboratories may want to pass through the testing requests to their respective reference laboratories.

5. **Safety requirements**—Serum samples can be handled on the open bench with appropriate precautions (e.g., wearing protective gloves) to mitigate against blood-borne virus infection. Safety goggles need to be worn if there is a risk of blood splashes during manipulations. When sputum samples suspected of containing *C. psittaci* are handled in the laboratory, they need to be handled as a potential hazard group 3 organism (UK Advisory Committee on Dangerous Pathogens) or biosafety level 3 in the USA. Hazard group 3 procedures are used with suspect agents that can cause severe human disease and may be serious.

6. **Nonhuman hosts**—*C. psittaci* is an intracellular bacterial species that may cause endemic avian chlamydiosis, epizootic outbreaks in mammals, and respiratory psittacosis in humans. Potential hosts include feral birds and domesticated poultry as well as cattle, pigs, sheep, and horses. *C. psittaci* is transmitted by inhalation (dried feces, feather dust and dander, or respiratory droplets), contact, or ingestion among birds and to mammals. Psittacosis in birds and in humans often starts with flu-like symptoms and becomes a life-threatening pneumonia. Many strains remain quiescent in birds until activated under stress. Birds are excellent, highly mobile vectors for the distribution of chlamydia infection because they feed on and have access to the detritus of infected animals of all sorts.

Birds can transmit *C. psittaci* to humans; the resulting infection is known as psittacosis (if the source of the infection is a member of the bird family *Psittacidae* such as parrots, parakeets, macaws, and cockatoos) or ornithosis (if infection is from another bird or animal source).

Infections in birds are important as they represent a biological hazard to human health as well as economic loss to the poultry industry and the pet bird retail trade. Birds can carry the organism without any signs of disease, or they can become mildly to severely ill.

Those at greatest risk of contracting the disease include bird fanciers and owners of pet birds. Pet shop employees and others whose occupation places them at risk of exposure (such as poultry slaughterhouse workers, veterinary surgeons, and zoo workers) are also at increased risk. Because human infection can result from brief, passing exposure to infected birds or their dried contaminated droppings, people with no identified bird contact can be infected but not identified in a higher risk group. A good example of this is contact with pigeons, which are common in the environment.

**7. Sample/specimen requirements**—If *C. psittaci* infection is suspected in a patient, the best sample to take is a sputum sample or lower respiratory tract sample, which should be tested by PCR.

Serological diagnosis can be achieved by taking a 10 ml clotted blood sample and testing for *C. psittaci* antibody by the CF test. A second convalescent sample taken at least 10–14 days after the onset of symptoms is recommended. This is more likely to have a higher CF antibody titer, but, more importantly, when the acute phase serum is tested in the CF with the convalescent phase serum, a 4-fold or greater rise in CF antibody titer gives a more secure diagnosis (rather than just 1 raised CF antibody titer).

**8. Testing requirements**—There are several different diagnostic PCR tests in use in specialist reference laboratories that are homemade tests using different primers and test methodologies, in use with appropriate controls. Although PCR tests are usually very sensitive, sensitivity and specificity data are not currently available. PCR tests can be designed to detect all *C. psittaci* organisms or can be tailored to detect specific serovars and genotypes.

The complement fixation test is not very sensitive, so false-negative results for psittacosis may occur especially when a serum sample is taken within the first 10–14 days after the onset of symptoms. Antibody titers as low as 8–16 may be significant, but at these low values, they may also be nonspecific. A 4-fold rise or greater in *C. psittaci* antibody titers has a high predictive value. All tests must incorporate appropriate controls.

**9. Reporting requirements**—In the UK, regulation 4 of the Health Protection (Notification) Regulations 2010 obliges the operators of diagnostic laboratories to notify Public Health England or other designated regional/national health authority if they diagnose a case of *C. psittaci* infection in a human patient.[1] Psittacosis is also a laboratory reportable disease in most other settings. Laboratory directors should determine whether it is reportable in their respective states, provinces, or countries.

**10. Referral network**—Since *C. psittaci* PCR and the complement fixation test for detecting *C. psittaci* antibody are only performed in a few specialist laboratories, local referral networks vary across the UK. *C. psittaci* testing may be restricted to specific laboratories depending on the country.

**11. Special considerations**—There is no human-to-human transmission of psittacosis. Human cases of *C. psittaci* infection are always acquired from birds or animals. Therefore, when a new human case is identified, the source of the infection needs to be investigated by public health authorities to prevent the occurrence of further cases from the identified source.

Psittacosis is an acute respiratory disease with an incubation period of 1 to 4 weeks. Symptoms range from asymptomatic illness to systemic illness with severe pneumonia. Severe disease usually presents as an atypical pneumonia. In the first week of psittacosis the symptoms often include debilitating high fevers, joint pains, diarrhoea, conjunctivitis, nose bleeds, and low level of white blood cells in the blood. Spleen enlargement is common toward the end of the first week. Headache can be so severe that it suggests meningitis. Toward the end of the first week, coma can be noted in severe cases. In the second week, patients often develop continuous high fevers, cough, and shortness of breath. X-rays often show patchy infiltrates or a diffuse whiteout of lung fields. Complications including hepatitis, myocarditis, and arthritis may occasionally occur. Psittacosis can be fatal (< 1% of cases), especially in older people.

Psittacosis is 1 of a group of diseases known as atypical pneumonias. The term was introduced in the 1930s and was created to describe the symptoms of those patients more likely to present with atypical generalized symptoms (i.e., fever, headache, sweating, and myalgia) and nonlobar bronchopneumonia, as opposed to those patients with the bacterial lobar pneumonia caused by bacteria such as Streptococcus pneumoniae. Other bacteria causing atypical pneumonia include *Coxiella burnetii* (Q fever), *Mycoplasma pneumoniae*, *Legionella pneumophila,* and *Chlamydia pneumoniae*.

## References

1. UK government. The Health Protection (Notification) Regulations 2010. Available at: http://www.legislation.gov.uk/uksi/2010/659/made. Accessed March 11, 2019.

[T. Wreghitt]

# Q FEVER

(query fever)

| DISEASE | ICD-10 CODE |
|---|---|
| Q FEVER | ICD-10 A78 |

**1. Clinical features**—Q fever is an acute febrile disease characterized by chills, headache, malaise, myalgia, and sweats. There is considerable variation in severity and duration; infections may be unapparent or present as a fever of unknown origin. A pneumonitis may be found on X-ray examination, although radiographic patterns are nonspecific and do not allow for differentiation from other etiologies. Abnormal liver function tests are common. Acute and chronic granulomatous hepatitis, which can be confused with tuberculous hepatitis, has been reported. Chronic Q fever manifests primarily as culture-negative endocarditis or vascular infection and occurs primarily in patients with preexisting risk factors such as valvular or vascular defects. Other rare clinical syndromes, including neurological syndromes, have been described. The case-fatality rate in untreated acute cases is usually less than 1%. Q fever endocarditis is fatal if untreated, whereas with treatment the 10-year mortality rate is 19%. A post-Q fever fatigue syndrome has been described.

**2. Causative agents**—*Coxiella burnetii*. The organism can be found in biological excreta of infected animals such as urine, feces, and milk, with the highest numbers of bacteria shed in birth products (e.g., placenta, amniotic fluid). The bacterium is highly resistant to many disinfectants and environmental conditions.

**3. Laboratory diagnosis**—Diagnosis of Q fever is facilitated by use of 2 antigenic preparations: (a) phase I, which represents the infectious agent, and (b) phase II, which is a laboratory-generated attenuated form of the infectious agent with truncated lipopolysaccharide. For acute Q fever, a demonstration of a 4-fold rise in phase II immunoglobulin class G (IgG) antibody between acute and convalescent serum taken 3–6 weeks apart is the standard for confirmed diagnosis. A single high serum phase II IgG titer may be considered evidence of probable acute infection in a clinically compatible patient. Laboratory diagnosis by polymerase chain reaction (PCR) of blood and serum can also be used in the first 2 weeks after symptom onset and prior to antibiotic administration. Diagnosis of chronic Q fever requires antiphase I IgG antibody titer greater than or equal to 1:1024 and a compatible clinical presentation. Anti-*C. burnetii* antibodies may be detectable for 10–15 years if sensitive methods such as immunofluorescence are used for detection. Bacteria may be identified in tissues (liver biopsy or heart valve) by immunohistochemistry (IHC) and electronic microscopy.

**4. Laboratory capability**—Serology and PCR can be performed in biosafety level 2 (BSL-2) laboratories. For culture and preparation of tissues such as heart valves, for diagnostics, BSL-3 is recommended owing to the extremely infectious nature of the *C. burnetii* organisms.

**5. Safety requirements**—Specialist BSL-3 laboratories are required for any work involving isolation and culture of the organism. Specialist culture involves either cell culture or culture in embryonated eggs, both of which pose extreme hazards. Egg culture, in particular, is a highly specialized technique requiring specialist facilities and experienced staff.

**6. Nonhuman hosts**—Q fever is a zoonotic infection acquired principally from contact with infected livestock, primarily cattle, sheep, and goats. Human Q fever is strongly associated with the management of domesticated animals. Infection has been confirmed in other animal species such as cats, dogs, rabbits, birds, and reptiles. The majority of animal infections are asymptomatic, and clinical illness is mainly associated with conception, stillbirth, abortion, birth, mastitis, and reproductive disorders such as infertility and endometriosis. Organisms are shed in large numbers in birth products and can also be shed in milk, urine, and feces of infected animals. Humans can be infected through inhalation of infectious aerosols either directly from animal products, particularly birth products, or from dust contaminated with dried secretions and body fluids. *C. burnetii* is extremely resilient and can persist in the environment from months to years.

**7. Sample/specimen requirements**—For acute infections, whole blood and serum samples should be taken before day 14 for PCR and up to day 21 for enzyme-linked immunosorbent assay (ELISA), immunofluorescence assay (IFA), or complement fixation. Convalescent serum for confirmation of rising titers should be taken 3–6 weeks after the acute sample. For chronic infections, whole blood, plasma, and serum for PCR and serology should be taken more than 6 weeks after acute infection. Samples from heart valves and other tissues can be taken from 6 weeks to years for PCR and culture, as chronic Q fever can manifest years after original exposure. All specimens for culture except whole blood should be stored at −80°C and transported on dry ice to the diagnostic laboratory. Ethylenediaminetetraacetic acid (EDTA) and sodium citrate blood can be used for PCR but not for culture. Whole blood, EDTA blood and sodium citrate blood should be stored at 4°C.

**8. Testing requirements**—For acute Q fever, serologic testing together with PCR is recommended, while for chronic Q fever, serology, PCR (for intermittent bacteremia), and culture of tissues such as heart valves (for infective endocarditis) are recommended.

1) Culture: detection of *C. burnetii* in clinical samples is indicative of infection, but culture, either in embryonated hens' eggs or cell culture, is time consuming and cumbersome and should be restricted to specialist laboratories. Culture can also lack sensitivity and is often negative if a patient is receiving antibiotic therapy but can be positive early in infection before a serological response can be detected. Sensitivity of culture has been reported to be as high as 88% from cardiac valves but as low as 40% from blood in chronic Q fever.
2) Serology: the main serological methods for diagnosis of Q fever are IFA and ELISA. Diagnosis for acute Q fever is based on a 4-fold rise in phase II IgG titers between serum samples taken from acute and

convalescent stages 3–6 weeks apart. Seroconversion takes place approximately 7–15 days following infection, and phase I IgM and IgG antibodies can be detected from the second week of acute illness. IgM and IgG antibodies to phase I antigens also increase but rarely exceed the titer of phase II antibodies during the acute phase. IgM antibodies typically have a much lower specificity than IgG, making IgM assays of limited diagnostic value as a standalone test. Cross-reactivity between *Coxiella*, *Legionella,* and *Bartonella* can occur, but usually at a much lower titer, and this does not usually result in misdiagnosis. Chronic Q fever is diagnosed by a high-titer IgG antibody response to phase I antigens by IFA or ELISA. Previous guidelines for Q fever diagnosis suggested a cutoff titer of 1:800 or greater, although more recent studies conducted following a large outbreak of Q fever in the Netherlands between 2007 and 2010 suggest a higher cutoff titer of 1:1,024 or greater is more accurate because a cutoff titer of 1:800 or greater can lead to a higher false-positive rate. The exact values vary among laboratories and the assay used, so local reference ranges should be used for interpretation of serology results. Persisting high antibody titers to phase II and phase I antigens are considered to be indicative of a risk of developing chronic Q fever due to persistent antigenic stimulation. IgA antibodies to phase I antigens are also used in the diagnosis of chronic Q fever. Other serological tests have been described, including complement-fixation tests, microagglutination, radioimmunoassay, dot immunoblotting, and Western blotting. IFA and ELISA are available as commercial assays. Sensitivity and specificity vary depending on the technique, but IFA, ELISA, and microagglutination are considered to be the most reliable for sensitivity, specificity, and positive-predictive values.

3) Molecular methods: a number of PCR assays have been described using various gene targets including 16S ribosomal ribonucleic acid (rRNA), 23S rRNA, superoxide dismutase, plasmid QpRS, plasmid QpH1, surface E protein gene (cbbe), and the htpAB-associated repetitive element IS1111. Such assays can vary in their sensitivity and specificity depending on the target used. Whole blood and serum can be used for PCR, as well as tissue samples for direct detection of *C. burnetii* in tissues. For diagnosis of acute Q fever, blood should be collected in the first 2 weeks of symptom onset and before or within 48 hours of antibiotic administration. Samples can be PCR positive before antibody can be detected using serology methods. For chronic Q fever, blood can be positive by PCR due to recurrent bacteremia, but the sensitivity of PCR in chronic Q fever

tends to be low, with sensitivity rates between 23%-64% being reported. The sensitivity of PCR on affected tissues such as cardiac valves is much higher, with sensitivities up to 100% being reported. PCR can be conducted on formalin-fixed and paraffin-embedded samples. PCR can also be conducted on cerebrospinal fluid, pleural fluid, bone marrow, bone biopsies, liver biopsies, milk, placenta, and foetal tissues.

4) Other methods: immunodetection methods such as IHC can be used to detect *C. burnetii* directly in tissue samples. This is particularly valuable for the diagnosis of chronic Q fever, even after antibiotic therapy has commenced. Samples can be tested fresh or after formalin fixation or paraffin embedding. The techniques tend to be specialized and conducted at a central reference laboratory.

**9. Reporting requirements**—Q fever can be a national notifiable disease in some countries such as the USA. Local guidelines for reporting confirmed Q fever cases should be followed.

**10. Referral network**—No specific international network or WHO collaborating center exists for Q fever. Twenty-six EU and European Economic Area countries provide epidemiological information to the European Centre for Disease Control, which collates and reports the information. Other local or regional referral networks may exist.

**11. Special considerations**—*C. burnetii* is considered to be a potential biothreat agent and is listed in the Select Agents and Toxins, 7 CFR Part 331, 9 CFR Part 121, and 42 CFR Part 73 (https://www.selectagents.gov). In the USA, confirmed isolates of select agents identified in a clinical or diagnostic laboratory must be reported. Each country may have specific registration requirements for laboratories working with *C. burnetii* for human or animal pathogen regulations, and these should be checked.

[J. Duggan]

# RABIES
(hydrophobia)

| DISEASE | ICD-10 CODE |
|---|---|
| RABIES | ICD-10 A82 |

**1. Clinical features**—Rabies is an acute viral zoonotic disease that causes a progressive viral encephalomyelitis that is nearly always fatal. Onset is generally heralded by a sense of apprehension, headache, fever, malaise, and sensory changes (paresthesia) at the site of an animal bite. Excitability and aerophobia and/or hydrophobia, often with spasms of swallowing muscles, are frequent symptoms. Delirium with occasional convulsions follows. Such classic symptoms of furious rabies are noted in two-thirds of cases, whereas the remaining present as paralysis of limbs and respiratory muscles with sparing of consciousness. Phobic spasms may be absent in the paralytic form. Coma and death ensue within 1–2 weeks, mainly due to cardiac failure.

**2. Causative agents**—Lyssaviruses, such as the classical rabies lyssavirus, are in the family *Rhabdoviridae* in the genus *Lyssavirus.* Genus *Lyssavirus* currently contains 14 species and is divided into 3 phylogroups. Only one of the species, classical rabies lyssavirus, is currently present in the Americas. Classical rabies lyssavirus is the most important for public health as it causes 99.9% of all human rabies cases worldwide. Lyssaviruses in Africa (Mokola and Duvenhage) and Eurasia (European bat lyssaviruses 1 and 2) and the Australian bat lyssavirus, which was first identified in 1996 in several species of flying foxes in Australia, have been associated with human deaths from rabies. All members of the genus are antigenically related, but use of monoclonal antibodies and nucleotide sequencing demonstrates differences according to animal species and/or geographical origin. Rabies caused by other lyssaviruses may be diagnosed by the standard direct fluorescent antibody (DFA) test on brain tissue or by suggested antemortem tests. Several other lyssaviruses (e.g., Aravan virus, Irkut virus, Khujand virus, Lagos bat virus, West Caucasian bat virus, Shimoni bat virus, Bokeloh bat lyssavirus, Ikoma lyssavirus, Lleida bat lyssavirus, and Gannoruwa bat lyssavirus) have been characterized as etiological agents of rabies in mammals but so far have not been identified in human infections.[1]

**3. Laboratory diagnosis**—Rabies can present in atypical forms, and medical personnel unfamiliar with the disease may misdiagnose it. Confirmatory diagnosis is made through specific postmortem fluorescent antibody (FA) staining of brain tissue or virus isolation in mouse or cell cultures. Antemortem diagnosis can be made by specific FA staining of viral antigens in frozen skin sections taken from the back of the neck at the hairline; detection of viral antibodies in serum and cerebrospinal fluid (CSF); and specific amplification of viral nucleic acids in saliva or skin biopsies by reverse transcription polymerase chain reaction (RT-PCR). Serological diagnosis is based on neutralization tests in cell culture or in mice. Viral shedding in body secretions is intermittent, and therefore the absence of virus or nucleic acids in those secretions does not exclude rabies as a diagnosis. A combination of tests for detection of rabies specific antibodies, antigens, and nucleic acids is therefore needed for conclusive antemortem diagnosis.

**4. Laboratory capability**—Antemortem testing for rabies is currently available at the following locations: CDC Poxvirus and Rabies Branch (https://www.cdc.gov/rabies/specific_groups/doctors/ante_mortem.html); Viral and Rickettsial Disease Laboratory, California Department of Public Health; and NY Department of Health, Wadsworth Center (https://www.wadsworth.org/programs/id/rabies/antemortem-human-testing). The WHO Reference Centers may also provide testing on humans to rule out rabies. Locations of WHO Collaborating Centers for Rabies can be found at: http://apps.who.int/whocc/List.aspx?tor=rabies&. Antemortem testing requires a high degree of expertise in performance and the interpretation of all the antemortem tests including indirect fluorescent antibody test for rabies-specific immunoglobulin class G (IgG); IgM antibodies in serum and CSF; rapid fluorescent focus inhibition test (RFFIT) for viral neutralizing antibodies in serum and CSF samples; DFA for rabies virus (RABV) antigen on cryosections of the nuchal (skin) biopsy; and real-time RT-PCRs on saliva and nuchal biopsy samples. Laboratories performing antemortem testing for rabies diagnosis in humans within the USA should be certified as compliant with the Clinical Laboratory Improvement Amendments of 1988 (CLIA). According to these regulations, only testing personnel who are competency assessed annually can test antemortem human samples to rule out rabies. In addition, laboratories are required to participate in 2 proficiency tests annually for each of the antemortem tests for rabies diagnosis according to CLIA regulations.

Postmortem testing for rabies in animals and humans may be performed at CDC, state public health laboratories, and some state veterinary diagnostic laboratories within the USA. Rabies testing in animals may be performed in a variety of different types of laboratories around the world. It is important to check which laboratories are qualified to perform such testing by checking with the country's ministry of health and the regional WHO office. Rabies testing personnel should be assessed to demonstrate competency annually, and the laboratory should enroll in a minimum of 2 semi-annual proficiency tests for DFA on brain tissues.

**5. Safety requirements**—All indigenous lyssaviruses in the Americas are RABVs (belong to phylogroup 1) and require a minimum handling at biological safety level 2 (BSL-2) conditions. Samples from international regions where phylogroup 2 and 3 lyssaviruses are enzootic require a minimum handling at BSL-3 level. Personnel working with RABV are required to have preexposure rabies prophylaxis and demonstrate a viral neutralizing antibody (VNA) titer of complete neutralization at 1:5 or 0.5 IU/ml before entering an area where rabies testing is performed. The general rules of laboratory safety should be followed, including appropriate personal protective equipment (PPE) such as safety glasses, laboratory coat, double gloves, and closed-toed shoes; use of pipetting devices (no mouth pipetting); and no eating, drinking, or smoking within the laboratory. All aerosol-generating procedures with potentially infectious materials need to be performed in a biological safety cabinet and require wearing of double gloves and closed-front gowns. All work surfaces, equipment, and disposable materials need to be decontaminated before use, reuse, or discarding. Work surfaces can be decontaminated with common disinfectants (1:256 quaternary ammonium compounds, 70% ethanol or isopropanol, 0.5% sodium hypochlorite, and some commercial iodophor). Instruments used in necropsy should be decontaminated by an autoclave cycle at 121°C for 60 minutes. Chemical disinfectants may not inactivate RABV on instruments contaminated with tissues. PPE should be removed and hands should be washed prior to leaving the laboratory.[2,3]

**6. Nonhuman hosts**—Rabies is a zoonotic disease and the only major disease in which diagnosis in an animal directly affects human prophylaxis. All mammals may be infected with lyssaviruses. The predominate rabies reservoir host species in the USA are bats; skunks in north central states, south central states and California; foxes in Alaska, Texas, and Arizona; raccoons in the eastern USA; and mongoose in Puerto Rico. Internationally, lyssavirus major reservoir host species include dogs, bats, skunks, mongoose, foxes, jackals, wild dogs, ferret badgers, wolves, and raccoon dogs. Nonreservoir domestic and wild mammals can be infected if bitten by a rabid animal. These animals can also transmit the disease to humans and other mammals.[4]

**7. Sample/specimen requirements**—The validity of diagnostic tests depends on the collection of the appropriate samples, maintenance of optimal storage temperatures, and appropriate packaging for samples in transit. Clinicians in the USA should consult with their state health department first and then the CDC rabies duty officer by phone (404-639-1050) prior to submission of antemortem samples for rabies diagnosis in humans. Four samples can be collected with minimum invasiveness (serum, CSF, saliva, and nuchal [skin] biopsy). All 4 are required. Serum and CSF (minimum of 0.5 ml each) can be collected and shipped without anticoagulants or preservatives for rabies serologic testing. These samples should be collected within a day of shipment to best reflect the patient's current antibody levels. Serum and CSF samples for rabies serologic testing may be kept for short intervals at 4°C prior to testing but should be stored long-term at −20°C or below. Saliva (minimum of 1 ml) should be collected aseptically using a transfer (dropper) pipet, kept cold, and stored at −70°C or below for real-time RT-PCR testing. Nuchal (skin) full-punch biopsy of 5–6 mm diameter is collected from the nape of the neck at the hairline and placed in a sterile container on gauze moistened with sterile water. The biopsy should contain a minimum of 10 hair follicles and should be kept cold (4°C) after collection, if possible stored and shipped at −70°C or below for real-time RT-PCR and antigen detection by DFA. The invasiveness and potential harmful sequelae related to brain biopsies and corneal impressions make collection of these samples for antemortem diagnosis unwarranted;

however, if available they should be stored at −70°C or below and can be tested by DFA or real-time RT-PCR.

Postmortem testing for rabies in humans and animals requires the appropriate central nervous system (CNS) tissues to test the maximum ascending and descending nerve tracts. The standard DFA protocol on fresh (unfixed) brain for diagnosis in the USA requires testing of a full cross-section of the brain stem from medulla, pons, or the midbrain and of the cerebellum from vermis, right and left lobes. If cerebellum is unavailable, testing of both hippocampi may be substituted, but rabies can only be ruled out if a full cross-section of brain stem is tested. The same CNS tissues may also be tested by real-time RT-PCR. Although samples for antigen detection by DFA may be stored for short intervals at 4°C (24–48 hours) or −20°C prior to testing, unfixed brain for rabies virus antigen detection, virus isolation, and RT-PCR require optimal and long-term storage at −70°C or below. If fresh frozen brain tissues are unavailable then formalin-fixed brain tissues may be suitable for rabies diagnosis. However, the same CNS tissues are required. The testing of fixed tissues requires tissue processing, embedding, sectioning, and immunohistochemistry (IHC) procedures, which can delay the final result as much as 1 week. Formalin-fixed samples should be stored and shipped at ambient temperature and never frozen or shipped on dry ice.

Antemortem human samples (saliva, skin, serum, CSF,) and unfixed postmortem CNS samples from animals or humans for rabies diagnosis, and rabies virus positive CNS tissues for confirmation and typing should be shipped as UN 3373 Biological Substance, category B, on dry ice. Please consult with the International Air Transport Association and the US Department of Transportation websites and resources for updated information on shipment of specimens and hazardous goods.[3]

Clinicians and laboratorians outside of the USA should consult with their respective ministry of health and regional WHO office to determine the availability of rabies testing in their location and the specimen collection guidelines that apply.

**8. Testing requirements**—Current laboratory tests for rabies include (a) antigen detection tests targeting primarily RABV nucleoprotein (DFA, direct rapid immunohistochemistry test [DRIT], IHC, and lateral flow assays [LFAs]); (b) serologic tests for rabies antibodies that bind to specific viral proteins, nucleoprotein, or glycoprotein (indirect fluorescent antibody test and enzyme-linked immunosorbent assay), and neutralizing antibody tests (rapid fluorescent foci inhibition test [RFFIT] and fluorescent antibody virus neutralization test [FAVN]); (c) virus isolation tests (inoculation of cell cultures [mouse neuroblastoma cells/MNA, baby hamster kidney/BHK] or mouse inoculation [3-week-old or neonatal mice]); (d) molecular tests for rabies virus nucleic acid (real-time RT-PCR, traditional RT-PCR or hemi-nested RT-PCR); and (e) antigenic typing with monoclonal antibodies and genetic typing by virus sequencing (Sanger, pyrosequencing, next-generation sequencing).[5]

1) Antigen detection tests: currently, the only WHO/OIE recognized test for rabies antigen detection is the DFA test. DFA is the standard protocol for diagnosis of rabies in postmortem brain tissues in humans and animals in the USA. Although the standard DFA test has a sensitivity and specificity of 99.9%, the reliability of the test depends on the quality assurance practices outlined in the procedure. Before performing the DFA test, the antirabies conjugates must be titrated to determine the optimal working dilutions by broad and narrow titrations against a minimum of 2 different RABV variants seen in the laboratory's geographical region. Although commercially available conjugates contain pan-reactive (monoclonal or polyclonal) antibodies, the affinity of conjugates may vary with different rabies variants. Use of 2 antirabies conjugates in every test ensures maximum epitope recognition. In addition, the protocol requires adequate sampling of brain tissues from the brainstem (cross-section through pons or medulla) and cerebellum (vermis, right and left lobes) to test maximum ascending and descending nerve tracts. The condition of the sample and criteria for acceptance are important. If tissue autolysis, substantial discoloration, or desiccation is present, then testing for antigen may be unreliable because the viral proteins antigens may be denatured. If the sample condition is unacceptable and no RABV antigen is detected, then the results must be reported as inconclusive. The protocol requires processing each sample in separate containers to avoid the possibility of cross-contamination. For quality assurance, 2 readers independently evaluate each set of test slides. If discrepant results occur between the reactions of the 2 conjugates or the interpretations of the 2 readers, then repeat testing is required. The standard DFA test protocol requires repeat testing of all weakly positive and inconclusive tests using 2 antirabies conjugates and a specificity (negative) control conjugate paired with 1 of the 2 antirabies conjugates in a confirmatory DFA test. Although the DFA is the only antigen detection test currently recognized by WHO and OIE, the DRIT has been used as a field test for surveillance purposes for over a decade and is recognized as an alternative test for RABV antigen detection. The test may be useful for field applications and in laboratories without a fluorescence microscope since only minimal equipment is required. The test is currently being reviewed by WHO and OIE as a diagnostic test for rabies. Sensitivity of the DRIT approximates that of the DFA test. Unlike the DRIT, the currently available commercial LFA kits have not demonstrated sufficient reliability to be used as a screening test especially when test results will be used to make postexposure prophylaxis recommendations.[6]

2) Serologic tests: rabies specific IgG and IgM antibodies in serum and CSF samples are detected by an indirect fluorescent antibody test. This is an in vitro procedure performed on 4-well slides coated with RABV infected MNA cell monolayers and can be completed in a few hours. The indirect fluorescent antibody test can detect the presence of both IgM (indicative of recent or primary infection) and IgG in serum and CSF against RABV proteins (primarily the nucleoprotein). The indirect fluorescent antibody test is valid if the positive and negative controls give the expected values. The endpoint titer is the last dilution of the sample (serum or CSF), which demonstrates 2+ specific fluorescence of rabies antigen within cells. The presence of rabies specific IgG and IgM antibodies in serum or CSF is indicative of a rabies infection.

   Neutralization tests are the standard tests for detection of antibodies to the RABV glycoprotein. The RFFIT, FAVN, and mouse neutralization (MNT) are highly specific tests which measure the ability of anti-RABV antibodies in serum or CSF samples to neutralize a known standard challenge virus dose. The RFFIT and FAVN (a modification of the RFFIT micro-neutralization test performed in microtiter plates instead of chamber slides) are most frequently used to determine the immunization status of vaccinated humans and animals.[7,8] Demonstration of complete neutralization at a 1:5 serum dilution, as required by the Advisory Committee on Immunization Practices (ACIP), or 0.5 IU/ml, by WHO, are considered indicators of an adequate adaptive immune response. The presence of RABV neutralizing antibodies in serum or CSF of patient with encephalitis without previous rabies postexposure prophylaxis or intravenous immunoglobulin is indicative of rabies infection. Monitoring of rabies VNA levels in serum and CSF of human rabies cases under experimental rabies antiviral treatment protocols is essential.

3) Nucleic acid detection: RT-PCR–based diagnostic methods have been used for decades for antemortem rabies diagnosis when brain tissues were unavailable. Although traditional primary RT-PCR tests have a sensitivity of detection of approximately 1 infectious unit, detection of RNA in antemortem samples such as saliva and nuchal biopsy samples or other antemortem fluids is very limited and often below the detection of primary RT-PCR. Nested or hemi nested RT-PCR, additional amplification using 1/10 of the primary RT-PCR using degenerate or short primers inside the original primers sets and an additional 40 cycles of PCR, have been used to produce specific amplicons when rabies virus RNA was extremely limited. Disadvantages of the method were the time required for hemi-nested or nested RT-PCR, low annealing temperatures used to

gain sensitivity cause nonspecific amplicons, the requirement to sequence all amplicons of the approximate target molecular weight adding additional time, and the possibility of contamination if extreme care was not taken during the nested PCR procedures. Recently, broadly reactive rapid real-time RT-PCR assays have been developed for the detection of all lyssaviruses.[9,10] A newly developed real-time RT-PCR assay named LN34, which uses a combination of degenerate primers and probes, has been developed and validated at CDC for antemortem human and confirmatory postmortem animal testing covered under CLIA. The testing has demonstrated sensitivity and specificity equal to that of the DFA in evaluations to date. The primers and probes of the LN34 assay target the highly conserved noncoding leader region and part of the nucleoprotein (N) coding sequence of the Lyssavirus genome and have broad reactivity with all known lyssaviruses.

4) Quality assurance: the fluorescence microscope hours used for immunofluorescence assays should be checked to make sure not to exceed the maximum lamp life. Pipettors should be calibrated annually at a minimum. Diagnostic test worksheets should be reviewed by a technical supervisor before reporting results. All routine quality assurance monitoring (e.g., daily, monthly, and annually) for environmental air-handling, biological safety cabinets, equipment (e.g., refrigerators, freezers, incubators, autoclaves, and microscopes), and reagents apply to the earlier diagnostic tests and the other rabies procedures.

**9. Reporting requirements**—Rabies in humans and animals is on the National List of Reportable Diseases in the USA. The National Notifiable Disease Surveillance System staff works with the CDC Rabies Program and the Council of State and Territorial Epidemiologists to account for all rabies cases in the USA. Timely reporting of rabies cases in humans and animals by the testing laboratory is essential in providing appropriate postexposure prophylaxis to individuals needing treatment.

Clinicians and laboratorians outside the USA should consult with their respective ministry of health to determine if rabies, including animal rabies, is a reportable disease.

**10. Referral network**—Within the USA, antemortem rabies testing is provided by the CDC Poxvirus and Rabies Branch, the New York State Department of Health Rabies Laboratory, and the California Department of Public Health Viral and Rickettsial Diseases Laboratory (see Laboratory Capability section in this chapter). CDC provides confirmatory testing and variant typing of all positive antemortem and postmortem laboratory-diagnosed human cases within the USA. In addition, confirmatory postmortem testing of indeterminate and positive tests in animals and variants typing is provided by CDC when unavailable in the states and on all positive canines and nonreservoir host species.

Laboratorians outside the USA should consult with their respective ministry of health and regional WHO office to determine the availability of rabies referral networks that serve their country or region.

**11. Special considerations**—For further information regarding rabies preexposure and postexposure rabies prophylaxis, the ACIP recommendations are available at: https://www.cdc.gov/mmwr/preview/mmwrhtml/rr5703a1.htm.

Similarly, further information is available as follows:

- Animal immunization: http://www.nasphv.org/Documents/NASPHVRabiesCompendium.pdf.
- Wisconsin human rabies treatment protocol: http://www.mcw.edu/Pediatrics/Infectious-Diseases/Patient-Care/Rabies.htm.
- Rabies surveillance in the USA: http://avmajournals.avma.org/doi/pdfplus/10.2460/javma.248.7.777.

The CDC rabies duty officer may be contacted by phone (404-639-1050) for consultation regarding rabies in humans and animals.

## References


1. Gunawardena PS, Marston DA, Ellis RJ, et al. Lyssavirus in Indian flying foxes, Sri Lanka. *Emerg Infect Dis*. 2016;22(8):1456–1459.
2. US Department of Health and Human Services, Centers for Disease Control and Prevention, National Institutes of Health. *Biosafety in Microbiological and Biomedical Laboratories*. 5th ed. 2009. Available at: https://www.cdc.gov/labs/pdf/CDC-BiosafetyMicrobiologicalBiomedicalLaboratories-2009-P.PDF. Accessed March 7, 2019.
3. Orciari LA, Hanlon CA, Franka R. Rabies virus. In: Jorgensen JH, Pfaller MA, Carroll KC, et al., eds. *Manual of Clinical Microbiology*. 11th ed. Washington, DC: ASM Press; 2015:1633–1643.
4. Xiaoyue M, Monroe BP, Cleaton JM, et al. Rabies surveillance in the United States during 2016. *J Am Vet Med Assoc*. 2018;252(8):945–957.
5. World Health Organization. WHO expert consultation on rabies: second report. 2013. Available at: http://www.who.int/iris/handle/10665/85346. Accessed March 11, 2019.
6. Eggerbauer E, de Benedictis P, Hoffmann B, et al. Evaluation of six commercially available rapid immunochromatographic tests for the diagnosis of rabies in brain material. *PLoS Negl Trop Dis*. 2016;10(6):e0004776
7. Smith JS, Yager PA, Baer GM. A rapid fluorescent focus inhibition test (RFFIT) for determining rabies virus neutralizing antibody. In: Meslin FX, Kaplan MM, Koprowski H, eds. *Laboratory Techniques in Rabies*. 4th ed. Geneva, Switzerland: World Health Organization; 1996:181–192.
8. Briggs DJ, Smith JS, Mueller FL, et al. A comparison of two serological methods for detecting the immune response after rabies vaccination in dogs and cats being exported to rabies-free areas. *Biologicals*. 1998;26(4):347–55.

9. Hoffmann B, Freuling CM, Wakeley PR, et al. Improved safety for molecular diagnosis of classical rabies viruses by use of a TaqMan real-time reverse transcription-PCR "double check" strategy. *J Clin Microbiol*. 2010;48(11):3970–3978.
10. Wadhwa A, Wilkins K, Gao J, et al. A pan-*Lyssavirus* Taqman real-time RT-PCR assay for the detection of highly variable rabies virus and other lyssaviruses. *PLoS Negl Trop Dis*. 2017;11(1):e0005258.

[L. A. Orciari, P. S. Satheshkumar]

# RAT-BITE FEVER

(streptobacillary fever, Haverhill fever, epidemic arthritic erythema, spirillary fever, sodoku)

| DISEASE | ICD-10 CODE |
|---|---|
| STREPTOBACILLOSIS | ICD-10 A25.1 |
| SPIRILLOSIS | ICD-10 A25.0 |

**1. Clinical features**—The general term "rat-bite fever" refers to 2 rare bacterial zoonoses—streptobacillosis and spirillosis—that have similar clinical features. In streptobacillosis, an abrupt onset of fever, headache, vomiting, and muscle pain is followed within 2–4 days by a maculopapular rash most marked on the extremities. The rash can also be petechial, purpuric, or pustular. A nonsuppurative polyarthritis can develop in more than half of cases. There is usually a history of a rodent bite, which healed normally within the previous 10 days. Bacterial endocarditis, pericarditis, parotitis, tenosynovitis, and focal abscesses of soft tissues or the brain can occur late in untreated cases. Symptoms usually resolve within 2 weeks without treatment, but relapses often occur, with an approximate case-fatality rate of 7%–10%. Spirillosis disease differs from streptobacillosis in the presence of an indurated or ulcerated lesion at the site of the bite when fever develops, in the rarity of arthritic symptoms, and in the presence of a distinctive rash of reddish or purplish plaques. Complications may resemble those of streptobacillosis. Untreated, the case-fatality rate is approximately 10%.

**2. Causative agents**—*Streptobacillus moniliformis* for streptobacillosis, *Spirillum minus* for spirillosis.

**3. Laboratory diagnosis**—Laboratory confirmation of streptobacillosis is through isolation of the organism by inoculating material from the primary lesion, lymph node, blood, joint fluid, or pus into the appropriate bacteriological medium enriched with 20% serum or ascitic fluid or into laboratory animals (guinea pigs or mice that are not naturally infected).

Subcultures will grow on agar supplemented with 5% sheep blood after 2–5 days in microaerophilic conditions (5%–10% $CO_2$) at 37°C. Addition of horse or rabbit blood/serum to the agar is equally successful. The organism is a fastidious, slow-growing organism; therefore, cultures should be maintained for 10 days following inoculation. Animal inoculation alone is used for isolation of *S. minus* since it has not been successfully cultured on artificial media. Serological tests are not available currently for either streptobacillary or spirillary rat-bite fever and were found to be unreliable.

**4. Laboratory capability**—Specialized laboratory facilities are not required for initial isolation and identification of the organism. However, *S. moniliformis* is rather fastidious, growing best in 10% carbon dioxide and will not grow in liquid media containing Liquoid (sodium polyethanol sulphonate [SPS]). Reference facilities for molecular methodology may be necessary to identify the organism from culture-negative specimens.

**5. Safety requirements**—Biosafety level 2 procedures are recommended. *S moniliformis* is not readily transmissible from samples, and cultures can be handled on the open bench, although aerosol generation should be avoided. Infected laboratory rats and mice have transmitted infection through bites or handling.

**6. Nonhuman hosts**—The natural host is the rat, but *S. moniliformis* has also been isolated from guinea pigs, gerbils, and squirrels, with reports of infection in koalas, cats, turkeys, and primates. Zoonotic transmission via rat, dog, and cat bites has been reported. Evidence of transmission from some of these animals to humans has been found in genotyping studies, although apart from bites and possibly exposure to urine or conjunctival secretions, the actual routes of transmission are obscure.

Sodoku (the Japanese term for the much rarer form of rat bite fever) is caused by *S. minus*, occurring mostly in Asia. *S. minus* cannot be cultured in the laboratory, necessitating animal inoculation.

**7. Sample/specimen requirements**—Alerting the laboratory to suspicion of the diagnosis enables appropriate sample handling and culture techniques.

Blood, tissue, and cerebrospinal and synovial fluids may be Gram-stained and cultured. SPS, an anticoagulant found in many aerobic bottles of commercial blood culture systems, inhibits growth; hence, *S. moniliformis* is usually first isolated in anaerobic blood–culture media.

**8. Testing requirements**—The organism is fastidious, nonmotile, and nonacid-fast. Depending on cultural age and conditions (e.g., whether from agar or liquid culture), *S. moniliformis* is usually Gram negative but can be highly pleomorphic. When appearing as single rods, arranged in chains, or unbranched filaments with occasional bulbar swellings, this string-of-beads appearance gives rise to species name (*moniliformis* = necklace).

*S. moniliformis* grows best in media with added serum, ascitic fluid, blood, and yeast extract. Subcultures will grow on agar supplemented with 5% sheep blood after 2–5 days in microaerophilic conditions (5%–10% $CO_2$) at 37°C.

Selective media incorporating colistin, sulfamethoxazole-trimethoprim, and nalidixic acid may aid growth from samples overgrown with contaminants.

Colonies of *S. moniliformis* are usually nonhemolytic, smooth, convex, and glistening, between 1–2 mm in diameter, although occasionally a fried-egg appearance may result from L forms. Using tryptone soy broth supplemented with horse serum or serum-supplemented thioglycolate broth, colonies resembling cotton wool balls or bread crumbs appear in 2–7 days.

Presumptive biochemical testing is affected by poor growth and weak reactions. *S. moniliformis* is not very active in routine biochemical testing, being negative for catalase, urea, nitrate reduction, Voges-Proskauer, and indole production.

Confirmatory testing with matrix-assisted laser desorption/ionization time-of-flight mass spectrometry has been found to be reliable for species identification. Reference laboratories have successfully used molecular methods including 16S ribosomal ribonucleic acid polymerase chain reaction–sequencing in tissues such as heart valves and synovial fluid.

Slow growth also affects sensitivity testing and minimum inhibitory concentration interpretation, although generally penicillin, tetracycline, gentamicin, and azithromycin have been effective.

Confirmation of diagnosis is by inoculating aspirates of pus or blood into mice, producing bacteremia in 5–15 days.

*S. minus* spirochetes stain poorly with Gram stain and are better visualized with Giemsa staining or dark ground microscopy of exudate from ulcers or blood. The coiled spiral rods measure 0.2–0.5 mm by 3–5 mm.

There are as yet no available molecular diagnostic methods reported to diagnose *S. minus* infection.

**9. Reporting requirements**—Rat-bite fever is not routinely reportable in most countries, but laboratories should determine if there are special circumstances such as zoonotic transmission where reporting is warranted.

**10. Referral network**—Reference laboratories for confirmation where available and necessary. Within the USA, molecular testing and identification available at the CDC Infectious Diseases Pathology Branch.

**11. Special considerations**—None.

[M. Morgan]

# RELAPSING FEVER

(borrelia recurrentis, louse-borne relapsing fever)

| DISEASE | ICD-10 CODE |
|---|---|
| RELAPSING FEVER | ICD-10 A68 |

**1. Clinical features**—A systemic louse-borne epidemic or tickborne sporadic spirochetal disease in which periods of fever lasting 2–7 days alternate with afebrile periods of 4–14 days; the number of relapses varies from 1–10 or more. Total duration of louse-borne relapsing fever (LBRF) averages 13–16 days; usually longer for tickborne relapsing fever (TBRF). Other nonspecific signs and symptoms include headache, myalgia, arthralgia, shaking chills, and gastrointestinal pain or illness. Patients with LBRF are more likely to have jaundice, central nervous system involvement, petechial rashes, blood-tinged sputum, and epistaxsis. By contrast, acute respiratory distress syndrome has been reported more frequently in TBRF. Predisposing factors (poor nutrition and thiamine or vitamin B deficiency) may lead to more severe disease and neurological involvement. The overall case-fatality rate in untreated cases is between 2%–10%.

**2. Causative agents**—Helical and motile spirochetes of the genus *Borrelia. Borrelia recurrentis* is the sole agent of human-specific LBRF and is spread from person to person by the human body louse. *Borrelia duttoni* also appears to be a human-specific pathogen but is 1 of more than 10 species that cause TBRF. All TBRF species are transmitted by soft-bodied (argasid) ticks except for *Borrelia miyamotoi,* which causes the only confirmed hard-tick transmitted TBRF. Both LBRF and TBRF spirochetes demonstrate antigenic variation in parallel with successive relapses. In North America, most human cases of TBRF are caused by *Borrelia hermsii* transmitted by the soft-bodied tick *Ornithodoros hermsi*. The classical agent of relapsing fever in Europe is *Borrelia hispanica*, also tickborne.

**3. Laboratory diagnosis**—The spiral shaped bacteria range in length from 7–30 μm and in width from 0.2–0.5 μm and stain poorly with Gram stain reagents. They are best detected in peripheral blood (febrile periods most sensitive) and visualized in wet mounts by dark-field microscopy (where corkscrew motility assists detection) or in Giemsa- or Wright-based stained smears with bright-field microscopy. Detection of spirochetes during afebrile and late-stage febrile periods is generally insensitive. Weanling mice and specialized liquid culture media (Barbour-Stoenner, Kelly [BSK]) may serve as amplifying environments to increase the sensitivity of subsequent microscopic detection but are normally impractical for the routine clinical laboratory.

Increasingly polymerase chain reaction (PCR) methods (e.g., based on 16S rRNA, *glpQ*, p41 and multilocus sequence typing [MLST]) are used that have a higher sensitivity compared with microscopic methods and enable species identification.

**4. Laboratory capability**—Laboratory facilities corresponding to biosafety level 2 (BSL-2) are required to work on *Borrelia* (see Safety Requirements section in this chapter). Most clinical and public health laboratories with trained microbiologists should be capable of providing diagnostic support for relapsing fever.

Laboratory personnel are required to be familiar with doing thin/thick blood smears; staining techniques (e.g., Giemsa, DAPI); light, immunofluorescence; and dark-field microscopy. Moreover, personnel familiar with PCR methods, sequencing, and sequence comparison, are recommended since these techniques are necessary for definite identification of the pathogens and most probably have a higher diagnostic sensitivity when compared with light microscopy. Experience in the difficult cultivation of *Borrelia* sp. causing relapsing fever is desirable.

**5. Safety requirements**—BSL-2 is required for handling patient samples or other material containing or suspected to contain these agents. Laboratory personnel must have specific training regarding handling of *Borrelia* sp. causing relapsing fever and must be supervised by a competent scientist. Access to the laboratory must be strictly limited during specific work. Because of a possibly high pathogen load, the handling of sharp items requires extreme precautions. Any procedures that pose a danger of infecting laboratory personnel (e.g., through aerosols) must be carried out in biological safety cabinets. For further information, see "Laboratory Safety Practices: Building a Strong Biosafety Program."

**6. Nonhuman hosts**—The only known host for *B. recurrentis* (louse-borne) is humans. Hosts for TBRF-*Borrelia* are rodents and, due to transovarial transmission, the ticks itself.

**7. Sample/specimen requirements**—Ethylenediaminetetraacetic acid (EDTA)-blood specimen is best taken at the beginning of or during a febrile episode. Blood taken between febrile episodes usually is negative by microscopic techniques. Cerebrospinal fluid should be collected in the case of neurological involvement. The laboratory should be informed about a suspected case of relapsing fever before any samples are sent. Transportation of samples should occur as soon as possible, and samples should be sent at ambient temperature. If sample processing is not possible the same day, samples should be held at 2°C–8°C.

**8. Testing requirements**—The screening for relapsing fever includes the direct detection of spirochetes in EDTA blood by dark-field or phase-contrast microscopy and/or on stained blood films (e.g., Giemsa, acridine orange). The lack of specificity of this procedure only allows for a report stating that spirochetes are detectable in blood. The sensitivity is estimated to be 70% and is highest in blood taken during a febrile period. There are no specific quality assurance measures required beyond those which are necessary for all diagnostic laboratory procedures.

Culture can be performed in specialized laboratories from EDTA blood using BSK or modified Kelly-Pettenkofer medium. The sensitivity is unclear. Successful culture must be confirmed by molecular biological methods (PCR and sequencing). Positive and negative control cultures are required to be run in parallel.

PCR testing is performed in specialized laboratories and includes sequencing of 16S rRNA, *glpQ*, and/or *flaB*. The sensitivity of PCR is estimated to be higher than microscopy. The specificity is high. Quality assurance must include positive, negative, and contamination controls.

Confirmatory testing is carried out using MLST. Quality assurance must include positive, negative, and contamination controls.

**9. Reporting requirements**—The required reporting of cases of relapsing fever by laboratories varies by country and region. Laboratories should determine what their reporting requirements are for their respective jurisdictions. Nevertheless, relapsing fever should immediately be reported to the responsible public health authorities to enable respective measures: search for additional cases, source of infection, and establishment of respective hygiene measures.

**10. Referral network**—There are no laboratory referral networks for relapsing fever; however, in case of suspect cases the primary testing laboratory may need to contact a reference laboratory with experience in tropical medicine and/or their national public health laboratory.

**11. Special considerations**—For LBRF, the fatality rate can reach more than 40% in untreated cases and even 2%–5% under treatment, mostly due to a Jarisch Herxheimer reaction. This reaction, which occurs within a few hours after start of treatment, is induced by a massive cytokine release resulting in a worsening of symptoms including generalized malaise, high fever, rigors, tachycardia, and initially hypertension, followed by hypotension and headache. Therefore, treatment of LBRF should be initiated in a setting with emergency equipment.

## Bibliography

Centers for Disease Control and Prevention. Tick-borne relapsing fever (TBRF). Available at: https://www.cdc.gov/relapsing-fever/index.html. Accessed March 11, 2019.

European Centre for Disease Prevention and Control. Facts about louse-borne relapsing fever. Available at: https://ecdc.europa.eu/en/louse-borne-relapsing-fever/facts. Accessed March 11, 2019.

European Centre for Disease Prevention and Control. Facts about tickborne relapsing fever. Available at: https://ecdc.europa.eu/en/tick-borne-relapsing-fever/facts. Accessed March 11, 2019.

[V. Fingerle]

# RICKETTSIOSES
(spotted fever group)

| DISEASE | CAUSATIVE AGENT | ICD-10 CODE |
|---|---|---|
| ROCKY MOUNTAIN SPOTTED FEVER (FIEBRE MACULOSA, SAO PAULO FEVER, BRAZILIAN SPOTTED FEVER ) | *Rickettsia rickettsii* | ICD-10 A77.0 |
| BOUTONNEUSE FEVER (MEDITERRANEAN SPOTTED FEVER, MARSEILLES FEVER, ISRAELI TICK TYPHUS, ASTRAKHAN FEVER, INDIAN TICK TYPHUS) | *Rickettsia conorii* and closely related organisms | ICD-10 A77.1 |
| AFRICAN TICK-BITE FEVER | *Rickettsia africae* | ICD-10 A77.8 |
| QUEENSLAND TICK TYPHUS | *Rickettsia australis* | ICD-10 A77.3 |
| NORTH ASIAN TICK TYPHUS (SIBERIAN TICK TYPHUS) | *Rickettsia sibirica* | ICD-10 A77.2 |
| TICKBORNE LYMPHADENOPATHY (TIBOLA), DERMACENTOR-BORNE NECROSIS AND LYMPHADENOPATHY (DEBONEL) | *Rickettsia slovaca, R. raoultii* | ICD-10 A77.x |
| FLINDERS ISLAND SPOTTED FEVER (THAI TICK TYPHUS) | *Rickettsia honei; Rickettsia honei* strain *marmionii* | ICD-10 A77.x |
| FAR-EASTERN SPOTTED FEVER | *Rickettsia heilongjiangensis* | ICD-10 A77.x |
| JAPANESE SPOTTED FEVER | *Rickettsia japonica* | ICD-10 A77.x |
| *RICKETTSIA PARKERI* RICKETTSIOSIS (TIDEWATER SPOTTED FEVER) | *Rickettsia parkeri* | ICD-10 A77.x |
| *RICKETTSIA FELIS* RICKETTSIOSIS (CAT FLEA-ASSOCIATED TYPHUS) | *Rickettsia felis* | ICD-10 A77.x |
| RICKETTSIALPOX (VESICULAR RICKETTSIOSIS) | *Rickettsia akari* | ICD-10 A79.1 |
| OTHER SPOTTED FEVER (multiple species newly recognized as causes of human illness) | *Rickettsia aeschlimanni, Rickettsia massiliae, Rickettsia monacensis,* and others | ICD 77.8 |

**1. Clinical features**—Spotted fever group rickettsial infections are a closely related group of primarily tickborne bacterial infections causing clinically similar diseases characterized by fever, rash, and vasculitis. Although clinical presentations and severity vary by species, some spotted fever infections can be associated with multiorgan involvement such as respiratory failure, hepatosplenomegaly, heart failure, renal failure, bleeding, and neurological complications.

1) Rocky Mountain spotted fever (RMSF) ranges greatly in severity and can be mild if treated early or rapidly fatal in some patients if appropriate treatment is not initiated before day 5 of symptoms. It is characterized by the sudden onset of moderate to high fever, significant malaise, deep muscle pain, severe headache, chills, and conjunctival injection. A maculopapular rash appears on the extremities on the third to fifth day in many patients; the rash includes the palms and soles in about 30% and spreads rapidly to the body trunk. A petechial exanthem generally occurs on or after the sixth day and is often associated with vascular and end organ damage. Every effort should be made to treat the disease before this time and prevent petechiae from developing. The case-fatality rate ranges from 20%–80% in different regions in the absence of treatment; with prompt recognition and treatment, death is uncommon. Median duration between symptom onset and death is 8 days in fatal cases, even in previously healthy people. The primary risk factor associated with more severe disease and death is delayed antibiotic therapy. Factors that make the disease more difficult to diagnose increase the risk of delayed treatment and therefore death. These factors include absence or delayed appearance of the typical rash, or failure to recognize it, especially in dark-skinned individuals; occurrence of the disease outside the typical seasonality; or occurrence of disease outside the established geographic distribution. Tick exposure reports are often misleading, as tick bites are typically painless and go unrecognized by patients. Low platelets, low sodium, and elevated liver enzymes are frequently observed in RMSF patients. The early stages of RMSF may be confused with ehrlichiosis, meningococcemia (see "Meningitis"), enteroviral infection, dengue, and many other febrile illnesses.
2) Mediterranean spotted fever (MSF) is a mild to severe febrile illness with abrupt onset; there may be a primary lesion or eschar at the site of a tick bite. This eschar (tache noire), often evident at the onset of fever, is a small ulcer 2–5 mm in diameter with a black center and red areola; regional lymph nodes are often enlarged. A generalized maculopapular erythematous rash occurs about the fourth to fifth day.

With appropriate antibiotic therapy, fever typically resolves within 48 hours. The case-fatality rate varies by region.

3) African tick-bite fever is similar to MSF but typically has a milder course. Fatalities are rarely reported. Abrupt onset of fever, nausea, headache, and myalgia are common and may be accompanied by 1 or multiple inoculation eschars. Regional draining lymphangitis and aphthous stomatitis may occur. Rash is noticed in only half the cases and may be maculopapular or vesicular. Complications are rare and symptoms typically resolve after 10 days but resolve more quickly with appropriate antibiotics.
4) Queensland tick typhus is clinically similar to MSF; the rash may be vesicular.
5) North Asian tick typhus is clinically similar to MSF; rash and lymphadenitis are common.
6) Tickborne lymphadenopathy is a mild rickettsiosis; main symptoms include an eschar, often found on the head; regional lymphadenopathy; low-grade fever; and, in some cases, alopecia at eschar site.
7) Flinders Island spotted fever is a mild disease with maculopapular rash; eschar and adenopathy are rare.
8) Far-Eastern tickborne rickettsiosis is characterized by eschar, faint macular or maculopapular rash, lymphadenopathy, and lymphangitis and conjunctival papulae may be present.
9) Japanese spotted fever similarly involves eschar, macular, or maculopapular rash (which may become petechial), lymphadenopathy, and enlarged lymph nodes; fatalities have been described.
10) *Rickettsia parkeri* rickettsiosis is a mild febrile illness with eschar and maculopapular-to-vesicular rash.
11) *Rickettsia felis* rickettsiosis is a relatively mild illness characterized by fever, headache, myalgia, and cutaneous manifestations (rash, eschar, ulcer). Lymphadenopathy, neurological manifestations, abdominal symptoms, and pneumonia may also be observed in these patients.
12) Rickettsialpox is an acute febrile illness characterized by an initial skin lesion (eschar) at the site of the mite bite, followed by fever; a disseminated vesicular skin rash appears, which generally does not involve the palms or soles and lasts only a few days. It may be confused with chickenpox. Death is uncommon. Acute hepatitis may be one of the leading symptoms after infection and before development of specific vesicular rash.

**2. Causative agents**—See the earlier table for rickettsial species associated with each disease entity. Species are distributed in distinct geographical regions, and histories of recent travel to or residence in these areas can be very helpful information. Specific rickettsioses are acquired by humans in areas consistent with the geographic distribution of their respective causative agents and their tick vectors.

1) RMSF: throughout the USA and in Argentina, Brazil, Canada, Colombia, Mexico, and Central America. In most of the USA infections occur primarily from April through September, mainly in the Southeast and south central regions; highest incidence rates are seen in North Carolina and Oklahoma. A focus of RMSF in the Southwest has cases occurring year-round with most cases reported March–November.
2) MSF: widely distributed throughout the African continent, in India, and in those parts of Europe and the Middle East adjacent to the Mediterranean and the Black and Caspian Seas, where genetically distinguishable strains may be related to differential pathogenetic and clinical features. In more temperate areas, the highest incidence is during warmer months when ticks are numerous; in tropical areas, disease occurs throughout the year. In some areas such as in the Negev, Israel; Astrakhan, Russia; and Portugal, tache noire lesions (eschars) are less frequently seen with MSF infections.
3) African tick-bite fever: sub-Saharan Africa, including Botswana, South Africa, Swaziland, and Zimbabwe; the Lesser Antilles and the West Indies. Outbreaks of disease may occur when groups of travelers (such as people on safari in Africa) are bitten by ticks. Cases are occasionally imported into the USA and are one of the most common infections imported into Western Europe.
4) Queensland tick typhus: Queensland, New South Wales, Tasmania, and coastal areas of eastern Victoria, Australia.
5) North Asian tick fever: North China, Mongolia, and Asiatic areas of Russia.
6) Tickborne lymphadenopathy: Europe and Asia.
7) Flinders Island spotted fever: Australia, Thailand, Flinders Island, and Tasmania.
8) Far-Eastern tickborne rickettsiosis: Far East of Russia, northern China.
9) Japanese spotted fever: Japan, China, South Korea, the Philippines, and Thailand.
10) *Rickettsia parkeri* rickettsiosis: coastal and inland grassland regions of eastern USA, a focus in Southern Arizona, southern South America including Argentina, Uruguay, and parts of Brazil.
11) *Rickettsia felis* rickettsiosis: the pathogen appears to occur worldwide, although human cases are less widespread.
12) Rickettsialpox is caused by *Rickettsia akari* and is found primarily in urban cities in the USA and other parts of the world.

**3. Laboratory diagnosis**—Diagnosis of spotted fever group rickettsiosis requires a combination of laboratory tests and clinical suspicion. The indirect immunofluorescence assay (IFA) is the gold standard for serological diagnosis confirmation. Serological diagnosis is confirmed by a 4-fold or greater rise in specific antibody (immunoglobulin class G [IgG]) titer when comparing a patient's acute and convalescent sera. The acute sample should be taken in the first week of illness, and the convalescent should be taken 3–4 weeks after the acute sample. IFAs become positive generally in the second to third week of illness. *Rickettsia akari* and *R. africae* infections may require an interval of at least 28 days for demonstration of seroconversion. Therefore, an acute titer taken in the first week of illness should be used as a baseline for comparison with the convalescent sample; a negative acute result does not rule out active infection, nor does a positive acute result confirm the diagnosis without a concomitant 4-fold titer increase. It is advocated that a simple change from a negative to positive result does not meet the strict definition of 4-fold titer increase; rather, a seroconversion/4-fold increase from a negative acute phase response should require a minimum convalescent titer 4-fold or more above the screening dilution. Older Weil-Felix tests using Proteus OX-19 and Proteus OX-2 antigens are less sensitive and less specific and are not recommended for modern diagnostics. During acute stages of infection and prior to doxycycline treatment, spotted fever group rickettsiae can sometimes be detected by polymerase chain reaction (PCR) assays in blood and serum. More frequently detection can be achieved in skin biopsies using immunostains or PCR assays. Culturing blood or buffy coat on cell culture monolayers permits isolation of the organisms and facilitates precise confirmatory diagnosis. See the later table.

**4. Laboratory capability**—Most clinical laboratory procedures should be conducted in a facility with biosafety level-2 (BSL-2) facilities and practices. Propagative procedures should be conducted at BSL-3 for more highly pathogenic species due to the potential for aerosolization. Test loads are often not sufficient to support testing at a local clinical laboratory, so most testing is done at commercial laboratories or public health laboratories. Testing for human diagnostics should be conducted at ISO 15189- or Clinical Laboratory Improvement Amendments–certified laboratories using established procedures. Personnel should be trained by experienced laboratorians, and annual proficiency testing should be conducted. Cultivation of rickettsial agents requires higher level containment and strict aseptic procedures, as antibiotics in cell culture can inhibit rickettsial growth. Laboratory animals are rarely used for diagnostic procedures but if used will require BSL-3 facilities and practices.

**5. Safety requirements**—BSL-2 is required for work with specimens from patients suspected of rickettsial disease. Cultivation of the organisms from clinical or autopsy specimens should be conducted at BSL-3. Prophylactic antibiotics are not recommended, and no vaccine is available for laboratorians working with spotted fever group rickettsiae. Consistent use of universal/standard precautions is necessary.

**Testing Method, Strategy, Sensitivity, Specificity, and Availability**

| Testing Method | Test Strategy | Sensitivity | Specificity | Availability |
|---|---|---|---|---|
| Indirect immunofluorescence assay (IFA) | Screening; confirmatory if tested in acute/convalescent pairs to demonstrate seroconversions (taken to be 4-fold or greater rises in IgG antibodies) | IgG: 85%–100% IgM: 83%–85% | IgG: 99%–100% IgM: 40%–100% | Common; commercial laboratories, public health laboratories, universities |
| Enzyme-linked immunosorbent assay (ELISA) | Screening; current commercial kits provide qualitative results | IgG: 83% IgM: 98% | IgG: 87%–96% IgM: ≤94% | Limited; some commercial laboratories, public health laboratories may provide as screening before IFA testing |
| Polymerase chain reaction (PCR) assay | Screening; confirmatory if adequately diverse genes are targeted by specific assays or product is sequenced | 23%–69% | ≥99% | Limited, but increasing; commercial laboratories; public health laboratories, university research centers |
| Culture in cell lines | Screening; confirmatory if cultivable strain and sustained isolates are obtained | unknown | 100% | Limited; public health laboratories and university research centers; require prior approval |
| Immunohistochemistry of affected tissues | Screening; confirmatory at spotted fever group level | 70%–90% | 91%–100% | Limited; public health laboratories and university research centers |

**6. Nonhuman hosts**—Most spotted fever group infections are vector-borne zoonoses, and the causative rickettsial organisms are maintained in nature among a variety of hard-bodied tick species Acari: Ixodidae by transovarial and transstadial passage. Other species utilize mites or fleas as host and vector. Vertebrate animals may serve as reservoirs in some cases but may act as amplifier hosts to infect additional arthropods that feed during rickettsemic periods. Humans are inadvertent hosts only.

Organisms that cause both RMSF and MSF can be transmitted to dogs, rodents, and other animals; animal infections can be subclinical and short-lived, but persistent infections in rodents and disease in dogs have been observed. Dogs are useful sentinels for spotted fever group rickettsiae, and clustered cases of RMSF in humans and dogs can occur. Rodents and reptiles are the reservoir for Flinders Island and Japanese spotted fevers; rodents and lagomorphs for Far-Eastern tickborne rickettsiosis. The reservoirs for Flinders Island spotted fever are suspected to be reptiles, migratory birds, and rodents. *Rickettsia felis* can be found in cats, opossums, and cat fleas. *Rickettsia akari* is found primarily in house mice (*Mus musculus*) and can also infect other commensal or wild rodents.

The pathogens can be monitored within arthropod hosts for ecological surveillance and prediction of human risk. Primary arthropod vectors are geographically distributed with their pathogens as follows:

1) RMSF: *Dermacentor variabilis* (American dog tick), *Dermacentor andersoni* (Rocky Mountain wood tick), *Rhipicephalus sanguineus* (brown dog tick), and *Amblyomma cajennense* s.l. (cayenne tick).
2) Mediterranean spotted fever: *R. sanguineus* (brown dog tick).
3) African tick-bite fever: *Amblyomma hebraeum* (African bont tick) and *Amblyomma variegatum* (tropical bont tick).
4) Queensland tick typhus: *Ixodes holocyclus* (paralysis tick).
5) North Asian tick fever: *Dermacentor* and *Haemaphysalis* spp. ticks.
6) Tickborne lymphadenopathy: *Dermacentor marginatus* (ornate sheep tick).
7) Flinders Island spotted fever: *Aponomma hydrosauri* (southern reptile tick), *Ixodes tasmanii* (common marsupial tick), and *Ixodes granulatus*.
8) Far-Eastern tickborne rickettsiosis: *Dermacentor silvarum*, *Haemaphysalis concinna* (relict tick) and *Haemaphysalis japonica douglasii*.
9) Japanese spotted fever: *Haemaphysalis flava, Haemaphysalis longicornis,* and *Ixodes ovatus.*
10) *Rickettsia parkeri* rickettsiosis: *Amblyomma maculatum* (Gulf Coast tick) in the USA; subtype of *R. parkeri* is found in *Dermacentor parumapertus* in the western states; *A. triste* in South America.
11) *Rickettsia felis* rickettsiosis: *Ctenocephalides felis* (cat flea).
12) Rickettsialpox: *Liponyssoides sanguineus* (house mouse mite).

**7. Sample/specimen requirements**—Clinical specimens should be collected early in the illness and before appropriate antibiotic therapy is initiated. Convalescent samples should be taken 3–4 weeks later for serologic confirmation. Antibodies are not generally detectable until 7–10 days of infection, thus paired analysis provides more diagnostic strength than single-sample determinations. *Rickettsia africae* requires at least 28 days to show seroconversion, and this delayed response can occur in other spotted fever group infections. A third sample taken 2 weeks after the convalescent could be needed. Sera can be stored for several days at 4°C but should be frozen at −20°C or lower for longer periods.

The most useful specimen for nucleic acid diagnosis of rickettsial infection is affected tissue. Skin biopsies (3-mm diameter) from the rash can be extremely valuable if rash is present. If an eschar is present, a swab or biopsy sample of the lesion can be evaluated by PCR assay and can provide a species-specific diagnosis. Acute phase whole blood (ethylenediaminetetraacetic acid- or sodium citrate-anticoagulated), buffy coat, plasma, and serum are rarely positive in PCR assays due to low bacteremia in the acute stage and their residence in endothelial cells. As the acute disease progresses, more organisms/infected cells are released into the bloodstream, and sensitivity is improved. If unable to process whole blood, plasma, buffy coat, or tissue for PCR within several days, specimens should be stored at −20°C or lower. Autopsy tissues (e.g., skin, spleen, kidney, lung, brain) are valuable samples that can be used to confirm fatal cases.

All specimens should be refrigerated at 4°C or for transport refrigerated on ice packs via overnight shipping services. Freezing tissues or whole blood limits the available testing options and is not recommended for some testing methods. Formalin-fixed, paraffin-embedded tissues should be shipped at ambient or refrigerated temperatures to avoid damage to the tissue architecture. All samples should be handled using universal/standard precautions in the clinical and laboratory settings.

**8. Testing requirements**—Rickettsial diseases often present with vague, undifferentiated clinical features, so the most effective testing strategy is to utilize multiple diagnostic methodologies to confirm cases. IgM class antibodies can rise just before or alongside IgG increases and remain elevated for prolonged intervals, limiting their use as an indicator of acute infection, and IgM use alone is not advocated. Seroconversion in the IgG class are used by public health officials for surveillance purposes, and 4-fold rises in antibody titer are strong evidence for infection. Nucleic acid amplification methods, such as PCR assays, are encouraged, but samples obtained during the acute infection and at or prior to antirickettsial therapy are critical to the effective use of these methods. Skin biopsies taken from the rash site, eschar, or eschar scab are rich sources of rickettsial pathogens in the acute stage before antibiotic treatment. After antibiotics are initiated, the ability to detect rickettsial pathogens by PCR assays, immunohistochemistry, or culture progressively and rapidly declines.

Positive and negative controls must be included in all testing runs and performance characteristics of reagents and controls must be documented. Limited reference reagents can be obtained from CDC, but commercial kits and services are increasingly available for these diseases. Serologic cross-reactions can occur across the spotted fever group (and periodically across the typhus group) rickettsiae, permitting group-level testing when specific antigens are not readily available or known. For instance, *Rickettsia akari* has been used with success as a surrogate antigen for *Rickettsia felis* infection. Test results should be interpreted in the context of the clinical presentation.

**9. Reporting requirements**—Spotted fever group rickettsioses are reportable conditions in the USA and thus notifiable under passive public health surveillance. The recognition of an increasing number of species causing human disease in the USA and the importation of rickettsial disease through travel resulted in a broadening of the case definition to include more than Rocky Mountain spotted fever (infection by *R. rickettsii*). Case reporting is conducted through electronic reports and case report forms to state health departments, which then report this information on the national level. These data are summarized weekly and annually in published morbidity and mortality reports. Internationally, case reporting is obligatory for many of the spotted fever group rickettsial diseases in some countries. It is the responsibility of laboratories located outside the USA to determine if rickettsial diseases are required to be reported by laboratories to the public health authorities within their respective jurisdictions.

CDC accepts deposition of *Rickettsia* spp. isolates into its CDC Rickettsial Isolate Reference Collection (see World Data Center for Microorganisms Collection 1093 available at: http://www.wdcm.org). CDC maintains and distributes strains to researchers globally. Call 1-404-639-1075 for further information on submission requirements.

**10. Referral network**—Referral as described in "Reporting requirements."

**11. Special considerations**—Because of the rapid nature of disease progression with certain spotted fever group rickettsioses, empiric treatment with doxycycline is warranted, although specimens should be taken for laboratory testing as treatment is initiated.

Rickettsial diseases often occur as sporadic cases or in small clusters of cases. Disease can be recognized in affected pets sharing the same peridomestic space that act as sentinels for human infection. Communication between veterinary and medical professionals can facilitate detection and response.

Further information on rickettsioses can be found in *CCDM20* and is available at: https://www.cdc.gov/mmwr/volumes/65/rr/rr6502a1.htm.

[W. L. Nicholson, J. S. Dumler]

# RIFT VALLEY FEVER

| DISEASE | ICD-10 CODE |
|---|---|
| RIFT VALLEY FEVER | ICD-10 A92.4 |

**1. Clinical features**—Rift Valley fever (RVF) is a viral zoonosis that primarily affects animals but also has the capacity to infect humans. RVF virus infection can be unapparent or characterized by a brief, self-limiting febrile illness with a sudden onset of fever, myalgia, chills, dizziness, and headache, lasting for 3–4 days. Recovery is usually without sequelae. In a small proportion of cases (1%), the clinical syndrome progresses to a severe disease of 3 forms: ocular, meningoencephalitis, or hemorrhagic with liver failure. The appearance of shock, multiorgan failure, and disseminated intravascular coagulation are of poor prognosis. Laboratory findings may include elevated liver enzyme levels, thrombocytopenia, leukopenia, anemia, and elevated blood urea nitrogen and creatinine. Variable neurological sequelae are observed in survivors of RVF encephalitis. In about 1%–5% of all RVF patients, unilateral or bilateral retinal hemorrhages occur, resulting in transitory or permanent scotoma visual field defects. The overall case-fatality rate is low (1%–5%) but can reach 50% in hospitalized patients.

**2. Causative agents**—RVF virus is a member of the genus *Phlebovirus* family *Bunyaviridae*.

**3. Laboratory diagnosis**—During the acute phase of disease, virus can be detected from blood or serum by conventional or real-time polymerase chain reaction (PCR), virus isolation, or by antigen detection enzyme-linked immunosorbent assays (ELISA). Serological diagnosis (immunoglobulin class M [IgM], IgG) is made by ELISA. RVF virus–specific neutralizing antibodies persist for years. Antibodies appear a few days post-onset, and virus is very rapidly cleared. In fatal cases, the virus can be detected in tissues (liver) by molecular techniques, virus isolation, or by immunohistochemistry (IHC).

**4. Laboratory capability**—Clinical specimens from suspect patients should always be collected and handled with universal/standard precautions. Diagnostic reagents are available only at select reference laboratories. Suspect RVF clinical specimens should be processed by trained personnel using appropriate biosafety level 3 (BSL-3) facilities.

**5. Safety requirements**—RVF virus is considered a BSL-3 or BSL-4 agent depending on different country regulations; the classification is dependent on whether the virus is endemic in the country. No human vaccines are currently commercially available. Collection should be done by trained personal with appropriate personal protective equipment (PPE) such as disposable caps, gowns, shoe covers, surgical gloves, and face masks (N99 or N100 [HEPA] filters). Handling of infectious or suspected infectious clinical specimens should be performed in a BSL-3 facility by trained personnel with appropriate personal protective equipment and protocols. Manipulation of and collection of specimens from sick or dead animals could be the source of human infection if not done properly. Procedures generating aerosols (e.g., centrifugation) should be minimized. The infectivity of samples may be greatly reduced, if not totally inactivated, by the addition of 0.5% Triton X-100 and heating at 56°C for 30 minutes, and the samples may then be safely tested by serologic or antigen capture assays in the field. Ribonucleic acid (RNA) extraction using commercial kits containing strong chaotropes will inactivate the specimen and can safely be carried out in a laminar-flow safety cabinet. Virus isolation attempts should always be performed at least in a BSL-3 facility.

**6. Nonhuman hosts**—RVF virus is maintained in nature in *Aedes* sp. mosquitoes. Virus has been isolated from male and female mosquitoes suggesting transovarial transmission. Hatching of infected *Aedes* eggs follows abnormally high rainfall and flooding; infected mosquitoes feed on susceptible wildlife species or livestock (e.g., sheep, goats, cattle, or camels) resulting in abortion storms and virus amplification. Horizontal transmission to other mosquito species (i.e., *Culex* sp.) is facilitated by the high viremia observed in domestic ruminants. RVF in ruminants is characterized by abortion in pregnant females, death in young animals, and severe clinical disease in adults.

**7. Sample requirements**—During acute febrile stages of disease, virus can be detected in serum, heparinized plasma, or whole blood, and serologic techniques can be performed on late acute or convalescent samples of the same type. Virus may also be detected or isolated in biopsy or autopsy specimens from various tissues in humans and animals. Diagnostic samples should be shipped and stored frozen, if possible, on dry ice or liquid nitrogen vapor. Formaldehyde-fixed tissue and paraffin-embedded blocks for viral antigen detection by IHC should be shipped and stored at room temperature. Livestock samples or mosquitoes collected in the field should be shipped and stored frozen for virus or RNA detection. Livestock or wildlife serum samples for antibody detection should ideally be shipped and stored frozen.

**8. Testing requirements**—RVF is rare in humans and usually diagnosed during large livestock epizootics; individual cases are rarely diagnosed. Diagnostic reagents are available only at select reference laboratories. There are no commercially available assays for human diagnosis. As for other infectious diseases, the diagnosis should always be based on the results of a combination of clinical and laboratory data. During acute febrile stages of disease, virus can be detected by conventional or real-time PCR or virus isolation, followed by sequencing or antigen detection ELISA. In late acute and convalescent stages, IgM or IgG antibodies can be detected by ELISA. Virus antigens can be detected by IHC in tissue samples collected post-mortem. Direct detection of virus, viral antigens, or IgM or IgG antibodies in an individual with a clinically compatible illness or an individual with a known high-risk exposure to the virus constitutes a confirmed case of infection. The same techniques can be used for livestock and wildlife specimens (ELISA assays for animals are commercially available). Virus can be detected in mosquitoes by reverse transcription PCR or virus isolation in cell cultures or suckling mice.

**9. Reporting requirements**—RVF should be reported to the local and national authorities according to country requirements. In some countries, isolation of the RVF virus needs to be reported immediately to biosecurity authorities (Select Agents regulations in the USA). Suspicion or confirmation of RVF in animals should be reported to the Office International des Epizooties, World Organisation for Animal Health. If RVF is suspected, contact the CDC Viral Special Pathogens Branch by phone (470-312-0094; 404-639-1115) or by e-mail (spather@cdc.gov).

**10. Referral network**—Testing can only be performed at select reference laboratories, usually WHO collaborative reference centers for human samples and OIE or Food and Agriculture Organization reference centers for animal samples. For shipping potentially infectious material, samples should be packaged and shipped by trained personal in accordance with current International Airline Transportation Association recommendations and forwarded, after consultation, to one of the facilities with diagnostic capability for these agents.

**11. Special considerations**—RVF virus has an extended geographical distribution. This virus is listed as an agent that must be assessed in terms of potential to cause Public Health Emergencies of International Concern under the 2005 International Health Regulations.

[P. E. Rollin, S. Nichol]

# ROTAVIRUS INFECTION

(rotavirus gastroenteritis, viral gastroenteritis)

| DISEASE | ICD-10 CODE |
|---|---|
| ROTAVIRUS INFECTION | ICD-10 A08.0 |

**1. Clinical features**—A sporadic, seasonal, often severe gastroenteritis of infants and young children, characterized by vomiting, fever, and watery diarrhea. Rotavirus infection is occasionally associated with severe dehydration and death in young children. Secondary symptomatic cases among adult family contacts can occur, athough subclinical infections are more common. Infection has occasionally been found in pediatric patients with a variety of other clinical manifestations, but the virus is probably coincidental rather than causative in these conditions. Rotavirus is a major cause of nosocomial diarrhea of newborns and infants. Although rotavirus diarrhea is generally more severe than acute diarrhea due to other agents, illness caused by rotavirus is not distinguishable from that caused by other enteric viruses for any individual patient.

**2. Causative agents**—Rotaviruses are members of the family *Reoviridae*, genus *Rotavirus*. There are currently 8 recognized groups within the genus: A, B, C, D, E, F, G, and H. Group A rotaviruses are the primary cause of gastroenteritis in humans, though groups B, C, and H have caused infrequent disease. Rotaviruses are nonenveloped viruses with a triple-layered capsid. The genome is composed of 11 segments of double-stranded ribonucleic acid (RNA) that encode 11 or 12 proteins. Two proteins make up the outer capsid layer: VP7, a glycosylated protein (G protein); and VP4, a protease-sensitive protein (P protein). Traditionally, rotaviruses have been typed by serological or genetic characterization of the G and P proteins, although the current typing system uses genetic information from all 11 segments. The rotavirus A genotypes that commonly cause disease in humans are G1P[8], G2P[4], G3P[8], G4P[8], G9P[8], and G12P[8]. The segmented genome of rotaviruses permits the viruses to undergo genetic reassortment when 2 strains infect the same cell.

**3. Laboratory diagnosis**—Antigen detection enzyme immunoassays (EIA) and lateral flow devices are most commonly used to diagnose rotavirus enteritis. Most devices use polyclonal or monoclonal antibodies recognizing epitopes on the VP6 inner capsid protein. Detection of rotavirus antigen in stool is considered diagnostic for rotavirus, but coinfections with other enteric viruses (e.g., norovirus) or bacterial pathogens can occur. Polymerase chain reaction (PCR)-based multiple pathogen detection assays also are used to diagnose rotavirus infection.

**4. Laboratory capability**—Testing can be performed by hospital, commercial, and public health laboratories. Laboratory personnel should be trained in biosafety level 2 (BSL-2) practices, EIA methods, and, if the laboratory is performing PCR-based multiple pathogen detection assays, nucleic acid extraction and PCR testing.

**5. Safety requirements**—Rotavirus samples and isolates are handled in BSL-2 laboratories. Manipulation of materials is carried out in class II biological safety cabinets. There are no vaccination requirements or recommendations for rotavirus. Rotavirus vaccines are recommended only for immunization of children younger than 24 weeks and 32 weeks for Rotarix and RotaTeq, respectively.

**6. Nonhuman hosts**—Group A rotavirus strains that infect humans are thought to have a human reservoir. Animal strains cause rare infections in humans. Genetic reassortment, in which human and animal rotaviruses exchange genomic segments, can result in chimeric strains that are able to cross the species barrier, adapt, and then establish themselves in human populations.

**7. Sample/specimen requirements**—Stool samples are the most appropriate type of sample for testing, though diaper elutions and rectal swabs also can be used. Samples should be collected as soon as possible after onset of disease; the peak of rotavirus shedding is 3–5 days after onset of symptoms. Stool samples can be stored at 4°C for days to weeks. For long-term storage, freezing of samples at −20°C or colder is recommended, and the number of freeze-thaws should be minimized. Stool samples should be shipped on cold packs or dry ice. Stool suspensions in buffered media are typically prepared prior to testing.

**8. Testing requirements**—Recommended laboratory practices include testing stool specimens by antigen detection EIA or lateral flow devices and/or PCR-based methods, so the laboratory must be equipped to perform these techniques. EIA methods require an enzyme-linked immunosorbent assays plate reader to determine optical density values. A 96-well plate washer is also useful. Lateral flow devices generally do not require additional equipment. PCR-based methods require thermal cyclers or other assay specific equipment and may require the resources to perform nucleic acid extraction from stool samples, though some instrumentation includes this step in the analytical procedure. PCR-based methods also require proper laboratory configuration and practices to avoid contaminating clean areas with PCR-amplified deoxyribonucleic acid. The sensitivity of antigen detection assays is typically 90% or higher, while specificity ranges from 97%–100%. PCR-based assays tend to have higher sensitivity, often 100%, and 99%–100% specificity. The FDA has approved both antigen detection and PCR-based multiple pathogen detection assays for in vitro diagnostic use. Unapproved tests are considered presumptive. Quality assurance for these tests includes inclusion of positive and negative controls in each test, regular calibration of instruments, regular assessment of competence of laboratory personnel in performing testing, and participation in a proficiency testing program.

**9. Reporting requirements**—In the USA, reporting of rotavirus enteritis cases is not compulsory, but rotavirus geotemporal activity is monitored through the National Respiratory and Enteric Virus Surveillance System, a passive, laboratory-based system that collects testing data from hospital, commercial, and public health laboratories.

**10. Referral network**—In the USA, no formal referral network exists currently, but CDC accepts samples for testing from state or local public health laboratories and other federal agencies. Specimens from hospitals and health care providers must be processed through state or local health department laboratories. CDC performs confirmatory diagnostic testing and strain typing.

**11. Special considerations**—CDC's New Vaccine Surveillance Network defines a confirmed case of rotavirus gastroenteritis as a child with diarrhea (3 or more loose stools in 24 hours) or vomiting (1 or more episodes in 24 hours) and with detection of rotavirus in a fecal specimen by a standard assay such as EIA. WHO's confirmed case definition is any child aged 0–59 months admitted for treatment of acute (≤14 days), watery, nonbloody diarrhea to a sentinel hospital conducting surveillance and in whose stool rotavirus antigen is detected by EIA.

[M. D. Bowen]

# RUBELLA

(German measles)

| DISEASE | ICD-10 CODE |
|---|---|
| RUBELLA | ICD-10 B06 |
| CONGENITAL RUBELLA SYNDROME | ICD-10 P35 |

**1. Clinical features**—Rubella is most often a mild febrile viral disease with a diffuse punctate and maculopapular rash. Clinically, rubella is indistinguishable from febrile rash illness due to measles, dengue, parvovirus B19, human herpesvirus 6, coxsackievirus, echovirus, adenovirus, or scarlet fever. Children usually present with few or no constitutional symptoms, but adults may experience a 1–5 day prodrome of low-grade fever, headache, malaise, mild coryza, and conjunctivitis. Postauricular, occipital, and posterior cervical lymphadenopathy is the most characteristic clinical feature and precedes the rash by 5–10 days. Thrombocytopenia can occur, but hemorrhagic manifestations are rare. Arthralgia and, less commonly, arthritis complicate a substantial proportion of infections, particularly among adult females. Encephalitis is seen in 1 out of 6,000 cases and occurs with a higher frequency in adults. Up to 50% of rubella infections are either without rash or subclinical. Rubella is important because it can produce a constellation of anomalies in the developing fetus, called congenital rubella syndrome (CRS). CRS may occur in up to 90% of infants born to women who are infected with rubella during the first 10 weeks of pregnancy. Fetuses infected early are at greatest risk of intrauterine death, spontaneous abortion, and CRS. Clinical manifestations of CRS include single or combined defects or symptoms such as hearing impairment, cataracts, microphthalmia, congenital glaucoma, microcephaly, meningoencephalitis, developmental delay, congenital heart defects (e.g., patent ductus arteriosus, atrial or ventricular septal defects), purpura, hepatosplenomegaly, jaundice, and radiolucent bone disease. Moderate and severe CRS is usually recognizable at birth; mild CRS with only slight cardiac involvement or hearing impairment may not be detected for months or even years after birth. Insulin-dependent diabetes mellitus is misrecognized as a frequent late manifestation of CRS. Congenital malformations and fetal death can also occur following inapparent maternal rubella. Defects are rare when maternal infection occurs after the 20th week of gestation. In patients with primary immune deficiencies, rubella vaccine virus can persist in skin, visceral organs, or brain for years after immunization and may cause granulomatous disease or encephalitis.

**2. Causative agents**—Rubella virus (genus *Rubivirus,* family *Togaviridae*). Only 1 serotype is known.

**3. Laboratory diagnosis**—Laboratory testing is required to confirm diagnosis of suspected clinical cases of rubella and CRS since the symptoms of postnatal rubella infection can be similar to other diseases and the birth defects may not be related to CRS (e.g., genetic disorders, environmental factors, or other teratogenic pathogens). Laboratory confirmation is usually based on a positive rubella-specific immunoglobulin class M enzyme-linked immunosorbent assay (IgM ELISA) test on a blood specimen. Rubella cases can also be confirmed by seroconversion or at least a 4-fold rise in rubella-specific IgG antibody titer in paired serum specimens by positive rubella reverse transcription polymerase chain reaction (RT-PCR) test or by virus isolation.

**4. Laboratory capability**—Laboratories performing confirmatory testing for rubella must be properly resourced in terms of staffing support, supplies, equipment, and training. Serologic testing for rubella requires training in handling blood specimens, while the molecular testing requires special training for processing nasopharyngeal fluid and/or urine specimens and experience and techniques for detecting viral ribonucleic acid (RNA). Laboratories performing virus isolation should be equipped with class II biosafety cabinets (BSC) and cell culture incubators. Rubella virus isolation requires training in cell culture techniques and knowledge of handling viral specimens.

**5. Safety requirements**—Rubella is classified as a biosafety level 2 agent. Inhalation of rubella-containing aerosols is a primary health hazard. Upon receiving clinical specimens, the shipping containers must be immediately unpacked in a designated class II BSC to reduce potential exposure of laboratory personnel to infectious agents. The laboratory workers should be familiar with standard microbiological techniques and be aware of potential health hazards when handling clinical specimens.

Laboratory coat, gloves, and eye protection must be used when handling clinical samples. In case breakage and leakage occur, the container and working area must be disinfected with 70% alcohol, 10% sodium hypochlorite solution (bleach), or 2% glutaraldehyde solution.

Live attenuated vaccine is available to prevent rubella. Rubella vaccine is commonly used in combination with measles and mumps vaccines (measles, mumps, rubella [MMR] vaccine). The most widely used RA27/3 vaccine strain is safe, has minimal side effects, and provides long-lasting immunity against all known rubella virus strains. MMR vaccine is contraindicated in pregnancy because it contains live viruses. Postexposure vaccination is not proven to be effective in preventing rubella. Vaccination of laboratory personnel or documentation of natural immunity through serological testing for rubella IgG is required to prevent laboratory acquired rubella infections.

**6. Nonhuman hosts**—Humans are the only natural reservoir for rubella virus.

**7. Sample/specimen requirements**—During postnatal infection, rubella-specific IgM antibodies may not be detectable within the first 5 days after rash onset, and thus optimal serum samples for detecting rubella IgM are those collected 5–7 days after rash. Timing of specimen collection from CRS infants is less critical because IgM antibody persists for up to 6 months after birth. Serum specimens can be stored at 4°C for short term (days) or at or below −20°C for long term (weeks).

For virus isolation and detection, throat and nasopharyngeal swabs or oral fluid are preferred clinical specimens. Occasionally, virus can also be detected in urine or blood. The best specimens are those collected within 3 days after rash onset in postnatal rubella cases or within the first month after birth in CRS cases. After collection, swabs should be immediately placed into 3–4 ml of viral transport media, isotonic fluid (e.g., PBS), or common tissue culture medium (e.g., MEM). The specimens should be stored at 4°C for short term (within 48 hours) or −70°C for long term (weeks). Freezing at −20°C is not recommended because it reduces rubella virus viability.

To confirm persistent rubella infection in tissues, fresh-frozen biopsy specimens or slides of formalin-fixed paraffin-embedded tissues should be submitted to the CDC Measles, Mumps, Rubella, and Herpesvirus Laboratory Branch for molecular or immunohistochemical testing, respectively. Availability of such testing in other countries and regions may vary.

In the preelimination and postelimination phase, both serum and virological specimens should be collected for all suspected rubella cases. As a rule, both virologic and serologic specimens should be sent to the laboratory as soon as possible by standard shipping methods at 4°C if the specimens are kept at 4°C prior to shipment. However, specimens should be shipped on dry ice if they are kept at −20°C or −70°C.

**8. Testing requirements**—Several strategies can be applied to confirm rubella infection, depending on the types and timing of specimens collected:

1) Serologic testing: detection of rubella specific IgM antibody is one of the commonly used diagnostic methods for recently acquired rubella infection and for congenital rubella infection in newborns. Commercial IgM ELISA for rubella-specific IgM antibody can differ substantially in diagnostic performance. An IgM capture ELISA typically performs better than indirect IgM ELISA, especially in regard to specificity. Although IgM ELISA is the fastest and most cost-effective diagnostic method, the result depends on the timing of specimen collection. False-negative results may be obtained for specimens collected close to the day of rash onset. In cases of postnatal infections, about 50% of the serum samples collected on the day of rash onset do not contain detectable IgM antibody, while most of the serum samples collected between 5–40 days after the rash onset are IgM antibody–positive. If negative results are obtained from specimens collected too soon after rash onset, a convalescent sample should be obtained 2–3 weeks later and tested in parallel with the acute serum sample. The timing of samples collection for CRS cases is not as critical as for postnatal infection since most CRS cases are IgM antibody positive at birth until 3–6 months of age. If the specimens collected at birth are IgM-negative, retesting for IgM using second samples collected a month later is recommended. The lack of rubella IgM in a specimen collected 1 month after birth unequivocally rules out CRS.

   Implementation of national immunization programs has led to the elimination of rubella or sharp decline in rubella incidence in many countries. Consequently, in these countries, the positive predictive value of IgM testing may be low. False-positive results for IgM testing may occur due to the presence of rheumatoid factor, other infections, or heterophile antibodies in a patient's serum. Therefore, IgM-positive serum samples from suspected cases without epidemiologically linked exposure should be confirmed by other tests such as IgG avidity testing. The IgM test is not recommended as a screening test for rubella immunity in pregnant women because IgM antibodies are not long-lasting. Thus, these tests are not the appropriate measure for documenting evidence of rubella immunity and because of the potentially serious consequences due to erroneous diagnosis based on false-positive or false-negative results.

   Rubella IgG is used as a measure of immunity against rubella virus. Rubella-specific IgG appears about a week after the onset of symptoms. IgG seroconversion or at least 4-fold rise in IgG antibody titer in convalescent serum samples taken at 2–3 weeks after rash onset relative to acute serum samples can be used to diagnose recent rubella infection. The 10 IU/ml antibody level was defined as sufficient for adequate protection from rubella disease. In addition to ELISA, other tests, such as latex agglutination (LA), hemagglutination inhibition (HAI), neutralization and indirect immunofluorescence assay (IFA), and bead-based immunoassays can be used to detect rubella-specific antibodies. Both ELISA and LA allow high throughput for prenatal screening, but ELISA is the most widely used assay that can be adapted to automated antenatal screening. Most clinical laboratories perform serologic testing and have trained and qualified proficient personnel to conduct these assays.

Level of IgG maturation, as indicated by avidity of antibodies, can also be used to differentiate recent infection from distant infection. In general, IgG of low avidity first appears after primary exposure and then the avidity increases as IgG matures 3–6 months later. The avidity test becomes an essential tool for confirmation of primary rubella infection in regions where rubella is eliminated. Because of its complexity, the avidity test should be performed by reference laboratories.

2) Detection of rubella virus: rubella viruses can be recovered from throat swabs taken up to 3–4 days after rash onset. These tests are usually conducted in reference laboratories because they require specific equipment, a well-controlled laboratory environment, and advanced training of laboratory personnel.

Rubella virus can infect many different cell types. To integrate measles virus isolation, Vero/hSLAM was chosen as the cell line for rubella virus isolation in the WHO measles and rubella laboratory network. Wild-type rubella virus does not produce significant cytopathic effect in most cell types, and thus detection of rubella proteins or RNA is necessary to confirm the presence of virus in the culture. This includes the detection of rubella virus antigens in infected cells by IFA or indirect immunocolorimetric assay using rubella-specific antibodies and/or detection of rubella virus RNA by RT-PCR. The latter also allows genotyping of virus to help identify the source of the virus.

Successful isolation of rubella virus depends on proper sample collection and adequate cold chain during transportation. If virus isolation in tissue culture fails, detection of rubella RNA directly from clinical specimens can be achieved by conventional end-point or real-time RT-PCR. RT-PCR tests can confirm cases within a day after receiving the specimens. Occasionally, genotyping of virus directly from the clinical specimens can be performed if a sufficient amount of viral RNA is present. In-house protocols used mostly by national or other qualified reference laboratories differ in sensitivity. Some of these assays can reliably detect 3–10 copies of viral RNA.

**9. Reporting requirements**—Rubella and CRS are reportable diseases in many countries. Health care providers and hospitals are required to immediately report to local public health authorities suspected, probable, or confirmed rubella and CRS cases. In general, all results of rubella-specific ELISA should be reported within 4–7 days of receipt of the serum sample. In situations where the laboratory results assist the control program in implementing a response, the laboratory should attempt to provide results within 24–48 hours after receiving the specimens.

**10. Referral network**—If suspected rubella and CRS cases are identified, the specimens including serum, throat swabs, and/or urine have to be sent to state health department and/or the CDC Measles, Mumps, Rubella, and Herpesvirus Laboratory Branch for confirmatory tests. In addition to providing services domestically, the CDC laboratory also serves as a regional reference laboratory in the Pan American Health Organization and a global specialized laboratory in the WHO Measles and Rubella Laboratory Network to provide technical assistance for laboratory diagnosis. Similar referral testing services for rubella may be available in most other regions.

**11. Special considerations**—WHO-recommended case definitions for surveillance purposes are as follows:

- Suspected rubella case is the illness caused by postnatal rubella infection characterized by fever, maculopapular rash, and lymphadenopathy.
- Suspected CRS case is defined as the illness in infants caused by in utero rubella infection that is characterized by either 2 symptoms from category A or 1 from category A and 1 from category B:
    - Category A: sensorineural deafness, ophthalmologic defects (cataract, glaucoma, microphthalmia, pigmentary retinopathy), cardiovascular defects (patent ductus arteriosus, pulmonary artery stenosis, ventricular septal defects).
    - Category B: neurologic defects (microcephaly, behavioral disorders, mental retardation, meningoencephalitis), thrombocytopenia with purpura, jaundice, hepatosplenomegaly, radiolucent bone disease.

[M. Chen, L. Perelygina]

# SALMONELLOSIS

(nontyphoidal *Salmonella*)

| DISEASE | ICD-10 CODE |
|---|---|
| SALMONELLOSIS | ICD-10 A02 |

This chapter is about illness caused by nontyphoidal *Salmonella* organisms. Illness caused by *Salmonella* serotypes Typhi and Paratyphi is described in "Typhoid Fever and Paratyphoid Fever."

**1. Clinical features**—A bacterial disease commonly manifested by sudden onset of diarrhea, abdominal pain, fever, nausea, and often vomiting. Diarrhea, which may be bloody, usually persists for several days. Dehydration, especially among infants and the elderly, may be severe. Deaths are uncommon, except in the very young, the frail elderly, the debilitated, and the immunosuppressed. Morbidity and costs from medical care and absenteeism may be high. More illness occurs than is confirmed by culture.

Infection may begin as acute enterocolitis and develop into septicemia or focal infection. In enterocolitis, fecal excretion of infectious organisms usually persists for days or weeks after illness has resolved; administration of antimicrobial agents may increase the duration of shedding. Occasionally, the agent localizes in a normally sterile site, producing abscess, septic arthritis, osteomyelitis, cholecystitis, endocarditis, meningitis, pericarditis, pneumonia, cystitis, or pyelonephritis. In the USA, 9% of laboratory-confirmed cases are extraintestinal infections. Severity of the disease is related to serotype, number of organisms ingested, and host factors; morbidity can be increased when the organism is resistant to antimicrobial agents used to treat the patient.

**2. Causative agents**—Nontyphoidal *Salmonella* bacteria. Approximately 2,600 serotypes have been identified. Most are spread from animal reservoirs, which are usually asymptomatic. In most areas, a small number of serotypes account for the majority of infections; nearly all *Salmonella* isolated from ill persons are serotypes of *Salmonella enterica* subsp. *enterica*. In most countries with surveillance for *Salmonella* infections, *S. enterica* subsp. *enterica* serotypes Typhimurium (*S.* Typhimurium) and Enteritidis (*S.* Enteritidis) are the most commonly reported. There is much variation in the relative prevalence of other serotypes from country to country, with *S.* Typhimurium and *S.* Enteritidis being the most commonly reported.

**3. Laboratory diagnosis**—In cases with diarrhea or septicemia, *Salmonella* may be isolated from feces or blood, respectively, on enteric media during acute stages of illness. *Salmonella* may also be isolated from other sites, such as cerebrospinal fluid and urine. Serological tests are not useful in diagnosis. Recently, rapid diagnostic testing using polymerase chain reaction (PCR) on stools and blood specimens have been reported with high specificity and sensitivity. In addition to microbiologic and serological identification, molecular methods such as multilocus sequence typing (MLST; based on sequencing analysis of 7 housekeeping genes located on the chromosome) have been used for identification and classification of *Salmonella,* and newer whole genome sequencing (WGS) methods such as high resolution single nucleotide polymorphism (SNP) typing have been used for outbreak detection and surveillance.

**4. Laboratory capability**—A contained, purpose-built, microbiological facility with the capacity to autoclave microbiological waste is required to handle this pathogen. Staff should be trained and shown to be competent to handle potentially hazardous biological agents and should be able to carry out molecular and basic microbiological techniques.

**5. Safety requirements**—Employers have a responsibility to protect their workers from the risks related to exposure to hazardous biological agents.[1] Most *Salmonella* spp. are hazard group 2 and should be handled within a biosafety level 2 (BSL-2) laboratory with exception of the enteric fever–causing agents (*S.* Typhi; *S.* Paratyphi A, B, and C), which are handled in a BSL-3 laboratory. *Salmonella* transmission is via the fecal-oral route, and therefore gloves should be worn when handling clinical samples (or cultures); the importance of good hand washing techniques must be emphasized to laboratory staff. In addition to gloves, other personal protective equipment should be worn including laboratory coat and laboratory safety glasses. Finally, it is recommended to use a class I or class II biosafety cabinet when handling this pathogen, particularly where there is a risk of aerosol production.

**6. Nonhuman hosts**—*Salmonella* bacteria are widely distributed in domestic and wild animals. These include food animals such as poultry, pigs, cattle; pets including cats, dogs, birds; and reptiles such as snakes, lizards, and tortoises. Chronic carriers are rare in humans but prevalent in animals and birds.

**7. Sample/specimen requirements**—*Salmonella* infection is diagnosed primarily through the testing of stool samples. Ideally a diarrheal stool sample should be collected within the first few days of a patient becoming symptomatic. Bacterial recovery will be improved if samples are taken before any antibiotic treatment is given. In resource-limited countries with few testing facilities, poor transport, and lack of storage facilities, rectal swabs can be used and ideally tested within a few days of a patient becoming symptomatic. Rectal swabs should be transported in a suitable medium (e.g., Cary Blair transport medium). In cases of bacteremia or invasive illness, the bacteria can also be detected in the blood and urine. Clinical samples should be placed into appropriate sterile containers and labeled with patient details (to ensure sample integrity). UN regulations stipulate that samples should be kept in appropriate containers to prevent leaking and transported according to the UN Transport of Infectious Substances Regulations.[2]

**8. Testing requirements**—Testing facilities must adhere to the quality standards set out to them by their accreditation body, and diagnostic laboratories must follow the manufacturer's instructions for any commercial assay being performed. Once a clinical sample (e.g., stool) has arrived at the testing facility, patient identifiers on the request form and sample container should be checked. Ideally samples will be tested on arrival. If this is not possible, fecal samples can be stored at refrigerated temperatures (4°C–8°C) to prevent overgrowing of other organisms.

Primary testing involves culture methods: plating the sample on blood and selective agar (e.g., MacConkey agar) to isolate pure colonies of *Salmonella*, followed by serology (agglutination test for *Salmonella*) to detect the antigenic structure of each of the 2,600 known serovars. Biochemical testing including urease, oxidase, and indole tests for confirmation should be carried out.

Rapid molecular methods have also recently been used for identification and subtyping (discrimination) for isolates from clinical samples. They include pulsed field gel electrophoresis, multiple-locus variable number tandem repeat analysis, MLST, and SNP assays using WGS. However, some of these methods remain accessible to reference laboratories only and are difficult to implement for routine bacterial identification in a clinical laboratory.

**9. Reporting requirements**—The notification of salmonellosis in humans is mandatory in many countries around the world. Surveillance systems and the legal basis for reporting *Salmonella* in human clinical diagnostic samples vary considerably from country to country. For example, in the UK, although the notification of food poisoning is mandatory, salmonellosis is not specifically designated as a notifiable disease. However, mandatory reporting of the isolation of *Salmonella* is a statutory requirement, and diagnostic laboratories must report the isolation of the organism from human samples to the relevant public health authorities. Public health officials and epidemiologists monitor the surveillance data derived from this system to detect and control outbreaks of salmonellosis at the local and the national level. Because it is a pathogenic gastrointestinal bacterium, it is important to consider the presence of this pathogen in patients with symptoms of food poisoning, particularly in those with a history of travel or residence in high incidence countries. International surveillance relies on the collaboration of international institutions such as WHO and the European Centre for Disease Control and reporting on international platforms such as the Epidemic Intelligence Information System (https://ecdc.europa.eu/en/publications-data/epidemic-intelligence-information-system-epis), Food- and Waterborne Diseases and Zoonoses (https://ecdc.europa.eu/en/food-and-waterborne-diseases-and-zoonoses), and Early Warming and Response System (https://ecdc.europa.eu/en/publications-data/early-warning-and-response-system-european-union-ewrs) to assess whether current and emerging public health threats have a potential impact in the EU and other registered countries.

**10. Referral network**—It is recommended to send pure isolates to the reference facilities for typing and characterization. If this is not possible, some facilities will offer PCR testing on fecal DNA extracts and primary isolation of *Salmonella* from stool samples.

**11. Special considerations**—The onset of disease symptoms occurs 6–72 hours (usually 12–36 hours) after ingestion of Salmonella, and illness lasts 2–7 days.

Outbreaks (particularly those in hospitals, nurseries, and other institutions) should be investigated by the local health protection teams, and enteric precautions should be followed for known or suspected cases. Good hand hygiene needs to be maintained. To determine how transmission is occurring, epidemiological investigations should be carried out with a focus on the number and type of cases, the geographical distribution of cases, the time period involved, and common exposures.

## References

1. EUR-Lex. Directive 2000/54/EC of the European Parliament and of the Council of 18 September 2000. Available at: https://eur-lex.europa.eu/legal-content/EN/ALL/?uri=CELEX%3A32000L0054. Accessed February 15, 2019.
2. International Air Transport Association. Dangerous goods regulations: division 6.2—infectious substances. 2017. Available at: https://www.iata.org/whatwedo/cargo/dgr/Documents/infectious-substance-classification-DGR56-en.pdf. Accessed April 2, 2019.

[S. Nair, D. Ready]

# SCABIES

(sarcoptic itch, sarcoptic acariasis)

| DISEASE | ICD-10 CODE |
|---|---|
| SCABIES | ICD-10 B86 |

**1. Clinical features**—A parasitic infestation of the skin caused by a mite whose presence is evident as papules, vesicles, or tiny linear burrows containing the mites and their eggs. Itching is intense, especially at night, but complications are limited to lesions secondarily infected by scratching.

Lesions are prominent around finger webs, anterior surfaces of wrists and elbows, anterior axillary folds, belt line, and thighs. Nipples, abdomen, and the lower portion of the buttocks are frequently affected in women as are external genitalia in men. In infants, the head, neck, palms, and soles may be involved; these areas are usually spared in older individuals.

In immunodeficient individuals and in senile patients, infestation often appears as a generalized dermatitis more widely distributed than the burrows with extensive scaling and sometimes vesiculation and crusting (Norwegian or crusted scabies); the usual severe itching may be reduced or absent. When scabies is complicated by beta-hemolytic streptococcal infection, there is a risk of acute glomerulonephritis.

**2. Causative agents**—*Sarcoptes scabiei* var. *hominis*, a mite of humans found worldwide. Other *Sarcoptes* spp. and other animal mites, including other variants of *S. scabiei*, can live but not reproduce on humans; such infestations are self-limiting.

**3. Laboratory diagnosis**—Typically done by clinical examination of papules. Diagnosis can be confirmed by recovery from a burrow and microscopic identification of the mites, their eggs, or their feces (scybala).

Adult female mites are subspherical and measure 350–450 μm long by 250–350 μm wide; males and nymphs are smaller. Adult and nymphal mites possess 8 legs (larvae only 6 legs), 2 pairs anterior and 2 pairs posterior from the ventral surface of the body. Spines are present on the dorsal surface.

Eggs are oval and measure 150 μm long by 100 μm wide and may contain a developing larva within.

Scybala appear as dark brown irregularly shaped granular objects.

**4. Laboratory capability**—Microscopy/morphologic testing should be available. Laboratorians should be trained in the morphologic identification of arthropod ectoparasites and undergo regular proficiency testing.

**5. Safety requirements**—Clinical specimens should always be collected and handled with standard precautions. *Sarcoptes scabiei* is a biosafety level 2 organism. Scabies is highly contagious and may be transmitted person-to-person or via fomites; clinical specimens submitted for diagnosis may be infectious. Specimens should be disposed of as infectious waste.

**6. Nonhuman hosts**—None.

**7. Specimen requirements**—Skin scrapings should be collected at the end of burrows in nonexcoriated and noninflamed areas. Scrapings should be performed using a sterile scalpel or glass microscopy slide with a drop of mineral or immersion oil applied to the surface (the oil helps the mites adhere to the blade or slide and facilitates transfer to a slide for microscopic examination). The skin should be scraped vigorously at an approximately 90° angle (vigorous meaning there should be some red blood cells on the slide but no obvious bleeding); the patient should be sampled at a minimum of 6 different sites. The scrapings can be pooled on a single slide or examined on individual slides; place a coverslip over the slide prior to examination. If the slides are to be transported to the laboratory, a clean slide can be used to cover the slide containing the scrapings and secured with a rubber band or similar fastener.

**8. Testing requirements**—Routine identification of gross (whole) arthropods. A calibrated ocular micrometer should be used to measure mites and their eggs. Diagnosis is confirmatory in specimens meeting morphologic criteria.

**9. Reporting requirements**—*Sarcoptes scabiei* can be identified to the species level. Scabies is not nationally reportable in the USA. Report to local health authority; official report not ordinarily justifiable. Reporting recommended for day care centers, group homes, and institutionalized living situations.

**10. Referral network**—None.

**11. Special considerations**—Epidemic measures are as follows:

1) Provide treatment and educate infested individuals and others at risk.
2) Cooperation of nonhealth authorities is often needed.
3) Coordinated mass treatment; soap and facilities for mass bathing and laundering are essential; Tetmosol soap may help prevent infestation.
4) Extend screening to whole families, military units, or institutions; segregate infested individuals if possible.

[B. Mathison]

# SCHISTOSOMIASIS

(bilharziasis, snail fever)

| DISEASE | ICD-10 CODE |
|---|---|
| SCHISTOSOMIASIS | ICD-10 B65 |

**1. Clinical features**—A blood fluke (trematode) infection with adult worms living within mesenteric veins or the venous plexus of the bladder of the host over a life span of many years. Mated female worms release eggs into the circulation; depending on the species, eggs make their way through the bowel or bladder wall and are shed in feces (*Schistosoma mansoni, Schistosoma japonicum*) or urine (*Schistosoma haematobium*). Eggs that fail to pass out of the body may produce granulomata and fibrosis in organs where they lodge.

Symptoms are related to host immune responses to schistosome eggs in the human host and vary by the number and location of the eggs. *S. mansoni* and *S. japonicum* give rise primarily to hepatic and intestinal pathology. Signs and symptoms include diarrhea, abdominal pain, and hepatosplenomegaly. Long duration and high intensity of infection can lead to liver fibrosis and portal hypertension. *S. haematobium* gives rise to urinary manifestations. Signs and symptoms include dysuria, urinary frequency, and hematuria at the end of urination; chronic infection can also cause hydronephrosis and inflammation in the female genital tract and has been associated with increased risk of bladder cancer in both sexes. Rarely, neuroschistosomiasis may develop when aberrant eggs lodge in the spinal cord (more common with *S. mansoni* or *S. haematobium*) or brain (more often *S. japonicum*).

Acute infection can cause systemic manifestations (Katayama fever), which have been reported in travelers to endemic countries. Signs and symptoms of acute schistosomiasis include fever, headache, myalgia, rash, diarrhea, and respiratory symptoms.

The larvae of certain schistosomes of birds and mammals may penetrate the human skin and cause dermatitis, sometimes known as swimmer's itch; these schistosomes do not mature in humans.

**2. Causative agents**—*S. mansoni*, *S. haematobium*, and *S. japonicum* are the major species causing human disease. *S. mansoni* is endemic in Africa, parts of the Middle East, Brazil, and Venezuela with some potential foci remaining in the Caribbean. *S. haematobium* infects people in Africa and the Middle East, with a recent transmission focus identified on Corsica. *S. japonicum* is found in some provinces of China, Indonesia, and the Philippines. *Schistosoma mekongi* (Cambodia and Laos), *Schistosoma guineensis* (Central Africa), and *Schistosoma intercalatum* (Central Africa) are only found in limited areas.

**3. Laboratory diagnosis**—Through demonstration of eggs in the stool by direct smear, the Kato-Katz technique, or formalin-ethyl acetate concentration of stool (*S. mansoni* or *S. japonicum*). *S. haematobium* infection is diagnosed by the microscopic examination of a urine sediment or Nucleopore filtration of urine. The optimal time for collecting urine for *S. haematobium* egg recovery is between 12 PM and 3 PM. Serologic testing is typically useful only for diagnosis of infections in residents of nonendemic settings who traveled to endemic areas; currently available methods do not distinguish between active and former infection. Useful immunologic tests include enzyme-linked immunosorbent assay with egg or adult worm antigen and confirmatory species-specific immunoblot analysis. Positive results on serologic antibody detection tests are indicative of ever having been infected and are not proof of current infection. Detection of circulating cathodic antigen (CCA) in urine using a commercially available point-of-care (POC) test is useful for population or outbreak surveillance for *S. mansoni* infection but has not undergone the necessary evaluation to be used for individual patient diagnosis. PCR to detect parasite deoxyribonucleic acid (DNA) in stool or urine is available in some specialized laboratories.

**4. Laboratory capability**—Laboratories with standard microscopy, serology, or molecular biology proficiency should be able to perform parasitologic, immunologic, or PCR detection of schistosome infection, respectively, with little additional training. Use of the POC circulating cathodic antigen test (POC-CCA; Rapid Medical Diagnostics, Pretoria, South Africa) requires no laboratory equipment or discipline-specific training.

**5. Safety requirements**—Safety requirements for performing testing for schistosome infection are the same universal/standard precautions as for handling any human sample. Schistosome eggs present in urine or stool are not infectious for human hosts.

**6. Nonhuman hosts**—*S. japonicum* is a zoonotic parasite that infects water buffalo, cattle, pigs, dogs, cats, and rodents. However, it is not possible for humans to become infected through animal contact. *S. mansoni* can infect nonhuman primates and rodents. Hybrids among the cattle schistosome, *Schistosoma bovis*, and *S. haematobium* have been reported to infect humans, but it is not clear how much this contributes to community infection levels.

**7. Sample/specimen requirements**—Fresh stool is used for smears or Kato-Katz detection of *S. mansoni* or *S. japonicum* eggs. Stool preserved in formalin, polyvinyl alcohol, and commercial fixatives can be used for concentration methods. Fresh or frozen stool that has been preserved in alcohol can be used for PCR, but other stool fixatives can inhibit the assay. Fresh or frozen urine can be used for *S. haematobium* egg detection or PCR. Fresh or frozen urine can also be tested using POC-CCA for *S. mansoni* antigen detection. Serum, plasma, or dried blood spots stored at −20°C can subsequently be used for antibody detection assays.

**8. Testing requirements**—Microscopic detection of schistosome eggs in stool or urine is a highly specific diagnostic test, but the sensitivity is affected by intensity of infection. The Kato-Katz method has poor sensitivity for light infections. Stool PCR sensitivity is similarly dependent on infection intensity as the DNA being detected is contained in eggs and not homogenously distributed in fecal contents; however, DNA from either species can be detected in urine. Detection of antischistosome antibodies is useful for diagnosing infection of travelers or recent immigrants but is not informative for control programs because the antibody response to antigens currently used in these tests persists for years after cure. The POC-CCA assay is more sensitive than Kato-Katz and rapidly becomes negative following successful cure but has mainly been used for screening purposes and has not yet been evaluated for individual diagnostic testing or incorporated into monitoring and evaluation of mass drug administration programs. The POC-CCA is also less reliable for detection of *S. haematobium* infections and may or may not be useful for *S. japonicum* testing.

**9. Reporting requirements**—Reporting requirements vary by country and region. In the USA, schistosomiasis is not a reportable disease.

**10. Referral network**—There is no laboratory referral network for schistosomiasis testing, but the diagnostic laboratory of the Division of Parasitic Diseases and Malaria of CDC offers serologic testing for schistosomiasis, including species-specific immunoblot testing.

**11. Special considerations**—There are no special laboratory-related considerations relevant for schistosomiasis. It is not possible to become infected with schistosomes through any of the diagnostic procedures.

[W. E. Secor, S. P. Montgomery]

# SHIGELLOSIS

(bacillary dysentery)

| DISEASE | ICD-10 CODE |
|---|---|
| SHIGELLOSIS | ICD-10 A03 |

**1. Clinical features**—An acute bacterial disease involving the distal small intestine and colon, characterized by loose stools accompanied by fever, nausea, and sometimes toxemia, vomiting, cramps, and tenesmus. Stools may contain blood and mucus (dysentery) resulting from mucosal ulcerations and confluent colonic crypt microabcesses caused by the invasive organisms; however, many cases present with nonbloody diarrhea. Convulsions may be an important complication in young children. Bacteremia is uncommon. Severity and case-fatality rate vary with the host (age and preexisting nutritional state) and serotype. *Shigella dysenteriae* type 1 (Shiga bacillus) spreads in epidemics and is often associated with serious disease and complications including toxic megacolon, intestinal perforation, and the hemolytic uremic syndrome; case-fatality rates have been as high as 20% among hospitalized cases even in recent years. Mild and asymptomatic infections occur. These are usually self-limited, lasting on average 4–7 days. Many infections with *Shigella sonnei* result in a short clinical course and almost negligible case-fatality rate except in immunocompromised hosts. Certain strains of *Shigella flexneri* can cause a reactive postinfectious arthropathy (formerly known as Reiter syndrome), especially in persons who are genetically predisposed by having HLA-B27 antigen.

**2. Causative agents**—*Shigella* strains are Gram-negative, facultatively anaerobic, nonmotile rods classified in the family *Enterobacteriaceae*. *Shigella* strains cause dysentery symptoms by invading and destroying the cells that line the large intestine. These symptoms are mediated by several invasion-related factors including *ipaC* and *ipaH*, which are encoded on a characteristic large 120- to 140-MDa plasmid. The *ipaH* factor is also chromosomally encoded. The severity of symptoms associated with infection by *Shigella dysenteriae* type 1 is thought to be related to its production of Shiga toxin type 1. Rarely, nontype 1 strains of *S. dysenteriae* and certain strains of *S. flexneri* also produce Shiga toxin type 1. With the exception of *Shigella boydii* serotype 13, *Shigella* and *Escherichia coli* represent a single genomospecies. *S. boydii* 13 has been determined to be a separate species, *Escherichia albertii*. There are 4 subgroups of *Shigella*, which have traditionally been regarded as separate species:

1) Group A: *S. dysenteriae*
2) Group B: *S. flexneri*
3) Group C: *S. boydii*
4) Group D: *S. sonnei*

Groups A, B, and C are further divided into 15, 8, and 19 serotypes, respectively, and *S. flexneri* serotypes 1 through 5 are further subdivided into 11 serotypes designated by numbers and lowercase letters (e.g., *S. flexneri* 2a). *S. sonnei* (group D) consists of a single serotype.

**3. Laboratory diagnosis**—Isolation of *Shigella* from feces or rectal swabs provides bacteriological diagnosis. Outside the human body, *Shigella* remains viable only for a short period, which is why stool specimens for culture must be processed rapidly after collection. *Shigella* isolates should be tested for antimicrobial susceptibility. Commercial rapid diagnostic tests or antigen detection assays are not available.

**4. Laboratory capability**—General clinical laboratories are sufficient for culture and identification. If typing or antimicrobial susceptibilities are not performed at the primary testing laboratory, then it may be necessary to submit an isolate for further work at a commercial or governmental reference laboratory.

**5. Safety requirements**—This agent should be handled under biosafety level 2 conditions, and all laboratorians must use personal protective equipment.

**6. Nonhuman hosts**—Humans and large nonhuman primates are the only natural reservoir. Infection may also occur from contaminated food or water, necessitating the use of food and water isolation methods.

**7. Sample/specimen requirements**—Fecal specimens should be collected in the early stages of illness. Whole stools or in some cases rectal swabs are acceptable. The use of commercially available transport media may be necessary (i.e., Aimes or Cary-Blair). Collection of multiple specimens can increase recovery rates. Testing specimens as soon as possible after collection increases the likelihood of isolating *Shigella.*

**8. Testing requirements**—*Shigella* are Gram-negative rods. Commercially available nucleic acid detection assays are possible with sensitivities and specificities ranging from >93%–100%. Enrichment for *Shigella* may use Gram-negative broth or Selenite broth. To optimize isolation, the use of multiple selective media should be considered. MacConkey, xylose-lysine-deoxycholate, Hektoen enteric, or deoxycholate-citrate agar are all acceptable options. Colonies suspected of being *Shigella* may be screened with Kligler iron agar or triple sugar iron agar. Production of an alkaline slant and acid butt (nonlactose fermenter) without production of gas or $H_2S$ is expected, although rare strains may produce gas. Motility and lysine decarboxylase tests are expected to be negative. Additionally, acetate utilization, mucate, and lactose are all negative as well. Serotyping is required for the identification of *Shigella*. Serotyping is generally performed using slide agglutination with a polyvalent somatic (O) antigen grouping sera. A monovalent antiserum is necessary for *S. dysenteriae* 1. Numerous typing systems (i.e., restriction fragment length polymorphism, pulsed-field gel electrophoresis, multiple-locus variable number tandem repeat analysis, whole genome single nucleotide polymorphism) are available if further characterization or epidemiological relationship studies are necessary. A preliminary report may be issued based upon consistent biochemical test results. Whenever serotyping is available, it should be included in reports. For the final reporting, isolates should be confirmed by both biochemical and serological methods.

**9. Reporting requirements**—New or unrecognized serotypes should be sent to public health reference labs for additional characterization. Public health authorities may require submission of either results or isolates. It is necessary to check the rules of the state/provincial or national public health bodies to ensure proper submission and reporting.

**10. Referral network**—When assistance with testing is required, reference labs may be contacted. If shipping of specimens is required, then all applicable International Air Transport Association regulations should be followed.

**11. Special considerations**—A high level of caution is recommended regarding automated identification instruments due to potential cross-reactivity with *E. coli* or *Salmonella*.

[M. Soehnlen]

# SMALLPOX AND OTHER POXVIRUS DISEASES

| DISEASE | ICD-10 CODE |
|---|---|
| SMALLPOX | ICD-10 B03 |
| VACCINIA | ICD-10 B08.0 |
| MONKEYPOX | ICD-10 B04 |
| ORF VIRUS DISEASE | ICD-10 B08.0 |

## I. SMALLPOX

The last naturally acquired case of smallpox in the world occurred in October 1977 in Somalia; global eradication was certified 2 years later by WHO in 1979 and by the World Health Assembly (WHA) in May 1980. Except for a limited outbreak after a laboratory accident at the University of Birmingham, UK, in 1978, no further cases have been identified. All known smallpox (variola) virus stocks are held under security in 2 places, CDC and the State Research Centre of Virology and Biotechnology (VECTOR), Koltsovo, Novosibirsk, Russia. In response to concerns that the world would not be equipped to respond to and contain the disease in the event that smallpox should reemerge as results of accidental or intentional release, the WHA authorized the retention of virus at the laboratories in Russia and the USA for the purposes of essential research, set up a biosafety inspection program for the 2 laboratories, and appointed a group of experts to oversee the research. Because few health care workers today have ever encountered smallpox or have ever managed cases of the illness, it is important that they become familiar with the clinical and epidemiological features of smallpox and how it can be distinguished from chickenpox and other rash illness. Laboratory confirmation of variola virus (VARV) from suspect patients is performed at the WHO Collaborating Centre laboratories where the virus stocks are held using appropriate biosafety containment practices.

**1. Clinical features**—Smallpox was a systemic viral disease generally presenting with a characteristic skin eruption. Preceding the appearance of the rash was a prodrome of sudden onset with high fever (40°C/104°F), malaise, headache, prostration, severe backache, and occasional abdominal pain and vomiting, a clinical picture that resembled influenza. After 2–4 days, the fever began to fall, and a deep-seated rash developed in which individual lesions containing infectious virus progressed through successive stages of macules, papules, vesicles, pustules, and then crusted scabs that fell off 3–4 weeks after the appearance of the rash. The lesions first appeared on the face and extremities, including the palms and soles, and subsequently on the trunk, the so-called centrifugal rash distribution. They were well circumscribed and at the same state of development in a given area.

Two types of smallpox were recognized during the 20th century: variola minor (including a genetically and biologically distinct subgroup described as alastrim), which had a case-fatality rate of less than 1%, and variola major, which had a case-fatality rate among unvaccinated populations of 20%–50% or more (30% on average). Fatalities normally occurred between the fifth and seventh day after onset of illness, occasionally as late as the second week. Fewer than 3% of variola major cases experienced a fulminant hemorrhagic course, characterized by a severe prodrome, prostration, and bleeding into the skin and mucous membranes; such hemorrhagic cases were rapidly fatal. In hemorrhagic smallpox, the usual vesicular rash did not appear, and the disease might have been confused with severe leukemia, meningococcemia, or idiopathic thrombocytopenic purpura. The rash of smallpox could also be significantly modified in previously vaccinated persons to the extent that only a few highly atypical lesions might be seen. In such cases, prodromal illness was not modified, but the maturation of lesions was accelerated with crusting by the 10th day.

Smallpox was most frequently confused with chickenpox (varicella), in which skin lesions commonly occur in successive crops with several stages of maturity visible at the same time. The chickenpox rash is more abundant on covered than on exposed parts of the body, is centripetal rather than centrifugal, and is usually intensely itchy. However, the appearance of the rash in the early florid stage of a very severe chickenpox case may generate diagnostic confusion for those unfamiliar with smallpox or monkeypox (MPXV). The smallpox vesicles are firm (bullet-like) and deep-seated, whereas the chickenpox vesicles are more superficial and easily deroofed.

**2. Causative agents**—Variola virus (VARV), a species of *Orthopoxvirus*.

**3. Laboratory diagnosis**—Smallpox was indicated by a clear-cut prodromal illness; the more or less simultaneous appearance of all lesions when the fever broke; the similarity of appearance of all lesions in a given area rather than successive crops; and deep-seated lesions with no surrounding inflammatory flare, often involving sebaceous glands and scarring of the pitted lesions. By contrast, chickenpox lesions are superficial, not well circumscribed, and manifest with irregular borders; the vesicle or pustule is surrounded by an inflammatory flare and chickenpox rash is usually pruritic. Smallpox lesions were virtually never seen at the apex of the axilla, and chickenpox lesions are rarely, if ever, seen on the palms and soles of the feet, a distribution characteristic of smallpox in many cases. Outbreaks of variola minor were recognized by low case-fatality rates in the late 19th century. Although the rash was like that seen in ordinary smallpox, patients generally experienced less severe systemic reaction, and hemorrhagic cases were virtually unknown.

Prior to eradication, laboratory confirmation of smallpox used isolation of the virus on chorioallantoic membranes or tissue culture from the scrapings of lesions, from vesicular or pustular fluid, from crusts, and sometimes from blood during the febrile prodrome. Electron microscopy or immunodiffusion technique often permitted a rapid provisional diagnosis, though eradication was made possible on the basis of clinical, not laboratory, diagnosis. It should be remembered that all orthopoxviruses look alike using electron microscopy, so it cannot distinguish smallpox from other orthopoxviruses that infect humans, such as vaccinia or monkeypox. Molecular methods, such as polymerase chain reaction (PCR), are now available for rapid diagnosis of smallpox and other orthopoxvirus infections. Should smallpox infection be suspected, immediate communication by national authorities to WHO is obligatory. Smallpox is a notifiable disease under the 2005 International Health Regulations. Guidance on appropriate laboratories to confirm the diagnosis and for guidance on management of the suspected case and follow-up of contacts can be provided.

4. **Laboratory capability**—In the USA, orthopoxvirus diagnostic specimens should be evaluated by public health laboratories, many of which are members of the Laboratory Response Network (LRN). Certain LRN laboratories are trained and capable of performing diagnostics on samples suspected of VARV infection. These laboratories are recommended to utilize biological safety level 3 (BSL-3) containment facilities with personnel vaccinated with smallpox vaccine. Laboratory studies utilizing live VARV are only permitted in the 2 WHO Collaborating Centres (CDC and VECTOR) within BSL-4 laboratory spaces. If a sample is suspected to contain VARV, propagation in vitro should NOT be attempted.

5. **Safety requirements**—Recommendations on biosafety and vaccination requirements for studies utilizing different orthopoxviruses (OPXV) can be found in *Biosafety in Microbiological and Biomedical Laboratories,* 5th Edition (*BMBL*) available at: https://www.cdc.gov/labs/pdf/CDC-BiosafetyMicrobiologicalBiomedicalLaboratories-2009-P.PDF. Certain OPXV such as monkeypox virus (MPXV) Congo Basin clade and VARV are classified as select agents by the Division of Select Agents and Toxins (DSAT) and require notification to DSAT upon identification (https://www.selectagents.gov/faq-reporting.html). VARV is a tier 1 select agent and should be handled only in the highest containment BSL-4 laboratory facilities at 1 of 2 approved WHO collaborating centers (CDC, VECTOR). The laboratory personnel are advised to get smallpox vaccination once every 3 years if working with VARV.

The current smallpox vaccine is live Vaccinia virus (VACV), ACAM2000, a clonal derivative of the previously used VACV DryVax vaccine. Vaccination is performed using a bifurcated needle and results in a major reaction termed "take" in primary vaccinees (progresses to vesicles and scab) or "immune take" in repeat vaccinees (erythematous). Smallpox vaccination of the general public is not recommended by WHO due to rare but serious adverse events or death (1/1,000,000 doses) in certain individuals. Also, this live vaccine is contraindicated in individuals with known immune disorders or certain skin diseases. A third generation, nonreplicating modified vaccinia ankara (MVA)-based vaccine is considered an alternate for vaccinating at risk contraindicated individuals but have not been approved yet by FDA. Treatment of vaccine adverse reactions/effects by prophylaxis using vaccinia immune globulin can be obtained for emergency use in the USA and other countries through respective public health agencies.

6. **Nonhuman hosts**—VARV is solely a human pathogen and no other natural reservoirs are known.

7. **Sample/specimen requirements**—Ideally during an active infection, collection of lesion materials (either swabs or cell infiltrates) is important for diagnostic assays (e.g., PCR, antigen capture, cell culture, electron microscopy). In addition, collection of serum particularly for suspect OPXV infections is required for confirmation by serological assays.

8. **Testing requirements**—The current diagnostic methods include molecular techniques utilizing real-time PCR. Serologic tests include enzyme-linked immunosorbent assays (ELISA) to determine the presence of immunoglobulin class M (IgM) or IgG antibodies. In addition, the presence of neutralizing antibodies in serum can be ascertained by traditional plaque reduction neutralization tests or by more recently developed reporter virus-based assays. Electron microscopy of lesion material or cell culture samples can positively identify poxviruses characterized by brick-shaped particles of size 300–400 nm (OPXV).

9. **Reporting requirements**—Surveillance for OPXV infections is conducted through the LRN laboratories within the USA. An algorithm was created by CDC to assist clinicians in discriminating OPXV infection from other commonly confused pustular rash disease differentials (see: https://www.cdc.gov/smallpox/clinicians/algorithm-protocol.html). Since smallpox has been eradicated, any infection with a high suspicion of smallpox after careful clinical evaluation must be immediately reported to the nearest government health department and FBI. Samples from the suspect patient should be sent simultaneously for VARV diagnostic testing at an approved LRN laboratory and the WHO Collaborating Centre at CDC. Confirmation of the initial smallpox case would require additional characterization of VARV at CDC (e.g., DNA sequence analysis). Further information can be found at: https://www.cdc.gov/smallpox/index.html. Both VARV and MPXV Congo Basin clade viruses are considered Select Agents by DSAT and require notification upon confirmation of identification (see: https://www.selectagents.gov/faq-reporting.html). National health authorities should inform WHO immediately. Notification of smallpox is mandatory under the International Health Regulations. Further information can be found at: http://www.who.int/csr/disease/smallpox.

10. **Referral network**—The LRN is responsible for conducting surveillance for OPXV disease within the USA. The LRN is a network of approximately 150 laboratories distributed throughout the USA and internationally. These public health laboratories are trained to perform diagnostic assays for the presence of OPXV within clinical samples and undergo routine proficiency testing on these diagnostic assays. Further information about LRN can be found at: https://emergency.cdc.gov/lrn/factsheet.asp.

**11. Special considerations**—Identification of select agents (e.g., MPXV Congo Basin clade, VARV) within diagnostic specimens requires notification of DSAT (see: https://www.selectagents.gov/faq-reporting.html). Since smallpox is eradicated, identification of a smallpox patient can have far-reaching impact. Therefore, immediate notification to the nearest government health department and the FBI is necessary. However, confirmation of the initial smallpox case would require additional characterization of VARV at CDC (e.g., DNA sequence analysis). Further information can be found at: https://www.cdc.gov/smallpox/index.html). National health authorities should inform WHO immediately. Notification of smallpox is mandatory under the International Health Regulations. Further information can be found at: http://www.who.int/csr/disease/smallpox.

## II. VACCINIA

Vaccinia virus (VACV) is the live, fully replicative orthopoxvirus-immunizing agent that was used to eradicate smallpox. Discovery of vaccinia variants causing human infection in the Indian subcontinent and in South America (Brazil) has led to the consideration that vaccine may have escaped into animal populations; alternatively, these occurrences may be indicative of the origins of VACV. VACV has been genetically engineered and biologically derived into candidate (some are in clinical trials) and approved vaccines with low potential for spread to nonimmune contacts.

Vaccination with licensed (fully replicative) smallpox vaccine is recommended for all laboratory workers at high risk of contracting infection, such as those who directly handle cultures or animals contaminated or infected with vaccinia or other orthopoxviruses that infect humans. It may also be considered for other health care personnel who are at lower risk of infection, such as doctors and nurses whose contact with these viruses would be limited to contaminated dressings. WHO does not recommend vaccination in the general public, because the risk of death (1/1,000,000 doses) or serious side effects are greater than the known risk of infection with smallpox. Vaccination is contraindicated in persons with deficient immune systems, persons with eczema or certain other dermatitis disorders, and pregnant women. Vaccine immune globulin can be obtained for laboratory workers in the USA through the CDC Drug Service (404-639-3670) and in other industrialized counties from public health agencies. Vaccination should be repeated unless a major reaction (one that is indurated and erythematous 7 days after vaccination) or take has developed. Booster vaccinations are recommended within 10 years in categories for which vaccine is recommended. WHO maintains a supply of the vaccine seed lot (vaccinia virus strain Lister Elstree) at the WHO Collaborating Center for Smallpox Vaccine at the National Institute of Public Health and Environmental Protection in Bilthoven, The Netherlands. WHO also maintains a stockpile of vaccine to be used if needed to control a confirmed outbreak of smallpox.

## III. MONKEYPOX

**1. Clinical features**—Human monkeypox is a sporadic zoonotic infection first identified in 1970 from remote rural villages in Central and West African rainforest countries, as smallpox disappeared. Clinically, the disease closely resembles ordinary or modified smallpox, but lymphadenopathy is a more prominent feature in many cases and occurs in the early stage of the disease. Pleomorphism and cropping similar to that seen in chickenpox are observed in 20% of patients, depending on strain. The case-fatality rate among children not vaccinated against smallpox ranges from 1%–14%.

**2. Causative agents**—Monkeypox virus (MPXV) is a species of the genus *Orthopoxvirus* with biological properties and a genome distinct from variola virus. At least 2 genetically distinct clades of monkeypox exist with different human clinical and epidemiologic manifestations. To date, West African clade monkeypox manifests without apparent human-to-human transmission and without human mortality, whereas the Congo Basin clade is associated with human-to-human transmission and case-fatality rates historically reported at an average of approximately 10% in unvaccinated persons.

**3. Laboratory diagnosis**—Ascertainment of a history of direct or indirect contact with animals of West and Central African origin and identification of the characteristic lesion through electron microscopy demonstration of poxvirions in the lesion; by growth of the virus in primate cell cultures or through positive molecular (e.g., PCR) or serological tests.

**4. Laboratory capability**—Poxvirus diagnostics can be performed in BSL-2 laboratories with proper precautions and procedures. Laboratory personnel should be trained adequately depending on the biosafety level required for performance of the diagnostic assays. Recommendations on laboratory requirements for studies utilizing different OPXV can be found in *BML5*.

**5. Safety requirements**—If vaccinated personnel are handling MXPV samples, BSL-2 laboratory facilities with BSL-3 precautions are recommended. Samples suspected to contain VACV, cowpox virus, or other OPXV can be manipulated within BSL-2 laboratories with proper precautions. Laboratory personnel are advised to obtain smallpox vaccination once every 3 years if manipulating MPXV or VARV, and every 10 years if handling less pathogenic OPXVs.

**6. Nonhuman hosts**—MPXV is primarily a zoonotic pathogen and is transmitted to humans by interaction with animals. Although particular reservoir hosts have not been identified for MPXV, it is most likely to be circulated in rodents and other species.

**7. Sample/specimen requirements**—Ideally during an active infection, collection of lesion materials (either swabs or cell infiltrates) are important for diagnostic assays (e.g., PCR, antigen capture, cell culture, electron microscopy).

In addition, collection of serum, particularly for suspect OPXV infections, is required for confirmation by serological assays.

**8. Testing requirements**—The current diagnostic methods include molecular techniques utilizing real-time PCR. Serologic tests include ELISA to determine the presence of IgM or IgG antibodies. In addition, the presence of neutralizing antibodies in serum can be ascertained by traditional plaque reduction neutralization tests or by more recently developed reporter virus-based assays. Electron microscopy of lesion material or cell culture samples can positively identify poxviruses characterized by brick-shaped particles of size 300–400 nm (OPXV).

**9. Reporting requirements**—MPXV Congo Basin clade viruses are considered Select Agents by DSAT and require notification upon confirmation of identification (see: https://www.selectagents.gov/faq-reporting.html).

**10. Referral network**—The LRN is responsible for conducting surveillance for OPXV disease within the USA. The LRN is a network of approximately 150 laboratories distributed throughout the US and internationally. These public health laboratories are trained to perform diagnostic assays for the presence of OPXV within clinical samples and undergo routine proficiency testing on these diagnostic assays. Further LRN information can be found at: https://emergency.cdc.gov/lrn/factsheet.asp.

**11. Special considerations**—Identification of select agents such as MPXV Congo Basin clade within diagnostic specimens requires notification to DSAT (see: https://www.selectagents.gov/faq-reporting.html).

## IV. ORF VIRUS DISEASE (contagious pustular dermatitis, human orf, ecthyma contagiosum)

**1. Clinical features**—A proliferative cutaneous viral disease in which the lesion, usually solitary and located on hands, arms, or face, is a red to violet vesiculonodule, macupapule, or pustule progressing to a weeping nodule with central umbilication. There may be several lesions, each up to 3 cm in diameter and lasting 3–6 weeks. With secondary bacterial infection, lesions may become pustular. Regional adenitis occurs in a few cases. A maculopapular rash may occur on the trunk. Erythema multiforme and erythema multiforme bullosum are rare complications. Disseminated disease and serious ocular damage have been reported but are uncommon. The disease has been confused with cutaneous anthrax and malignancy.

**2. Causative agents**—Orf virus, a deoxyribonucleic acid (DNA) virus belonging to the genus *Parapoxvirus* of poxviruses (family *Poxviridae*). The agent is closely related to other parapoxviruses that can be transmitted to humans as occupational diseases, such as milkers' nodule virus of dairy cattle and bovine popular stomatitis virus of beef cattle. Contagious ecthyma parapoxvirus of domesticated camels may infect people on rare occasions.

**3. Laboratory diagnosis**—Presentation of the characteristic lesion and ascertainment of a history of contact with sheep, goats, or wild ungulates, in particular their young. Identification through electron microscopy demonstration of ovoid parapoxvirions in the lesion or by growth of the virus in ovine, bovine, or primate cell cultures; or through positive molecular (i.e., PCR) or serological tests.

**4. Laboratory capability**—Suspect parapoxvirus infected samples can be handled in a BSL-2 laboratory for processing and diagnostic assays. Laboratory personnel should be trained adequately depending on the biosafety level required for performance of the diagnostic assays. Recommendations on laboratory requirements for studies utilizing different OPXV can be found in *BML5*.

**5. Safety requirements**—There are no specific vaccination requirements for handling parapoxvirus suspect samples, but in general any work should be performed in BSL-2 facilities with standard personnel protective equipment deemed necessary by the laboratory.

**6. Nonhuman hosts**—Parapoxvirus infections are common after interaction with infected livestock or wild ungulates. The virus is very resistant to physical factors, except ultraviolet light, and may persist for months in soil and on animal skin and hair.

**7. Sample/specimen requirements**—Parapoxvirus infections are determined primarily by PCR-based molecular diagnostic tests of lesions.

**8. Testing requirements**—The current diagnostic methods include molecular techniques utilizing real-time PCR. Electron microscopy of lesion material or cell culture samples can positively identify poxviruses characterized by ovoid particles with crisscross spindles (*Parapoxvirus*).

**9. Reporting requirements**—Local reporting requirements should be followed. Case report to local health authority is not usually required but may be desirable when a human case occurs in areas not previously known to have the infection.

**10. Referral network**—The LRN is responsible for conducting surveillance for poxvirus disease within the USA. Further LRN information can be found at: https://emergency.cdc.gov/lrn/factsheet.asp.

**11. Special considerations**—None.

[P. S. Satheshkumar, V. A. Olson]

# SPOROTRICHOSIS

| DISEASE | ICD-10 CODE |
|---|---|
| SPOROTRICHOSIS | ICD-10 B42 |

**1. Clinical features**—A fungal disease, usually of the skin, often of an extremity. It begins as a nodule. As this grows, lymphatics draining the area become firm and cord-like and form a series of nodules, which in turn may soften and ulcerate. Osteoarticular, pulmonary, and multifocal infections occur but are relatively rare, except multifocal disseminated infections in human immunodeficiency virus patients. Fatalities are uncommon.

**2. Causative agents**—*Sporothrix schenckii* spp. complex, consisting of *S. schenckii*, *Sporothrix mexicana*, *Sporothrix globosa*, and *Sporothrix brasiliensis*. *Sporothrix luriei*, *Sporothrix albicans*, and *Sporothrix inflata* are genetically different species.

**3. Laboratory diagnosis**—Culture of a biopsy, pus, or exudate confirms the diagnosis in skin lesions. Organisms are rarely visualized by direct smear. Biopsied tissue should be examined with fungal stains. Serologic testing is available for detection of antibodies.

**4. Laboratory capability**—Specimens and cultures must be handled within a biosafety level 2 (BSL-2) facility equipped with a class II biosafety cabinet (BSC). Laboratory personnel must be specifically trained in handling and recognition of *Sporothrix* spp., supervised by scientists with advanced training in mycology.

**5. Safety requirements**—*Sporothrix* spp. are classified within risk groups 1 and 2, with *S. schenckii* being risk group 2. Specimens and cultures should be handled with BSL-2 precautions. Culture material must only be manipulated in a BSC, and contact with skin should be avoided.

**6. Nonhuman hosts**—Cats are particularly susceptible and cat-to-cat and cat-to-human transmission has been documented. In particular, sporotrichosis caused by *S. brasiliensis* is predominantly zoonotic, and to date has only been found in certain regions of South America. Armadillos may be another source of zoonotic transmission, and, rarely, other warm-blooded vertebrates and even arthropods (fire ants, spiders) have carried the infection.

**7. Sample/specimen requirements**—Biopsies, pus, or exudate in appropriate sterile containers should be transported to the laboratory and processed as soon as is practical. Although delays should be avoided, samples may be held refrigerated (4°C–8°C) for up to several days without appreciably affecting organism viability.

**8. Testing requirements**—Histopathology may demonstrate cigar-shaped yeast-like cells, but is less sensitive than culture and does not permit specific identification of the etiological agent. Isolation of the causative agent is diagnostic, although standard bacteriology testing alone typically fails to culture the organism. Laboratory requests should include fungal-specific microscopy and culture, as well as bacterial and mycobacterial testing for differential diagnosis of other infectious agents. Obtaining a clinical history is useful, specifically noting activities that might expose the patient to potentially contaminated plant material. As sporotrichosis is rare in many localities, laboratories should take care not to ignore melanized fungal isolates that might be easily overlooked as contaminants. Referral to a reference laboratory is advised. Care should be taken to exclude non-pathogenic *Sporothrix* spp. and the *Sporothrix*-like basidiomycete *Quambalaria cyanescens*. Identification may be made on the basis of thermal dimorphism, ability to grow at 30°C, 35°C, and 37°C, morphological features; assimilation of sucrose, raffinose, and ribitol; and sequencing of the internal transcribed spacer regions of the ribosomal DNA. Protocols for identification of *S. schenckii* using matrix-assisted laser desorption/ionization have also been described. Serological testing may be performed, where available, by latex agglutination (IMMY, Norman, OK); this test requires 1 mL (minimum volume 0.2 mL) serum. Sensitivity varies from 56%–100% depending on disease presentation (disseminated > articular > pulmonary > cutaneous).

**9. Reporting requirements**—Sporotrichosis is not known to be a reportable disease, although laboratories should always confirm what is reportable to their respective public health authorities.

**10. Referral network**—Laboratories without the expertise to handle or identify *Sporothrix* spp. should refer suspected cases/cultures to a state or national mycology reference laboratory.

**11. Special considerations**—Outside of South America, infection is usually acquired by direct contact or penetrating injury from contaminated plant material including hay, wood, and sphagnum moss. Thus infections often have an association with certain occupational or gardening activities. Sporadic outbreaks occur where environmental factors amplify the growth of the fungus on relevant organic substrates.

[S. E. Kidd, I. Arthur]

# STAPHYLOCOCCAL DISEASES

| DISEASE | ICD-10 CODE |
|---|---|
| BOILS, CARBUNCLES, FURUNCLES, ABSCESSES | ICD-10 L02<br>B95.6–95.8 |
| IMPETIGO | ICD-10 L01 |
| CELLULITIS | ICD-10 L03 |
| STAPHYLOCOCCAL SEPSIS | ICD-10<br>A41.0–A41.2 |
| STAPHYLOCOCCAL PNEUMONIA | ICD-10 J15.2 |
| ARTHRITIS | ICD-10 M00.0 |
| OSTEOMYELITIS | ICD-10 M86 |
| ENDOCARDITIS | ICD-10 I33.0 |
| IMPETIGO NEONATORUM | ICD-10 L00 |
| ABSCESS OF THE BREAST | ICD-10 P39.0 |
| STAPHYLOCOCCAL DISEASE ON HOSPITAL, MEDICAL, AND SURGICAL WARDS | ICD-10 T81.4 |
| TOXIC SHOCK SYNDROME | ICD-10 A48.3 |
| Staphylococcal food poisonings (see "Foodborne Intoxications") | |

Members of the genus *Staphylococcus* are found widely as commensals in humans and animals. *Staphylococcus aureus* is the major pathogenic species; it is an important cause of disease in human and veterinary medicine, responsible for considerable morbidity and mortality.

Its propensity to produce a broad range of virulence factors (including toxins, enzymes, and adhesins) means *S. aureus* can cause a diverse range of clinical and epidemiological manifestations including (a) community-acquired disease, (b) hospital-acquired disease of newborns, (c) hospital-acquired disease in medical-surgical wards, and (d) toxic shock syndrome.

**1. Clinical features—**

1) Community-acquired staphylococcal disease: common skin lesions include impetigo, folliculitis, furuncles (boils), carbuncles, abscesses, and infected wounds. The basic lesion of impetigo is described in this chapter. (For further information, see Clinical Features section under Staphylococcal Disease in Hospital Nurseries in "Staphylococcal Disease" in *CCDM20*.) A distinctive scalded skin syndrome is associated with certain strains of *S. aureus*, which produce 1 or more epidermolytic toxins. Other skin lesions are more localized and discrete. Constitutional symptoms are unusual. If lesions extend or are widespread, fever, malaise, headache, and

anorexia may develop. Usually, lesions are uncomplicated, but seeding into the deeper tissues and/or bloodstream may lead to necrotizing lesions, necrotizing fasciitis, lung abscess, osteomyelitis, arthritis, endocarditis, or meningitis. In addition to primary skin lesions, staphylococcal conjunctivitis can occur, particularly in newborns and the elderly. Staphylococcal pneumonia is a well-recognized complication of influenza. Staphylococcal endocarditis and other complications of staphylococcal bacteraemia may result from parenteral use of illicit drugs or nosocomially from intravenous catheters and other devices. Embolic skin lesions are frequent complications of endocarditis due to *S. aureus*. Coagulase-negative staphylococci can also cause sepsis, meningitis, endocarditis, or female urinary tract infections. These are reported with increasing frequency, are commonly multiply resistant, and are difficult to treat.

2) Staphylococcal disease in hospital nurseries: impetigo or pustulosis of the newborn and other purulent skin manifestations are the staphylococcal diseases most frequently acquired in nurseries. Characteristic skin lesions develop secondary to colonization of the nose, umbilicus, circumcision site, rectum, or conjunctivae. Staphylococci commonly colonize these sites asymptomatically; their presence does not necessarily imply disease. Lesions most commonly occur in diaper and intertriginous areas. They are initially vesicular, rapidly turning seropurulent, surrounded by an erythematous base. Rupture of pustules favors their spread. Complications are unusual, although lymphadenitis, furunculosis, breast abscess, pneumonia, arthritis, osteomyelitis, and others have been reported. Though uncommon, staphylococcal scalded skin syndrome (Ritter disease, pemphigus neonatorum) may occur. Clinical manifestations range from diffuse scarlatiniform erythema to generalized bullous desquamation. Like bullous impetigo, it is caused by strains of *S. aureus,* which produce an epidemolytic toxin.

3) Staphylococcal disease on hospital medical and surgical wards: lesions vary from simple furuncles or stitch abscesses to extensively infected bedsores or surgical wounds, septic phlebitis, acute or chronic osteomyelitis, pneumonia, meningitis, endocarditis, or sepsis. A toxic state can complicate infection if the organism produces toxins. This is an ever-present risk.

4) Toxic shock syndrome: toxic shock syndrome is a severe illness characterized by sudden onset of high fever, vomiting, profuse watery diarrhea, and myalgia, followed by hypotension and—in severe cases—shock. More than three-fourths of cases occur in females. An erythematous sunburn-like rash is present during the acute phase, about 1–2 weeks after onset, with desquamation of the skin, especially

of palms of hands and soles of feet. Fever is usually high (39°C [102F]), with hypotension and multiple organ system involvement.

**2. Causative agents**—Various *Staphylococcus* spp. can cause disease in humans and animals, but *S. aureus* is the most prominent human pathogen. Two new species closely related to *S. aureus* were described in 2015: *Staphylococcus argenteus* and *Staphylococcus schweitzeri*. Collectively, these 3 species compose the *S. aureus*-related complex (SAC). *S. argenteus* has been identified predominantly in humans causing a similar spectrum of disease to *S. aureus*, while the primary host for *S. schweitzeri* appears to be animals, including bats and primates.

Across the One Health landscape, antibiotic resistant strains, most notably methicillin-resistant *S. aureus* (MRSA), are a particular public health concern. Three epidemiological groups of MRSA encoding the methicillin resistance gene (*mecA*) are recognized: health care associated, community-associated, and livestock-associated MRSA detected primarily in hospitals, the community, and livestock, respectively. In 2011, another group of MRSA with a different methicillin resistance gene (*mecC*) was identified in humans and diverse wildlife species. More recently (in 2018), there has been a single report of *mecB* plasmid-mediated methicillin resistance in *S. aureus*.

Microscopically, members of the SAC are Gram-positive spherical bacteria (cocci) that occur as clusters resembling grapes and are often hemolytic when grown on blood agar. They are nonmotile, non–spore-forming, coagulase positive, oxidase negative, facultatively anaerobic, have a broad temperature range (10°C–45°C), are salt tolerant (5%–15% sodium chloride), and can survive drying for many months.

**3. Laboratory diagnosis**—Many of the clinical manifestations of *S. aureus* disease can be caused by a range of other bacterial pathogens; therefore, the primary tool for differential diagnostic purposes is identification of the etiological agent by culture of clinical material (e.g., blood, sputum, wound exudate). *S. aureus* grows well on standard culture media such as nutrient or blood agar. Various enrichment media and chromogenic agars are available where selective screening for particular strains such as MRSA is required.

Following culture, presumptive identification is frequently based on colonial morphology. Variation in colony pigmentation and the possible emergence of small colony variants (SCVs) especially in chronic or relapsing infections mean that some form of confirmatory testing is advisable. Coagulase testing is used widely as a primary diagnostic test to distinguish *S. aureus* from more than 40 species of coagulase-negative staphylococci commonly found in humans and animals. Differentiation from other coagulase-positive staphylococci found less frequently in humans (e.g., *S. argenteus*, *S. schweitzeri*, *Staphylococcus schleiferi* subsp. *coagulans*, *Staphylococcus pseudintermedius*, and *Staphylococcus hyicus*) requires additional testing (e.g., biotyping or matrix-assisted laser desorption/ionization time-of-flight mass spectrometry

[MALDI-TOF]). Aside from coagulase testing, other phenotypic tests commonly used for identification purposes include screening for catalase and/or thermostable deoxyribonuclease activity, commercial latex agglutination kits, biotyping, and MALDI-TOF.

Molecular methods such as polymerase chain reaction (PCR), microarray, or whole genome sequencing are being employed increasingly for identification purposes with the benefit of affording a more comprehensive analysis of the isolate including typing, virulence, and antimicrobial resistance (AMR) gene profiling to support diagnostic and micro-epidemiological investigations.

For non–culture-based diagnosis, various commercial PCR-based systems approved for clinical diagnostic use are available enabling the identification of *S. aureus* directly in clinical material (e.g., nasal swabs, blood) and can provide a rapid result within 2–4 hours to help guide patient management.

4. **Laboratory capability**—Patient samples should be handled in a clinical microbiology diagnostic laboratory accredited to an internationally recognized standard (currently ISO 15189). Similarly, laboratory personnel should be registered with an appropriate accredited regulatory body according to their role (clinical, scientific, technical, or medical).

Routine diagnostic microbiology laboratories should have the capability to undertake primary isolation of the etiological agent followed by identification and susceptibility testing to support and guide patient treatment. For the rapid identification of MRSA-positive patients for isolation/cohorting purposes, various molecular methods can be used to detect the organism directly in clinical material.

Depending on the clinical and epidemiological context, detailed characterization of isolates may be required (e.g., phenotypic detection of unusual resistances, determination of toxin and AMR gene status, identification of high-risk clones, assessing strain relatedness to assist with outbreak investigations). Such analyses are most often undertaken in specialist regional or national reference laboratories with multidisciplinary public health teams (e.g., microbiologists, epidemiologists, infection prevention and control specialists, research scientists, and bioinformaticians) working in partnership to provide expert advice and support.

5. **Safety requirements**—All staphylococci belong to hazard group 2 (i.e., a biological agent that can cause human disease and may be a hazard to employees but is unlikely to spread to the community, and for which there is usually effective prophylaxis or treatment available) and should be handled at biosafety level/containment level 2. Where laboratory procedures are likely to generate airborne droplets, such work should be risk-assessed and, where appropriate, conducted in a biosafety cabinet. If it is suspected that a specimen may contain hazard group 3 biological agents, all work on that specimen must be conducted at biosafety level/containment level 3.

To comply with health and safety law, any risks associated with the laboratory work being undertaken must be identified and appropriate control procedures implemented. Laboratory standard operating procedures should be in place detailing how the work may be conducted safely and stipulating the personal protective equipment required for the procedures being undertaken (e.g., disposable gloves, protective laboratory coat or gown, eye protection).

6. **Nonhuman hosts**—Although humans are a major source of *S. aureus*, the species is also found in a broad range of wild and domestic animals and birds, including food-producing animals (e.g., pigs, poultry, cows) and their products (e.g., meat, milk, cheese). *S. aureus* can be shed by colonized and infected hosts via skin scales and aerosols, resulting in contamination of other niches such as the environment, soil, vegetation, water, and air.

Some lineages of *S. aureus* display a high degree of host specialization, while others have a broad host spectrum across the One Health landscape. *S. aureus* can be transmitted from animals to humans (zoonosis) or from humans to animals (reverse zoonosis or anthroponosis). Recent genomic studies have provided evidence of the adaptability of *S. aureus* with some human strains adapting and becoming successful in animals and vice versa. Consequently, animals in close contact with humans can acquire human-adapted strains. Similarly, certain occupational groups are at increased risk of exposure to animal-associated lineages (e.g., veterinarians, farmers). These aspects are of particular public health concern for those working in settings where AMR strains such as MRSA may be prevalent (e.g., health care workers, veterinarians, and farmers).

7. **Sample/specimen requirements**—Specimens should be taken as soon as possible after the onset of clinical symptoms and, where possible, before the initiation of antimicrobial therapy. The nature of the sample will depend on the clinical context and may be from a sterile site (e.g., blood, joint fluid, cerebrospinal fluid) or a contaminated site (e.g., sputum, wound exudate, skin swab). In cases of suspected food poisoning, suitable specimens include vomit, feces, or food samples.

Clinical material should be transported promptly to the testing laboratory and processed as soon as possible, ideally within 4–24 hours of being taken, to avoid deterioration or overgrowth with other microorganisms that may be present.

The sample must be labeled and placed in a transport bag; where necessary, absorbent material should be used to contain any leakage that may occur. A request form outlining the relevant clinical information and the nature of the microbiological testing required should be put in a pocket attached to the transport bag. The sample and form should then be placed into an appropriate (i.e., in Europe, CE marked) leak-proof container and transported to the laboratory in an approved secondary container. If a specimen is to be mailed, the packaging must comply with local postal regulations.

8. **Testing requirements**—The recovery of *S. aureus* as the sole organism from a sterile or contaminated site in the presence of relevant clinical signs

and symptoms should be regarded as diagnostic. As polymicrobial infections can occur, recovery of *S. aureus* along with other microbial species from a sterile or contaminated site requires investigation and clinical review to determine whether it is likely to be the primary pathogen. Subsequent identification and characterisation of the cultured organism affords confirmatory testing.

Screening samples from various body sites such as the nose, throat, axilla, or groin are commonly used to determine the carriage status of an individual for a variety of reasons such as (a) patient management purposes (therapeutic treatment and/or isolation), (b) identification of possible transmission events as part of outbreak investigations, or (c) assessing the efficacy of decolonization therapy.

The sensitivity and specificity of cultural techniques may be reduced in the case of (a) prior antimicrobial therapy, (b) infection with fastidious or slow growing variants such as SCVs, (c) a low bioburden, (d) delays in sample processing, or (e) heavily contaminated material (e.g., feces, foods). To maximize recovery of *S. aureus* in such situations, the use of selective media, broth enrichment, and/or prolonged incubation periods should be considered.

Where staphylococcal disease is strongly suspected but cultures are negative, molecular methods applied directly to clinical material can be used as a presumptive diagnostic tool. Molecular methods enable rapid identification of the target pathogen, including variants that are slow to grow or are unculturable, particularly in time-critical situations (e.g., emergency surgery, patient fatalities, possible ward closure). Alternative techniques such as the application of 16S ribosomal ribonucleic acid gene sequencing directly to clinical material can provide a presumptive diagnosis. Metagenomics is being increasingly explored and may provide a further option for presumptive diagnostics. The detection of *S. aureus*-specific antigens (including toxins) in clinical material such as blood, pleural fluid, food, and feces is available in some specialized centers. Such tests are generally not commercially available and are mostly licensed for research purposes only.

For quality assurance purposes, clinical diagnostic laboratories must control their analytical processes in accordance with the ISO 15189 framework. Laboratories should participate in relevant external quality assessment schemes and undertake appropriate internal quality control procedures to ensure that all commercial and in-house tests have been validated and shown to be fit for purpose. In some countries, compliance with ISO is audited through inspection by an independent national organization. Documents outlining national standards for microbiological investigations help promote a good standard of practice and serve as a valuable resource in some countries.

**9. Reporting requirements**—Both MRSA colonization and infection are notifiable conditions (i.e., a legal requirement) in some regions of the world. In other areas, notification is restricted to invasive disease (e.g., bacteremia). Monitoring of MRSA rates is valuable for informing trends, the need for interventions, assessing the efficacy of control measures, and for monitoring performance against national infection prevention goals. In some instances, data are captured across regions and countries via organizations such as European Centres for Disease Control and CDC.

Various reporting initiatives provide insights into changes in the epidemiology of MRSA and/or staphylococcal disease via ad hoc surveys of, for example, postsurgical site infection, food poisoning incidents, AMR in zoonotic incidents, and indicator bacteria in humans, animals, and food.

Resistance to antibiotics is a public health concern internationally, especially where it may limit utility of certain antibiotics of last resort (e.g., vancomycin, linezolid). Such exceptional resistances are subject to public health monitoring and are notifiable in some countries (e.g., vancomycin-resistant *S. aureus*).

**10. Referral network**—Testing laboratories can be categorized as local, regional, or national according to their role and the level of public health service they provide. Individual institutions may be responsible for the processing of samples from different ecological niches (e.g., food, animals, humans) while in others processing may be the responsibility of a single overarching organization.

The referral of isolates to a specialist/reference laboratory should be in accordance with local policies and regulatory requirements. This can vary from mandating the referral of isolates from all newly identified cases of MRSA or invasive isolates only to the voluntary referral of selected isolates that require testing not available in routine diagnostic laboratories (e.g., phenotypic detection of unusual resistances, determination of toxin and AMR gene status, identification of high-risk clones, assessing strain relatedness to assist with outbreak investigations).

**11. Special considerations**—Staphylococcal enterotoxin B (SEB) is a category B select agent, an important toxin threat in warfare. At low concentrations, it can cause multiorgan system failure and death, making it a biological agent of concern to both military and civilian target populations. Testing for SEB needs to be conducted by specialist laboratories with appropriate expertise and containment facilities.

In response to the increasingly serious threat posed by AMR to the effective prevention and treatment of *S. aureus* infections, alternative therapeutic strategies have been sought. Despite extensive developmental research and clinical trials of vaccines and antivirulence therapeutics for staphylococcal disease, none have been successfully licensed for human use.

Factors such as increasing interaction between humans, animals, diverse ecological niches, migration, international travel, and selective pressures (e.g., the widespread use of antimicrobials) have contributed to the adaptation and emergence of multidrug resistant *S. aureus* clones, including MRSA. In response to this, key agencies such as the United Nations and WHO seek to monitor for changes in disease incidence, molecular epidemiology,

AMR, and zoonotic potential across the One Health landscape through international collaborative efforts. For further information on One Health, see "Animal, Food, and Environmental Testing in Support of Communicable Disease Control: A One Health Approach."

[A. Kearns]

# STREPTOCOCCAL DISEASES

| DISEASE | ICD-10 CODE |
|---|---|
| STREPTOCOCCAL SORE THROAT | ICD-10 J02.0 |
| IMPETIGO | ICD-10 L01.0 |
| ERYSIPELAS | ICD-10 A46 |
| SCARLET FEVER | ICD-10 A38 |
| PUERPERAL FEVER | ICD-10 O85 |
| OTHER GROUP A STREPTOCOCCAL INFECTIONS | ICD-10 A49.1 |
| GROUP B STREPTOCOCCAL SEPSIS OF THE NEWBORN | ICD-10 P36.0 |
| STREPTOCOCCAL DENTAL CARIES IN EARLY CHILDHODD | ICD-10 K02 |
| STREPTOCOCCAL TOXIC SHOCK SYNDROME | ICD-10 B95.0 |
| Streptococcus pneumoniae infections (see "Pneumonia") | |

## I. GROUP A STREPTOCOCCAL INFECTIONS

**1. Clinical features**—The most frequently encountered group A streptococcal (GAS) conditions are pharyngitis/tonsillitis and superficial skin infections such as impetigo or pyoderma. Other acute infections include scarlet fever, puerperal fever, septicemia, erysipelas, cellulitis, mastoiditis, otitis media, pneumonia, peritonsillitis, wound infections, and, rarely, necrotizing fasciitis and a toxic shock-like syndrome. One or other form of clinical disease often predominates during outbreaks. Acute glomerulonephritis may develop after pharyngeal or skin infection with a limited number of (nephritogenic) strains of GAS associated with specific types of M protein (M-types).

1) Streptococcal sore throat: patients with streptococcal sore throat typically exhibit sudden onset of fever, exudative tonsillitis, or pharyngitis (sore throat), and tender, enlarged anterior cervical lymph nodes. The pharynx, the tonsillar pillars, and soft palate may be injected and edematous; petechiae may be present against

a background of diffuse redness. Coincident or subsequent otitis media or peritonsillar abscess may occur. Possible nonsuppurative complications include acute rheumatic fever (an average of 19 days following pharyngitis) and acute glomerulonephritis (an average of 10 days following pharyngitis or ≥3 weeks after skin infection). Rheumatic heart (valvular) disease occurs days to weeks after acute streptococcal infection, and Sydenham chorea (in the past, often referred to as Saint Vitus' Dance) several months following infection.

2) GAS skin infection (pyoderma, impetigo): usually superficial and may proceed through vesicular, pustular, and encrusted stages. Glomerulonephritis may occur later, usually 3 weeks after the skin infection.

3) Scarlet fever: a form of GAS infection characterized by a skin rash, occurring when the infecting strain produces a pyrogenic exotoxin (erythrogenic toxin) and the patient is sensitized, but not immune, to the toxin. Clinical characteristics may include all symptoms associated with a streptococcal sore throat (or with a streptococcal wound, skin, or puerperal infection) as well as enanthem, strawberry tongue, and exanthem. The rash is usually a fine erythema, commonly punctate, blanching on pressure, often felt (like sandpaper) better than seen, and appearing most often on the neck, chest, folds of the axilla, elbow, groin, and inner surfaces of the thighs. Typically, the scarlet fever rash does not involve the face, but there is flushing of the cheeks and circumoral pallor. High fever, nausea, and vomiting often accompany severe infections. During convalescence, skin peeling occurs at the tips of fingers and toes and less often over wide areas of trunk and limbs, including palms and soles; it is more pronounced where the exanthem was severe. The case-fatality rate in some parts of the world has occasionally been as high as 3%. Scarlet fever may be followed by the same sequelae as streptococcal sore throat.

4) Erysipelas: an acute skin infection characterized by fever, constitutional symptoms, leukocytosis, and a red, tender, edematous spreading lesion of the skin, typically with a definite raised border. The central point of origin tends to clear as the periphery extends. Face and legs are common sites. Recurrences are frequent and disease is more common among persons with underlying skin conditions. The disease has a good prognosis with early diagnosis and treatment but may be especially severe in patients suffering from debilitating disease. Erysipelas due to GAS is to be distinguished from erysipeloid caused by *Erysipelothrix rhusiopathiae*, a localized cutaneous infection (typically without fever or systemic

symptoms) seen primarily as an occupational disease of people handling freshwater fish or shellfish; infected swine or turkeys or their tissues; or, rarely, sheep, cattle, chickens, or pheasants.

5) Perianal cellulitis (due to GAS): recognized more frequently in the past decade and, though it occurs among all ages, is primarily a disease of early childhood. It can also result in disease outbreaks.

6) GAS puerperal fever: an acute disease, usually febrile, with local and general symptoms and signs of bacterial invasion of the genital tract and sometimes the bloodstream in the postpartum or post-abortion patient. Case-fatality rate is low when streptococcal puerperal fever is adequately treated. Puerperal infections may be caused by organisms other than hemolytic streptococci; they are clinically similar but differ bacteriologically and epidemiologically (see "Staphylococcal Diseases").

7) Streptococcal toxic shock syndrome (STSS) and necrotizing fasciitis: the most severe forms of invasive GAS infection. Although the incidence of these manifestations of GAS likely increased in the late 1980s and early 1990s, active surveillance in the USA indicates that rates of STSS and necrotizing fasciitis due to GAS have been fairly stable during the last 15 years. Necrotizing fasciitis (sometimes known as flesh-eating bacteria) can be caused by multiple pathogens, but the most common etiology is GAS. It is a rapidly progressive disease that destroys muscles, fat, and skin tissue. Patients often present with skin that is erythematous, edematous, and hot to the touch. The pain is often described as out of proportion to what is expected by physical exam. Patients often have fever and chills, fatigue, vomiting, and diarrhea. In the USA, the mortality rate is approximately 25%. STSS clinical features include hypotension and 1 or more of the following: renal impairment, thrombocytopenia, disseminated intravascular coagulation, serum glutamic oxaloacetic transaminase or bilirubin elevation, adult respiratory distress syndrome, a generalized erythematous macular rash, or soft-tissue necrosis (necrotizing fasciitis). STSS may occur with either systemic or focal (throat, skin, lung sites) group A streptococcal infections, and mortality rates are as high as 35%–40%. For both necrotizing fasciitis and STSS, rapid diagnosis, aggressive management, and early use of appropriate antibiotics are critical.

**2. Causative agents**—*Streptococcus pyogenes*, or GAS, are Gram-positive, β-hemolytic bacteria. While the critical virulence factor, the M protein, generates type-specific immunity, distinct GAS serotypes are increasingly being identified through *emm* typing—a system that determines the *emm* gene encoding the M-protein. Over 240 distinct *emm* types that vary by geographic and time distributions have been recognized. Skin infections caused by GAS usually differ serologically from GAS-associated with throat infections. In scarlet fever, 3 immunologically different types of erythrogenic toxin (pyrogenic exotoxins A, B, and C) have been demonstrated. In STSS, 80% of isolates produce pyrogenic exotoxin A. Phenotypically mucoid strains have been involved in recent outbreaks of rheumatic fever.

**3. Laboratory diagnosis**—Provisional laboratory findings are based on the isolation of the organisms from affected tissues (e.g., blood, wounds) using blood agar or other appropriate media, or on identification of GAS antigen in pharyngeal secretions (the rapid antigen detection test). Colony morphology and the production of clear beta-hemolysis on blood agar made with sheep's blood identify streptococci on cultures; inhibition by special antibiotic discs containing bacitracin (0.02–0.04 units) constitutes tentative identification.

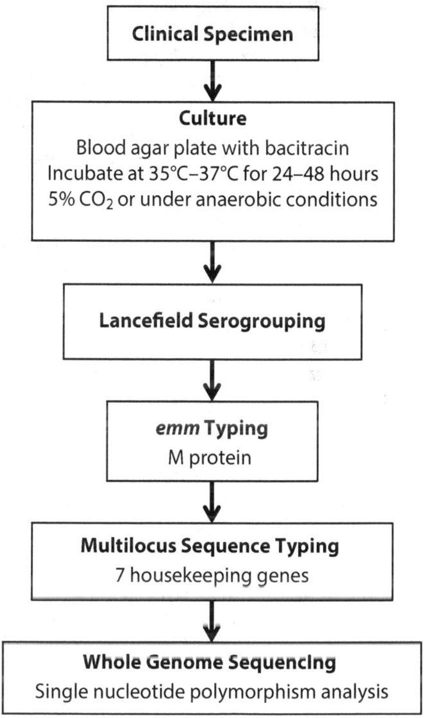


Algorithm for Laboratory Diagnosis of Group A Streptococci

Specific serogrouping procedures provide definitive identification. Antigen detection tests also allow rapid identification, demonstrating a rise in serum antibody titer (antistreptolysin O, antihyaluronidase [not commercially available], anti-DNA [deoxyribonucleic acid]-ase B) between acute and convalescent stages of illness; high titers may persist for several months.

In many industrialized countries, current recommended practice for diagnosis of strep pharyngitis is to first do a rapid antigen detection test (high specificity but low sensitivity) or a throat culture and, if this is positive, assume the patient has a GAS infection. If the result of a rapid test used in a child or adolescent is negative or equivocal, a throat culture should be done to guide management and prevent superfluous use of antibiotics. The first figure describes the algorithm for laboratory diagnosis of group A streptococci.

**4. Laboratory capability**—Suspected *S. pyogenes* clinical samples are usually processed by local or regional laboratories and isolates are sent to a specialized reference laboratory to confirm identification and further characterization of *S. pyogenes* strains. The main aim of the laboratory is to provide rapid, robust, and specific methods to confirm a clinical diagnosis of *S. pyogenes* so that clinicians can provide the appropriate treatments. Ideally laboratories should have adequate space and equipment to safely perform all activities. Personnel should have received specialized training in *S. pyogenes* diagnostics. Guidelines for the laboratory diagnosis of group A streptococcal infections have been published by WHO.[1]

**5. Safety requirements**—*Streptococcus pyogenes* is categorized as a human pathogen hazard group 2 and requires containment level 2 facilities, equipment, and operational practices for work involving infectious or potentially infectious clinical samples or cultures.

Laboratory safety procedures required for working with *S. pyogenes* include a laboratory safety manual, risk assessments, and standard operating procedures (SOPs). New staff should be aware of the laboratory safety manual, which describes safe laboratory practice for *S. pyogenes*, biosafety, chemical, fire, and electrical safety requirements as well as handling waste disposal and spillages.

Laboratory-acquired infections can result from inhalation and hand-to-mouth contact, through skin punctures, cuts, or abrasions, or by liquids splashing onto mucus membranes. Personal protective equipment (PPE) should be used where required to minimize these risks in addition to safe methods of working. All staff must wear a clean laboratory coat and gloves when direct skin contact with infected materials may occur. Eye protection must be used where there is a known or potential risk of exposure to splashes.

All procedures that may produce aerosols, or involve high concentrations or large volumes, should be conducted in a class I or II biosafety cabinet (BSC). The use of needles, syringes and other sharp objects should be strictly limited. Care must be taken to minimize the production of aerosols. All work likely to cause aerosols from potentially infected material or culture must be carried out in a BSC. Risk of exposure is considered to be low using PPE (laboratory coat, gloves and safety glasses) and BSC used for all tests that involve suspensions of live cultures (e.g., preparation of broth suspensions for serotyping, storage of cultures in glycerol blood broths, recovery of organisms from freeze-dried cultures, preparing cell pellets for DNA extraction). Such samples should be centrifuged in sealed buckets and loaded or unloaded in a BSC.

For the purposes of transportation, potentially infected clinical samples or cultures of *S. pyogenes* are classified as a biological substance, category B, packed to full UN3373 specification. For international transportation, samples must be transported via a specialist courier service. Some countries may require an import permit, shipper's declaration, and other relevant documents.

**6. Nonhuman hosts**—Humans are the primary reservoir for this bacterium, although cattle can also act as a reservoir. Cows infected by humans are intermediate hosts (although a rare occurrence) and can pass the bacterium in their milk, which, if consumed unpasteurized, can infect other humans.

**7. Sample/specimen requirements**—Clinical samples such as respiratory specimens, skin lesions, blood, sputum and wound exudates may contain the infectious agent. Commercially available Dacron or Rayon swabs with an aluminum or plastic shaft with either Stuart or Amies liquid medium are recommended for collecting specimens from the throat, nose, skin lesions, wounds, or other affected body sites.

Any delay between collection of a specimen and its examination in the laboratory increases the likelihood of false-negative results. For specimens that cannot be immediately cultured, the use of a transport medium (e.g., Stuart's or Amies liquid medium) is recommended to prevent loss of viability of *S. pyogenes*. Specimens are transported to the laboratory at room temperature and can be stored at 4°C for 48 hours (once received) if sample processing is delayed. If there are considerable delays, which may occur in field studies for example, the use of a silica gel transport system is recommended as described in the WHO manual.[1]

Laboratory diagnosis of *S. pyogenes* infections primarily relies on culturing the bacteria from clinical specimens (sterile sites) and superficial and environmental samples (non-sterile sites). To detect *S. pyogenes* in clinical specimens, the material is often cultured on blood agar plates, which facilitates an easy preliminary screen for β-hemolytic colonies.

**8. Testing requirements**—To identify *S. pyogenes* in clinical samples, blood agar plates (5% sheep or horse blood) are screened for the presence of β-hemolytic colonies. The typical appearance of *S. pyogenes* colonies, after 24 hours of incubation at 35°C–37°C in the presence of 5% $CO_2$ or under anaerobic conditions, is a white greyish color with a diameter of 0.5 mm or greater, surrounded by β-hemolysis that is often 2–4 times larger than the colony diameter. Negative results can be confirmed after a total culture time of 48 hours. For presumptive identification of *S. pyogenes*, cultures should be tested for bacitracin susceptibility and pyrrolidonyl arylamidase (PYR) activity. A definitive diagnosis should include a positive Lancefield group A antigen test.

There are a number of conventional identification tests that can be used including Lancefield antigen determination, PYR test, Bacitracin susceptibility test, species determination using automated identification systems (e.g., matrix-assisted laser desorption/ionization time-of-flight [MALDI-TOF]), direct antigen detection from throat specimens, nucleic acid detection techniques, and serologic tests. Since each of these tests has limitations, the most reliable identification can be achieved by combining some of these methods described later. To further characterize *S. pyogenes* strains, the gold standard *emm* typing method is performed by a reference laboratory. During an outbreak investigation, other molecular typing methods such as multilocus sequence typing (MLST) or whole genome sequencing (WGS) can be implemented (see the first figure earlier).

Automated bacterial identification systems have become more widely accessible in clinical laboratories within the last decade. These commercially available systems generally perform well at identifying commonly isolated pathogenic streptococci, such as *S. pyogenes* and *S. agalactiae*. Although automated bacterial identification by MALDI-TOF has limitations in misidentifying several streptococcal species such as. *dysgalactiae* subsp. *equismilis* as *S. pyogenes*, the results for *S. pyogenes* correspond well to species identification by conventional tests.

Although numerous assays for direct detection of the group A-specific carbohydrate antigen in throat swabs by agglutination methods or immunoassays (enzyme, liposome, or optical) have become commercially available, culturing throat swabs for *S. pyogenes* remains the gold standard. The specificity of rapid antigen tests is generally high, even though false-positive antigen results can be seen from patients previously diagnosed and/or treated for *S. pyogenes* or patients colonized with non-*S. pyogenes* streptococcal species that carry the Lancefield group A antigen. Despite the obvious advantages of a rapid diagnosis, it must be noted that the positive predictive value of rapid group A antigen tests is currently low in the adult population and can frequently result in unnecessary antimicrobial therapy.

The diagnosis of post-streptococcal diseases, such as glomerulonephritis, acute rheumatic fever, and cerebral disorders relies on the determination of specific antibodies (e.g., antistreptolysin O and anti-DNase B). Antibody levels against streptolysin O (ASO) start rising after 1 week of infection and reach maximum levels at about 3–6 weeks of infection. About 20% of infected individuals do not respond by an increase in ASO titer, thus negative ASO titer alone cannot be used to rule out rheumatic fever or other streptococcal sequelae, and an additional antibody test is required (e.g., anti-DNase B). DNase B titers start appearing 2 weeks after the onset of infection and may not reach maximum titers for 6–8 weeks. Anti-DNase B titers tend to remain elevated longer than the ASO titers and are more reliable than ASO for the confirmation of a preceding streptococcal skin infection. Moreover, since only 80%–85% of patients with rheumatic fever will present with elevated ASO titers, additional DNase titers may be helpful. The classic ASO and anti-DNase B assays are both based on neutralization assays, although less standardized assay techniques such as latex agglutination tests are also commercially available.

For further strain characterization, epidemiological studies and outbreak investigations, different typing methods have been developed and performed by reference laboratories. Conventional typing of *S. pyogenes* is based on the antigenic specificity of the surface expressed T and M proteins. Currently, 20 T-types and 83 M serotypes are validated and internationally recognized. However, these typing methods do not offer high discriminatory power and are no longer used by reference laboratories. The M protein, encoded by the *emm* gene, acts as a major virulence factor and is an important epidemiological marker used globally to characterise *S. pyogenes* strains. With more than 200 different M-protein genes sequence types (*emm* types) identified, the *emm*-typing scheme is the current gold standard for *S. pyogenes* molecular typing and is based upon the DNA sequence of the 5' end 150 nucleotides of the *emm* gene. Subtypes can be assigned by sequencing 150 nucleotides that encode the N terminal 50 residues of the mature M protein (see: http://www.cdc.gov/ncidod/biotech/strep/emmtypes.htm).

An MLST scheme based on 7 housekeeping genes has been developed to study the molecular epidemiology and population genetic structure of *S. pyogenes.* Although several *emm* types can be shared between different clonal complexes, MLST does not provide a highly discriminatory typing method for *S. pyogenes* (see: https://pubmlst.org/spyogenes).

Typing of *S. pyogenes* is crucial for infection control and epidemiology. While WGS is revolutionizing the way that bacterial organisms are typed, it is necessary to provide backward compatibility with currently used typing schemes to facilitate comparisons and understanding of epidemiological trends. Using this approach, not only *emm* types and MLST and clonal lineages can be identified rapidly and efficiently (< 10 days), the presence or absence of specific virulence and antibiotic resistance genes as well as mutations in transcriptional regulators of virulence and in genes encoding for antibiotic targets can also be assessed. Although WGS is a robust and powerful typing tool, there is a need for global standardisation of this methodology as well as analysis and interpretation of single nucleotide polymorphism (SNP) data during an outbreak investigation.

The maintenance of a quality management system is crucial to laboratories for providing the correct test results every time. Internal and external quality assurance procedures should also be in place. An external quality assessment (EQA) scheme is an important element of a quality management system as it aims to analyse the accuracy of the entire testing process from receipt of sample and testing of sample to reporting of results (also known as proficiency testing). International EQA programs for *S. pyogenes* have been performed under the auspices of WHO, and it is imperative to continuously improve and assess laboratory performance and offer training to any laboratories that have technical difficulties.[2]

**9. Reporting requirements**—To confirm identification and for further characterization and typing of strains, pure cultures of *S. pyogenes* should be submitted to the reference laboratory. Laboratory results are reported to the clinician responsible for the case, the public health physician, and the local and national health protection teams (in an outbreak investigation). The reporting of streptococcal testing results by laboratories to the public health authorities is required in most settings globally. Laboratories should check the applicable regulations in their specific location to assure compliance.

**10. Referral network**—There is no defined international referral network for group A streptococcal infections. However, ad-hoc workshops and expert meetings are occasionally commissioned by WHO. There is an International Lancefield Society that meets every 3 years to update on the current status of these and other streptococcal infections.

**11. Special considerations**—Local or state public health officials may investigate clusters or outbreaks of invasive group A *Streptococcus* (group A strep) infections. The most common clusters investigated tend to be those occurring in long-term care facilities. Other types of outbreak investigations include clusters of pharyngitis (strep throat) among school-aged children, health care–associated infections such as postpartum and postsurgical infections, and, rarely, foodborne outbreaks of pharyngitis. In these clusters, urgent public health action is often indicated. There is currently no vaccine to prevent group A strep infections, although several vaccines are in development.

## II. GROUP B STREPTOCOCCAL SEPSIS OF THE NEWBORN

**1. Clinical features**—Human subtypes of group B streptococci (*Streptococcus agalactiae*) produce invasive disease in the newborn of 2 distinct forms. Early onset disease (from 1–7 days) with sepsis, pneumonia, and less frequently meningitis, osteomyelitis, or septic arthritis is acquired in utero or during delivery. Late onset disease (7 days to several months) is acquired in about half the cases through person-to-person contact and presents mostly as meningitis or sepsis. Advances in neonatal care have led to a fall in the case-fatality rate from 50%–4%. Survivors may have speech, hearing, and/or visual problems; psychomotor retardation; or seizure disorders if there has been meningeal involvement

**2. Causative agents**—*S. agalactiae* or group B streptococci (GBS) is the cause of sepsis in newborns. GBS harbours an important number of virulence factors including the capsular polysaccharide (rich in sialic acid) and a pore-forming toxin, β-haemolysin. The GBS capsule is probably the key virulence factor because it helps GBS escape from the host defence mechanisms interfering with phagocytic killing of GBS by human phagocytes.

**3. Laboratory diagnosis**—Culture and isolation of GBS from blood, cerebrospinal fluid, or other normally sterile body fluid.

GBS grows readily on blood agar plates as microbial colonies surrounded by a narrow zone of β-haemolysis. Haemolytic GBS strains also produce an

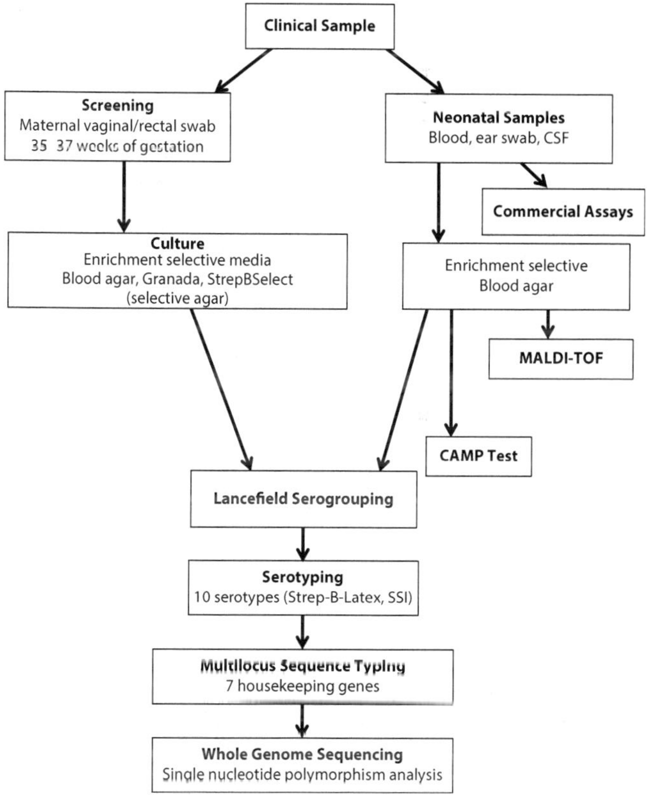


Algorithm for Laboratory Diagnosis of Group B Streptococci

orange-brick-red nonisoprenoid polyene pigment (ornythinrhamnododecaene [granadaene] when cultivated on selective media such as, granada medium. GBS is characterized by the presence of the capsular polysaccharide Lancefield group B antigen that can be detected directly in intact bacteria using commercial latex agglutination tests. Many local laboratories can now identify GBS (from culture) using MALDI-TOF mass spectrometry, and direct detection of GBS from neonatal samples can be achieved using commercially available real-time polymerase chain reaction (PCR)-based assays; however, such tests require specialist equipment and trained staff. The second figure earlier describes the algorithm for laboratory diagnosis of group B streptococci.

GBS can be differentiated into 10 distinct capsular polysaccharide serotypes (Ia, Ib, and II–IX) and their distribution varies worldwide. Approximately, 10% of GBS strains are nontypeable and can be further tested using multiplex PCR assays for capsular typing of GBS. Other typing methods such as MLST, based on ~500 bp fragments of 7 housekeeping genes, and, more recently, WGS can also be used to investigate the clonal population structures and genetic lineages of GBS strains.

**4. Laboratory capability**—Suspected GBS maternal or neonatal clinical samples and swabs are usually processed by local or regional laboratories and GBS isolates are sent to specialized reference laboratories for identification, confirmation, and further characterization and typing. The main aim of the laboratory is to provide rapid, robust, and specific methods to confirm a clinical diagnosis of neonatal GBS infection so that clinicians can provide the appropriate treatments. Ideally laboratories should have adequate space and equipment to safely perform all activities. Personnel should have received specialized training in *S. agalactiae* diagnostics and should follow national guidelines and SOPs.

**5. Safety requirements**—*Streptococcus agalactiae* are categorized as a human pathogen hazard group 2 and require containment level 2 facilities, equipment, and operational practices for work involving infectious or potentially infectious clinical samples or cultures.

Laboratory safety manual, risk assessments, and SOPs should be available for each laboratory. New staff should be aware of the laboratory safety manual which describes safe laboratory practice for *S. agalactiae*, biosafety, chemical, fire, and electrical safety requirements, as well as handling waste disposal and spillages.

Infections can be acquired by inhalation and hand-to-mouth contact, through skin punctures, cuts, or abrasions, or by liquids splashing onto mucus membranes. PPE, in addition to safe methods of working, should be used where required to minimize these risks. All staff must were a clean laboratory coat and gloves. Eye protection should be used where there is a known or potential risk of exposure to splashes.

All procedures that may produce aerosols or involve high concentrations or large volumes should be conducted in a class I or II BSC. The use of needles, syringes and other sharp objects should be strictly limited. Care must be taken to minimise the production of aerosols. All work likely to cause aerosols from potentially infected material or culture must be carried out in a BSC. Risk of exposure is considered to be low using PPE (laboratory coat, gloves, and safety glasses) and BSCs for all tests that involve suspensions of live cultures. All pregnant staff must take extra care when handling suspected *S. agalactiae* clinical samples or cultures.

For transportation, potentially infected clinical samples or cultures of *S. agalactiae* are classified as a biological substance, category B, packed to full UN3373 specification. For international transportation, samples must be transported via a specialist courier service. Some countries may require an import permit, shipper's declaration, and other relevant documents.

**6. Nonhuman hosts**—Invasive disease due to *S. agalactiae* is not limited to humans as it is also a common veterinary pathogen because it can cause bovine mastitis (inflammation of the udder) in dairy cows. Other species affected include terrestrial mammals such as dogs and cats and aquatic or semi-aquatic species such as sea mammals, crocodiles, bullfrogs, and fish.

**7. Sample/specimen requirements**—Maternal low vaginal/rectal swabs should be taken between 35–37 weeks of gestation for culture. Rayon or Dacron swabs should be used with commercially available non-nutritive transport media (e.g., Amies or Stuart's without charcoal). This preserves the viability of the organism by providing moisture and buffering to maintain the pH. Samples from neonates with clinical symptoms of sepsis include surface swabs (ear swabs), blood, or cerebrospinal fluid (CSF).

Vaginal and rectal swabs placed in transport medium and/or neonatal specimens should be immediately submitted to the local laboratory (within the day); if any delay is expected, specimens should be refrigerated (2°C–8°C) for a maximum of 48 hours. In these conditions, GBS can remain viable.

Initially swabs for GBS prenatal screening cultures should be inoculated into commercially available selective enrichment broth medium such as Lim broth, which consists of Todd Hewitt broth supplemented with colistin (10 mg/L) and nalidixic acid (15 mg/L). If both a vaginal and rectal swab is submitted from 1 patient, both swabs may be placed into an enrichment broth and incubated at 35°C–37°C in 5%–10% $CO_2$ (caps should be kept loose during incubation). After 18–24 hours of incubation, subculture with a sterile loop and inoculate a Columbia blood agar. Selective chromogenic agar such as Granada or StrepBSelect agar plates may also be used. Neonatal samples can also be tested at local laboratory by culture and or directly using a commercial antigen system or MALDI TOF.

**8. Testing requirements**—Laboratories should follow their national guidelines and standard procedures for processing maternal and neonatal samples. To improve sensitivity and predictive values of GBS antenatal screening, culture techniques that maximize the likelihood of GBS recovery are required for prenatal screening. Important factors that influence the accuracy of detection of GBS maternal colonization are the choice of culture media, the body sites sampled, and the timing of the sample. The yield of GBS-positive culture is increased by sampling the anorectum in addition to the lower vaginal area because the gastrointestinal tract is a major reservoir of GBS.

After collection, maternal vaginal/rectal swabs must be placed in a non-nutrient transport medium (e.g., Amies or Stuart). Swabs should then be inoculated into selective broth medium such as Todd-Hewitt broth with nalidixic acid and colistin (e.g., commercially available Lim broth). After incubation (18–24 hours, 35°C–37°C), the enrichment broth should be subcultured to blood agar plates. On blood agar, suggestive colonies of GBS are gray, translucent, with a surrounding zone of β-hemolysis (or no hemolysis, very rare). Use of selective and differential media for subcultures can improve screening sensitivity as well as shorten the turnaround time and is already recommended in some European countries for antenatal GBS-screening cultures.

The current gold standard for diagnosis of neonatal sepsis, namely blood culture method, has low sensitivity and is time consuming (48–72 hours). Rapid detection of sepsis and institution of antimicrobial therapy may improve patient outcomes. Alternative GBS detection methods in clinical samples have been developed, including methods based on nucleic acid amplification tests, such as PCR tests, and DNA hybridization probes. These tests can also be used to detect GBS directly from broth media, after the enrichment step, avoiding the subculture of the incubated enrichment broth to an appropriate agar plate.

The genetic diversity of GBS population has been studied using various typing methods, and GBS strains can be subdivided into genetic (sequence) types using molecular methods such as MLST based on 7 housekeeping genes (see: https://pubmlst.org/sagalactiae); however, very little is known about the diversity of these types from carriage and disease.

The performance of standard methods depends on the quality of reagents, equipment, and commercial and in-house test procedures. Laboratories should ensure that these have been validated and shown to be fit for purpose. Internal and external quality assurance procedures should also be in place. The maintenance of a quality management system is crucial to laboratories for providing the correct test results every time. An EQA scheme is an important element of a quality management system as it aims to analyse the accuracy of the entire testing process from receipt of sample and testing of sample to reporting of results (also known as proficiency testing). International EQA programs for GBS have been performed previously; however, it is imperative to continuously improve and assess laboratory performance and offer training to any laboratories that have technical difficulties.[3]

**9. Reporting requirements**—To confirm identification and for further characterization and typing of strains, pure GBS cultures should be submitted to the reference laboratory. Laboratory results are reported immediately to the clinician (neonatologist, pediatrician, and/or gynecologist) responsible for the case, the public health physician, and the local and national health protection teams (in an outbreak investigation). The reporting of streptococcal testing results by laboratories to the public health authorities is required in most settings globally. Laboratories should check the applicable regulations in their specific location to assure compliance.

**10. Referral network**—There is no defined international referral network for group B streptococcal infections. However, ad-hoc workshops and expert meetings are occasionally commissioned by national institutes of health. An ad-hoc consortium was established in 2008 under the auspices of the European Commission to support vaccine development.[4] There is also the International Lancefield Society that meets every 3 years to update the current status of these and other streptococcal infections.

**11. Special considerations**—Various policies are in place for prevention of GBS neonatal infections, with a screening-based policy amongst pregnant women being the most widely used and effective strategy. A risk-based GBS prevention strategy continues to be recommended in many countries as being the most clinically and cost-effective method; however, there are significant differences in incidence rates within countries using the different strategies with universal screening being the most effective.[5] There is currently no vaccine to prevent group B strep infections, although several vaccines are in various stages of development.

## References

1. Johnson DR, Kaplan E.L, Sramek J, et al. *Laboratory Diagnosis of Group A Streptococcal Infections*. World Health Organization. 1997. Available at: http://apps.who.int/iris/bitstream/10665/41879/1/9241544953_eng.pdf. Accessed March 14, 2019.
2. Neal S, Beall B, Ekelund K, et al. International quality assurance study for characterization of *Streptococcus pyogenes*. *J Clin Microbiol*. 2007;45(4):1175–1179.
3. Afshar B, Broughton K, Creti R, et al. International external quality assurance for laboratory identification and typing of *Streptococcus agalactiae* (group B streptococci). *J Clin Microbiol*. 2011;49(4):1475–1482.
4. Rodriguez-Granger J, Alvargonzalez JC, Berardi A, et al. Prevention of group B streptococcal neonatal disease revisited, The DEVANI European project. *Eur J Clin Microbiol Infect Dis*. 2012;31(9):2097–2104.
5. Verani JR, McGee L, Schrag SJ; Division of Bacterial Diseases, National Center for Immunization and Respiratory Diseases, Centers for Disease Control and Prevention (CDC). Prevention of perinatal group B streptococcal disease–revised guidelines from CDC, 2010. *MMWR Recomm Rep*. 2010;59(RR-10):1–36

[B. Afshar, A. Efstratiou]

# STRONGYLOIDIASIS

| DISEASE | ICD-10 CODE |
|---|---|
| STRONGYLOIDIASIS | ICD-10 B78 |

**1. Clinical features**—An often asymptomatic helminthic infection with clinical manifestations that include transient dermatitis when larvae of the parasite penetrate the skin on initial infection; cough, rales, and sometimes demonstrable pneumonitis when larvae pass through the lungs; or abdominal symptoms caused by adult worms in the intestinal mucosa. Symptoms of chronic infection may be mild or severe, depending on the intensity of infection. Classic symptoms of chronic infection include abdominal pain (usually epigastric, often suggesting peptic ulcer), diarrhea, and urticaria; and sometimes also nausea, weight loss, vomiting, weakness, and constipation. Intensely pruritic dermatitis (larva currens) radiating from the anus may occur, as can stationary wheals lasting 1–2 days, as well as a migrating serpiginous rash moving several centimeters per hour across the trunk. Rarely, intestinal autoinfection with increasing worm burden (hyperinfection) may lead to disseminated strongyloidiasis with wasting, pulmonary involvement, and death, particularly, but not exclusively, in the immunocompromised host. In these cases, secondary Gram-negative sepsis is common. Eosinophilia is usually moderate (10%–25%) in the chronic stage but may be normal or low with dissemination. Immunosuppressed persons, including those with human T-cell lymphotrophic virus, those on oral or intravenous steroids, those receiving chemotherapy for malignancies, or transplant patients, are at increased risk for disseminated or hyperinfection strongyloidiasis..

**2. Causative agents**—*Strongyloides stercoralis* (worldwide in tropical and subtropical regions), *Strongyloides fuelleborni* subsp. *fuelleborni* (Africa, also reported from Surinam), and *S. fuelleborni* subsp. *kellyi* (Papua New Guinea).

**3. Laboratory diagnosis**—No single method is capable of detecting all cases of *S. stercoralis* infection. Conventional microscopic methods of analysis have poor sensitivity; direct microscopy of fresh stool for motile rhabditiform larva has only 21% sensitivity, while standard formol-ethyl acetate concentration is 48% sensitive. Concentration of larva in a Baermann apparatus is more sensitive (83.6%) but is surpassed by Koga agar plate culture (89% sensitivity).[1] Harada-Mori culture is less effective than agar plate culture for *Strongyloides* spp.[1] No molecular methods for the detection of *S. stercoralis* are currently FDA-approved, but 1 research study found the sensitivity of a commonly used polymerase chain reaction method to vary between 16%–100%, proportional to the intensity of larval output. The sensitivity of microscopy, culture, and molecular methods is increased by the analysis of multiple stool specimens. In cases of systemic strongyloidiasis, larval output is very high, easily detectable upon direct microscopy, and adult parasitic females as well as eggs may be encountered in fecal samples. Filariform larva will often be seen in sputa from such cases.

*S. stercoralis* rhabditiform larvae are differentiated from those of the hookworms based upon their short buccal cavity and prominent rhomboid genital primordium. Filariform larva of *S. stercoralis* are more slender than those of hookworms and have a 1:1 esophagus:intestine ratio and a notched tail. Adult parasitic female Strongyloides are only passed in severe infections. Adult free-living males and females may be seen after several days in culture.

Serology remains the simplest and, depending on the antigen used, the most sensitive single method for the diagnosis of *S. stercoralis* infection. Definitive determination of sensitivity and specificity of serologic methods is difficult as there is no universal reference standard for determining *S. stercoralis* infection. Antigens employed include crude larval antigen of both *S. stercoralis* and *S. ratti* recombinant antigens, particularly the 32 kD recombinant immunodiagnostic antigen NIE.[1] These antigens have been used variously in immunofluorescence antibody testing (IFAT), enzyme-linked immunosorbent assays (ELISA), and luciferase immunoprecipitation system (LIPS) formats.[1] There are 2 available commercial ELISA kits, 1 using a *Strongyloides ratti* crude antigen and another employing a *S. stercoralis* crude antigen.[2,3] Neither kit is FDA approved. Comparison of the sensitivity and specificity of 5 methods was undertaken in 1 recent trial, using a reference of agar culture, direct microscopy, and a composite of concordant results in at least 3 of 5 of the serological tests assayed. Results were as follows: Bordier ELISA (sens. 90.8%, spec. 94.1%), IVD-ELISA (sens. 92.3%, spec. 97.4%), NIE-ELISA (sens. 70.8%, spec. 91.1%), IFAT using *S. stercoralis* larval crude antigen (sens. 94.6%, spec. 87.4%), and NIE-LIPS (sens. 83.8%, spec. 99.6%). Relative sensitivity and specificity will vary. Serological titers often drop following successful treatment, but in some cases positive results may occur due to residual antibody titer long after treatment or cross-reaction in other nematode infections. Furthermore, negative serological results cannot definitively exclude strongyloidiasis, particularly in long-term infected and immunosuppressed patients.

*S. fuelleborni* differs from *S. stercoralis* in that eggs are passed in feces rather than rhabditiform larva. Eggs are oval, with a thin shell. They are larvated on passage and are 45–55 μm in breadth by 30–35 μm in width. Eggs will hatch almost immediately on contact with water or saline but remain intact in iodine-stained preparations.

4. **Laboratory capability**—Clinical diagnostic laboratories with trained fecal parasitic microscopists are needed. Culture and microscopy methods are required for the laboratory diagnosis of strongyloidiasis. Serological tests are available through reference laboratories. Laboratories performing microscopy and/or serology should participate in regular external quality assessment.

**5. Safety requirements**—Biosafety level 2 conditions are required to work with fecal samples and larval cultures. Infective larva in culture are capable of transdermal migration, and standard precautions should be followed at all times. Particular care should be taken when undertaking culture-based methodologies. Testing waste and residual specimens should be disposed of as infectious waste. Formalin used in stool concentration should be only used in a well-ventilated space or preferably in a chemical fume hood. Formalin containing waste should be disposed of as chemical waste following local regulations.

**6. Nonhuman hosts**—*S. stercoralis* may be found infecting humans or dogs.

**7. Sample/specimen requirements**—For microscopic detection, fresh feces (within 24 hours of passage) are required; feces are preserved in 10% formalin, sodium acetate formalin, polyvinyl alcohol, or other commercial fixatives. For culture, fresh, unrefrigerated, unpreserved feces are required. Up to 3 fecal samples collected on separate days should be analyzed to exclude infection. For serology, either serum, plasma in EDTA, or plasma in lithium heparin may be used.

**8. Testing requirements**—Morphological identification of larva in feces or larva/adults in agar plate culture, with differentiation from hookworm larva, is both diagnostic and confirmatory for *S. stercoralis*. Morphological identification of eggs in feces, with differentiation from other hookworm like eggs by size and morphology, or adult females in agar plate culture is both diagnostic and confirmatory for *S. fuelleborni*. Individual providers will include *Strongyloides* larva in external quality assurance programs for the morphological identification of intestinal parasites.

**9. Reporting requirements**—Report larva of *S. stercoralis*, including whether rhabditiform or filariform stage. If eggs or parasitic female adult stage are seen in feces, this should be reported, as this finding indicates severe systemic disease. Report eggs of *S. fuelleborni* from feces. The detection and species of free-living adults recovered from cultures should be reported without commenting on life stages. Serology reports should include the method and antigen used, serological titer, and cutoff for positive infection. Disseminated strongyloidiasis is a notifiable disease in the Northern Territory of Australia.

**10. Referral network**—Networks vary among countries. First-line laboratories may identify eggs or larva in culture, stool, or sputum. Reference laboratories may perform morphological species identification of the parasitic female worm. CDC DPDx service in the USA will identify adult worms to species level and assist with identification of eggs of *S. fuelleborni* or free-living adult nematodes and other stages in cultures. Reference laboratories in many countries will perform *Strongyloides* serology.

**11. Special considerations**—In regard to disinfection of larvae following laboratory procedures or following laboratory occupational exposure, infective (L3) larvae of *S. stercoralis* instantly killing by exposure to 1% tincture of iodine has been demonstrated. However, the larvae are relatively resistant to hypochlorite.

## References

1. Requena-Méndez A, Chiodini P, Bisoffi Z, Buonfrate D, Gotuzzo E, Muñoz J. The laboratory diagnosis and follow up of strongyloidiasis: a systematic review. *PLoS Negl Trop Dis*. 2013;7(1):e2002.
2. Bordier Affinity Products. ELISA kit for the diagnosis of strongyloidiasis in humans. Available at: http://www.bordier.ch/9450%20Strongylo%C3%AFdes%20ratti. Accessed August 23, 2018.
3. IVD Research. ELISA. Available at: https://ivdresearch.com/elisa. Accessed August 23, 2018.

[R. S. Bradbury]

# SYPHILIS

(lues)

| DISEASE | ICD-10 CODE |
|---|---|
| SYPHILIS | ICD-10 A50–A52 |

**1. Clinical features**—Syphilis is a systemic treponemal infection characterized by 3 possible clinical stages and variable periods of latency. The primary stage is characterized by an indurated, painless ulcer known as a chancre. About 3 weeks after contact with another person's infectious lesions, the primary chancre develops at the site of exposure. Chancres can appear anywhere on the skin or mucous membranes. Although they commonly occur on the penis, vulva, mouth, or perianal skin, they might occur internally on the cervix or anus and go unnoticed. Firm, nonfluctuant, painless, regional lymphadenopathy frequently develops with the primary lesion. Without treatment, the chancre involutes in 4–6 weeks.

Within several weeks to months of the primary lesion, and occasionally at the same time as the primary lesion, a secondary skin eruption appears. Symmetric macular-to-papulosquamous skin lesions develop, classically occurring on the trunk, palms, and soles. Mucous patches (glistening, white-to-red patches) are seen in the mouth or on other mucous membranes, and condyloma lata (white, smooth papules or plaques) are seen in the genital area. The secondary stage is often accompanied by fever, sore throat, malaise, and generalized lymphadenopathy. Secondary manifestations resolve without treatment in weeks to 12 months; all untreated cases will go on to latent infection. In the early years of latency, there might be recurrences of lesions of the skin and mucous membranes. Up to one-third of untreated patients will eventually exhibit signs and symptoms of tertiary syphilis.

In the primary and secondary stages, treponemal invasion of the central nervous system (CNS) and abnormalities in the cerebrospinal fluid (CSF) are common. Patients are most often asymptomatic, but some might develop acute syphilitic meningitis with cranial nerve palsies and deafness. CNS disease in the form of meningovascular syphilis might develop 5–12 years after initial infection, and paresis or tabes dorsalis might develop 15–20 years after initial infection.

Most untreated patients do not go on to develop tertiary syphilis but remain in the latent period for the rest of their lives. In 5–20 years after initial infection some untreated patients develop gummas of the skin, musculoskeletal system, or internal organs; syphilitic endarteritis with aortic and coronary artery disease; or CNS disease described earlier. The widespread use of antimicrobials has decreased the frequency of these tertiary manifestations.

Concurrent human immunodeficiency virus (HIV) infection might change the appearance and behavior of the primary and secondary mucocutaneous lesions and increase the risk of CNS disease in patients with syphilis. Neurosyphilis must be considered in the differential diagnosis of HIV-infected individuals with CNS symptoms and ocular and otologic complaints.

A woman with untreated early (primary, secondary, or early latent) syphilis during pregnancy has a very high risk of transmitting the infection to her fetus. Congenital syphilis can cause stillbirth, prematurity, neonatal death, or a live-born infant with a spectrum of clinical manifestations of congenital syphilis. Although these infants often appear normal at birth, early manifestations of congenital syphilis appear by 2 months of age and include failure to thrive, mucocutaneous abnormalities similar to those seen in secondary syphilis, organomegaly, anemia, bony lesions, and CNS abnormalities. Congenital infection might also result in late manifestations that appear by 2 years of age. These late manifestations include CNS abnormalities, such as interstitial keratitis, deafness, and bony or dental abnormalities such as notched incisors, saddle-nose deformities, or saber shins.

**2. Causative agents**—*Treponema pallidum* subsp. *pallidum*, a spirochete.

**3. Laboratory diagnosis**—Using the traditional algorithm, testing begins with a nontreponemal serologic test such as the rapid plasma reagin (RPR) or Venereal Disease Research Laboratory (VDRL). If that test is positive, the patient should have a confirmatory treponemal serologic test, such as the

*T. pallidum* particle agglutination (TP-PA). When both tests are positive, and the patient has never been treated for syphilis, the diagnosis is confirmed. For patients with a history of treatment for syphilis, reinfection is determined by a 4-fold increase in nontreponemal test titer compared with previous titers.

Using the reverse algorithm, testing begins with a treponemal test, such as an enzyme immunoassay (EIA) or a chemiluminesence immunoassay (CIA). Patients who test positive should be tested with a nontreponemal test. When both are positive, results are interpreted as earlier. If only the treponemal test is positive, and the patient has never been treated for syphilis, the patient might have old untreated syphilis or early primary syphilis. In that case, a second treponemal test can be done, and if positive (or no second test is available), the patient should be treated. Patients do not require additional treatment if they have a positive treponemal test, a negative nontreponemal test, and a history of treatment for syphilis.

Patients in the early stage of disease with primary lesions may have nonreactive serologic tests. Smears of lesion exudate from primary and secondary syphilis can be examined for spirochetes using dark-field microscopy (DF) or polymerase chain reaction (PCR).[1,2] Although no commercial PCR tests for *T. pallidum* are available in the USA, some laboratories provide locally developed and validated PCR tests. Paraffin embedded tissue sections from the brain, placenta, umbilical cord, or skin (except primary lesions) can be tested by immunohistochemistry (IHC) or silver staining to observe spirochetes.

Infants should be screened by testing the mother's serum. This is because the infant's serum may be nonreactive if the mother's serologic test result is of low titer or if the mother was infected late in pregnancy. If maternal serum is not available, infant serum is preferred to cord blood. Syphilis patients with neurologic abnormalities or evidence of treatment failure may have neurosyphilis and should have CSF testing performed.

Reactive treponemal and nontreponemal test results are consistent with current or past syphilis infection; however, if the titer is lower than 1:4 this could be associated with a serofast condition of early syphilis where nontreponemal titers neither increase nor decrease 4-fold after treatment. If the treponemal test is nonreactive, then there is no laboratory evidence of syphilis infection. If the nontreponemal test is reactive but the treponemal test is nonreactive, then it is most likely a biological false positive. If the first treponemal test in the reverse algorithm is reactive and the nontreponemal test is nonreactive but the second (supplemental) treponemal test is reactive, then this is consistent with past or potential early syphilis infection. If nonreactive, it is inconclusive for syphilis infection or a false positive. Quantitative nontreponemal test titers are used to monitor response to treatment with a treatment response in syphilis patients defined by resolution of disease manifestations, a 4-fold decline in nontreponemal titers (or a change in 2 dilutions; e.g., from 1:16 to 1:4) using the same assay, or seroreversion of a nontreponemal test to a nonreactive test. Nontreponemal test titers usually decline after treatment and can become nonreactive with time; however, in some treated persons, nontreponemal antibodies can persist for a long period of time, a response referred to as the serofast reaction.

4. **Laboratory capability**—Serological testing can be performed in laboratories with standard equipment and basic scientific and technical knowledge, but the high throughput tests require automation, which are usually found in clinical or reference laboratories. Rapid syphilis tests (RSTs) can be performed by staff with minimal laboratory training and can be used at all levels of health care facilities, even those without a laboratory. RSTs are available as treponemal only (e.g., Uni-Gold Syphilis Treponemal, Trinity Biotech, Bray, Ireland), treponemal/nontreponemal (e.g., DPP Syphilis Screen & Confirm Assay, Chembio, Medford, NY), or HIV/syphilis (e.g., Alere HIV/Syphilis Duo, Abbott, Chicago, IL). The Trinity Biotech Syphilis Health Check is the only FDA-cleared Clinical Laboratory Improvement Amendments-waived treponemal RST for use in the USA. Specialized scientific and technical knowledge including a sophisticated facility and equipment are essential for performing PCR testing.

5. **Safety requirements**—Biosafety level 2. Standard precautions are required when working with blood or clinical specimens.

6. **Nonhuman hosts**—Humans are the only known reservoir for *T. pallidum* subsp. *pallidum*.

7. **Sample/specimen requirements**—Serum is the specimen of choice for treponemal and nontreponemal serological tests, but plasma can be used for some tests. Serum or CSF can be used for the VDRL test. RSTs use whole blood obtained through a finger stick. Serum, plasma, and CSF should be stored at 4°C if testing cannot be performed within 4 hours and at −20°C or lower if testing will be done later than 5 days from collection. Serous exudate from moist lesions of primary and secondary syphilis are amenable to DF, immunofluorescent staining (IS), and PCR. Lymph node aspirates and amniotic fluid can be tested by DF, IS, or PCR, although these specimen types are rarely obtained. Specimens for DF must be tested within 20 minutes of collection. Oral lesions should not be examined by DF because commensal spirochetes cannot be distinguished from *T. pallidum* subsp. *pallidum*. Slides with air-dried lesion exudates or touch preparations for IS can be stored at 4°C–29°C for up to 2 weeks or fixed with acetone and stored at −20°C until testing. Tissue biopsies of clinical manifestations of neurosyphilis, secondary and tertiary disease, and placenta or umbilical cord can be used for silver staining, IHC or PCR. A 3–4 cm section of the cord closer to the baby's end should be obtained for testing. Tissue for silver staining and IHC should be fixed in 10% buffered formalin as soon as possible at ambient temperature and then paraffin embedded and sectioned for staining. PCR can be performed on either fixed or unfixed tissue, although unfixed tissue is

preferred. All samples for PCR should be stored at −70°C if testing cannot be performed immediately.

**8. Testing requirements**—A quantitative nontreponemal test is used for assessing response to therapy. Serological tests are recommended for antenatal screening. Automated treponemal tests are used in screening applications such as blood donors. Participation in the WHO/CDC Syphilis Serology Proficiency Testing Programme or the use of a commercial proficiency testing provider is recommended for maintaining proficiency in treponemal and nontreponemal testing. The sensitivity of treponemal tests (e.g., microhemagglutination assay for antibodies to *T. pallidum*; TP-PA; fluorescent treponemal antibody-absorption test) ranges from 45.9%–100% for primary syphilis, 90%–100% for secondary, 94.4%–100% for early latent syphilis, 84.5%–100% for late latent syphilis, and 94%–96% for tertiary syphilis. The sensitivity of nontreponemal tests (RPR, VDRL) ranges from 57.7%–78.4% for primary syphilis, 100% for secondary syphilis, 85%–100% for early latent syphilis, 63.6%–76.8% for late latent syphilis, and 47%–63.8% for tertiary syphilis. The specificity of treponemal tests is about 99% and nontreponemal tests is about 98%. The sensitivity of treponemal EIAs/CIAs (e.g., TrepSure, Trinity Biotech; LIAISON, DiaSorin, Saluggia, Italy; Captia, Trinity Biotech) ranges from 53.8%–100% for primary syphilis, 100% for secondary, and 91.7%–100% for latent syphilis (LIAISON and Captia). The sensitivity of treponemal RSTs ranges from 69.7%–97.3%, and specificity ranges from 91.5%–99.7%. The sensitivity of the treponemal component of dual treponemal/nontreponemal RSTs ranges from 90.7%–98%, and specificity ranges from 97.2%–99.6%, while the nontreponemal component sensitivity ranges from 85.5%–94.6%, and specificity ranges from 94.4%–97.3%.

PCR is recommended over DF for moist lesions of primary and secondary syphilis; however, PCR tests are not widely available, and currently none are FDA approved for use in the USA. Detection of specific *T. pallidum* deoxyribonucleic acid (DNA) targets by PCR or observation of a single motile spirochete with the characteristic corkscrew movement by DF is definitive of syphilis infection. In the absence of a gold standard, the sensitivity of PCR on lesion swabs is 87% compared with DF and about 95% versus serology. PCR sensitivity in secondary syphilis ranges from 50%–84% on specimens from mucous patches, condyloma lata, and maculopapular rash and from 36%–57% in blood. Sensitivity varies for other specimen types such as CSF, lymph node aspirate, amniotic fluid, and tissue. Compared with PCR, the sensitivity of DF is about 88%. IHC, silver stain, or PCR is used for tissue biopsies. Use of a hematoxylin counterstain with IHC allows tissue structure to be observed with localization of treponemes. The sensitivity of silver staining is low because it is prone to staining artifacts, and it cannot distinguish *T. pallidum* from other spirochetes such as *Borrelia burgdorferi*. A real time multiplex PCR assay or a combination of PCR and sequencing can be used to detect the 2 mutations

(A2058G, A2059G) in the 23S ribosomal ribonucleic acid genes associated with azithromycin resistance in *T. pallidum*.[3,4]

**9. Reporting requirements**—Laboratories are required to report cases of early infectious syphilis and congenital syphilis in most countries. Confidentiality of the individual must be ensured. Molecular tests should be reported as DNA of *T. pallidum* subsp. *pallidum* detected or not detected. Where a molecular assay for azithromycin resistance has been performed, this should be reported as positive or negative for the presence of mutations conferring azithromycin resistance. Laboratories should report treponemal and nontreponemal test results together to the clinician if feasible.

**10. Referral network**—No specific referral networks exist.

**11. Special considerations**—International measures are as follows:

1. Examine groups of adolescents and adults who emigrate from areas of high prevalence for syphilis and endemic treponematoses (e.g., bejel, yaws, pinta), as none of the currently available serologic tests can distinguish venereal syphilis from the endemic treponematoses.
2. Adhere to international agreements concerning records, provision of diagnostic and treatment facilities, and contact interviews at seaports for foreign merchant seamen (e.g., Brussels Agreement).
3. Provide for rapid international exchange of information about contacts.

## References


1. Chen CY, Chi KH, George RW, et al. Diagnosis of gastric syphilis by direct immunofluorescence staining and real-time PCR testing. *J Clin Microbiol.* 2006;44(9):3452–3456.
2. Chen CY, Ballard RC. The molecular diagnosis of sexually transmitted genital ulcer disease. *Methods Mol Biol.* 2012;903:103–112.
3. Chen CY, Chi KH, Pillay A, Nachamkin E, Su JR, Ballard RC. Detection of the A2058G and A2059G 23S rRNA gene point mutations associated with azithromycin resistance in *Treponema pallidum* by use of a TaqMan real-time multiplex PCR assay. *J Clin Microbiol.* 2013;51(3):908–913.
4. Lukehart SA, Godornes C, Molini BJ, et al. Macrolide resistance in *Treponema pallidum* in the United States and Ireland. *N Engl J Med.* 2004;351(2):154–158.


[A. Pillay, C. Y. Chen]

# TAPEWORM

| DISEASE | ICD-10 CODE |
|---|---|
| DWARF TAPEWORM | ICD-10 B71.0 |
| RAT TAPEWORM | ICD-10 B71.0 |
| DOG TAPEWORM | ICD-10 B71.1 |
| BROAD OR FISH TAPEWORM | ICD-10 B70.0 |
| TAENIASIS | ICD-10 B68 |
| *TAENIA SOLIUM* TAENIASIS | ICD-10 B68.0 |
| *TAENIA SAGINATA* TAENIASIS | ICD-10 B68.1 |
| TAENIASIS, UNSPECIFIED | ICD-10 B68.9 |
| CYSTICERCOSIS | ICD-10 B69 |
| Echinococcosis (see "Echinococcosis") | |

## I. DWARF TAPEWORM (hymenolepiasis due to *Hymenolepis nana*); RAT TAPEWORM (hymenolepiasis due to *Hymenolepis diminuta*)

**1. Clinical features**—An intestinal infection with small tapeworms; usually an infection of children. Infections with *H. diminuta* and light infections with *H. nana* are usually asymptomatic. Massive numbers of *H. nana* worms may cause enteritis with or without diarrhea, abdominal pain, and other nondescript symptoms such as pallor, loss of weight, and weakness.

**2. Causative agents**—*H. nana* (dwarf tapeworm) and *H. diminuta* (rat tapeworm). *H. nana* is the only intestinal human tapeworm without an obligatory intermediate host. Both species occur worldwide, although human cases with *H. diminuta* are less-commonly reported.

**3. Laboratory diagnosis**—The diagnosis can be made by the microscopic finding of eggs in stool. Proglottids (tapeworm segments) are rarely observed macroscopically in stool. There are no serologic nor molecular tests available for routine clinical diagnosis.

Eggs of *H. nana* are 30–47 µm in diameter and subspherical in shape; the shell is thin and hyaline; the internal oncosphere contains 6 refractile hooklets and 4–8 polar filaments that arise from opposite ends of the oncosphere into the space between the oncosphere and outer shell.

Eggs of *H. diminuta* are 70–85 µm in diameter and subspherical in shape; the shell is thick and textured; the internal oncosphere contains 6 refractile hooklets and lacks polar filaments.

**4. Laboratory capability**—Microscopy and stool concentration/centrifugation capabilities should be available. Laboratorians should be trained in the microscopic/morphologic detection of parasites and undergo regular proficiency testing.

**5. Safety requirements**—Clinical specimens should always be collected and handled with standard precautions. *Hymenolepis* spp. are biosafety level 2 (BSL-2) organisms. Eggs of *H. nana* are infective to the human host. Formalin should only be used in a well-ventilated area, preferably in a chemical fume hood. Unpreserved and preserved stools should be disposed of as infectious waste.

**6. Nonhuman hosts**—Rodents are the natural definitive host for *Hymenolepis* spp., and insects, usually granary beetles, are the natural intermediate hosts. While the intermediate host is not necessary with *H. nana*, insects containing infective cysticercoid larvae of both species are infectious to humans if ingested.

**7. Sample/specimen requirements**—Stool should be promptly preserved in an appropriate liquid medium, such as 10% buffered formalin or sodium acetate-acidic acid-formalin (SAF). Single-vial systems for ova and parasite (O&P) collection are also adequate. Specimens in the appropriate preservatives are acceptable for concentration of direct examination indefinitely. To maximize O&P sensitivity, up to 3 stool specimens should be collected.

**8. Testing requirements**—Routine concentration (sedimentation) procedures for stool. A calibrated ocular micrometer should be used to measure egg size. No additional confirmatory testing is needed when eggs meeting morphological criteria are identified in stool specimens.

**9. Reporting requirements**—*Hymenolepis* spp. are identifiable to the species level based on egg morphology. Hymenolepiasis is not nationally reportable in the USA. Report to local health authority; official report not ordinarily justifiable.

**10. Referral network**—None.

**11. Special considerations**—Outbreaks of *H. nana* in schools and institutions can best be controlled through treatment of infected persons and special attention to personal and group hygiene.

## II. DOG TAPEWORM (dipylidiasis)

**1. Clinical features**—Infected children are usually asymptomatic, but parents may be alarmed by motile, seed-like proglottids at the child's anus or on the surface of the stool.

**2. Causative agents**—*Dipylidium caninum* (dog tapeworm), a parasite of dogs and cats worldwide.

**3. Laboratory diagnosis**—The diagnosis is usually made by the finding of proglottids in feces, less commonly egg packets or individual eggs during routine O&P examinations of stool. There are no serologic nor molecular tests available for routine clinical diagnosis.

Mature proglottids are 5–23 mm long, white in color, and have 2 genital pores, 1 on each lateral margin. Proglottids from the human host are often smaller than those from the natural definitive hosts and resemble grains of rice or seeds. Internally, proglottids are divided into many compartments, each containing an egg packet that contains 8–15 eggs. Clearing proglottids in lactophenol may enhance the observation of egg packets contained therein.

Individual eggs are usually contained within packets and are 25–40 μm in diameter, have a thin shell, and have an oncosphere containing 6 refractile hooklets.

**4. Laboratory capability**—Microscopy and stool concentration/centrifugation capabilities should be available. Laboratorians should be trained in the microscopic/morphologic detection of parasites and undergo regular proficiency testing.

**5. Safety requirements**—Clinical specimens should always be collected and handled with standard precautions. *D. caninum* is a BSL-2 organism. Formalin and lactophenol should only be used in a well-ventilated area, preferably in a chemical fume hood. Unpreserved and preserved stools and proglottids should be disposed of as infectious waste.

**6. Nonhuman hosts**—Dogs and cats are the natural definitive hosts, and insects, usually fleas, are the natural intermediate hosts. Fleas containing infective cysticercoid larvae are infectious to humans if ingested.

**7. Sample/specimen requirements**—Stool should be promptly preserved in an appropriate liquid medium, such as 10% buffered formalin or SAF. Single-vial systems for O&P collection are also adequate. Proglottids and chains of proglottids should also be placed in a liquid preservative such as 10% formalin or 70% laboratory-grade ethanol as soon as possible after collection to avoid desiccation and alteration of morphologic features. Specimens in the appropriate preservatives are acceptable for concentration of direct examination indefinitely. To maximize O&P sensitivity, up to 3 stool specimens should be collected.

**8. Testing requirements**—Routine concentration procedures for stool (eggs, egg packets) and routine examination of gross helminths (proglottids). A calibrated ocular micrometer should be used to measure egg size. No additional confirmatory testing is needed when eggs meeting morphological criteria are identified in stool specimens.

**9. Reporting requirements**—*D. caninum* is reportable to the species level based on proglottid and egg packet morphology. Dipylidiasis is not nationally reportable in the USA. Report to local health authority; official report not ordinarily justifiable.

**10. Referral network**—None.

**11. Special considerations**—None.

## III. BROAD OR FISH TAPEWORM (dibothriocephaliasis, diphyllobothriasis)

**1. Clinical features**—An intestinal tapeworm infection of long duration. Symptoms are commonly trivial or absent; some patients, however, develop vitamin B12 deficiency anemia (*Diphyllobothrium latum* infections). Massive infections may be associated with diarrhea, obstruction of the bile duct or intestine, and toxic symptoms.

**2. Causative agents**—Cestodes in the genera *Dibothriocephalus, Diphyllobothrium*, and *Adenocephalus*, including *Dibothriocephalus latus* (Holarctic), *Dibothriocephalus nihonkaiensis* (Asian Pacific and the Pacific Northwest), *Diphyllobothrium cordatum* (Arctic), *Diphyllobothrium lanceolatum* (Holarctic), *Dibothriocephalus dendriticus* (Holarctic), *Dibothriocephalus ursi* (North America), *Dibothriocephalus dalliae* (Alaska and Siberia), *Diphyllobothrium klebanovskii* (Russian Far East), and *Adenocephalus pacificus* (southern South America, southern Asia and Australia). Diphyllobothriasis is more common in the Northern Hemisphere than many other helminthic infections.

**3. Laboratory diagnosis**—The diagnosis is usually made by microscopic examination of eggs or macroscopic examination of proglottids in feces. There are no serologic nor molecular tests available for routine clinical diagnosis. Molecular methods may be used for epidemiologic purposes.

Mature proglottids are typically (but not always) wider than long, on average measure 3 mm long by 11 mm wide, have a rosette-shaped centrally placed uterus, and have a single genital pore that is located on the midventral surface. Clearing proglottids in lactophenol may enhance the observation of eggs contained therein.

Individual eggs are 58–75 μm long by 40–50 μm wide and are unembryonated when shed in feces. The eggs are operculate and need to be distinguished from the eggs of trematodes. There is usually a small knob at the abopercular end of the eggs. The different species of *Diphyllobothrium* and related cestodes cannot be separated based on egg morphology.

**4. Laboratory capability**—Microscopy and stool concentration/centrifugation capabilities should be available. Laboratorians should be trained in the microscopic/morphologic detection of parasites and undergo regular proficiency testing.

**5. Safety requirements**—Clinical specimens should always be collected and handled with standard precautions. Diphyllobothriid cestodes are BSL-2 organisms. Formalin and lactophenol should only be used in a well-ventilated area, preferably in a chemical fume hood. Unpreserved and preserved stools and proglottids should be disposed of as infectious waste.

**6. Nonhuman hosts**—Fish-eating mammals and birds are the natural definitive hosts for diphyllobothriid cestodes. The first intermediate host is a microcrustacean, such as a copepod, that harbors the procercoid larva. The second intermediate host is a fish that harbors the infective plerocercoid larva; larger fish usually serve as paratenic hosts. Fish containing plerocercoid larvae are infectious to the human host.

**7. Sample/specimen requirements**—Stool should be promptly preserved in an appropriate liquid medium, such as 10% buffered formalin or SAF. Single-vial systems for O&P collection are also adequate. Proglottids and chains of proglottids should also be placed in a liquid preservative such as 10% formalin or 70% laboratory grade ethanol as soon as possible after collection to avoid desiccation and alteration of morphologic features. Specimens in the appropriate preservatives are acceptable for concentration of direct examination indefinitely. To maximize O&P sensitivity, up to 3 stool specimens should be collected.

**8. Testing requirements**—Routine concentration procedures for stool (eggs) and routine examination of gross helminths (proglottids). A calibrated ocular micrometer should be used to measure egg size. No additional confirmatory testing is needed when eggs meeting morphological criteria are identified in stool specimens.

**9. Reporting requirements**—Diphyllobothriid cestodes are usually reported as a group (*Diphyllobothrium, Dibothriocephalus, Adenocephalus*) or at a broad genus-level identification (e.g., *Diphyllobothrium* spp.) unless molecular data allow for a species-level identification. Identification to the genus or species level is not needed for patient management. Diphyllobothriasis is not nationally reportable in the USA. Report to local health authority; official report not ordinarily justifiable. Report is indicated if a commercial source is implicated.

**10. Referral network**—None.

**11. Special considerations**—None.

## IV. TAENIASIS

**1. Clinical features**—Taeniasis is an intestinal infection with the adult stage of large tapeworms in the genus *Taenia*; *Taenia solium* can also cause cysticercosis (see Cysticercosis section later in this chapter). Clinical manifestations of infection with the adult worm, if present, are variable and may include nervousness, insomnia, anorexia, weight loss, abdominal pain, and digestive disturbances. Except for the annoyance of having segments of worms emerging from the anus, many infections are asymptomatic.

**2. Causative agents**—Cestodes in the genus *Taenia*, including *T. solium* (pork tapeworm), *Taenia saginata* (beef tapeworm), and *Taenia asiatica* (Asian tapeworm). *T. asiatica* has historically been considered a subspecies of *T. saginata* but is now generally given species-level rank. *T. saginata* and *T. solium* occur nearly worldwide, while *T. asiatica* occurs in Taiwan, the People's Republic of China, Korea, Malaysia, Indonesia, Vietnam, Thailand, and the Philippines.

**3. Laboratory diagnosis**—Infection with an adult tapeworm is diagnosed by the macroscopic identification of proglottids (segments) or microscopic examination of eggs in the feces; examination of several specimens may be necessary to detect eggs. Antigen testing is not routinely used for clinical diagnosis. Eggs of *Taenia* spp. cannot be differentiated morphologically. Specific diagnosis is based on the morphology of the scolex (head) and/or gravid proglottids. There are no serologic nor molecular tests available for routine clinical diagnosis of intestinal taeniasis.

Eggs of *Taenia* spp. are 31–43 μm in diameter and have a thick striated shell. The internal oncosphere contains 6 refractile hooklets.

Mature proglottids of *Taenia* spp. are longer than broad and have a single, prominent lateral genital pore. Mature proglottids of *T. saginata* and *T. asiatica* have 12–30 primary uterine branches coming off each side of the central uterine stem, while proglottids of *T. solium* have only 7–13 primary uterine branches. Visualization of the uterine branches can be enhanced by clearing proglottids in lactophenol by itself or by clearing followed by India ink injection.

The scoleces of *T. solium* and *T. asiatica* have an armed rostellum with rows of hooklets, while the scolex of *T. saginata* has a retracted, unarmed rostellum.

Coproantigen testing, which detects parasite-specific antigens released in the feces of *Taenia* spp. carriers, is currently the most reliable approach for surveillance of human taeniasis. This test is an ELISA only available for research and not for routine clinical diagnostics. Coproantigen testing is a good way to identify *Taenia* worm carriers and to confirm purging of the parasite. Coproantigen testing cannot differentiate between *T. solium* and *T. saginata*, however.

**4. Laboratory capability**—For morphologic identification of worms and eggs, microscopy and stool concentration/centrifugation capabilities should be available. Laboratorians should be trained in the microscopic/morphologic detection of parasites and undergo regular proficiency testing.

For serologic and coproantigen testing, routine serologic capabilities should be available. Parasite serology and coproantigen testing are likely to only be available at specialized reference labs. Laboratorians should be trained in the serologic diagnosis of parasitic diseases and undergo regular proficiency testing.

**5. Safety requirements**—Clinical specimens should always be collected and handled with standard precautions. *Taenia* spp. are BSL-2 organisms. Eggs of *T. solium* are infectious to the human host, and all unknown proglottids should be handled as possible *T. solium* until proven otherwise. Formalin and lactophenol should only be used in a well-ventilated area, preferably in a chemical fume hood. Unpreserved and preserved stools and proglottids should be disposed of as infectious waste.

**6. Nonhuman hosts**—For all 3 species, humans are the only definitive hosts. Pigs are the natural intermediate hosts for *T. solium* and *T. asiatica*, dogs act as an alternative intermediate host for *T. solium* in some areas, and cattle are the natural intermediate hosts for *T. saginata*.

**7. Sample/specimen requirements**—Stool should be promptly preserved in an appropriate liquid medium, such as 10% buffered formalin or SAF. Single-vial systems for O&P collection are also adequate. Proglottids and chains of proglottids should also be placed in a liquid preservative such as 10% formalin or 70% laboratory-grade ethanol as soon as possible after collection to avoid desiccation and alteration of morphologic features. Specimens in the appropriate preservatives should remain intact indefinitely. To maximize O&P sensitivity, up to 3 stool specimens should be collected.

**8. Testing requirements**—Routine concentration procedures for stool (eggs) and routine examination of gross helminths (proglottids). A calibrated ocular micrometer should be used to measure egg size. Diagnosis is confirmatory in specimens meeting morphologic criteria.

**9. Reporting requirements**—*Taenia* is reported at the genus level when only eggs are observed. It is important to attempt a species-level identification in all cases of intestinal taeniasis due to the risk of cysticercosis in patients and the contacts of patients harboring *T. solium*.

Taeniasis is selectively reportable in the USA. Report to state and local health authority. Any patient from which *Taenia* eggs are recovered should be advised to use good hygiene practices.

**10. Referral network**—None.

**11. Special considerations**—Investigation of contacts and source of infection. Evaluate symptomatic contacts. Ensure good sanitation and human waste disposal.

## V. CYSTICERCOSIS (infection with larval *Taenia solium*)

**1. Clinical features**—Cysticercosis may produce serious somatic disease when larvae localize in the muscles, eye, or central nervous system (CNS). Clinical manifestations of cysticercosis depend on the number, location, and stage (viable, degenerating, or calcified) of the cysticerci and the intensity of the inflammatory response. The most important clinical manifestations occur when cysticerci are located in the brain. Seizures are the most common CNS manifestation; encephalitis, intracranial hypertension, hydrocephalus, chronic meningitis, and cranial nerve abnormalities are less frequent. CNS cysticercosis, or neurocysticercosis, may cause serious disability but with a relatively low case-fatality rate.

**2. Causative agents**—The larval stage (cysticercus) of *Taenia solium*.

**3. Laboratory diagnosis**—Specific serological tests should support the clinical diagnosis of cysticercosis. Subcutaneous cysticerci may be visible or palpable; microscopic examination of an excised cysticercus confirms the diagnosis. Cysticercosis in intracerebral and other tissues may be recognized by computerized axial tomography scan or magnetic resonance imaging. Standard radiography is of limited use for detection of calcified cysticerci.

A serological immunoblot (Western blot [WB]) assay may complement in the diagnosis of neurocysticercosis (laboratory-developed test, CDC). The reference serologic assay for detecting neurocysticercosis is a lentil-lectin purified glycoprotein (LLGP) WB. The sensitivity of the assay varies from 97% for multiple lesions in the brain to 52% for single viable cyst. Specificity is 97%.

The QuickELISATM assays (Immunetics, Boston, MA) utilize the T24H, GP50, and Ts18var 1 antigens with a sensitivity and specificity of 96.3% and 99.2%, 93.5% and 98.6%, and 89.8% and 96.4%, respectively.

**4. Laboratory capability**—Routine serologic capabilities should be available. Serologic testing for parasitic diseases is usually performed at specialized reference laboratories. Laboratorians should be trained in the serologic diagnosis of parasitic diseases and undergo regular proficiency testing. Automated plate readers used for ELISA should have annual maintenance performed. Known positive and negative controls should be tested with each run.

**5. Safety requirements**—Clinical specimens should always be collected and handled with universal precautions. Clinical specimens submitted for diagnosis of cysticercosis should be handled under BSL2 parameters. Blood, sera, and CSF should be disposed of as infectious waste.

**6. Nonhuman hosts**—Pigs are a natural part of the life cycle for *T. solium* but do not play a direct role in acquiring cysticercosis as the infectious sources are food and fomites contaminated with human feces containing *T. solium* eggs.

**7. Sample/specimen requirements**—Blood collected with or without anticoagulant should be collected for serological detection. If available, CSF could be submitted for diagnosis of neurocysticercosis. Spun serum can be shipped at room temperature; whole blood and CSF should be kept chilled during transport. A minimum of 500 μL of serum or CSF should be submitted for testing.

**8. Testing requirements**—Testing laboratories should be equipped and have expertise to perform and interpret WB assays. Diagnosis is confirmatory on specimens meeting serologic criteria.

**9. Reporting requirements**—The LLGP WB is reported as positive or negative based on the observation of 6 or more of the diagnostic bands for cysticercosis at 50, 42–39, 24, 18, 14, or 13 kDa. Cysticercosis is selectively reportable in the USA. Report to state and local health authority.

**10. Referral network**—None.

**11. Special considerations**—Public health investigation of contacts and source of infection. Evaluate symptomatic contacts. Ensure good sanitation and human waste disposal for contacts harboring *Taenia* eggs.

[B. Mathison, I. T. McAuliffe, S. Handali]

# TETANUS
(lockjaw)

| DISEASE | ICD-10 CODE |
|---|---|
| TETANUS | ICD-10 A35 |
| OBSTETRICAL TETANUS | ICD-10 A34 |
| TETANUS NEONATORUM | ICD-10 A33 |

**1. Clinical features**—Tetanus is an acute disease that is caused by an exotoxin produced by the anaerobic bacterium *Clostridium tetani* at the site of an injury. However, history of an injury or an apparent portal of entry may be lacking. Four clinical types of disease are often described: generalized, localized, cephalic, and neonatal. Generalized tetanus is characterized by painful muscular contractions, primarily of the masseter and neck muscles (trismus), and secondarily of trunk muscles. Generalized spasms are frequently induced by sensory stimuli; typical features of the tetanic spasm are extreme hyperextension of the body, in which the head and heels are bent backward and the spine arches forward (opisthotonos), and the facial expression known as risus sardonicus. A common first sign suggestive of tetanus in older children and adults is abdominal rigidity, though rigidity is sometimes confined to the region of injury (localized tetanus). Infected wounds of the head and neck area can lead to cranial nerve dysfunction or cephalic tetanus.

Tetanus neonatorum (neonatal tetanus) is typified by a newborn infant who sucks and cries well for the first few days after birth but who subsequently develops progressive difficulty and then inability to feed because of trismus—generalized stiffness with spasms or convulsions and opisthotonos.

The case-fatality rate of tetanus ranges from 10% to more than 80% depending on age, the quality of care available, and the length of the incubation period. Case-fatality rates for neonatal tetanus are highest, exceeding 80% among those with short incubation periods. Neurological sequelae including cognitive delay occur in 5% to more than 20% of those infants who survive. The case-fatality rate is also high in the elderly and varies inversely with the availability of experienced intensive care unit personnel and resources and with the length of the incubation period.

**2. Causative agents**—*C. tetani*, the tetanus bacillus.

**3. Laboratory diagnosis**—Tetanus is normally diagnosed clinically as there are no readily available laboratory tests to help diagnose tetanus. Attempts at laboratory confirmation do not help establish the diagnosis. A negative culture does not rule out the diagnosis as the organism is rarely recovered from the site of infection, and antitetanus antibodies are undetectable in most cases.

**4. Laboratory capability**—If *C. tetani* isolation is attempted, clinical specimens should be handled with standard precautions within a laboratory that handles biosafety level 2 (BSL-2) pathogens. The laboratory should be capable of standard anaerobic microbiology methods. Most clinical laboratories are unable to measure antitetanus antibodies, and these samples should be sent to a regional or national reference laboratory. Clinical waste from suspect cases should be disposed of in accordance with local and national protocols for the management of biohazardous waste.

**5. Safety requirements**—*C. tetani* is a BSL-2 pathogen. There is a vaccine available to prevent the disease. Clinical and laboratory staff should be vaccinated against tetanus. For those who are vaccine naïve, human tetanus immunoglobulin should be accessible. Standard personal protective equipment is required when handling suspect specimens. Any procedure performed that may generate an aerosol should be performed in a biological safety cabinet.

**6. Nonhuman hosts**—There are no direct nonhuman hosts. Tetanus spores are commonly found in the soil as well as human and animal feces.

**7. Sample/specimen requirements**—The diagnosis of tetanus is normally based on clinical features. Isolation of *C. tetani* from tissue samples or swabs from contaminated wounds may be supportive of the diagnosis when clinical tetanus is suspected. The samples should be obtained on presentation to a health care provider. Specimens of at least 2 mL of serum are preferred for testing for the presence of *C. tetani* neurotoxin. This optimally should be collected within 3 days of the onset of symptoms and sent to a regional or national reference laboratory capable of performing tetanus toxin testing.

**8. Testing requirements**—*C. tetani* is difficult to culture as it is a strict anaerobe. *C. tetani* is a Gram-positive rod and has a characteristic drumstick appearance due to the presence of a terminal spore. Specimens should be cultured in anaerobic conditions on blood agar for 40–48 hours at 35°C–37°C. *C. tetani* has a fine swarming growth pattern which may be beta-hemolytic on blood agar. In the UK, the National Gastrointestinal Reference Unit offers toxin gene PCR testing on all pure growths of *C. tetani* and tissue samples from suspected cases. *C. tetani* neurotoxin can be detected in serum and may aid in the diagnosis of tetanus. Serum antitoxin antibody levels can be measured and used in conjunction with the clinical features to assist with the diagnosis of tetanus. The samples must be obtained before the administration of antitoxin. If tetanus toxin antibody levels are low or undetectable, this may support a clinical diagnosis of tetanus as symptoms are much more likely to develop if the patient does not have preexisting immunity. The minimum protective level is a level greater than 0.1 IU/mL.

**9. Reporting requirements**—In the USA, tetanus is reportable to National Notifiable Diseases Surveillance System. A probable diagnosis is defined as follows:

1) In the absence of a more likely diagnosis, an acute illness with (a) muscle spasms or hypertonia and (b) diagnosis of tetanus by a health care provider; or
2) Death, with tetanus listed on the death certificate as the cause of death or a significant condition contributing to death.

There are no case definitions for confirmed tetanus. If a case meets the criteria in the USA, then the local state public health service must be notified. Tetanus is similarly a statutory notifiable disease within most European countries.

**10. Referral network**—In order to transport BSL-2 pathogens to a reference laboratory, all potentially infectious samples should be packaged in accordance with current recommendations (International Airline Transportation Association). The national reference laboratory in the UK is the Gastrointestinal Reference Unit at Colindale.

**11. Special considerations**—Tetanus is an infectious disease that is not communicable. In the event of an outbreak, as defined by local guidelines, then it is important to search for contaminated sources such as contaminated street drugs. Outbreaks of tetanus have been reported following armed conflict and natural disasters such as the tsunami affecting Aceh in Indonesia. Following such incidents, it is important to ensure high levels of vaccination as well as access to large stocks of human tetanus immunoglobulin. If human tetanus immunoglobulin is not available, intravenous human normal immunoglobulin may be used instead (not approved by FDA in the USA).

[S. D. Woolley, N. J. Beeching]

# TOXOPLASMOSIS

| DISEASE | ICD-10 CODE |
|---|---|
| TOXOPLASMOSIS | ICD-10 B58 |
| CONGENITAL TOXOPLASMOSIS | ICD-10 P37.1 |

**1. Clinical features**—A systemic coccidian protozoan disease in which infections are frequently asymptomatic, present as acute disease with lymphadenopathy only, or resemble infectious mononucleosis with fever, lymphadenopathy, and lymphocytosis persisting for days or weeks. Development of an immune response decreases parasitemia, but *Toxoplasma gondii* cysts remaining in the tissues contain viable organisms. These cysts may reactivate if the immune system becomes compromised. Among immunodeficient individuals, including human immunodeficiency virus-infected patients, primary or reactivated infection may cause a maculopapular rash, generalized skeletal muscle involvement, cerebritis, chorioretinitis, pneumonia, myocarditis, and/or death. Cerebral toxoplasmosis is a frequent component of acquired-immunodeficiency syndrome (AIDS).

Infections with genetically distinct subtypes have been described, predominantly in South America, with fatal outcome in otherwise immunocompetent patients. An increased occurrence of chronic chorioretinitis in acquired toxoplasmosis has also been described in this region.

A primary infection during early pregnancy may lead to fetal infection with death of the fetus or manifestations such as chorioretinitis, brain damage with intracerebral calcification, hydrocephaly, microcephaly, fever, jaundice, rash, hepatosplenomegaly, xanthochromic cerebrospinal fluid (CSF), and convulsions evident at birth or shortly thereafter. Later in pregnancy, maternal infection results in milder or subclinical fetal disease with delayed manifestations, such as recurrent or chronic chorioretinitis. In immunosuppressed pregnant women who are *Toxoplasma*-seropositive, a reactivation of latent infection may result in congenital toxoplasmosis, though this is thought to be a rare event.

**2. Causative agents**—*Toxoplasma gondii*, an intracellular coccidian protozoan that completes its sexual life cycle phase in cats and belongs to the family *Sarcocystidae*, in the class *Sporozoasida*.

**3. Laboratory diagnosis**—Diagnosis is based on clinical signs and supportive serological results, demonstration of the agent in body tissues or fluids by biopsy or autopsy, or isolation in animals or cell culture. Rising antibody titers are indicative of active infection; the presence of specific immunoglobulin class M (IgM) and/or rising IgG titers in sequential sera of newborns is conclusive evidence of congenital infection. The presence of IgA is also helpful in determining infection in newborns. High IgG antibody levels may persist for years with no relation to active disease. Reference laboratories may use the IgG avidity test, differential agglutination test, and IgA- and IgE-specific antibody tests to help determine the timing of infection. In addition, polymerase chain reaction (PCR) assays of body fluids have been used to assist with the diagnosis.

Because clinical or biopsy-proven specimens from patients with toxoplasmosis are difficult to obtain, the true sensitivity and specificity of serologic tests is difficult to ascertain. Commercial test kit reported sensitivity and specificity may be based on a comparison with results obtained by another approved test kit. In addition, the assessment of test parameters is affected by the particular population being evaluated and the prevalence of *T. gondii*. The Sabin-Feldman dye test, which measures total *Toxoplasma*-related immunoglobulin (primarily IgG antibodies), has long been thought to be the gold standard *T. gondii* serologic test and is also useful for evaluation of IgG antibody kits; however, it is relatively expensive and requires a higher level of technical expertise, so it is only offered at a few reference laboratories. *T. gondii* antibodies are generally detected within the first several weeks after infection. Unless it is a very recent infection, a negative Sabin-Feldman dye test can be considered to rule out *T. gondii* infection. The commercial *Toxoplasma* IgG tests available vary over time, but many approved in the USA are enzyme immunoassay (EIA) tests (91%–100% sensitive and 72%–100% specific when compared with the Sabin-Feldman dye test in selected past studies) with several other types offered (examples: chemiluminescent immunoassay, indirect immunofluorescence assay [IFA], agglutination tests). In a recent evaluation of common commercial IgG immunoassays compared with a national reference laboratory using the dye test or IFA, sensitivities ranged from 97.1%–100%, and specificities ranged from 99.5%–100%.

There is no gold standard test for IgM or IgA antibodies to *T. gondii*; commercial tests are primarily EIAs, IFAs, immunochemiluminometric assays, and the IgM immunosorbent agglutination assay (ISAGA, often used for infants younger than 6 months). One study in the 1990s of 6 commercial IgM test kits found sensitivities of 93%–100% and specificities of 78%–99%

when these kits were compared with the double-sandwich IgM enzyme-linked immunosorbent assay (ELISA) from the Toxoplasma Serology Laboratory at Palo Alto Medical Foundation (the US reference laboratory). A more recent evaluation of automated commercial IgM immunoassays found sensitivities that ranged from 65.0%–97.9% and specificities from 92.6%–100% compared with IFA or ISAGA IgM tests performed in a national reference laboratory. To aid in the detection of recent infection, IgM and IgA tests have been multiplexed on a gold chip along with an IgG test and, when compared with tests at the Toxoplasma Serology Laboratory, found to have sensitivities of 97.6% and 90.9% for IgM and IgA, respectively, and specificities of 96.9% and 95.2% for IgM and IgA, respectively; the IgG test in this platform had a 100% correlation with the Sabin-Feldman dye test.

In infants, transplacental maternal *Toxoplasma* IgG antibodies can last up to a year. In congenitally infected infants, *Toxoplasma* IgM antibodies may be present but may have disappeared before birth in early fetal infections and are often absent when anti-*Toxoplasma* treatment has been given. The sensitivity of *Toxoplasma* IgM for detecting congenital infection in infants is generally less than 75%. The *Toxoplasma* IgA test can assist in detecting congenital infection. Clinicians should be aware that placental leak can cause a low-level false-positive *Toxoplasma* IgM or IgA test shortly after birth; these tests should be repeated after 10 days to verify if antibodies produced by the infant are present.

There is no standardized or FDA approved procedure for *Toxoplasma* PCR detection. Kits are available commercially and are often used for research purposes. The most common targets are 18s ribosomal deoxyribonucleic acid (DNA), B1, AF146257, and Rep-529. Testing is available for numerous body fluids, including amniotic fluid, bronchoalveolar lavage, CSF, ocular fluids, serum, urine, and whole blood. PCR is often done on the CSF, peripheral blood, and urine in infants suspected of having congenital toxoplasmosis. The sensitivity of PCR varies with the specific procedure, type of sample, and expertise of the laboratory (for example, blood: sensitivity 15%–85%, specificity >95%). Reference laboratories have reported good results for testing of amniotic fluid with PCR for evidence of congenital infection (in 1 study at a reference laboratory in women with ≥18 weeks gestation: 92% sensitivity, with the occasional false-negatives occurring in the last trimester; and 100% specificity); other evaluations have found sensitivities of 80%–97% during the second trimester and 68%–88% during the third trimester with specificities of generally 100% in expert laboratories. Also see Testing Requirements section in this chapter for further information about PCR.

**4. Laboratory capability**—Routine or reference diagnostic capabilities are necessary depending on the diagnostic testing that will be performed. Laboratorians should be trained to perform morphological, serologic, or molecular diagnosis and undergo regular proficiency testing. Known positive and negative controls should be tested in each run.

**5. Safety requirements**—Clinical specimens should always be collected and handled with standard precautions. *Toxoplasma gondii* is a biosafety level 2 organism. Blood specimens should be disposed of as infectious waste.

*T. gondii* oocysts are highly resistant to environmental influences, including freezing. Chlorine treatment will not inactivate *T. gondii* oocysts; however, tincture of iodine (2%) will inactivate *T. gondii* oocysts with a long (3 hours) exposure. Ammonia (5.5% solution) with a 3-hour exposure can also inactivate *T. gondii* oocysts. Filtering water (absolute 1 micron filter) or boiling will eliminate *T. gondii* oocysts.

Bradyzoites in meat tissue cysts can be killed by heating to 150°F (66°C) or freezing meat for several days at subzero (0°F, −18°C) temperatures.

**6. Nonhuman hosts**—Infection occurs worldwide in mammals and birds. The definitive hosts of *T. gondii* are cats (felines), which acquire infection mainly from eating infected mammals (especially rodents) or birds and probably also from oocysts in soil contaminated with cat feces (acquired during licking/grooming). Felines alone harbor parasites in the intestinal tract, where the sexual stage of the protozoan life cycle occurs, resulting in excretion of oocysts in the feces for 10–20 days and, rarely, longer. Intermediate hosts include sheep, goats, rodents, swine, cattle, chickens, and other birds; all may carry an infective stage encysted in tissue, especially muscle and brain. Tissue cysts remain viable for long periods, perhaps lifelong. Cattle seem to be only minimally affected by natural *T. gondii* infection.

**7. Sample/specimen requirements**—The diagnosis of toxoplasmosis is typically made by serologic testing. Serum or plasma (collected with ethylenediaminetetraacetic acid [EDTA], heparin or citrate) should be separated from the clot or red cells as soon as possible to avoid any hemolysis. The sera can be stored at 2°C–8°C for up to 48 hours; beyond that, store at −20°C. Serologic testing is also available for CSF and ocular fluid. PCR testing is available for CSF, amniotic fluid, bronchoalveolar lavage, pleural, ascitic, peritoneal and ocular fluids, serum, solid tissues, whole blood, and urine. Parasite isolation is available for whole blood (EDTA or citrate preferred), amniotic fluid, placenta, and other tissues. The Toxoplasma Serology Laboratory indicates the following: (a) Specimens must not be frozen or placed in formalin or other fixative, (b) inoculations are recommended within 48 hours of specimen collection date, and (c) results are available in 6 weeks.

**8. Testing requirements**—Sera can be tested for the detection of antibodies (IgM, IgG, IgA, and IgE) by ELISA, agglutination test, chemiluminescent, avidity, dye, and immunofluorescence assays. For the Toxoplasma Serotology Laboratory, a list of the available tests and sample requirements can be found at: http://www.pamf.org/serology/testinfo.html. See the later table.

PCR assays of body fluids can be used to assist with the diagnosis. *T. gondii* PCR testing of amniotic fluid is used for prenatal diagnosis of congenital infection. Peripheral blood, CSF, and urine can be examined by PCR in newborns suspected to have congenital disease

Algorithm for Immunodiagnosis of Toxoplasmosis

| IgG Result | IgM Result | Report/Interpretation for Humans[a] |
|---|---|---|
| Negative | Negative | No serological evidence of infection with *Toxoplasma*. |
| Negative | Equivocal | Possible early acute infection or false-positive IgM reaction. Obtain a new specimen for IgG and IgM testing. If results for the second specimen remain the same, the patient is probably not infected with *Toxoplasma*. |
| Negative | Positive | Possible acute infection or false-positive IgM result. Obtain a new specimen for IgG and IgM testing. If results for the second specimen remain the same, the IgM reaction is probably false-positive. |
| Equivocal | Negative | Indeterminate: obtain a new specimen for testing or retest this specimen for IgG in a different essay. |
| Equivocal | Equivocal | Indeterminate: obtain a new specimen for both IgG and IgM testing. |
| Equivocal | Positive | Possible acute infection with *Toxoplasma*. Obtain a new specimen for IgG and IgM testing. If results for the second specimen remain the same or if the IgG becomes positive, both specimens should be sent to a reference laboratory with experience in diagnosis of toxoplasmosis for further testing. |
| Positive | Negative | Infected with *Toxoplasma* for 6 months or more. |
| Positive | Equivocal | Infected with *Toxoplasma* for probably more than 1 year or false-positive IgM reaction. Obtain a new specimen for IgM testing. If results with the second specimen remain the same, both specimens should be sent to a reference laboratory with experience in the diagnosis of toxoplasmosis for further testing. |
| Positive | Positive | Possible recent infection within the last 12 months or false-positive IgM reaction. Send the specimen to a reference laboratory with experience in the diagnosis of toxoplasmosis for further testing. |

[a]Except for infants.

*T. gondii* PCR is also used to assist in confirming the diagnosis of toxoplasmic encephalitis in immunocompromized persons by testing CSF or in patients with suspected disseminated toxoplasmosis by testing other body fluids (for example, blood [buffy coat], bronchoalveolar lavage, urine, pleural, ascitic, peritoneal, or ocular fluids). PCR of vitreous or aqueous fluid is helpful to establish diagnosis in patients who present with atypical retinal lesions, who show a suboptimum response to appropriate antitoxoplasma treatment, or who are immunocompromised.

Conventional PCR, nested-PCR, real-time PCR, and loop-mediated isothermal amplification (LAMP) have all been used for *T. gondii* testing of human specimens. Real-time PCR can be used to assess disease progression and treatment efficacy because it can estimate the intensity of *T. gondii* infection. In a Brazilian study real-time PCR with the B1 gene was considered the best-performing technique for diagnosis of congenital toxoplasmosis compared with conventional PCR and nested-PCR. LAMP allows visual detection of amplification and can be useful in the field in resource-poor settings.

The Toxoplasma Serology Laboratory uses a PCR assay based on amplification of the B1 gene of *T. gondii*. The minimum sample requirements for PCR in this laboratory can be found at: http://www.pamf.org/serology/requirements.html. PCR based on the *T. gondii* Rep-529 target is often the preferred method in France. In a French study qPCR based on the Rep-529 target was superior to qPCR based on the B1 target.

Direct observation of the parasite can be done on stained tissue sections, CSF, biopsy, necropsy or isolation in animals, or cell culture. Giemsa and haematoxylin and eosin staining are generally used. Immunologic techniques can be used to identify parasites in tissue sections or tissue cultures (fluorescein isothiocyanate- or peroxidase-labeled antisera are useful in detecting tachyzoites in tissue sections).

An algorithm for the immunodiagnosis of toxoplasmosis for individuals older than 1 year is shown in the earlier table. The EIA and IFA tests for IgG and IgM antibodies are the tests most commonly used today.

Persons should be initially tested for the presence of *Toxoplasma*-specific IgG antibodies to determine their immune status. A positive IgG titer indicates infection with the organism at some time. If more precise knowledge of the time of infection is necessary, then an IgG-positive person should have an IgM test performed by a procedure with minimal nonspecific reactions, such as IgM-capture EIA. A negative IgM test essentially excludes recent infection, but a positive IgM test is difficult to interpret because *Toxoplasma*-specific IgM antibodies may be detected by EIA for as long as 18 months after acute acquired infection.

A major problem with *Toxoplasma*-specific IgM testing is lack of specificity. Two situations occur frequently: (a) persons with a positive IgM but negative IgG, and (b) individuals with positive IgG and IgM results. In the first situation, a positive IgM result with a negative IgG result in the same specimen should be viewed with great suspicion; the patient's blood should be redrawn 2 weeks after the first blood draw and tested together with the first specimen. If the first specimen was drawn very early after infection, the patient should have highly positive IgG and IgM antibodies in the second sample. If the IgG is negative and the IgM is positive in both specimens, the IgM result should be considered to be a false positive and the patient should be considered to be not infected. In the second situation, a second specimen should be drawn and both specimens submitted together to a reference laboratory which employs a different IgM testing system for confirmation.

If the patient is pregnant, and IgG/IgM positive, an IgG avidity test should be performed. A high avidity result in the first 12–16 weeks of pregnancy (time dependent upon the commercial test kit) essentially rules out an infection acquired during gestation. A low IgG avidity result should not be interpreted as indicating recent infection because some individuals have persistent low IgG avidity for many months after infection. Suspected recent infection in a pregnant woman should be confirmed prior to intervention by having samples tested at a toxoplasmosis reference laboratory. If the patient has clinical illness compatible with toxoplasmosis but the IgG titer is low, a follow-up titer 2–3 weeks later should show an increase in antibody titer if the illness is due to acute toxoplasmosis, assuming the host is not severely immunocompromised.

**9. Reporting requirements**—*T. gondii* may be reported back to the requesting clinical authority at the species level based on laboratory results. It is not generally required that *T. gondii* infections are reported to public health authorities by laboratories but, given the importance and significance of infections with *T. gondii*, laboratories should verify any requirement for reporting positive findings with their local or regional public health authority.

**10. Referral network**—The US reference laboratory for toxoplasmosis is the Toxoplasma Serotology Laboratory at the Palo Alto Medical Foundation (http://www.pamf.org/serology). Currently in the USA, referrals go directly to this laboratory. In other countries it is recommended that primary testing laboratories ascertain whether there is a toxoplasmosis referral network in the public or private sector.

**11. Special considerations**—Newborn infants suspected of congenital toxoplasmosis should be tested by both an IgM- and an IgA-capture EIA. Detection of *Toxoplasma*-specific IgA antibodies is more sensitive than IgM detection in congenitally infected infants. None of the current commercial assays offered in the USA have been cleared by FDA for in vitro diagnostic use for infants; consequently, all specimens from neonates suspected of having congenital toxoplasmosis should be sent to the Palo Alto Medical Foundation *Toxoplasma* Serology Laboratory, which has the most experience with infant testing.

Serological determination of active central nervous system toxoplasmosis in immunocompromised patients is not possible at this time. *Toxoplasma*-specific IgG antibody levels in AIDS patients often are low to moderate, but occasionally no specific IgG antibodies can be detected. Tests for IgM antibodies are usually negative.

[J. L. Jones, H. Rivera, R. S. Bradbury]

# TRACHOMA

| DISEASE | ICD-10 CODE |
|---|---|
| TRACHOMA | ICD-10 A71 |
| Pneumonia due to *Chlamydia trachomatis* (see "Pneumonia") | |

**1. Clinical features**—A chlamydial conjunctivitis of insidious or abrupt onset; the infection may persist for a few weeks if untreated and tends to resolve with no consequence. Conjunctivitis (active disease) is characterized by the presence of lymphoid follicles and diffuse conjunctival inflammation (papillary hypertrophy), particularly on the tarsal conjunctiva lining the upper eyelid. The inflammation can produce superficial vascularization of the cornea (pannus) and scarring of the conjunctiva, which increases with the severity and duration of inflammatory disease. The marked conjunctival scarring causes lid deformities and in-turning of eyelashes (entropion and trichiasis), which later in adult life cause chronic abrasion of the cornea and opacity in some individuals, resulting in visual impairment and blindness. Secondary bacterial infections frequently occur in populations with endemic trachoma and may contribute to the communicability and severity of the disease. Active trachoma in some developing countries is an endemic early childhood disease. It may be clinically indistinguishable from conjunctivitis caused by other bacteria (including genital strains of *Chlamydia trachomatis*). Differential diagnosis includes molluscum contagiosum nodules of the eyelids, toxic reactions to chronically administered eye drops, and chronic staphylococcal lid-margin infection. An allergic reaction to contact lenses (giant papillary conjunctivitis) may produce a trachoma-like syndrome with tarsal nodules (giant papillae), conjunctival scarring, and corneal pannus.

**2. Causative agent**—*C. trachomatis* serovars A, B, Ba, and C.

**3. Laboratory diagnosis**—While the diagnosis is primarily made though clinical observation, confirmation of the causative organism can be made through polymerase chain reaction (PCR), Giemsa-stained smears for the detection of intracellular chlamydial elementary bodies in epithelial cells of conjunctival scrapings, immunofluorescence examination after methanol fixation of the smear, detection of chlamydial antigen by enzyme immunoassay, detection of deoxyribonucleic acid by probe, or isolation of the agent in special cell culture.

**4. Laboratory capability**—Most clinical and public health laboratories should have the capability to test for trachoma. Laboratory staff must be competently trained and experienced in the detection of *C. trachomatis*.

Ongoing competency is performed through sufficient training, education, audits, and quality assurance.

Laboratories must enroll in quality assurance programs and meet all regulated quality requirements in accordance with their respective national regulations. Laboratory accreditation is normally performed by approved accrediting organizations.

Quality assessment and quality control is an ongoing comprehensive approach to monitor and ensure true results are obtained. It is a way to ensure each platform is used in accordance with guidelines and only by properly qualified and appropriately trained laboratory staff. Quality control must be performed regularly to ensure the test is working according to the manufacturer's protocol.

Quality control also ensures that *C. trachomatis* testing methods maintain high sensitivity and specificity for detection. *C. trachomatis* PCR testing capability should be maintained in order to monitor and support surveillance and epidemiology. This is particularly necessary in a setting where there could be variant *C. trachomatis* circulating such as the variant described in Sweden in 2007.[1]

**5. Safety requirements**—Biosafety level 2 practices, personal protective equipment, containment equipment, and facilities are recommended for laboratory staff working with clinical specimens, cultures, or materials known to contain or that may contain ocular *C. trachomatis*. Risk assessments for processes and substances relating to *C. trachomatis* assays should be performed before implementing an assay and when a deviation from the normal method is implemented. The goal of performing risk assessments is to consider all hazards and risks associated with processing and testing and to reduce the risk. Risks for *C. trachomatis* testing include cross-contamination and carryover contamination, specimen mix-up, and use of dangerous chemicals and reagents for testing.

Contamination and specimen mix-up could occur at the specimen collection preanalytical stage, during testing at the analytical stage, or at the postanalytical stage during analysis, interpretation and reporting. The most critical steps of testing require risk assessments to determine ways of reducing and eliminating contamination.

Good management and use of adequate personal protective equipment at all stages of *C. trachomatis* testing is required to minimize risk.

**6. Nonhuman hosts**—*C. trachomatis* has only been identified as a pathogen of humans.

**7. Sample/specimen requirements**—Adult conjunctivitis and neonatal conjunctivitis: Eye swabs should be collected and then rolled over a slide. After the fixative has been applied, the slide can be stored or transported at ambient temperature. The laboratory should process the slide within 7 days of specimen collection.

For PCR testing, swab specimens can be stored for up to 6 days at 2°C–27°C or 30 days at 2°C–8°C. Specimens can be frozen at −70°C and tested within 60 days after collection.

**8. Testing requirements—**

1) Direct fluorescent antibody tests (DFA): direct fluorescent antibody tests are currently the only FDA-cleared tests for ocular *C. trachomatis* infections.
2) Culture: where available, involves culturing *C. trachomatis* in tissue culture medium followed by detection using fluorescent antibody.
3) Nucleic acid amplification tests (NAAT): although most commercial NAATs are not validated for *C. trachomatis* testing in extragenital sites, eye swabs for *C. trachomatis* PCR have been used with satisfactory performance.[2]

**9. Reporting requirements—**The requirement for laboratory-based reporting of cases of trachoma varies by country. Laboratories must determine what diseases are required to be reported by laboratories within their respective jurisdictions.

**10. Referral network—**

1) International Agency for the Prevention of Blindness (IAPB): IAPB's mission is to eliminate the main causes of avoidable blindness and visual impairment. IAPB is made up of a consortium of governments, non-governmental organizations and national committees from more than 60 countries established to facilitate sustainable national eye care programs. In 2013, the Universal Eye Health: A Global Action Plan was approved to commit governments to reducing visual impairment by 2019.[3]
2) National Trachoma Surveillance and Reporting Unit (NTSRU): NTSRU provides surveillance reports on trachoma statistics in Australia.[4]
3) SAFE strategy: SAFE strategy refers to surgery (for trichiasis), antibiotics (to clear infection), facial cleanliness (to reduce transmission) and environmental improvement (especially water and sanitation) to reduce transmission.

These WHO interventions are part of the Global Elimination of Trachoma (GET 2020), utilized by primary health care systems globally.[5]

**11. Special considerations—**Importing or transporting *C. trachomatis* may require importation permits.

Mass treatment campaigns have been successful in eliminating trachoma as a public health concern in regions of high prevalence.[6,7] This has been particularly effective when associated with improvement in personal and environmental hygiene.

WHO/Alliance for the Global Elimination of blinding Trachoma and associated WHO Collaborating Centres provide technical and coordination support.

## References


1. Unemo M, Olcen P, Agne-Stadling I, et al. Experiences with the new genetic variant of Chlamydia trachomatis in Orebro county, Sweden-proportion, characteristics and effective diagnostic solution in an emergent situation. *Euro Surveill.* 2007; 12(4):E5–6.
2. Butcher R, Houghton J, Derrick T, et al. Reduced-cost Chlamydia trachomatis-specific multiplex real-time PCR diagnostic assay evaluated for ocular swabs and use by trachoma research programmes. *J Microbiol Methods.* 2017;139:95–102.
3. The International Agency for the Prevention of Blindness. Website. Available at: https://www.iapb.org. Accessed June 24, 2018.
4. Australian Government Department of Health. Trachoma surveillance reports. Available at: http://www.health.gov.au/internet/main/publishing.nsf/content/health-oatsih-pubs-trachreport. Accessed June 24, 2018.
5. World Health Organization. Trachoma - Strategy. 2018. Available at: http://www.who.int/trachoma/strategy/en. Accessed June 24, 2018.
6. Hammou J, El Ajaroumi H, Hasbi H, Nakhlaoui A, Hmadna A, El Maaroufi A. In Morocco, the elimination of trachoma as a public health problem becomes a reality. *Lancet Glob Health.* 2017;5(3):e250–e251.
7. Pan American Health Organization. Mexico eliminates trachoma, leading infectious cause of blindness. 2017. Available at: https://www.paho.org/hq/index.php?option=com_content&view=article&id=13179%3Amexico-eliminates-trachoma-leading-infectious-cause-blindness&catid=740%3Apress-releases&Itemid=1926&lang=pt. Accessed June 24, 2018.


[A. G. Costa]

# TRICHINELLOSIS

(trichiniasis, trichinosis)

| DISEASE | ICD-10 CODE |
|---|---|
| TRICHINELLOSIS | ICD-10 B75 |

**1. Clinical features**—A roundworm disease in which clinical illness is highly variable and can range from inapparent infection to a fulminating, fatal disease, depending on the number of larvae ingested. These are sometimes followed by subconjunctival, subungual, and retinal hemorrhages; pain; and photophobia. Thirst, profuse sweating, chills, weakness, prostration, and rapidly increasing eosinophilia may follow shortly after the ocular signs.

Gastrointestinal symptoms, such as diarrhea due to the intra-intestinal activity of the adult worms, may precede the ocular manifestations. Remittent fever is usual, sometimes as high as 40°C (104°F); fever terminates after 1–6 weeks, depending on intensity of infection. Cardiac and neurological complications may appear in the third to sixth week; in the most severe cases, death due to myocardial failure may occur in either the first to second week or between the fourth and eighth weeks.

**2. Causative agents**—*Trichinella spiralis* and other *Trichinella* spp.; nematodes. *T. spiralis* has a cosmopolitan distribution and broad host range in primarily temperate areas of the world. Separate taxonomic designations have been accepted for isolates found in carnivorous and omnivorous animals of the Arctic and subarctic (*Trichinella nativa*) and Palaearctic (*Trichinella britovi*), wild animals in temperate North America (*Trichinella murrelli*), in Africa (*Trichinella nelsoni*), in mammals and birds (*Trichinella pseudospiralis*), and in omnivorous and carnivorous animals (*Trichinella papuae, Trichinella zimbabwensis*, and T6, T8, T9, T12 genotypes) in several specific regions of the world.

**3. Laboratory diagnosis**—Marked peripheral eosinophilia combined with elevated muscle enzymes (creatine phosphokinase and lactate dehydrogenase) in infected patients may aid in initial clinical suspicion. Serology is a noninvasive first line of testing for trichinellosis. Circulating immunoglobulin class G (IgG) antibodies may be detected from 12–60 days after infection. Anti-*Trichinella* IgG enzyme-linked immunosorbent assay (ELISA) has been shown to have a sensitivity of up to 100% for biopsy-confirmed *T. spiralis* at 50 days postinfection and 90% for outbreak-associated clinically diagnosed cases. Sensitivity may vary for infections with other *Trichinella* spp., with a sensitivity of only 87% being reported for *T. nativa* infections 70 days postinfection during 1 outbreak. ELISA tests based on the 49 kDa *T. spiralis* excretory/secretory (E/S) antigen rather than crude larval extracts are considered to be more specific (reported 88%) for the detection of *Trichinella* infection and allow earlier detection of disease. Western blot employing the E/S antigens of *T. spiralis* has been found to be the most specific test. Western blot is generally used as a confirmatory test due to the expense and difficulty in its performance compared with ELISA. Some cross-reaction with *Schistosoma* spp. and *Onchocerca volvulus* antibodies has been noted.

Biopsy of skeletal muscle, typically from the deltoid region, allows microscopic visualization and further molecular analysis of the larvae. Biopsies should be taken later than 10 days after infection and are most often positive more than 1 month after infection. Stained histological sections or muscle squash preparations following tissue digestion frequently provide conclusive evidence of infection by demonstrating an uncalcified, encapsulated, coiled nematode larva in the interfibrillar region of the biopsy. *T. pseudospiralis*, *T papuae*, and *T. zimbabwensis* larvae are unencapsulated in muscle but retain the coiled morphology of other *Trichinella* spp. The sensitivity of muscle biopsy for the detection of trichinellosis is dependent on the intensity of larval infestation in that muscle. In the absence of larva visualization, the basophilic transformation of haematoxylin- and eosin- (H&E) stained muscle fibers in histological section may be an indicator of trichinellosis. Recovery of larvae in biopsy allows for definitive species identification through genotyping via multiplex polymerase chain reaction (PCR) and sequencing of either the large subunit 5S ribosomal ribonucleic acid region, expansion segment 5 (ES5) region, or internal transcribed spacer regions (ITS1 and ITS2) of the nematode.

**4. Laboratory capability**—Regional or district level clinical diagnostic laboratory with trained parasitic microscopists for morphological detection. Microscopic identification of species from larval worms requires reference laboratory level skills. Serological detection requires reference laboratory level skills. No PCR for *Trichinella* has been FDA approved, although some reference laboratories will run such assays as research-only tests.

**5. Safety requirements**—All clinical specimens should be collected and handled using universal/standard precautions. *Trichinella* spp. parasites are categorized as risk group 2 agents; therefore, specimens should be handled in a biosafety level 2 laboratory. Accidental ingestion of *Trichinella* larvae from fresh or digested specimens could cause infection.

**6. Nonhuman hosts**—Any carnivorous mammal may act as a reservoir host of *Trichinella* spp. Important reservoir hosts for specific species of *Trichinella* are for *T. spiralis*: pigs and rodents; *T. nativa*: bears, foxes, and walruses; *T. britovi*: pigs; *T. nelsoni*: wild animals; *T. pseudospiralis*: pigs and birds; and for *T. papuae* and *T. zimbabwensis*: pigs and reptiles.

**7. Sample/specimen requirements**—Skeletal muscle tissue is required for histological analysis and morphological identification. For molecular diagnosis, larvae in muscle biopsies may be examined provided the tissue has not been fixed in formalin. Serum or plasma are required for serology and should be transported to the laboratory at 4°C within 48 hours or frozen at −80°C if longer storage or transportation times are necessary.

**8. Testing requirements**—Morphological identification of *Trichinella* spp. larvae from a muscle biopsy is both diagnostic and confirmatory. Histological specimens may be examined using squash preparation following tissue digestion or by using H&E-stained sections. If available, the suspected animal meat may also be examined for the presence of *Trichinella* spp. larvae. However, detection of larvae in animal meat is not definitively diagnostic; therefore, infection in the patient should be confirmed through serologic testing. Serologic testing is the preferred method for diagnosing *Trichinella* spp. infections as it is more sensitive and less invasive than muscle biopsy analysis. An anti-*Trichinella* IgG ELISA test for *Trichinella* spp. is available at the CDC. Although species identification is not required to diagnose or treat *Trichinella* spp. infections and is not FDA approved, molecular genotyping can be used to determine the species of larvae recovered from biopsy tissue or infected animal meat for epidemiological purposes.

**9. Reporting requirements**—Trichinellosis is a nationally notifiable disease in the USA as well as some other countries. Report all positive serologic tests and cases in which *Trichinella* spp. larvae have been identified in a patient tissue specimen.

**10. Referral network**—Networks vary among countries. CDC offers E/S antigen ELISA testing, morphological identification, and genotyping. The International *Trichinella* Reference Centre (Istituto Superiore di Sanita) in Rome, Italy, also offers services for the full identification of *Trichinella* spp. and genotypes.

**11. Special considerations**—Following any case of trichinellosis, a thorough epidemiological investigation should be conducted to determine the source and scope of the outbreak and to prevent further infections. Dispose of any remaining infected meat. Any confirmed cases should be reported to CDC for further investigation.

[R. S. Bradbury, K. J. Kines]

# TRICHOMONIASIS

| DISEASE | ICD-10 CODE |
|---|---|
| TRICHOMONIASIS | ICD-10 A59 |

**1. Clinical features**—Asymptomatic infection in about 70% of infected persons. Symptoms include mild-to-moderate genital inflammation, pruritus, vaginitis, urethritis, or prostatitis. Affected persons may notice pain during urination or sexual intercourse and malodorous genital discharge that can appear clear, white, yellow, or green. Infection can increase the risk of acquiring other sexually transmitted infections, including the human immunodeficiency virus.

**2. Causative agents**—*Trichomonas vaginalis*, a flagellated protozoan parasite.

**3. Laboratory diagnosis**—Infection has been most commonly diagnosed by identifying the motile parasite in genital secretions viewed on a microscope slide (wet mount) within 20 minutes of collection. Culture in modified Diamond's media is more sensitive than wet mount, and there is now a commercial product (InPouch TV, BioMed Diagnostics, White City, OR) having the ability to culture parasites in a format that facilitates microscopic assessment of growth. A point-of-care lateral flow antigen detection test (OSOM Trichomonas Rapid Test, Sekisui Diagnostics, San Diego, CA) provides results within 10 minutes and is Clinical Laboratory Improvement Amendments (CLIA)-waived. A number of commercially available nucleic acid detection methods have been developed and are being used more regularly: ribonucleic acid probe hybridization (Affirm VP III Identification Test, Becton Dickinson, Franklin Lakes, NJ); transcription mediated amplification (APTIMA *Trichomonas vaginalis* assay, Hologic, San Diego, CA); polymerase chain reaction (PCR) coupled with oligonucleotide probe detection (cobas TV/MG, Roche Diagnostics, Rotkreuz, Switzerland); strand displacement amplification with fluorescence detection (BD Probe Tec Trichomonas Vaginalis Qx, Becton Dickinson); and real-time PCR (Xpert TV Assay, Cepheid, Sunnyvale, CA).

**4. Laboratory capability**—Laboratory requirements and training for wet mount, culture, or antigen detection methods are relatively minimal. Only a microscope is needed for wet mounts. Culture requires a 37°C incubator and microscope. Antigen detection requires no specialized laboratory equipment or discipline-specific training. Specialized equipment is needed for the nucleic acid detection assays, but the different commercial systems have specific apparatus, processing reagents, and training protocols that facilitate their use. This includes automated sample preparation for some of the tests.

**5. Safety requirements**—Safety requirements for performing testing for *T. vaginalis* infection are the same universal and standard precautions as for handling any human sample. Laboratory workers are not at risk of infection.

**6. Nonhuman hosts**—Although other trichomonad species can be found in animals, *T. vaginalis* only infects humans.

**7. Sample/specimen requirements**—Both men and women are infected with *T. vaginalis*, but symptoms and pathology are much more common in women, with men often having self-limiting infections. For culture and wet mount, vaginal secretions or swabs of the vagina or endocervix are the preferred specimen type for women. For men, urethral swabs, semen, or sediments from urine are used. Multiple sampling increases sensitivity. For antigen detection, vaginal swabs expressed in test buffer or the saline solution remaining from a wet mount are tested. Antigen testing is not FDA-approved for men. The Xpert TV real-time PCR is approved for testing *T. vaginalis* in both women and men, but the other nucleic acid detection tests are approved for women only. Vaginal or endocervical swabs are appropriate samples for these tests.

**8. Testing requirements**—Wet mount testing is widely available for any clinic or laboratory with a microscope and is fairly inexpensive, but it has poor sensitivity (51%–65%) that decreases with the amount of time between when a sample is collected and when it is read. Culture is more sensitive (75%–96%) and both wet mount and culture approach 100% specificity when performed by trained readers. The antigen detection test has 82%–95% sensitivity and 97%–100% specificity. The Affirm VP III test is less sensitive (63%–83%) than the nucleic acid amplifications tests (NAATs, 95%–100%) because it is based on direct hybridization, but it is considered a point-of-care test as results are available within 45 minutes, which can facilitate provision of treatment. Nucleic acid testing also has high specificity, and samples collected based on suspicion of 1 sexually transmitted infection (STI) can be tested for multiple pathogens. As a result, testing for *T. vaginalis* is becoming more common in the absence of characteristic symptoms of trichomoniasis.

**9. Reporting requirements**—In the USA, trichomoniasis is not a reportable disease.

**10. Referral network**—There is no referral network for *T. vaginalis* infections.

**11. Special considerations**—For trichomoniasis that fails to resolve following standard nitroimidazole treatment, drug susceptibility testing and treatment recommendation are available from CDC. This testing requires obtaining the isolate from the infected individual. Because NAAT for multiple STIs is highly sensitive, persistent *T. vaginalis* can be detected even in the absence of symptoms even if the parasite numbers are so low that it is difficult to acquire a viable isolate for susceptibility testing. Future guidelines will need to consider the implications and procedures for treating NAAT-detected persistent asymptomatic infections.

[W. E. Secor]

# TRICHURIASIS

(whipworm disease)

| DISEASE | ICD-10 CODE |
|---|---|
| Trichuriasis | ICD-10 B79 |

**1. Clinical features**—A nematode infection of the large intestine, usually asymptomatic. Heavy infections may cause bloody, mucoid stools and diarrhea, and at times rectal prolapse, clubbing of fingers, hypoproteinemia, and anemia with growth retardation.

**2. Causative agents**—*Trichuris trichiura*, or human whipworm, a nematode, soil-transmitted helminth that occurs worldwide.

**3. Laboratory diagnosis**—Made through demonstration of eggs in feces, or observation of worms attached to the wall of the lower colon during a sigmoidoscopic examination. There are no molecular or serologic tests available for routine clinical diagnosis of trichuriasis.

Eggs of *T. trichiura* are 50–55 μm long by 22–24 μm wide, are barrel-shaped, have a thick shell, and possess bipolar hyaline plugs at each end. Eggs are unembryonated when shed in feces. Eggs should be differentiated from those of *Capillaria philippinensis*, due to the possibility of autoinfection with the latter.

Adult worms have a very distinctive morphology. Males are 30–45 mm in length while the females are slightly larger at 35–50 mm. The anterior end contains the esophagus and stichosome and is very long and whip-like; the posterior end contains the rest of the digestive tract and reproductive tract and is short and thick. The posterior end of the male is curved. Sometimes, worms break at the juncture of the thick and thin portions when removed via colonoscopy. This can create challenges in identification, and manipulation of the specimen may result in liberation of eggs (if a female) or the characteristic spicule (if a male).

**4. Laboratory capability**—Microscopy and stool concentration/centrifugation capabilities should be available. Laboratorians should be trained in the microscopic/morphologic detection of parasites and undergo regular proficiency testing.

**5. Safety requirements**—Clinical specimens should always be collected and handled with standard precautions. *T. trichiura* is a biosafety level 2 organism. Formalin should only be used in a well-ventilated area, preferably in a chemical fume hood. Unpreserved and preserved stools should be disposed of as infectious waste.

**6. Nonhuman hosts**—None.

**7. Sample/specimen requirements**—Stool should be promptly preserved in an appropriate liquid medium such as 10% buffered formalin or sodium acetate-acetic acid-formalin. Single vial systems for ova and parasites (O&P) collection are also adequate. Adult worms should also be placed into a liquid preservative such as 10% formalin or 70% laboratory grade ethanol as soon as possible after collection to avoid desiccation and alteration of morphologic features. Specimens in the appropriate preservatives should remain intact indefinitely. To maximize O&P sensitivity, up to 3 stool specimens should be collected.

**8. Testing requirements**—Routine concentration procedures for stool (eggs) and routine examination of gross helminths (adults). A calibrated ocular micrometer should be used to measure egg size. Diagnosis is confirmatory in specimens meeting morphologic criteria.

**9. Reporting requirements**—Positive cases are reported as *T. trichiura*. Trichuriasis is not nationally reportable in the USA. Follow national, regional/state, and local regulations for reporting to public health authorities; official report not ordinarily justifiable.

**10. Referral network**—None.

**11. Special considerations**—Advise school health authorities of unusual frequency in school populations. It is important to notify public health officials if a positive patient is a resident of a long-term care facility.

[B. Mathison]

# TRYPANOSOMIASIS

| DISEASE | ICD-10 CODE |
|---|---|
| AFRICAN TRYPANOSOMIASIS | ICD-10 B56, B56.1 |
| AMERICAN TRYPANOSOMIASIS | ICD-10 B57 |

## I. AFRICAN TRYPANOSOMIASIS (sleeping sickness)

**1. Clinical features**—The 2 forms of human African trypanosomiasis (HAT; the West African and East African forms) occur in different regions of sub-Saharan Africa, are caused by different subspecies of the protozoan parasite *Trypanosoma brucei*, and progress at different rates from the hemolymphatic stage of infection (first stage), to the meningoencephalitic stage (second stage), and, if untreated, to death. West African HAT is endemic in parts of western and central Africa, is caused by *T. brucei* subsp. *gambiense*, and progresses gradually until eventual death (on average, ~3 years after acquisition of infection). By contrast, East African HAT is endemic in parts of eastern and southern Africa, is caused by *T. brucei* subsp. *rhodesiense*, and typically progresses to the second stage within a few weeks and to death within 6 months after acquisition of infection.

In *T. b. gambiense* infection, posterior cervical lymphadenopathy (Winterbottom's sign) is a common clinical finding. During the first 2–3 weeks of *T. b. rhodesiense* infection, some patients have a lesion (chancre) at the site of the infective bite; the lesion may evolve from an erythematous, tender swelling to an indurated nodule, which may ulcerate. In first-stage HAT, patients may have various nonspecific manifestations such as fever, headache, lymphadenopathy, pruritus, dermatologic eruptions, local edema, musculoskeletal pain, hepatosplenomegaly, and cardiac involvement. Patients with second-stage HAT (after parasites have crossed the blood-brain barrier into the central nervous system [CNS]) also have neuropsychiatric manifestations such as sleep, sensory, motor/movement, and mood disorders; behavioral changes; seizures; lethargy; and coma. Although both East African HAT and West African HAT typically are fatal if not treated, potential cases of asymptomatic and self-resolving first-stage *T. b. gambiense* infection have been reported.

**2. Causative agents**—The gambiense or chronic form of HAT is caused by the protozoan parasite *T. brucei* subsp. *gambiense* in western and central Africa. The rhodesiense or acute form of HAT is caused by the protozoan parasite *T. brucei* subsp. *rhodesiense* in eastern and southern Africa. Both occur in humans as a hemoflagellate (trypomastigote).

**3. Laboratory diagnosis**—Trypanosomes may be detected in the blood, when present, by examination of thick and thin films and buffy-coat preparations stained with Giemsa, Field's, Wright-Giemsa, or Wright's stain. The motile trypanosomes may be detected in buffy-coat preparations after capillary (microhematocrit) centrifugation or after use of the triple centrifugation tube technique or the miniature anion exchange centrifugation technique (mAECT), which is the most sensitive method for the detection of bloodstream trypanosomes by light microscopy. Examination of smears of lymph node aspirates may sometimes yield positive results, as may examination of cytospin preparations of cerebrospinal fluid (CSF).

Several polymerase chain reaction (PCR) and loop mediated isothermal amplification (LAMP) tests for both *T. brucei* subspp. that cause HAT have been described. Concerns have been raised about the sensitivity of PCR for the diagnosis of HAT; validation of sensitivity and specificity has been difficult because of the absence of a suitable comparison standard diagnostic method, particularly for *T. b. gambiense* infection. Positive molecular test results for parasite deoxyribonucleic acid (DNA) or ribonucleic acid in CSF specimens that otherwise have normal laboratory parameters should be interpreted with care.

As both microscopy and PCR for the detection of *T. b. gambiense* infection may be insensitive due to the very low numbers of circulating trypanosomes, serologic testing often is performed. Two available rapid antibody test kits for *T. b. gambiense* have varying sensitivity and specificity, depending in part on specimen storage and the geographic region in which the infection was acquired. In patients with *T. b. gambiense* infection, the sensitivities of 2 available card agglutination test for trypanosomiasis (CATT) assays were 99.6% for the SD BIOLINE HAT test and 99.1% for the HAT Sero-K-SeT test; the specificities in healthy controls were, respectively, 87.9% and 88.3%. No available serologic test differentiates between current and past infection.

**4. Laboratory capability**—CATT and microscopy services should be available at first-line laboratories. Laboratorians should be trained in the appropriate techniques used for detection of parasites and should undergo regular proficiency testing. Specific equipment is required for PCR (thermocycler) and LAMP (hot block or water bath with temperature monitoring).

**5. Safety requirements**—Clinical specimens should always be collected and handled with universal/standard precautions. *T. brucei* subspp. are biosafety level 2 organisms. Blood and other clinical specimens should be disposed of as infectious waste.

**6. Nonhuman hosts**—Infected tsetse flies (genus *Glossina*) transmit both *T. brucei* subspp. that cause HAT. *T. b. gambiense* infection is predominantly anthroponotic. *T. b. rhodesiense* is zoonotic, with cattle and various antelope species being the primary reservoir hosts.

**7. Sample/specimen requirements**—Ethylenediaminetetraacetic acid (EDTA) blood, CSF, or lymph node (or chancre) aspirate for morphologic and molecular diagnosis. Whole blood, serum, or plasma for CATT testing for evidence of *T. b. gambiense* infection. Specimens for morphologic diagnosis should be prepared and examined within 1–2 hours of collection, before the trypanosomes lyse, unless stained slides are prepared, which may be examined later following fixation.

**8. Testing requirements**—In first-stage disease, morphological diagnosis may be carried out on thick and thin blood smears as well as buffy-coat smears. Smears should be stained with Giemsa, Field's, Wright-Giemsa, or Wright's stain. To increase sensitivity, mAECT has been used, as has capillary centrifugation (see Laboratory Diagnosis section in this chapter); CSF specimens should be centrifuged before examination for trypanosomes. The level of parasitemia in *T. b. rhodesiense* infection is often high but varies from case to case. For *T. b. gambiense*, bloodstream trypomastigotes are often not readily detected after the acute phase of infection, and their recovery in CSF in second-stage disease may be difficult. The subspecies of *T. brucei* are morphologically indistinguishable. They are spindle-shaped, motile, serpentine organisms from 14–33 (average 23) μm in length.

The trypanosomes have a central nucleus and a small kinetoplast close to the posterior end. A prominent undulating membrane is present. Three forms may be seen: a short, broad form without a flagellum; an intermediate form; and a long thin flagellated form. In *T. b. rhodesiense* infection, the long, thin form predominates. Staining of blood films or CSF cytospin preparations can be helpful in identifying the characteristic cellular features of the trypomastigote stage found in humans. The finding of Mott cells (large morula-like plasma cells with many vacuoles) in the CSF is indicative of *T. brucei* subsp. infection.

**9. Reporting requirements**—Reporting requirements/criteria vary by country and local jurisdiction. Laboratories are responsible for determining whether HAT is reportable by laboratories in their respective setting.

**10. Referral network**—CATT testing for evidence of infection with *T. b. gambiense* and PCR testing for *T. brucei* subspp. are available through McGill University, Canada, and the Institute for Tropical Medicine, Antwerp, Belgium.

**11. Special considerations**—Confirmation of the diagnosis by a reference laboratory is encouraged.

## II. AMERICAN TRYPANOSOMIASIS (Chagas disease)

**1. Clinical features**—The acute disease, with variable fever, lymphadenopathy, malaise, and hepatosplenomegaly, generally occurs in children, although the majority of infections are asymptomatic or paucisymptomatic. In 20%–30% of infections, irreversible chronic manifestations generally appear later in life. An inflammatory response at the site of infection (chagoma) may last up to 8 weeks. Unilateral bipalpebral edema (Romaña's sign) occurs in a small percentage of acute cases. Life-threatening or fatal manifestations of acute infection include myocarditis and meningoencephalitis. Chronic irreversible sequelae include myocardial damage with cardiac dilatation; arrhythmias and major conduction abnormalities; and intestinal tract involvement with megaesophagus and megacolon. Megavisceral manifestations are recognized mainly in central Brazil. The prevalence of megaviscera and cardiac involvement varies according to regions; the latter is not as common north of Ecuador as in southern areas. In AIDS patients, acute myocarditis and severe multifocal or diffuse meningoencephalitis with necrosis and hemorrhage occur as relapses of chronic infection. Reactivation of chronic Chagas disease may also occur with non-AIDS immunosuppression and is characterized by skin lesions, blood parasitemia, and, often, acute myocarditis. CNS involvement is not usually seen.

Infection with *T. rangeli* may occur in some foci of endemic Chagas disease; prolonged parasitemia occurs, sometimes coexisting with *T. cruzi* flagellates (with which *T. rangeli* shares reservoir hosts). No clinical manifestations attributable to *T. rangeli* infection have been noted.

**2. Causative agents**—*T. cruzi* is a protozoan that occurs in humans as a hemoflagellate (trypomastigote) and as an intracellular parasite (amastigote) without an external flagellum.

**3. Laboratory diagnosis**—Trypomastigotes of *T. cruzi* may be detected in Giemsa-, Field's-, Wright-Giemsa-, or Wright's-stained blood films during the acute phase of the infection and in specimens from immunosuppressed patients with reactivated infection. Serological tests to detect antibody to *T. cruzi* include enzyme-linked immunosorbent assay, immunofluorescence antibody test, and indirect hemagglutination test. In the chronic phase, the infection typically is diagnosed by demonstrating seroreactivity to parasite antigens, taking into account the epidemiologic (and clinical, if applicable) plausibility of *T. cruzi* infection. To date, no one serologic assay is sufficiently sensitive and specific to be relied on alone; typically, at least 2 assays, based on different antigens and principles (assay formats), are used; use of a third assay may be warranted if the results with the other 2 assays are discrepant.

PCR-based methods can be used to directly detect *T. cruzi* DNA in acute cases, including infections caused by exposure to feces from infected triatomine bugs, laboratory accidents, congenital transmission, oral ingestion, and blood transfusions or organ transplants from donors with chronic Chagas disease. PCR is also useful for monitoring immunosuppressed patients to detect reactivation (e.g., after solid-organ transplantation). The sensitivity of PCR has been found to be higher in buffy coat (46.5%) than whole blood (40%). The most commonly used PCR targets are a *T. cruzi* nuclear minisatellite region and *T. cruzi* minicircle DNA from the kinetoplast. These PCR assays are highly sensitive but will amplify other *Trypanosoma* spp.

Antibodies to *T. rangeli* are not detected in *T. cruzi* crude antigens-based serological tests. Infection with both species may be diagnosed by detection of the pertinent trypomastigotes in blood films stained with Giemsa, Field's, Wright-Giemsa, or Wright's stain.

**4. Laboratory capability**—Microscopy services as well as molecular and serological techniques are required. Laboratorians should be trained in the appropriate techniques for detection of parasites and should undergo regular proficiency testing. Specific equipment is required for molecular and serological testing.

**5. Safety requirements**—Clinical specimens should always be collected and handled using universal/standard precautions. *T. cruzi* is a biosafety level 2 organism. Blood specimens should be disposed of as infectious waste.

**6. Nonhuman hosts**—The insect vectors are triatomine bugs (also known as kissing bugs, assassin bugs, cone-nosed bugs, and blood suckers). Infected mammals serve as reservoir hosts for the parasite.

**7. Sample/specimen requirements**—EDTA blood for morphologic and molecular diagnosis. Serum or plasma for serology.

**8. Testing requirements**—Specimens from patients with suspected acute infection, within the first few months of inoculation, can be tested by PCR and blood smears examined morphologically for the parasite. Serology can be performed for a baseline. PCR testing for evidence of acute or reactivated infection and morphological identification of trypanosomes to the species level are available at reference diagnostic laboratories in many countries, including the CDC. Patients with suspected chronic phase Chagas disease (infections acquired more than several months before) can be diagnosed by serologic testing; PCR is not sufficiently sensitive to diagnose chronic Chagas disease.

Trypomastigotes are approximately 15–24 (average 20) μm in length and spindle shaped. Long and broad or short and slender forms may be seen; *T. cruzi* trypomastigotes often curl into a C-shape in the blood film. *T. cruzi* may be further differentiated morphologically from *T. brucei* and *T. rangeli* by its much larger kinetoplast at the anterior end of the trypomastigote and by its less prominent undulating membrane. During the chronic phase of the infection, trypomastigotes are generally not readily detectable by laboratory testing of blood specimens, but amastigotes may be found in a wide range of tissues. Amastigotes of *T. cruzi* are 1.5–4 μm in diameter and morphologically indistinguishable from those of *Leishmania* spp.

Trypomastigotes of *T. rangeli* are 20–100 (average 30) μm in length and spindle shaped; they have a very long, pointed posterior end; a very small kinetoplast, which is situated internally at the posterior end; and a prominent undulating membrane. Trypomastigotes often have a corkscrew appearance in blood films.

**9. Reporting requirements**—Reporting requirements/criteria vary by country and local jurisdiction. Laboratories are responsible for determining whether trypanosomiasis is reportable by laboratories in their respective setting.

**10. Referral network**—*T. cruzi* serology is available in many commercial diagnostic laboratories in the USA, Canada, Mexico, Central America, South America, and elsewhere. PCR is less widely available. In the USA, PCR for *T. cruzi* currently is available at 2 public health laboratories: CDC and Wadsworth Center, NY State Department of Health.

**11. Special considerations**—The transmission of *T. cruzi* via blood transfusion is a recognized risk. Blood-donor screening is conducted in multiple countries (including the USA), but the approaches used vary among countries. Confirmation of the diagnosis by a reference laboratory is encouraged.

[R. S. Bradbury, T. Benedict, H. Rivera]

# TUBERCULOSIS AND OTHER MYCOBACTERIAL DISEASES

| DISEASE | ICD-10 CODE |
|---|---|
| TUBERCULOSIS | ICD-10 A15–A19 |
| DISEASES DUE TO OTHER MYCOBACTERIA | ICD-10 A31 |
| Buruli ulcer (see "Buruli Ulcer") | |
| Leprosy (Hansen's disease; see "Leprosy") | |

## I. TUBERCULOSIS (TB, TB disease)

**1. Clinical features**—There are 2 forms of tuberculosis (TB), latent and active (pulmonary and/or extrapulmonary). Latent TB infection can be established following exposure to an infectious patient expelling aerosolized particles containing viable bacilli. Initial infection generally causes no outward clinical manifestations and is called latent TB. It is characterized by microscopic lesions in the lungs that commonly heal, leaving no residual changes other than occasional small pulmonary or tracheobronchial lymph node calcifications.

Active TB disease can develop following infection and be facilitated by certain risk factors. It can be pulmonary and/or extrapulmonary. Active pulmonary TB may arise from reactivation of a latent focus originating from the initial subclinical infection or from reinfection. Extrapulmonary TB occurs in 15%–30% of cases and may affect any organ or tissue as follows: lymph nodes (33%); pleura (20%); genitourinary tract (5%–10%); bones and joints (5%–10%); meninges (5%); gastrointestinal tract and peritoneum (3.5%); and pericardium (2%–3%).

Cough, fatigue, fever, night sweats, and weight loss are common symptoms associated with active pulmonary TB. In most cases, cough is initially nonproductive and later accompanied by purulent sputum.

Symptoms such as hemoptysis and hoarseness associated with laryngeal TB are sometimes prominent in advanced stages. Chest radiography reveals pulmonary infiltrates and cavitations in the upper segments of the lung lobes. In prolonged disease, fibrotic changes with volume loss are seen.

**2. Causative agents**—*Mycobacterium tuberculosis* complex includes *M. tuberculosis*, *Mycobacterium bovis* (bovine tubercle bacillus, historically an important cause of TB transmitted through unpasteurized milk), *Mycobacterium africanum*, and *Mycobacterium canettii*. The latter 2 are the causes of a small number of infections in Africa. Occasionally, *Mycobacterium microti*, *Mycobacterium caprae*, *Mycobacterium pinnipedii*, *Mycobacterium mungi*, and *Mycobacterium orygis*, rarely isolated members of *M. tuberculosis* complex, produce disease clinically indistinguishable from tuberculosis.

**3. Laboratory diagnosis**—The classification of active pulmonary TB has been traditionally based primarily on the presence or absence of acid-fast bacilli (AFB) in the microscopic examination of the sputum. At least 2 sputum specimens (1 early morning) should be obtained. Specimens should undergo AFB smear microscopy; good quality microscopy of 2 consecutive sputum specimens identifies the vast majority of smear-positive TB patients. Fluorescence microscopy using auramine staining is preferred over Ziehl-Neelsen staining; Kinyoun staining is not recommended.

Since 2010, a molecular cartridge-based method has been recommended by WHO for rapid diagnosis of pulmonary and extrapulmonary TB in adults and children, including in settings where human immunodeficiency virus (HIV) is highly prevalent and where multidrug-resistant TB (MDR-TB) is potentially present. This method also detects rifampin resistance as a proxy of MDR-TB. In all instances, isolation of *M. tuberculosis* on culture confirms diagnosis and permits determination of antimicrobial susceptibility. Persons suspected of having TB disease should have a full diagnostic evaluation, including a chest radiograph. In the absence of bacteriological confirmation (AFB smear microscopy, molecular assay, and/or culture), active disease can be presumed if clinical, histological, or radiological evidence is suggestive of TB and other likely diseases can be ruled out. Diagnosis of TB among HIV-positive persons may be complicated by the tendency to yield negative AFB smears. Current serological tests have no role in diagnosis of active TB.

Extrapulmonary TB is diagnosed by AFB microscopy, molecular assay, culture, and histopathological examination on specimens from the involved sites. Ultrasound, computerized tomography scan, and magnetic resonance imaging facilitate diagnosis.

All TB isolates, especially from previously treated patients, should be submitted for culture and antimicrobial susceptibility testing. Rapid molecular tests such as cartridge-based and line-probe assays result in more rapid diagnosis and treatment of drug-resistant TB.

**4. Laboratory capability**—Diagnostic testing should be aligned and appropriate for the capacity for patient evaluation and treatment in each location. AFB smears may be the only practicable diagnostic test. As clinics become larger and have access to improved diagnostic testing, introduction of rapid diagnostic molecular tests such as line-probe or cartridge-based assays become feasible. In larger municipal or regional laboratories, mycobacterial cultures may be feasible, although many do not have the capacity to perform antimicrobial susceptibility tests. Lastly, laboratories in teaching hospitals and large private hospitals, and national public health laboratories, often have the capacity to provide the full scope of mycobacterial diagnostic testing.

**5. Safety requirements**—The most important biosafety issue for diagnostic testing of specimens that could contain mycobacteria is the potential presence of *M. tuberculosis* complex. Protection of workers from laboratory transmission requires using laboratory universal/standard precautions, good laboratory practices, safety devices, personal protective equipment (PPE), and appropriate decontamination and disposal of biological hazards.

Because the scope and scale of testing varies widely among laboratories, every laboratory should perform a risk assessment and stratification that can be used to guide development of a biosafety program specific for that laboratory. Laboratories can be divided into low-, moderate-, and high-risk categories. Low-risk laboratories such as biosafety level 2 (BSL-2) laboratories typically only manipulate specimens to perform AFB smears with or without use of a molecular assay. Moderate-risk laboratories (BSL-3) process specimens for inoculation onto culture media and may perform direct antimicrobial susceptibility testing. High-risk laboratories (BSL-3) process mycobacterial cultures to identify *M. tuberculosis* complex and may perform indirect antimicrobial susceptibility testing.

**6. Nonhuman hosts**—*M. bovis* causes TB in warm-blooded animals including cattle, deer, and elk and can be transmitted to primates and humans. In the early 20th century, up to 30% of TB cases in Europe were caused by *M. bovis*; these were largely transmitted to humans via inhalation of infectious droplets from infected cattle and consumption of contaminated, unpasteurized dairy products. Some members of the *M. tuberculosis* complex are found primarily in animals including *M. caprae* (goat), *M. pinnipedii* (seal), *M. microti* (vole), *M. orygis* (oryx), and *M. mungi* (mongoose).

**7. Sample/specimen requirements**—Most specimens will be from the respiratory tract, especially expectorated and induced sputum (optimal volume is 5–10 mL), bronchial aspirates, and bronchoalveolar lavages. Other specimen types that are also acceptable for processing for AFB include body fluids such as urine, peritoneal, pleural, synovial, and pericardial, plus tissue biopsies such as lung, liver, and kidney. Fluids, tissues, and lavages (gastric and bronchoalveolar) are much better for AFB recovery than specimens collected on swabs; swab specimens should be discouraged.

Blood collection tubes should contain sodium polyanethol sulfonate (SPS), heparin, or citrate anticoagulants and be transported expeditiously to the laboratory. Ethylenediaminetetraacetic acid (EDTA) tubes should not be used.

**8. Testing requirements**—

1) AFB smear: despite major advances in the diagnosis of mycobacterial infections, microscopic examination for AFB remains a primary tool because it identifies highly infectious AFB smear–positive cases rapidly and inexpensively. Although reported to have more than 80% sensitivity compared with culture for identifying cases of pulmonary TB in some settings, AFB sensitivity has also been reported to be lower and variable in other reports; of note, AFB smear microscopy is of limited utility in paucibacillary disease such

as in pediatric patients, persons living with HIV, and extrapulmonary infections. Also, the specificity of AFB smear microscopy is limited where nontuberculous mycobacterial infections are prevalent since these patients can also present with AFB smear-positive specimens. Nucleic acid amplification test (NAAT): algorithms for testing specimens from patients suspected of having TB should include a nucleic acid amplification test. This is especially important if a diagnosis of TB has not yet been made and the test result would alter patient care or TB control. It is important to note that NAAT should not replace or delay routine microbiologic methods including AFB smear; NAAT are approximately 75% sensitive in AFB smear-negative and TB culture-positive sputum samples.

Due to the slow growth of *M. tuberculosis* complex, molecular techniques are well-suited to not only detect *M. tuberculosis* complex directly from patient specimens but also screen for mutations associated with antimicrobial resistance. Line-probe and cartridge-based assays detect rifampin resistance as rifampin resistance can be a marker for MDR-TB. In addition, line probe assays may detect the more common isoniazid resistance and other antimicrobial resistance (fluoroquinolones, aminoglycosides and cyclic peptides).

2) Processing and growth detection: due to the lengthy incubation times required for growth of most *Mycobacterium* spp., methods should be employed to eliminate nonmycobacterial bacteria and fungi before plating of the specimens. Sterile tissues and body fluids may not need such decontamination; however, sputum, bronchoalveolar lavage, stool, urine, skin, and many other specimens that usually contain contaminating microbes need to be decontaminated to allow for growth of mycobacteria.

   A combination of broth and solid media should be included for inoculation. Broth media is essential to recover *Mycobacterium* spp. in as short an incubation time as possible. There are many types of broth media, many of which are included in automated mycobacterial detection systems; most are based on Middlebrook 7H9 broth. Solid media (egg-based and agar-based) are included to assure recovery of rare strains that may not grow in broth.

3) Identification: commercially available probes for culture confirmation are available for *M. tuberculosis* complex and have increased accuracy and decreased turnaround time relative to conventional biochemical methods. Immunochromatography-based lateral flow assays using monoclonal antibody against the MPB64 protein secreted by the *M. tuberculosis* complex are reported to be a reliable, rapid, and simple tool to identify the *M. tuberculosis* complex and differentiate its members from nontuberculous

mycobacteria in growth-positive solid or liquid cultures. A commercially available line probe assay can differentiate species within the *M. tuberculosis* complex such as *M. tuberculosis*, *M. bovis*, *M. bovis* BCG, and some other mycobacterial species.

4) Antimicrobial susceptibility testing: the determination of antimicrobial resistance in mycobacteria is important for patient treatment and, with *M. tuberculosis* complex, is essential not just for individual patient treatment but for TB control. Antimicrobial susceptibility testing results guide treatment, which is especially vital with the emergence of drug-resistant strains and for estimating prevalence of drug resistance in a community. Phenotypic, culture-based techniques for antimicrobial susceptibility testing rely on isolation of the organism, and although there are some molecular methods available, phenotypic testing must still be performed.

   In the USA, CDC offers a molecular detection of drug resistance (MDDR) service to rapidly identify multidrug-resistant TB. This service utilizes DNA sequencing for detection of mutations most frequently associated with rifampin and isoniazid drug resistance. Additional testing is conducted to identify mutations associated with resistance to the most effective second-line drugs; fluroquinolones, amikacin, kanamycin, and capreomycin.

**9. Reporting requirements**—Report active pulmonary or extrapulmonary TB to local public health authorities when diagnosis is suspected; case reports are obligatory in most countries. Reports should state whether the case is bacteriologically confirmed (AFB smear-positive, culture-positive, or molecular detection [NAAT]), whether diagnosis was based on clinical and/or radiographic findings, and whether the case was previously treated.

**10. Referral network**—For mycobacteriology services to be effective, they must be integrated with systems for clinical care and public health programs; this is in part because they focus primarily on TB and not on other mycobacteria but also because detection of drug resistance is of paramount concern. Rapid test turnaround time also is a critical issue because many patients are from low-resource settings, such as rural areas, and have only limited access to health care facilities.

Since 1994, the TB Supranational Reference Laboratory Network is an important technical resource for laboratory scale-up and capacity development in high-burden TB countries. Center of Excellence is a new category of laboratory specifically designed to recognize well-performing laboratories in large middle-income countries. A designated center primarily works to build in-country laboratory capacity.

In the USA, the submission of initial isolates from culture-confirmed TB patients to the respective public health laboratory for genotyping at the CDC Tuberculosis Genotyping Program is required. The program provides funding and support for universal genotyping with the goal of typing all *M. tuberculosis* complex culture-positive cases in the USA. The methods routinely used include spoligotyping and mycobacterial interspersed repetitive units analysis and, since 2018, whole genome sequencing. This technology can help target public health interventions and identify new drug-resistant TB strains as they emerge.

**11. Special considerations**—The live, attenuated Bacille Calmette-Guérin (BCG) strain of *M. bovis* is used for TB vaccination. Instillation of BCG into the bladder can also be used to treat bladder cancer. However, some individuals treated for bladder cancer can develop infections with *M. bovis* BCG in different organs. Rapid differentiation of *M. bovis* and *M. bovis* BCG diseases, and their differentiation from *M. tuberculosis*, is crucial for optimizing treatment, contact tracing, and additional control measures.

In 2015, FDA cleared a cartridge-based assay to aid physicians in determining if patients with suspected TB can be removed from airborne infection isolation. In a consensus statement by the US National TB Controllers Association and the Association of Public Health Laboratories, it is noted that the process described in the company's statement is not to be used alone to rule out TB. Clinical decisions regarding the need for continued airborne infection isolation should be made in conjunction with other clinical and laboratory data, and not solely on negative cartridge-based test results.

## II. DISEASES DUE TO OTHER MYCOBACTERIA (mycobacterioses, nontuberculous mycobacterial disease, NTM disease)

**1. Clinical features**—Nontuberculous mycobacteria (NTM), comprised of mycobacteria other than *M. tuberculosis* complex organisms, *Mycobacterium leprae* (see "Leprosy"), and *Mycobacterium ulcerans* (see "Buruli ulcer"), are ubiquitous environmental microorganisms that can be recovered from soil, freshwater, and seawater (natural and treated). Clinical syndromes associated with the NTM can be classified broadly as follows:

1) Disseminated disease, often in the presence of severe immunodeficiency such as that determined by HIV/acquired immunodeficiency syndrome, can be caused by *Mycobacterium avium* complex (MAC), *Mycobacterium kansasii*, *Mycobacterium haemophilum*, and *Mycobacterium genavense*. *Mycobacterium abscessus* and *Mycobacterium fortuitum* can infect intravenous catheters and indwelling lines, causing disseminated disease. In the presence of disseminated NTM, symptoms include fever, weight loss, and fatigue. Diagnosis can be obtained through isolation in blood, liver, or bone marrow culture.

2) Pulmonary disease resembling tuberculosis, caused by MAC, *M. kansasii*, *M. abscessus*, *Mycobacterium xenopi*, *Mycobacterium simiae*, and *Mycobacterium malmoense*, should be suspected in cases of prolonged respiratory symptoms, especially in patients with underlying chronic pulmonary disease.
3) Lymphadenitis (primarily cervical) caused by MAC and *M. kansasii*.
4) Skin ulcers caused by *M. fortuitum*, *Mycobacterium chelonae*, *M. abscessus*, and *Mycobacterium marinum*. These infections may appear as nodular or ulcerating; at times, they spread along the lymphatics.
5) Posttraumatic wound infections caused by *M. fortuitum*, *M. chelonae*, *M. abscessus*, *M. marinum*, and MAC.
6) Nosocomial disease such as surgical wound infections and catheter-related infections (bacteremia, peritonitis, postinjection abscesses) caused by *M. fortuitum*, *M. chelonae*, and *M. abscessus*.

Until recently there was no evidence of human-to-human or animal to human transmission of NTM. However, 2 recent findings investigating outbreaks in cystic fibrosis patients by using thorough conventional epidemiologic and state-of-the-art molecular typing investigations such as whole genome sequencing suggest potential transmission of *M. abscessus* subsp. *massiliense* and *M. abscessus* subsp. *abscessus* between these patients. Since NTM may be found in both natural and man-made reservoirs, human infections are suspected to be acquired from these environmental sources. However, the identification of the specific source of infection is usually not possible.

**2. Causative agents**—The NTM are often classified based on their growth characteristics after subculture onto solid media. Some grow rapidly, within 7 days (e.g., *M. abscessus, M. chelonae, M. fortuitum, M. peregrinum*). Others grow more slowly, requiring more than 7 days to form visible colonies (e.g., MAC, *M. kansasii*, *M. marinum*). From 41 valid species in 1980, currently the genus *Mycobacterium* encompasses almost 200 recognized species and 14 subspecies.

**3. Laboratory diagnosis**—In general, specimens for NTM are processed for AFB smear and culture in the laboratory the same way as for *M. tuberculosis* complex with the exception of specimens collected from cystic fibrosis patients with a history of *Pseudomonas* infections. A single isolation from sputum or gastric washings can occur in the absence of signs or symptoms of clinical disease. Multiple isolations of NTM from respiratory specimens, in the absence of illness or other specific pathology, may be evidence of colonization (e.g., with *Mycobacterium gordonae*), with no clinical significance. A single positive culture from a wound or tissue is generally considered diagnostic. In general, the diagnosis of disease requiring treatment is based on repeated isolations of many colonies from symptomatic patients with progressive illness. Where human infections with NTM are prevalent, cross-reactions may interfere with the interpretation of tuberculin skin testing for *M. tuberculosis* complex infection, but less so if interferon-gamma release assays are used.

**4. Laboratory capability**—Laboratories testing for TB often isolate NTM as part of their routine testing algorithm. Once NTM organisms have been isolated and identified, their clinical significance needs to be determined. Accurate identification and antimicrobial susceptibility of NTM may be beyond the scope of laboratories focusing on TB only.

**5. Safety requirements**—The most important biosafety issue for diagnostic testing of specimens that could contain mycobacteria is that of *M. tuberculosis* complex. Protection of workers from laboratory transmission requires using universal/standard precautions, good laboratory practices, safety devices, PPE, and appropriate decontamination and disposal of biological hazards.

Because the scope and scale of testing varies widely among laboratories, every laboratory should perform a risk assessment and stratification that can be used to guide development of a biosafety program for that laboratory. Laboratories can be divided into low-, moderate-, and high-risk categories. Low-risk laboratories (BLS-2) typically only manipulate specimens to perform AFB smears with or without use of a molecular assay. Moderate-risk laboratories (BSL-3) process specimens for inoculation onto culture media and may perform direct *M. tuberculosis* complex antimicrobial susceptibility testing. High-risk laboratories (BSL-3) process mycobacterial cultures to identify *M. tuberculosis* complex and may perform indirect antimicrobial susceptibility testing. Once TB has been ruled out, NTM isolates are considered BSL-2 organisms.

**6. Nonhuman hosts**—Environmental sources (i.e., water and soil) are the reservoir for most human infections caused by MAC, which is also present in tap water. Water is also the likely source of infection for numerous other NTM species including *M. marinum* (salt and fresh water, fish tanks and swimming pools), *M. kansasii*, nosocomial outbreaks or pseudo-outbreaks due to rapidly growing mycobacteria (including tap water and ice), *M. xenopi*, and *M. simiae*. *M. xenopi* is an obligate thermophile that requires temperatures of 28°C or above to grow and has been recovered almost exclusively from hot water and hot water taps within hospitals. Since 2013, more than 100 cases of *Mycobacterium chimaera* prosthetic valve endocarditis and disseminated disease were reported in Europe and the USA, linked to contaminated heater–cooler units used during cardiac surgery. *M. genavense* has not been recovered from soil or water, but it has been recovered from a dog and a variety of pet birds including psittacine birds.

Much less is known about the environmental epidemiology and sources of infection for most of the other NTM.

**7. Sample/specimen requirements**—Most specimens will be from the respiratory tract, especially expectorated and induced sputum (optimal volume is 5–10 mL), bronchial aspirates, and bronchoalveolar lavages. Other specimen types that are also acceptable for processing for AFB include body fluids such as urine, peritoneal, pleural, synovial and pericardial; plus tissue biopsies including those from lung, liver, lymph nodes, and skin. Fluids, tissues, and lavages (gastric and bronchoalveolar) are much better for AFB recovery than specimens collected on swabs; swab specimens should be discouraged.

Blood collection tubes should contain SPS, heparin, or citrate anticoagulants and be transported expeditiously to the laboratory. EDTA tubes should not be used.

**8. Testing requirements**—Methods used for AFB smear and growth detection of *M. tuberculosis* are acceptable for NTM; for further information see TB section earlier in this chapter. Some NTM have a different temperature incubation requirement or require supplements. Examples include *M haemophilum*, a fastidious mycobacterium with an optimal growth temperature of 28°C–30°C that grows better on solid medium and requires hemin or hemoglobin as an iron source. *M. genavense* is a fastidious, slowly growing mycobacterium that shows a better recovery in liquid medium supplemented with mycobactin J, especially at an acidic pH (pH 5.5). *M. marinum* is a photochromogenic, slowly growing (8–12 days) organism that optimally grows between 30°C–33°C.

1) Identification: for frequently encountered NTM species, there are several commercially available assays for identification including DNA probes, line probes, high-performance liquid chromatography, and most recently matrix-assisted laser desorption/ionization time-of-flight. The gold standard, however, is considered sequencing. Biochemicals are no longer sufficient to identify NTM accurately.
2) Antimicrobial susceptibility testing: the role and relevance of in vitro antimicrobial susceptibility testing of NTM to guide the treatment and clinical management of patients with NTM disease is under continuous debate. The basis of this debate is that, in contrast with *M. tuberculosis* complex, clinical response to antituberculosis drugs or antibiotics has been shown to correlate only with some compounds and only in some NTM (e.g., MAC and macrolides and amikacin, or *M. kansasii* and rifampin), whereas similar correlation for several other clinically significant NTM (e.g., *M. abscessus*) were not established. On the other hand, most clinically significant NTM isolates already show intrinsic resistance.

Additionally, determination of antimicrobial susceptibility testing in NTM can be method-and species-dependent.

**9. Reporting requirements**—NTM diseases are usually not mandatory to report since they are not generally communicable; however, reporting is required in a few US states. In 2017, the US Council of State and Territorial Epidemiologists developed a Standardized Case Definition for Extrapulmonary Nontuberculous Mycobacteria Infections. Further information is available at: https://c.ymcdn.com/sites/www.cste.org/resource/resmgr/2017PS/2017PSFinal/17-ID-07.pdf

**10. Referral network**—For final identification (including subspeciation) and antimicrobial susceptibility testing, laboratories often rely on expert reference NTM laboratories. Isolates from suspected NTM outbreaks are best handled by expert reference NTM laboratories.

**11. Special considerations**—There are geographic differences in rates of isolation for certain mycobacteria, such as *M. xenopi* in northern countries, including Europe and Canada.

In a recent study in Ontario, Canada, of pulmonary NTM disease, the 5-year prevalence increased from 29.3 cases per 100,000 persons in 1998–2002 to 41.3 per 100,000 in 2006–2010. A similar study in the USA among adults 65 years or older found that from 1997–2007 the annual incidence significantly increased from 20–47 cases per 100,000 persons, or 8.2% per year. Women were 1.4 times more likely to be diagnosed with pulmonary NTM than men. Relative to whites, Asians/Pacific Islanders were twice as likely to be infected, whereas blacks were half as likely.

For further information, see:

- http://www.who.int/tb/features_archive/policy_statement.pdf
- http://apps.who.int/iris/bitstream/10665/44586/1/9789241501545_eng.pdf
- https://www.cdc.gov/biosafety/publications/bmbl5
- http://www.who.int/tb/areas-of-work/laboratory/srl-network/en
- https://www.cdc.gov/tb/programs/genotyping/default.htm
- https://www.aphl.org/programs/infectious_disease/tuberculosis/Documents/NTCA_APHL_GeneXpert%20Consensus%20Statement_Final.pdf
- https://clsi.org/standards/products/microbiology/documents/m24
- http://www.bacterio.net/mycobacterium.html

## Bibliography

Clinical and Laboratory Standards Institute. *M24: Susceptibility Testing of Mycobacteria, Nocardiae, and Other Aerobic Actinomycetes*, 3rd ed. Wayne, PA; 2018.

Forbes BA, Hall GS, Miller MB, et al. Practice guidelines for clinical microbiology laboratories: mycobacteria. *Clin Microbiol Rev*. 2018;31(2):e00038-17.

[M. Salfinger]

# TULAREMIA

(rabbit fever, deerfly fever, Ohara's disease, Francis disease)

| DISEASE | ICD-10 CODE |
|---|---|
| TULAREMIA | ICD-10 A21 |

**1. Clinical features**—A bacterial zoonotic infection that causes 1 of 6 clinical syndromes depending on the site of inoculation and virulence of the infecting organism. The most common syndrome is ulceroglandular tularemia, characterized by a skin ulcer and regional lymphadenopathy. Glandular tularemia is similar but lacks an obvious skin ulcer. Oropharyngeal tularemia presents with painful pharyngitis (with or without ulceration) and marked cervical lymphadenopathy, which may be unilateral. Pneumonic tularemia may be primary following inhalation of the organism, or secondary due to hematogenous spread to the lungs from other parts of the body. Although not readily distinguished from other forms of community-acquired pneumonia, pneumonic tularemia is often accompanied by a transudative pleural effusion that yields the organism if cultured. Purulent conjunctivitis, punctate palpebral ulcers, and periauricular lymphadenopathy characterize oculoglandular tularemia. The sixth syndrome, typhoidal tularemia, refers to patients who lack localizing symptoms. Sudden high fever, chills, fatigue, general body aches, headache, and nausea accompany all forms of tularemia. Pneumonic tularemia can be life threatening; however, the overall case fatality is less than 5% with proper treatment. Differential diagnosis includes anthrax, brucellosis, plague, staphylococcal and streptococcal infections, cat scratch fever, and tuberculosis.

**2. Causative agents**—*Francisella tularensis* is a highly infectious, small, faintly staining, pleomorphic Gram-negative coccobacillus. The majority of human infections are caused by 2 subspecies that differ in distribution and virulence: *F. tularensis* subsp. *tularensis* (Jellison type A, generally the more virulent) and *F. tularensis* subsp. *holarctica* (Jellison type B). A third subspecies, *F. tularensis* subsp. *mediasiatica*, has been isolated from animals in central Asia but has not been linked to human illness. Related species *Francisella novicida*, *Francisella philomiragia*, and *Francisella hispaniensis* are rare causes of human illness.

**3. Laboratory diagnosis**—The diagnosis of tularemia is generally established serologically by demonstrating a 4-fold rise in specific antibody titers between acute and convalescent sera using tube or microagglutination. Cross-reactions with *Brucella* spp. have been observed when using tube agglutination. In some instances, a sufficiently high titer in a single specimen is considered positive. Enzyme-linked immunosorbent assay (ELISA) assays for tularemia have also been used. Culture can provide a conclusive diagnosis but must be attempted only with appropriate biosafety conditions. Appropriate specimens include swabs or scrapping of skin lesions, lymph node aspirates or biopsies, pharyngeal swabs, sputum, bronchial/tracheal washings, sputum, or pleural fluid, depending on the form of illness. Blood cultures should also be collected, although yield is low.

When tularemia is suspected, it should be communicated to laboratory personnel beforehand because of the need to select the most appropriate specimens and the requirement for using special isolation procedures. A presumptive diagnosis of tularemia may be made through the testing of suspected isolates using direct fluorescent antibody, immunohistochemical staining, or polymerase chain reaction (PCR) assays. In some jurisdictions *F. tularensis* has been identified as a select agent, and therefore only registered laboratories are allowed to work with the organism.

**4. Laboratory capability**—For *F. tularensis* subsp. tularensis (type A), specialist biosafety level 3 (BSL-3) laboratories are required for isolation and growth of the organism. *F. tularensis* subsp. *holartica* (type B) and other *Francisella* spp. can be handled in BSL-2 laboratories. Since it may not always be clear what subspecies of *Francisella* one is working with, it is advisable to use a higher level of containment pending speciation (see Safety Requirements section in this chapter).

**5. Safety requirements**—*F. tularensis* subsp. *tularensis* (type A) is 1 of the most infectious organisms known with an extremely low infectious dose for humans (estimated at 10 organisms for subcutaneous injection and 25 organisms for aerosol exposure). For this reason, extreme care must be taken when handling samples from suspected tularemia cases, and all manipulations of samples either known to contain *F. tularensis* type A, or where the index of suspicion is very high, should be handled inside a microbiological safety cabinet in a BSL-3 laboratory. Confirmation of suspected *F. tularensis* isolates (especially type A) should only be conducted in specialized laboratories with trained personnel.

**6. Nonhuman hosts**—Tularemia is an arthropod-borne disease that is maintained in arthropod-mammalian-arthropod cycles. Humans are dead-end hosts and acquire infection either through the bite of an infected arthropod or by contact with infected animals. The main mammalian hosts of tularemia are rabbits, hares, ground squirrels, and prairie dogs for *F. tularensis* type A and beavers, muskrats, lemmings, voles, and mice for *F. tularensis* type B.

**7. Sample/specimen requirements**—For culture, samples should ideally be taken before antibiotic therapy is given. The best samples for culture and PCR include whole blood, respiratory secretions, swabs from lesions, aspirates from lymph nodes or lesions, and tissue biopsies particularly from lymph nodes and postmortem samples. Ideally, samples must be transported to the laboratory within 24 hours and preferably within 2 hours and transported at ambient temperature. If transport is likely to take longer than 24 hours, the sample should be chilled to 4°C. For serology, paired sera taken a few weeks apart are the best samples, although single serum and plasma samples can be used for diagnosis. Sera can be frozen if there is likely to be a delay of more than 24 hours in transporting the samples to the laboratory.

**8. Testing requirements**—Tularemia can be detected using direct pathogen detection methods (culture, PCR, antigen capture immunoassays) or by using serology. Serology is the most commonly used method for diagnosis.

1) Culture: while culture provides a definitive diagnosis for tularemia, it is not recommended for routine microbiology laboratories due to the extreme hazard for laboratory workers. If tularemia is strongly suspected, the specimens should ideally be sent to specialist laboratories for culture. *F. tularensis* grows on a number of cysteine/cystine supplemented agars including enriched chocolate agar, cystine heart agar with 9% chocolatized blood (CHAB), thyoglycollate-glucose blood agar, buffered charcoal yeast extract, Thayer-Martin agar (a Mueller-Hinton agar with 5% chocolate sheep blood and antibiotics), and GC agar II with 1% haemoglobin and 1% IsoVitale X. When grown on CHAB media, *F. tularensis* presents as green, opalescent shiny, raised colonies after 24–48 hours incubation. *F. tularensis* can be isolated from blood cultures from patients with septicaemia. For samples where there is likely to be a mixed flora, for example respiratory samples, isolation on CHAB with added antibiotics (CHAB-A) is recommended.
2) Molecular methods: a number of PCR assays have been described in the literature. Conventional PCR assays targeting the FopA and Tul4 genes for outer surface proteins have been described. Real-time PCR assays including multiplex assays to detect the different subtypes of *F. tularensis* have been developed targeting Tul4, *23kDa*, IS*Ftu2* element, and 16S RNA. Multitarget assays capable of differentiating between pathogenic *F. tularensis* (Types A and B) and *F. philomiragia* have been described. Real time assays are generally more sensitive and specific than conventional PCR assays. Genetic typing systems, such as multiple-locus variable number tandem repeat analysis, canonical single polymorphisms, and pulsed-field gel electrophoresis typing can be used to

characterise outbreak strains and for epidemiological tracking. 16S RNA sequencing can detect *F. tularensis* in pure or mixed cultures, the latter when using *Francisella*-specific 16S rRNA primers.

3) Serology: the most common methods for serology include microagglutination, ELISA, and Western blotting. Antibodies first appear 2–3 weeks after infection and can last for years following recovery. In general, a rise in titer between acute and convalescent stages is indicative for tularemia infection. Microagglutination is easy to perform and cheap but can lack sensitivity (particularly early in disease when antibody titres are low) and specificity. The most commonly performed assays are indirect ELISAs, which are considered to be sensitive. A number of commercial assays are available (ELISAs and immunochromatic assays) with reported good performance regarding sensitivity, specificity, and positive predictive value. Proteome-based microarrays are in development but are not yet widely available, and little is known of their sensitivity and specificity.
4) Other diagnostic methods: matrix-assisted laser desorption/ionization time-of-flight mass spectrometry (MALDI-TOF MS) can be used to detect and speciate *F. tularensis* following cultivation. However, MALDI-TOF MS is only likely to be available in large, well-funded specialist microbiology laboratories. While MALDI-TOF MS can be rapid (10–30 minutes to result) and does not need a high level of staff training, culture is still required, which could delay the time to a diagnostic result by 24–48 hours after receipt of the sample at the laboratory.

**9. Reporting requirements**—Tularemia can be a national notifiable disease in some countries such as the USA and the UK. Local guidelines for reporting confirmed tularemia cases should be followed. Following positive diagnosis, public health should be notified according to local procedures. It is important that an investigation is performed to ensure that there was not exposure of laboratory staff to the pathogen (particularly in a laboratory that may have subsequently sent it to a reference laboratory where it was finally identified).

**10. Referral network**—The WHO Collaborating Centre for Bacterial Vector-Borne Diseases, which include tularemia, is the CDC Bacterial Diseases Branch, Division of Vector Borne Infectious Diseases, Fort Collins, CO. Each country may have separate guidelines for referral of specimens, cultures, and reported cases, and these should be referred to individually.

**11. Special considerations**—*F. tularensis* is considered to be a potential biothreat agent and is listed in the Select Agents and Toxins,

7 CFR Part 331, 9 CFR Part 121, and 42 CFR Part 73 (http://www.selectagents.gov). In the USA, confirmed isolates of select agents identified in a clinical or diagnostic laboratory must be reported. Each country may have specific registration requirements for laboratories working with *F. tularensis* for human or animal pathogen regulations, and these should be checked. *F. tularensis* is on the World Organisation for Animal Health-listed notifiable disease.

[J. Duggan]

# TYPHOID FEVER AND PARATYPHOID FEVERS

| DISEASE | ICD-10 CODE |
|---|---|
| TYPHOID FEVER | ICD-10 A01.0 |
| PARATYPHOID FEVER | ICD-10 A01.1–A01.4 |

**1. Clinical features**—Typhoid fever is a systemic human disease transmitted by the fecal-oral route that continues to be a significant clinical and public health problem in some low-middle-income countries, with children disproportionately affected. Patients generally present with a pattern of intermittent fevers, which become more persistent over the first few days of infection. Close monitoring of the patient's temperature may allow detection of this incremental progression of fever. It is common to have fever (or rigors) and headaches; other reported symptoms include malaise, anorexia, relative bradycardia, splenomegaly, nausea, vomiting, abdominal cramps, nonproductive cough, and rose spots (visible on the trunk of ~25% of Caucasian patients). Interestingly, patients may experience diarrhea (more common in children or those with human immunodeficiency virus [HIV]) or constipation (more common in adults). Peyer patches present in the ileum can become ulcerative with hemorrhage or perforation of the intestine. Mild disease is frequently seen in endemic areas and patients may simply present with gastroenteritis. Given this range of clinical presentations, it is important to consider patients of having typhoid if they have specific risk factors associated with travel to, or residence in, an endemic country, a history of contact with a known case; or ingestion of suspected food products. The incubation period for typhoid is generally longer than that seen for cases of salmonellosis and is usually 7–14 days ranging from 3–60 days. The incubation period for paratyphoid ranges from 1–10 days. Family contacts may be transient or permanent carriers. A carrier state may follow acute illness or mild or even subclinical infections. In most parts of the world, short-term fecal carriers are more common than urinary carriers. The chronic carrier state is most common (2%–5%) among persons infected during middle age, especially women; carriers frequently have biliary tract abnormalities including gallstones, with *Salmonella* Typhi located in the gallbladder.

**2. Causative agents**—The bacterium causing typhoid fever is *Salmonella enterica* subsp. *enterica* serovar Typhi (commonly *S.* Typhi); and for paratyphoid fever, *Salmonella enterica* subsp. *enterica* serovar Paratyphi A, Paratyphi B, and Paratyphi C (commonly *S.* Paratyphi A, *S.* Paratyphi B, and *S.* Paratyphi C).

**3. Laboratory diagnosis**—In cases with diarrhea or septicemia, *Salmonella* may be isolated from feces and frequently via blood cultures on enteric media during acute stages of illness. *Salmonella* are able to grow in the presence of sodium selenite, which is inhibitory to enterococci and *Escherichia coli*, and the diagnostic yield can be improved by using this fluid enrichment if carried out at low oxygen tension in Selenite F medium. It is important to carefully control the quality of this medium as the level of inhibition may vary from batch to batch. Stool culture may be negative in up to half of cases, in particular, if samples are collected in the first week of infection. The positivity rate can be increased if samples are collected from the second week of illness. Blood culture is positive in approximately 75% of cases, and an increased positivity rate can be obtained by culturing bone marrow samples even if cases have commenced antimicrobial therapy. *S.* Typhi can also be cultured from urine, which can lead to confusion if the patient has a suspected urinary tract infection. The Widal test, which was established in the 1950s, relies on infected patients producing detectable serum antibodies to *S.* Typhi and *S.* Paratyphi O and H antigens. Although this test is relatively easy to carry out, interpretation of the result is far more challenging. It requires the detection of a rise in titer in paired acute and convalescent samples combined with an understanding of the limitations of the test, the patient's country of residence, vaccination, travel, and clinical history. It should be noted that some patients will have high H antibody titers due to historical infection or vaccination, and infection with other Salmonella serovars can give positive results due to cross-reactivity. It may be possible to accommodate for this by the addition of a nonspecific *Salmonella* antigen in the testing panel. Finally, it should be noted that some patients with typhoid do not produce a detectable rise in titer in the presence of infection.

Recently rapid diagnostic testing using real-time polymerase chain reaction (PCR) with deoxyribonucleic acid (DNA) extracts from fecal samples, along with blood specimens, have been reported with high specificity and sensitivity.

**4. Laboratory capability**—A contained, purpose-built, microbiological facility with the capacity to autoclave microbiological waste is required to handle this pathogen. Staff should be trained and shown to be competent to handle potentially biosafety level 3 (BSL-3) hazardous biological agents and should be able to carry out a range of molecular and phenotypic techniques.

**5. Safety requirements**—Employers have a responsibility to protect their workers from the risks related to exposure to hazardous biological agents.[1] *S.* Typhi, *S.* Paratyphi A, B, and C should be handled in either a BSL-2 or BSL-3 laboratory, depending on the country-specific regulations and the kind of risk that is created by the specific procedures being used. All laboratories must operate under the biosafety requirements of their respective jurisdictions and countries. *Salmonella* transmission is via the fecal–oral route, and therefore gloves should be worn when handling clinical samples (or cultures). The importance of good hand washing techniques must be emphasized to laboratory staff. In addition to gloves, other personal protective equipment should be worn including laboratory coat and laboratory safety glasses. Finally, it is recommended to use a class I or class II biosafety cabinet when handling this pathogen, particularly where there is a risk of aerosol production.

**6. Nonhuman hosts**—Humans are the key reservoir for both typhoid and paratyphoid; rarely, domestic animals for paratyphoid. Transmission may occur from ingestion of food and water contaminated by feces and urine of patients and carriers. Important vehicles in some countries include shellfish (particularly oysters) from sewage-contaminated beds, raw fruit, vegetables fertilized by night soil and eaten raw, contaminated milk/milk products (usually through hands of carriers), and missed cases. Flies may contaminate foods in which the organism then multiplies to infective doses (those are lower for typhoid than for paratyphoid bacteria). Epidemiological data suggest that, while waterborne transmission of *S.* Typhi usually involves small inocula, foodborne transmission is associated with large inocula and high attack rates over short periods.

**7. Sample/specimen requirements**—A blood culture is the main sample of choice for acute infections. Human fecal samples can also be used for diagnosis and are useful for determining carriage state and fecal clearance. Bacterial recovery will be improved if samples are taken before any antibiotic treatment is given. Human fecal samples should be placed into appropriate sterile containers and labeled with patient details (to ensure sample integrity). Cary-Blair, Amies, and Stuart transport media may be used to support the transport of fecal species for isolation of *Salmonella*. UN stipulates that *S.* Typhi and *S.* Paratyphi culture is a category A (UN 2814) infectious substance, which is an infectious substance in a form capable of causing permanent disability or life-threatening or fatal disease in otherwise healthy humans or animals when exposure to the substance occurs.[2]

**8. Testing requirements**—Testing facilities must adhere to the quality standards set out to them by their accreditation body, and diagnostic laboratories must follow the manufacturer's instructions for any commercial and noncommercial assay being performed. Once a clinical sample has arrived at the testing facility, patient identifiers on the request form and sample container should be checked. Ideally samples will be tested on arrival; if this is not possible, fecal samples can be stored at refrigerated temperatures (between 4°C–8°C) to prevent overgrowing of other organisms. A blood culture set (1 aerobic and 1 anaerobic bottle), collected early after onset of symptoms, should be incubated as soon as possible after collection. Primary test involves culture methods: plating the sample on blood and selective agar (MacConkey, xylose lysine deoxycholate) to isolate pure colonies of *Salmonella*, followed by serology (agglutination test for *Salmonella*) to detect the antigenic structure of each of 2,600 known serovars. Biochemical tests (e.g., urease, oxidase, indole) for confirmation can be carried out.

**9. Reporting requirements**—Infections with *S.* Typhi, *S.* Paratyphi A, B, and C are notifiable in most countries, and it is important to consider the presence of this pathogen and provide appropriate public health advice, control, and surveillance of these infections.

**10. Referral network**—It is recommended to send pure isolates to the reference facilities for typing and characterization. If this is not possible, some facilities will offer PCR testing on fecal DNA extracts and primary isolation of *S.* Typhi and *S.* Paratyphi from stool samples. This would usually be carried out when other tests have ruled out the presence of another pathogen. Rapid molecular methods have also recently been used for identification and sub-typing (discrimination) for isolates from clinical samples. They include pulsed field gel electrophoresis, multiple-locus variable number tandem repeat analysis, multilocus sequence typing (MLST), and single nucleotide polymorphism (SNP) assays using whole genome sequencing (WGS). However, some of these methods remain accessible to reference laboratories only and are difficult to implement for routine bacterial identification in a clinical laboratory.

In addition to microbiological and serological identification, molecular methods such as MLST (based on sequencing analysis of 7 housekeeping genes located on the chromosome) have been used for identification and classification of *Salmonella,* and newer WGS methods such as high resolution SNP typing have been used for outbreak detection and surveillance. Full characterization for public health surveillance and typing can be carried out using a whole-genome sequencing-based methodology.

**11. Special considerations**—Worldwide estimates suggest that there are approximately 21 million cases and 220,000–600,000 typhoid-related deaths annually, predominately in children of school-age or younger, with the highest burden of disease in less economically developed countries. It has been estimated that 90% of deaths occur in Asia, and while it is largely an endemic disease, outbreaks of typhoid will occur periodically in nonendemic countries. Infection with multidrug-resistant strains of *S.* Typhi, resistant to chloramphenicol, ampicillin, and co-trimoxazole is associated with more severe illness and a higher rate of complications and death. Immunization is advised for international travellers to typhoid-endemic areas, especially if travel is likely to involve exposure to unsafe food and water or close contact in rural areas to indigenous populations. Infants and young children are a significant risk group for infection, with malnourished children living in developing countries particularly at risk of infection. Other groups to consider are HIV-infected persons and international travellers to developing countries. In endemic countries a combined program should be implemented to control enteric fever, including making improvements to water quality and sanitation, sewage disposal, improving access to diagnosis and treatment, ensuring that training is delivered to health care professionals, active surveillance programs (particularly for preschool and school-aged children), and health education for all at-risk populations. These control measures should be combined with a targeted vaccination program. Two typhoid vaccines are currently recommended by WHO for use.[3] One is an injectable polysaccharide vaccine based on purified Vi antigen (Vi-PS) for people aged 2 years and older, and the other is in capsule form and is a live-attenuated oral Ty21a vaccine suitable for those older than 5 years. WHO recommended use of these new vaccines in 1999 for school-aged children in areas with high incidence and/or antibiotic resistance to control endemic disease and also for the control of outbreaks. As typhoid incidence varies considerably within and between countries, control measures can focus on high-risk populations to provide the maximum benefit to the health of the affected communities. Other Vi polysaccharide-protein conjugate vaccines are nationally licensed or under development, and these are expected to be available in the future for infant immunisation. Reduced access to clean water supplies and sewage disposal will promote the transmission of enteric fever. Displaced communities may have limited availability to food, shelter, and health care, and the presence of any active typhoid cases or carriers within these conditions will allow for the rapid spread of disease. It is essential to rapidly provide safe drinking water and sewage removal (sanitation). A directed immunization program to support these other public health measures may be helpful for defined groups (school children, prisoners, health care staff, and international relief personnel).

## References


1. EUR-Lex. Directive 2000/54/EC of the European Parliament and of the Council of 18 September 2000. Available at: https://eur-lex.europa.eu/legal-content/EN/ALL/?uri=CELEX%3A32000L0054. Accessed February 15, 2019.
2. International Air Transport Association. Dangerous goods regulations: division 6.2—infectious substances. 2017. Available at: https://www.iata.org/whatwedo/cargo/dgr/Documents/infectious-substance-classification-DGR56-en.pdf. Accessed April 2, 2019.
3. World Health Organization. Typhoid vaccines: WHO position paper. February 8, 2008. Available at: https://www.who.int/wer/2008/wer8306.pdf?ua=1. Accessed April 5, 2019.


[D. Ready, S. Nair]

# TYPHUS

| DISEASE | ICD-10 CODE |
|---|---|
| EPIDEMIC LOUSE-BORNE TYPHUS FEVER | ICD-10 A75 |
| BRILL-ZINSSER DISEASE | ICD-10 A75.1 |
| ENDEMIC FLEA-BORNE TYPHUS FEVER | ICD-10 A75.2 |
| SCRUB TYPHUS | ICD-10 A75.3 |
| Queensland tick typhus (see "Rickettsioses") | |

## I. EPIDEMIC LOUSE-BORNE TYPHUS (louse-borne typhus, typhus exanthematicus, classical typhus fever)

**1. Clinical features**—A rickettsial disease with variable onset; often with sudden onset of headache, chills, malaise, fever, and general pains. A macular eruption appears on the fifth or sixth day, initially on the upper trunk, followed by spread to the entire body, but usually not to the face, palms or soles. The eruption is often difficult to observe on patients with darkly pigmented skin and is absent in up to 40% of patients. Cough and tachypnea may be present, and neurological signs are common, including confusion, drowsiness, coma, seizures, and hearing loss. The case-fatality rate increases with age and varies from 10%–40% in the absence of treatment. Less severe infections may occur without eruption, especially in children. The disease can recrudesce years after the primary attack as Brill-Zinsser disease; this form of disease is typically less severe, has fewer complications, and has a lower case-fatality rate.

**2. Causative agents**—*Rickettsia prowazekii*.

**3. Laboratory diagnosis**—Moderate thrombocytopenia and elevated hepatic transaminase levels are common and may aid in making a diagnosis. Laboratory confirmation of a diagnosis typically occurs late in the disease process and is therefore not useful for making initial treatment decisions. The indirect immunofluorescence assay (IFA) is the most accurate serological method for laboratory confirmation and requires a 4-fold increase in antibody titers when comparing a patient's acute and convalescent sera. An acute serum sample should be collected during the first week of symptoms and a convalescent serum sample obtained 3–4 weeks after convalescence. Antibody tests usually become positive in the second to third week of illness. Therefore, the primary sample taken in the acute stage of illness is used to obtain a baseline titer for comparison with the convalescent sample. A negative acute result does not rule out active infection, nor does a positive acute result confirm the diagnosis. Because antigens of *R. prowazekii* are cross-reactive with those of *Rickettsia typhi*, the agent of flea-borne typhus, serologic tests cannot discriminate between louse-borne and flea-borne typhus unless the sera are differentially absorbed with the respective rickettsial antigen prior to testing by IFA (i.e., a cross-adsorption assay). Other diagnostic methods include enzyme immunoassays, complement fixation, polymerase chain reaction (PCR), and immunohistochemistry (IHC) staining of tissues. In many regions of the world, the Weil-Felix agglutination reaction is a commonly used and widely available assay but lacks sensitivity and specificity and is not currently recommended as a confirmatory method for any rickettsial disease. Skin biopsy samples of rash sites can be tested by IHC or PCR, but only PCR and sequence analysis provide definitive agent identification. Sending lice to a reference laboratory for PCR testing may help detect an outbreak.

4. **Laboratory capability**—Routine diagnostic procedures, including processing of clinical specimens for serological, IHC, and PCR assays, can occur in biosafety level-2 (BSL-2) laboratories equipped with a class II biological safety cabinet (BSC). BSL-3 practices, containment equipment, and facilities should be used for all propagative techniques, including inoculation, incubation, and harvesting of infected cell cultures or embryonated chicken eggs, and all aerosol-generating procedures involving concentrates of live organisms, to include sonicating, vortexing, blending, or centrifuging. When evaluating human samples for clinical purposes, tests should occur in a Clinical Laboratory Improvement Amendments (CLIA)-certified laboratory that routinely performs proficiency testing of established techniques and competency assessments of laboratory personnel. Facilities should be equipped with a validated method for decontaminating all laboratory waste such as autoclaving or chemical disinfection. Animal BSL-3 (ABSL-3) facilities and practices are required if laboratory animals are used for diagnostic procedures.

5. **Safety requirements**—Laboratory-acquired infections with *R. prowazekii* have been described, and personal protective equipment (PPE) that includes goggles or safety glasses and disposable gloves and gowns is recommended for all manipulations of clinical specimens. Consistent adherence to universal/standard precautions is required. Aliquoting blood or serum samples, initial inactivation of materials for deoxyribonucleic acid (DNA) extraction, and inoculation and subsequent manipulation of cell cultures should occur in a class II BSC. All equipment that could produce infective aerosols should be fitted with aerosol-resistant lids and must be contained in spaces that exhaust air through high-efficiency particulate air filtration or other equivalent technology. Applicable local, state, or national regulations could require enhanced environmental and personal protection. Prophylactic antibiotic treatment following a potential exposure is discouraged in the absence of clinically compatible signs and symptoms and could only delay onset of disease. No vaccine is currently available for louse-borne typhus.

6. **Nonhuman hosts**—The human body louse, *Pediculus humanus corporis,* is the vector of epidemic typhus, and transmission occurs by

contamination of bite sites, conjunctivae, or mucous membranes with the feces or crushed bodies of infectious lice. Lice infected with *R. prowazekii* die within 2 weeks from extensive multiplication of bacteria in the midgut epithelium. Consequently, humans represent the reservoir for epidemic louse-borne typhus and are responsible for maintaining *R. prowazekii* during inter-epidemic periods. The only other well-documented extra-human host of *R. prowazekii* is the southern flying squirrel, *Glaucomys volans,* which occurs throughout most of the eastern USA. Sporadic cases of classical typhus fever have been identified in a small number of persons across the recognized range of *G. volans*, possibly following inhalation of aerosolized, infectious ectoparasite feces. *R. prowazekii* is isolated rarely from other sources, including livestock and various species of hard ticks in North Africa, but a definite epizootiological role for these associations has not been established.

**7. Sample/specimen requirements**—Antibodies reactive with *R. prowazekii* are not generally detectable until 7–10 days of infection, and most serological tests are typically insensitive during the first week of the illness. Paired serum samples, comprising a specimen collected during the acute stage of the illness and a second sample collected 2–4 weeks after convalescence, should be tested in tandem. Whole blood anticoagulated in citrated, heparinized, or ethylenediaminetetraacetic acid-treated tubes are standard specimens for molecular assays and cell culture isolation. A minimum of 1 mL is desirable, but larger volumes (3–5 mL) are generally preferred. A cutaneous punch biopsy specimen (≥ 3 mm in diameter) obtained from a rash lesion represents another important sample for these analyses and for IHC staining. Molecular and cell culture assays are most sensitive during the first week of illness and before the initiation of specific antibiotic therapy. Sensitivity of molecular detection generally diminishes within 1 week of sample collection in refrigerated specimens. When transporting specimens to a referral laboratory, refrigerate at 4°C and attempt overnight delivery.

**8. Testing requirements**—Cross-reactions can occur between antigens of *R. prowazekii* and *R. typhi*, and cross-adsorption assays are required to determine conclusively the specific agent responsible for the serological response. Increased titers of immunoglobulin class G (IgG) antibodies do not allow differentiation between a primary infection with *R. prowazekii* and Brill-Zinsser disease; however, specific IgM antibodies are characteristically absent in patients with recrudescent typhus. Include positive and negative controls in all test runs and document performance characteristics of reagents and controls. Always interpret serologic test results in the context with clinical and epidemiological circumstances.

**9. Reporting requirements**—The last outbreak of louse-borne typhus in the USA occurred in 1921; contemporary US cases of infection with

*R. prowazekii* are rare, associated almost exclusively with flying squirrel typhus or Brill-Zinsser disease, and are not nationally notifiable. Nonetheless, foci of infected people exist worldwide, particularly among impoverished populations in rural highlands of Central and Eastern Africa, as well as mountainous regions of Central and South America, and explosive outbreaks can occur in certain settings. In these situations, outbreaks should be reported expeditiously to WHO (see: http://www.who.int/ihr/alert_and_response/outbreak-network/en).

**10. Referral network**—In the USA, serological and molecular assays used to detect infections with *R. prowazekii* are available at CDC as well as approximately 30 Laboratory Response Network (LRN) reference laboratories. Positive results identified by a LRN laboratory should be reported to and verified by CDC (see: https://emergency.cdc.gov/lrn/index.asp).

**11. Special considerations**—The rapid and potentially life-threatening progression of louse-borne typhus warrants empiric treatment with doxycycline in those patients who present with features that are clinically and epidemiologically compatible with this disease. Therapy should not be delayed pending results of a confirmatory laboratory assay. Because infection with *R. prowazekii* can occur following inhalation of aerosolized louse feces, the nurses, physicians, and other health care providers caring for or obtaining clinical samples from louse-infested patients are at increased risk of infection. PPE that includes eye protection and a filtering face-piece is recommended for attending field staff during epidemic settings. *R. prowazekii* is a category B potential biological terrorism agent, as well as a select agent, and its possession, use, storage, and transfer to other laboratories are strictly regulated (see: http://www.selectagents.gov). Non-select agent laboratories should not attempt to cultivate or molecularly confirm clinical specimens suspected to contain *R. prowazekii*; instead, these samples should be transferred to select agent-registered laboratories for further evaluation and testing. Further information about louse-borne typhus can be found at: https://www.cdc.gov/typhus/epidemic/index.html.

## II. ENDEMIC FLEA-BORNE TYPHUS (murine typhus, shop typhus, flea-borne rickettsiosis)

**1. Clinical features**—The course of flea-borne typhus resembles that of louse-borne typhus but is generally less severe. The illness begins with an abrupt onset of fever, headache, and myalgia. Rash occurs in 50%–80% of patients; however, it typically is not present at initial presentation. Abdominal signs and symptoms such as nausea, vomiting, and abdominal pain may occur and are more common in children. Complications can include acute renal failure, myocarditis, respiratory failure, neurologic manifestations, and hemophagocytic syndrome, but occur relatively infrequently. The case-fatality rate for all ages is less than 5% but increases with age. Presence of fleas and absence of louse infestation, geographic and seasonal distribution, and sporadic occurrence of the disease help differentiate it from louse-borne typhus. Flea-borne rickettsiosis (caused by infection with *Rickettsia felis*) is similar clinically to murine typhus and most commonly manifests as fever and generalized maculopapular rash. No deaths have been attributed to flea-borne rickettsiosis.

**2. Causative agents**—*R. typhi, R. felis.*

**3. Laboratory diagnosis**—Moderate thrombocytopenia and elevated hepatic transaminase levels are common and may aid in making a diagnosis. Laboratory confirmation of a diagnosis typically occurs late in the disease process and is therefore not useful for making initial treatment decisions. The IFA assay is the most accurate serological method for laboratory confirmation and requires a 4-fold increase in antibody titers when comparing a patient's acute and convalescent sera. An acute serum sample should be collected during the first week of symptoms and a convalescent serum sample obtained 3–4 weeks after convalescence. Antibody tests usually become positive in the second to third week of illness. Therefore, the primary sample taken in the acute stage of illness is used to obtain a baseline titer for comparison with the convalescent sample. A negative acute result does not rule out active infection, nor does a positive acute result confirm the diagnosis. Because antigens of *R. typhi* are cross-reactive with those of *R. prowazekii*, serologic tests cannot discriminate between flea-borne typhus and louse-borne typhus unless the sera are differentially absorbed with the respective rickettsial antigen prior to testing by IFA (i.e., a cross-adsorption assay). Patients infected with *R. felis* generally produce antibodies that cross-react with antigens of spotted fever group rickettsiae rather than typhus group rickettsiae. Other diagnostic methods include enzyme immunoassays, complement fixation, PCR, and IHC staining of tissues. In many regions of the world, the Weil-Felix agglutination test, which uses the OX-19 and OX-2 strains of *Proteus vulgaris* as antigen, is a commonly used and widely available assay but lacks sensitivity and specificity and is not currently recommended as a confirmatory method for any rickettsial disease. Skin biopsy samples of rash sites can be tested by IHC or PCR, but only PCR and sequence analysis provide definitive agent identification.

**4. Laboratory capability**—Routine diagnostic procedures, including processing of clinical specimens for serological, IHC, and PCR assays can occur in BSL-2 laboratories equipped with a class II BSC. BSL-3 practices, containment equipment, and facilities should be used for all propagative techniques, including inoculation, incubation, and harvesting of cell cultures or embryonated eggs, and all aerosol-generating procedures involving concentrates of live organisms, to include sonicating, vortexing, blending, or centrifuging. When evaluating human samples for clinical purposes, tests should occur in a CLIA-certified laboratory that routinely performs proficiency testing of established techniques and competency assessments of laboratory personnel. Facilities should be equipped, preferably within the laboratory, with a validated method for decontaminating all laboratory waste, such as autoclaving or chemical disinfection. BSL-3 facilities and practices are required if laboratory animals are used for diagnostic procedures.

**5. Safety requirements**—Laboratory-acquired infections with *R. typhi* have been described, and PPE that includes goggles or safety glasses and disposable gloves and gowns should be used for all manipulations of clinical specimens. Consistent adherence to universal/standard precautions is required. The initial processing of blood or serum samples for serology, inactivation of materials for DNA extraction, and inoculating and subsequently manipulation of cell cultures should occur in a class II BSC. Equipment that could produce infective aerosols should be fitted with aerosol-resistant lids and contained in spaces that exhaust air through HEPA filtration or other equivalent technology. Applicable local, state, or national regulations could require enhanced environmental and personal protection. Person-to-person transmission of flea-borne typhus has not been reported. Prophylactic antibiotic treatment following a potential exposure is discouraged in the absence of clinically compatible signs and symptoms and could only delay onset of disease. No vaccines are currently available for infections caused by *R. typhi* or *R. felis*.

**6. Nonhuman hosts**—For most areas of the world, *R. typhi* is a zoonosis maintained in a transmission cycle that involves predominantly the Oriental rat flea, *Xenopsylla cheopis*, and commensal and urban *Rattus* spp., particularly *Rattus rattus* and *Rattus norvegicus.* In Texas and California, another epidemiologically relevant transmission cycle involves opossums (*Didelphis virginianus*) and cat fleas (*Ctenocephalides felis*). Natural infections with *R. typhi* have been detected in many other species of wild and domesticated animals and several other flea species around the world; nonetheless, these have not been demonstrated as important routes of transmission of the pathogen to humans. *R. felis* has been detected in more than 20 species of fleas, ticks, and mites around the world; nonetheless, the cat flea is the most commonly recognized vector. Recent evidence suggests that *Anopheles gambiae* might also serve as a potential vector in some regions of Africa.

**7. Sample/specimen requirements**—Antibodies reactive with *R. typhi* or *R. felis* are not generally detectable until 7–10 days of infection, and most serological tests are typically insensitive during the first week of the illness. Paired serum samples, comprising a specimen collected during the acute stage of the illness and a second sample collected 2–3 weeks after convalescence, should be tested in tandem. Whole blood anticoagulated in citrated, heparinized, or ethylenediaminetetraacetic acid (EDTA)–treated tubes are standard specimens for molecular assays and cell culture isolation. A minimum of 1 ml is desirable, but larger volumes (3–5 ml) are generally preferred. A cutaneous punch biopsy specimen (≥ 3 mm in diameter) obtained from a rash or eschar lesion represents another important sample for these analyses and represents the optimal specimen for IHC staining. Molecular and cell culture assays are most sensitive during the first week of illness and before the initiation of specific antibiotic therapy. Sensitivity of molecular detection generally diminishes within 1 week of sample collection in refrigerated specimens. When transporting specimens to a referral laboratory, refrigerate at 4°C and attempt overnight delivery.

**8. Testing requirements**—Cross-reactions can occur between antigens of *R. typhi* and *R. prowazekii*, and cross-adsorption assays are required to determine conclusively the specific agent responsible for the serological response. Positive and negative controls should be included in all test runs and document performance characteristics of reagents and controls. Low levels of IgG or IgM antibodies may persist in some patients for months or years after primary exposure. In this context, the rigorous application of at least a 4-fold titer rise is required for serological confirmation of acute infection. Molecular and cell culture assays are most sensitive during the first week of illness and before the initiation of specific antibiotic therapy. Sensitivity of molecular detection generally diminishes within 1 week of sample collection in refrigerated specimens. Isolation of *R. typhi* or *R. felis* in cell culture can be a time-consuming process that requires 1 to several weeks.

**9. Reporting requirements**—Flea-borne typhus is not a nationally notifiable disease in the USA; nonetheless, it is currently reportable in 14 US states: CA, HI, IL, IN, MI, MN, MS, NE, NH, OH, OR, PA, TX, and WA. Laboratories outside the USA should determine if flea-borne typhus is a reportable disease within their respective jurisdictions.

**10. Referral network**—In the USA, serological and molecular assays to detect infections with *R. typhi* are available at CDC, as well as some public health department laboratories where the disease occurs with highest frequency, including CA, HI, and TX.

**11. Special considerations**—The rapid and potentially life-threatening progression of flea-borne typhus warrants empiric treatment with doxycycline in those patients who present with features that are clinically and epidemiologically compatible with this disease. Therapy should not be delayed pending results of a confirmatory laboratory assay. Further information about flea-borne typhus can be found at: https://www.cdc.gov/typhus/murine/index.html.

## III. SCRUB TYPHUS (Tsutsugamushi disease, mite-borne typhus fever)

**1. Clinical features**—A rickettsial disease often characterized by a primary punched-out skin ulcer (eschar) corresponding to the site of attachment of an infected mite (chigger). Not all patients with scrub typhus have an eschar, and the frequency of this symptom varies by region. An acute febrile onset follows within several days, along with headache, profuse sweating, conjunctival injection, and lymphadenopathy. A transient maculopapular rash appears on the trunk in about half of patients around day 7 of fever. Cough and X-ray evidence of pneumonitis are common and may progress to acute respiratory distress syndrome (ARDS) and respiratory failure. Neurological findings such as confusion or hearing loss may occur. This disease may cause spontaneous abortions in pregnant women. Without antibiotic therapy, fever lasts for about 14 days. The case-fatality rate in untreated cases varies from 1%–60% according to area, strain of infectious agent, and previous exposure to disease; it is consistently higher among older people.

**2. Causative agents**—*Orientia tsutsugamushi,* with multiple, serologically distinct strains; *Orientia chuto.*

**3. Laboratory diagnosis**—Laboratory confirmation of a diagnosis typically occurs late in the disease process and is therefore not useful for making initial treatment decisions. The IFA is the reference method for serological confirmation and requires a 4-fold increase in antibody titers when comparing a patient's acute and convalescent sera. An acute serum sample should be collected during the first week of symptoms and a convalescent serum sample obtained 3–4 weeks after convalescence. Antibody tests usually become positive in the second to third week of illness. Therefore, the primary sample taken in the acute stage of illness is used to obtain a baseline titer for comparison with the convalescent sample. A negative acute result does not rule out active infection, nor does a positive acute result confirm the diagnosis. Other serological methods include indirect immunoperoxidase and complement fixation assays. In some resource-limited regions of the world, a presumptive diagnosis of scrub typhus is made with the Weil-Felix agglutination reaction using the OX-K strain of *Proteus mirabilis* as antigen; nonetheless, this assay is non-specific and does not provide definitive laboratory evidence of infection with *O. tsutsugamushi*. Reinfections with different strains can occur, and serologic diagnosis may need to include testing for multiple *O. tsutsugamushi* strains to improve assay sensitivity and specificity. Five major serotypes have been identified (Kato, Karp, Boryong, Kawasaki, and Gilliam). Antigens of *Orientia* generally do not cross-react with those of *Rickettsia* spp. Commercially available immunochromatographic tests (dipstick and immunodot assays) follow a simple protocol, do not require sophisticated ancillary equipment, and provide rapid results, but the cost of these kits may be prohibitive in some areas. PCR assays of eschar biopsy specimens and swabs of eschar lesions are highly sensitive and specific techniques to establish a diagnosis.

**4. Laboratory capability**—Routine diagnostic procedures, including processing of clinical specimens for serological, IHC, and PCR assays can occur in BSL-2 laboratories equipped with a class II BSC. BSL-3 practices, containment equipment, and facilities should be used for all propagative techniques, including inoculation, incubation, and harvesting of cell cultures or embryonated eggs, and all aerosol-generating procedures involving concentrates of live organisms, to include sonicating, vortexing, blending, or centrifuging. When evaluating human samples for clinical purposes, tests should occur in a CLIA-certified laboratory that routinely performs proficiency testing of established techniques and competency assessments of laboratory personnel techniques. Facilities should be equipped, preferably within the laboratory, with a validated method for decontaminating all laboratory waste, such as autoclaving or chemical disinfection. ABSL-3 facilities and practices are required if laboratory animals are used for diagnostic procedures.

**5. Safety requirements**—Laboratory-acquired infections with *O. tsutsugamushi* have been described, and PPE that includes goggles or safety glasses and disposable gloves and gowns should be used for all manipulations of clinical specimens. Consistent adherence to universal/standard precautions is required. Aliquoting blood or serum samples, initial inactivation of materials for DNA extraction, and inoculation and subsequent manipulation of cell cultures should occur in a class II BSC. All equipment that could produce infective aerosols should be fitted with aerosol-resistant lids and must be contained in spaces that exhaust air through HEPA filtration or other equivalent technology. Applicable local, state, or national regulations could require enhanced environmental and personal protection. Person-to-person transmission of scrub typhus has not been reported. Prophylactic antibiotic treatment following a potential exposure is not recommended in the absence of clinically compatible signs and symptoms and could delay onset of disease. No vaccine is currently available for scrub typhus.

**6. Nonhuman hosts**—More than 50 species of trombiculid mites have been identified as vectors or potential vectors of *O. tsutsugamushi*, although members of the genus *Leptotrobidium* are most often identified as epidemiologically important. Mites maintain *O. tsutusgamushi* through transovarial and transtadial transmission. Although infected mites can transmit *O. tsusugamushi* to many different species of wild rodents, typically only few uninfected mites will acquire the infection during feeding from an infected rodent, and mites that acquire the infection in this manner neither develop a generalized infection nor transmit the pathogen transovarially to the subsequent generation. The vectors and reservoirs of *O. chuto* are unknown.

**7. Sample/specimen requirements**—Paired serum samples comprising a specimen collected during the acute stage of the illness and a second sample collected approximately 2–4 weeks after convalescence should be tested in tandem. Whole blood anticoagulated in citrated, heparinized, or EDTA-treated tubes are standard specimens for molecular assays and cell culture isolation. A minimum of 1 ml is desirable, but larger volumes (3–5 ml) are generally preferred. A cutaneous punch biopsy specimen (≥3 mm in diameter) obtained from an inoculation eschar or rash lesion represents another important sample for these analyses and represents the optimal specimen for IHC staining. PCR of eschar crusts or eschar material sampled by swabbing can provide a highly sensitive method for establishing the diagnosis. When transporting specimens to a referral laboratory, refrigerate at 4°C and attempt overnight delivery.

**8. Testing requirements**—Positive and negative controls should be included in all test runs, and performance characteristics of reagents and controls should be documented. Antibodies reactive with *Orientia* are not generally detectable until 7–10 days of infection, and most serological tests are typically insensitive during the first week of the illness. Low levels of IgG or IgM antibodies reactive with *O. tsutsugamushi* may persist in some patients for months or years after primary exposure, and background seropositive rates in areas where *O. tsutsugamashi* is endemic can be very high. In this context, the rigorous application of at least a 4-fold titer rise is required for serological confirmation of acute infection. Molecular and cell culture assays are most sensitive during the bacteremic phase of the disease, which occurs characteristically during the first 8 days of fever, and before the initiation of specific antibiotic therapy. Buffy coat specimens obtained from anticoagulated whole blood can provide increased sensitivity. Sensitivity of molecular detection generally diminishes within 1 week of sample collection in refrigerated specimens. Isolation of *O. tsutsugamushi* in cell culture can be a time-consuming process that requires 1 to several weeks.

**9. Reporting requirements**—Scrub typhus is not a nationally notifiable illness in the USA; nonetheless, national surveillance for this disease exists in several countries where scrub typhus is endemic, including Bhutan, China, Japan, South Korea, Taiwan, and Thailand.

**10. Referral network**—Commercially available tests for scrub typhus in the USA are limited predominantly to serological assays. Molecular tests can be performed at CDC.

**11. Special considerations**—The rapid and potentially life-threatening progression of scrub typhus warrants empiric treatment with doxycycline in those patients who present with features that are clinically and epidemiologically compatible with this disease. Therapy should not be delayed pending results of a confirmatory laboratory assay. Further information about scrub typhus can be found at: https://www.cdc.gov/typhus/scrub/index.html.

[C. Paddock]

# WEST NILE VIRUS DISEASE

| DISEASE | ICD-10 CODE |
|---|---|
| WEST NILE FEVER | ICD-10 A92.3 |
| WEST NILE VIRUS ENCEPHALITIS | ICD-10 A83.8 |
| WEST NILE VIRUS MENINGITIS | ICD-10 A87.8 |
| WEST NILE VIRUS ACUTE FLACCID PARALYSIS | ICD-10 A88.8 |
| KUNJIN | ICD-10 A83.4 |

**1. Clinical features**—Approximately 70%–80% of human West Nile virus (WNV) infections are asymptomatic. Most symptomatic people experience an acute systemic febrile illness that often includes headache, myalgia, or arthralgia; gastrointestinal tract symptoms and a transient maculopapular rash also are commonly reported. Less than 1% of infected people develop neuroinvasive disease, which typically manifests as meningitis, encephalitis, or acute flaccid paralysis. WNV meningitis is indistinguishable clinically from aseptic meningitis caused by most other viruses. Patients with WNV encephalitis usually present with seizures, mental status changes, focal neurologic deficits, or movement disorders. WNV acute flaccid paralysis often is clinically and pathologically identical to poliovirus-associated acute flaccid paralysis, with damage of anterior horn cells and may progress to respiratory paralysis requiring mechanical ventilation. WNV-associated Guillain-Barré syndrome has also been reported and can be distinguished from WNV acute flaccid paralysis by clinical manifestations and electrophysiologic testing. Cardiac dysrhythmias, myocarditis, rhabdomyolysis, optic neuritis, uveitis, chorioretinitis, orchitis, pancreatitis, and hepatitis have been described rarely after WNV infection.

Most patients with WNV nonneuroinvasive disease (i.e., West Nile fever) or meningitis recover completely, but fatigue, malaise, and weakness can linger for weeks or months. Patients who recover from WNV encephalitis or acute flaccid paralysis often have residual neurologic deficits. Among patients with neuroinvasive disease, the overall case-fatality rate is approximately 10% but is significantly higher in WNV encephalitis and acute flaccid paralysis than in WNV meningitis.

WNV disease should be considered in the differential diagnosis of acute neurologic or febrile illnesses associated with recent exposure to mosquitoes, blood transfusion, or organ transplantation and of illnesses in neonates whose mothers were infected with WNV during pregnancy or while breastfeeding. In addition to other more common causes of aseptic meningitis and encephalitis (e.g., herpes simplex virus and enteroviruses), other arboviruses should also be considered in the differential diagnosis (see "Arboviral Diseases").

**2. Causative agents**—WNV, of the family *Flaviviridae* and genus *Flavivirus*.

**3. Laboratory diagnosis**—Identifying anti-WNV immunoglobulin class M (IgM) antibodies in serum or cerebrospinal fluid (CSF) is the most common way to diagnose WNV infection. The presence of anti-WNV IgM in serum is usually good evidence of recent WNV infection but may indicate infection with another closely related flavivirus. Because anti-WNV IgM can persist in serum in some patients for longer than a year, a positive test result occasionally may reflect past infection. IgM antibody to WNV develops in a majority of WNV-infected patients by the fourth day after symptom onset; 95% of infected patients develop IgM antibody within 7 days of symptom onset. Detection of WNV IgM in CSF is diagnostic of neuroinvasive disease. For patients in whom serum collected within 10 days of illness lacks detectable IgM, testing should be repeated on a convalescent-phase sample. IgG antibody generally is detectable shortly after IgM and can persist for years.

Plaque-reduction neutralization tests can be performed to measure virus-specific neutralizing antibodies and to discriminate between cross-reacting antibodies in primary flavivirus infections. A 4-fold or greater increase in virus-specific neutralizing antibodies between acute- and convalescent-phase serum specimens collected 2–3 weeks apart may be used to confirm recent WNV infection. In patients who have been immunized against or infected with another flavivirus in the past (i.e., who have secondary flavivirus infections), cross-reactive antibodies in IgM, IgG, and neutralization assays may make it difficult to identify which flavivirus is causing the patient's illness. Immunization history, date of symptom onset, and information regarding other flaviviruses known to circulate in the geographic area that may cross-react in serologic assays should be considered when interpreting results.

Viral culture and WNV nucleic acid amplification tests (including reverse transcription polymerase chain reaction [RT-PCR]) can be performed on acute-phase serum, CSF, or tissue specimens. However, by the time most immunocompetent patients present with clinical symptoms, WNV ribonucleic acid (RNA) is usually no longer detectable, thus RT-PCR is not recommended for diagnosis in immunocompetent patients. The sensitivity of these tests is likely to be higher in immunocompromised patients. Immunohistochemical staining can detect WNV antigens in fixed tissue, but negative results are not definitive.

**4. Laboratory capability**—The standard commercially available assays for detection of IgG and IgM by enzyme immunoassay (EIA) or immunofluorescence assay (IFA) can be used in routine diagnostic laboratories provided they follow the manufacturer's instructions. Reliable performance of IFAs requires a good quality fluorescence microscope and an experienced operator. IgG avidity EIA is available to help distinguish between recent and past infection. Competitive EIAs using WNV specific monoclonal antibodies significantly improve specificity. Where the diagnosis is uncertain and/or there is concern about the presence of cross-reacting antibodies, then further testing should be conducted in a reference laboratory that can test for other flaviviruses and carry out specific assays. Isolation of the virus, testing for WNV-RNA and testing of tissue samples are generally conducted in reference laboratories.

**5. Safety requirements**—Clinical samples may be handled under routine biosafety level 2 (BSL-2) laboratory conditions. WNV, with the exception of the Kunjin strain (KUNV), is classified as a BSL-3 agent, and therefore live virus must be handled in a BSL-3 facility. Inactivated virus (e.g., following nucleic acid extraction) is safe and can be handled in BSL-2 facilities. Due to its lower pathogenicity, KUNV is a BSL-2 organism.

**6. Nonhuman hosts**—WNV has a range of mammalian and avian hosts and is maintained primarily in a cycle between birds, either perching birds or ardeid birds depending on the country, and mosquitoes. The primary vector species are *Culex* spp., especially *Culex pipiens*, *Culex quinquefasciatus*, *Culex tarsalis*, and for KUNV, *Culex annulirostris*. Some bird species such as crows and geese develop clinical disease but are not thought to have an important role in maintenance of the virus. Horses develop clinical disease but are dead-end hosts. Chickens become infected by WNV but are asymptomatic, and sentinel flocks have been used for monitoring WNV activity by regular testing for antibody in the chickens.

**7. Sample/specimen requirements**—Serum should be collected for antibody testing, including acute and convalescent samples, collected 10–14 days apart. Where meningoencephalitis is suspected, CSF should also be collected for IgM testing and nucleic acid amplification of RNA. Samples should be stored and transported at 4°C–8°C. If testing is delayed by more than 3–4 days, samples should be frozen, preferably at or below −20°C. Tissue samples should be placed in virus transport medium (VTM) or kept moist in saline if VTM is not available or if the sample has to be divided for other tests such as histopathology or immunochemistry. Do not place samples for culture or RNA detection in fixatives such as formalin or alcohol.

**8. Testing requirements**—Detection of WNV, WNV RNA, or WNV antigen in blood or tissues is regarded as definitive evidence of infection, provided the tests have been conducted properly. Nucleic acid amplification tests such as PCR are particularly at risk of false-positive results if the laboratory does not have strict measures for preventing cross-contamination. Antigen detection tests on tissues such as brain are carried out by some reference laboratories. They are less sensitive than RNA detection, though they do provide information about the location of the virus within tissues. Diagnosis is usually made by detection of IgM in serum and or CSF by EIA or

IFAs, confirmed by a rise in specific antibodies between acute and convalescent samples. As for all flaviviruses, IgG and, to a lesser extent, IgM will cross-react with other flavivirus antigens. In areas where there are other potential infecting flaviviruses, such as Japanese encephalitis virus or dengue, cross-reacting IgM can occur, and testing for IgM to these other viruses should be undertaken to exclude that. IgM commonly persists for several months and therefore does not necessarily indicate recent infection. IgG avidity testing by EIA measures the strength of binding of the patient's antibody, which increases with time after onset. Therefore, high avidity IgG in the presence of IgM indicates recent past infection, while low avidity antibody suggests acute infection.

The specificity of IgG is classically determined by neutralization assays, requiring the WNV titer to be at least 4-fold higher than that of other flaviviruses that may have infected the person. Antibody formed within the early convalescent period may not be specific as the antibody response may not have matured sufficiently. Repeat testing at least a month after onset may be needed. Competitive EIAs are available that measure the ability of the patient's serum to block the binding of a WNV-specific monoclonal antibody. This is usually sufficient to indicate WNV infection, but cross-reactions can occur occasionally, so that testing for IgG antibodies to other likely infecting flaviviruses is still recommended where very high specificity is required. None of the antibody tests are able to distinguish between antibodies to the different WNV types and subtypes.

Patients who have had previous flavivirus infections or vaccination may have attenuated IgM responses in both serum and CSF and a rapid rise in IgG, with the initial response being to the previously infecting virus, the so-called original antigenic sin. Convalescent serum should show a rise in specific antibody to the recently infecting virus.

Laboratories should participate in quality assurance activities for any testing they undertake. Preferably this should be part of a recognized external quality assurance program, such as the European Network for the Diagnostics of "Imported" Viral Diseases-Collaborative Laboratory Response Network and the Royal College of Pathologists of Australasia Quality Assurance Program. Both are distributed internationally. Other programs may be available locally or supplied by reference laboratories. Where there is no external quality assurance program available, then alternatives such as specimen exchanges should be undertaken.

**9. Reporting requirements**—Infection with WNV is a notifiable disease in most countries and should be reported promptly to public health authorities. As WNV may infect animals, notification to the agricultural/animal health authorities is also recommended. Responses may include enhanced vector control measures, enhanced case detection, and public health monitoring.

**10. Referral network**—Samples for testing and/or confirmation can be sent to state, national, or regional reference laboratories, or to one of the relevant WHO Collaborating Centres.

**11. Special considerations**—None.

[D. W. Smith, J. S. Mackenzie]

# YAWS
(framboesia topica)

| DISEASE | ICD-10 CODE |
|---|---|
| YAWS | ICD-10 A66 |

**1. Clinical features**—Yaws is a chronic relapsing nonvenereal treponematosis. It is characterized by highly contagious primary and secondary cutaneous lesions (early yaws) and noncontagious tertiary destructive lesions (late yaws).

The typical initial lesion (mother yaw) is a papilloma on the face or extremities (usually the leg) that persists for weeks or months and is painless unless secondarily infected. This proliferates slowly and may form a framboesial (raspberry) lesion or ulcerate (ulcero papilloma).

Secondary disseminated or satellite papillomata and/or papules and squamous macules appear before, or shortly after, healing of the initial lesion. These appear in successive crops, often accompanied by periostitis of the long bones (saber shin) and fingers (polydactylitis), with mild constitutional symptoms. In the dry season, papillomatous crops are usually restricted to the moist skinfolds, and papules or macular lesions predominate. Painful, and usually disabling, papillomata and hyperkeratosis on palms and soles may appear in early and in late stages. Lesions heal spontaneously; relapses may occur after periods of latency. Early yaws can last up to 5 years after initial infection.

The late stage, with destructive lesions of skin and bone, occurs in about 10%–20% of untreated patients, usually 5 or more years after infection. Unlike in syphilis, the brain, eyes, heart, aorta, and abdominal organs are not involved. The infection is rarely, if ever, fatal but can be very disfiguring and disabling, resulting in social stigma and economic impact.

Almost all cases of yaws occur in children younger than 15 years, with the peak incidence in children aged 6–10 years. The incidence is about the same in males and females.

**2. Causative agents**—*Treponema pallidum* subspecies *pertenue*, a spirochete.

**3. Laboratory diagnosis**—Based on clinico-epidemiological findings in the field. Confirmed through dark-field or direct fluorescent antibody microscopic examination of exudates from primary or secondary lesions. Molecular methods using polymerase chain reaction (PCR) and deoxyribonucleic acid (DNA) sequencing have been developed to detect *T. pallidum* subsp. *pertenue*-specific sequences in lesion exudate. Nontreponemal serological tests for syphilis (e.g., venereal disease research laboratory [VDRL] and rapid plasma reagin [RPR]) become reactive during the initial stage, remain so during the early infection, and tend to become nonreactive after many years of latency, even in the absence of specific treatment; in some patients, they remain reactive at a low titer for life. Treponemal serological tests (e.g., *T. pallidum* particle agglutination [TP-PA] and microhemagglutination assay for *T. pallidum* antibodies [MHA-TP]) usually remain reactive for life despite adequate treatment. A nontreponemal test should be confirmed by treponemal testing. Yaws, bejel, and venereal syphilis cannot be distinguished on the basis of serological testing.

**4. Laboratory capability**—Serological testing can be performed in laboratories with standard equipment and minimal scientific and technical knowledge, but the high throughput tests require automation, which are usually found in more sophisticated laboratories. Point-of-care serological tests can be performed by staff with minimal laboratory training and can be used at all levels of health care facilities, even those without a laboratory. Specialized scientific and technical knowledge including sophisticated laboratory equipment is essential for performing PCR testing.

**5. Safety requirements**—Biosafety level 2 conditions are required. Standard precautions should be taken when working with blood or clinical specimens as other infectious agents may also be present.

**6. Nonhuman hosts**—Disease caused by *T. pallidum* has been identified in a range of nonhuman primates. Sequencing data suggests these organisms are closely related and possibly identical to human *T. pallidum* subsp. *pertenue*. Experimental evidence suggests that nonhuman primate strains are infectious to humans, but evidence of zoonotic transmission in the field has not been demonstrated.

DNA of *T. pallidum* subsp. *pertenue* has been identified in flies, but whether flies are involved in transmission is unclear.

**7. Sample/specimen requirements**—Serum is the specimen of choice for treponemal and nontreponemal serological tests, but plasma can be used for some tests. Rapid point-of-care tests use whole blood obtained through a finger stick. Serum and plasma should be stored at 4°C if testing cannot be performed within 4 hours and at −20°C or lower if testing will be done more than 5 days from collection. Serous exudate from moist lesions of primary and secondary yaws are amenable to dark-field microscopy (DF) and PCR.

Specimens for DF must be tested within 20 minutes of collection. Tissue for silver staining and immunohistochemistry (IHC) should be fixed in 10% buffered formalin as soon as possible at ambient temperature and then paraffin embedded and sectioned for staining. PCR can be performed on either fixed or unfixed tissue, although unfixed tissue is preferred. All samples for PCR should be stored at −70°C if testing cannot be performed immediately.

**8. Testing requirements**—Serology is the mainstay for diagnosis of yaws, although serological tests may be negative in early primary yaws. Treponemal antibody tests (e.g., TP-PA or MHA-TP) and fluorescent treponemal antibody absorption remain positive for life. Quantitative nontreponemal tests become positive following infection and the titer then falls following successful treatment.

Traditionally samples were screened using a nontreponemal test (e.g., RPR or VDRL), and if this test was positive a confirmatory treponemal test was performed. Many labs have now adopted an alternative algorithm (the reverse syphilis screening algorithm). Using this approach, the initial test is a treponemal antibody test. When this test is positive a quantitative nontreponemal test is then performed. If the nontreponemal test is negative a second treponemal test (preferably antibodies against different *T. pallidum* antigens using a different test platform) can be performed.

Point-of-care serological tests are now available. The majority detect only treponemal antibodies (commonly referred to as rapid syphilis tests). Point-of-care tests that detect both treponemal and nontreponemal antibodies are now available. When using a point-of-care test it is important to ensure the kit meets appropriate quality standards.

It should be noted that serological assays cannot distinguish yaws from other endemic treponematoses or syphilis. When both treponemal and nontreponemal tests are positive, the diagnosis is confirmed. A quantitative nontreponemal test is required for assessing response to therapy. Participation in the WHO/CDC Syphilis Serology Proficiency Programme is recommended for maintaining proficiency in treponemal and nontreponemal testing.

Detection of specific *T. pallidum* subsp. *pertenue* DNA targets by PCR or observation of spirochetes is definitive of yaws infection. Lesion samples should be initially screened with a pan-treponemal PCR (such as polA or tp47). In samples that are positive, PCR may allow differentiation of *T. pallidum* subsp. *pertenue* from other subspecies. IHC, silver stain, or PCR is used for tissue biopsies. Use of a hematoxylin counterstain with IHC allows tissue structure to be observed with localization of treponemes. On molecular testing many clinically suspicious lesions will not have detectable treponemal DNA present. In a proportion of these samples an alternative organism, most commonly *Haemophilus ducreyi*, may be identified.

**9. Reporting requirements**—Reactive treponemal and nontreponemal test results are consistent with current or past yaws infection but cannot distinguish from other treponemal infections (most importantly syphilis). If the nontreponemal titer is less than 1:4 this could be associated with a serofast state where nontreponemal titers neither increase nor decrease 4-fold after treatment. If the treponemal test is nonreactive, then there is no laboratory evidence of yaws infection. If the nontreponemal test is reactive but the treponemal test is nonreactive, then it is most likely a biological false positive. If the first treponemal test in the reverse algorithm is reactive and the nontreponemal test is nonreactive but the second/supplemental treponemal test is reactive, then this is consistent with past or potential early infection with yaws or an alternative treponemal infection. If nonreactive, it is inconclusive for yaws infection or a false positive.

Molecular tests should be reported as DNA of *T. pallidum* subsp. *pertenue* detected or not detected. Where a molecular assay for azithromycin resistance has been performed this should be reported as positive/negative for the presence of mutations conferring azithromycin resistance.

In some endemic areas, yaws may be a reportable disease. Laboratories should determine if yaws is reportable to the public health authorities in their specific setting.

**10. Referral network**—No specific referral networks exist.

**11. Special considerations**—

1) Differentiation of venereal and nonvenereal treponematoses, with proper reporting of each, has particular importance in the evaluation and consolidation of mass campaigns.
2) International measures: examine groups of children and adults who emigrate from areas of high prevalence for treponemal infections.

[A. Pillay, M. Marks]

# YELLOW FEVER

| DISEASE | ICD-10 CODE |
|---|---|
| YELLOW FEVER | ICD-10 A95 |

**1. Clinical features**—Majority of infected persons are asymptomatic. Clinical disease varies from mild febrile illness to severe disease with jaundice and hemorrhage. Initial symptoms include sudden onset of fever, chills, headache, backache, general muscle pain, prostration, nausea, and vomiting. The pulse may be slow and weak, out of proportion to the elevated temperature (Faget sign). Leukopenia appears early and is most pronounced about the fifth day; however, leukocytosis is often seen in the second week of the disease. Most symptoms resolve at this stage.

In approximately 15% of cases, there is a brief remission of hours to a day, followed by recurrence of initial symptoms with progression to jaundice and hemorrhagic symptoms, including epistaxis, gingival bleeding, hematemesis, or melena. Elevated liver enzymes, abnormal clotting factors, albuminuria, and anuria may occur as a result of liver and renal failure. The overall case-fatality rate for severe cases is 20%–50%. Recovery from yellow fever results in lifelong immunity.

**2. Causative agents**—Yellow fever virus, of the family *Flaviviridae* and genus *Flavivirus*.

**3. Laboratory diagnosis**—In acute disease, laboratory diagnosis often can be made through (a) isolation of virus from blood by inoculation into suckling mice, mosquitoes, or cell cultures; (b) demonstration of viral antigen in tissues, especially liver, by use of labeled specific antibodies; or (c) demonstration of viral ribonucleic acid (RNA) in blood or tissue by reverse transcription polymerase chain reaction (RT-PCR). RT-PCR can also be used to distinguish acute infections with yellow fever virus from recent vaccination. Serological diagnosis includes demonstrating virus-specific immunoglobulin class M (IgM) in early sera or a 4-fold or greater rise in titer of virus-specific antibodies in paired acute and convalescent sera. Serological cross-reactions occur with other flaviviruses. In natural infections, antibodies appear in the blood within the first week.

**4. Laboratory capability**—Isolation of yellow fever virus (YFV) should only be carried out in laboratories specializing in virus isolation and with the capacity and expertise to work with biosafety level 3 (BSL-3) pathogens. Serological testing can be carried out in most clinical and public health laboratories. Enzyme-linked immunosorbent assay (ELISA) tests and immunofluorescence assay (IFA) slides are available commercially for detection of YF IgG and IgM by IFA and should be performed according to the manufacturer's instructions. These include antigens for other flaviviruses, so that IgG and IgM cross-reactions can be assessed. Due to the significance of a diagnosis of YF, positive results from patients infected in areas without known local activity should be confirmed by a reference laboratory, or the primary sample should be referred for testing. Isolation of the virus, testing for YFV-RNA, identifying vaccine and wild-type strains, testing of tissue samples, and performing YFV-specific neutralising antibody titers are generally conducted in reference laboratories.

**5. Safety requirements**—Clinical samples may be handled by trained individuals using standard precautions under routine BSL-2 laboratory conditions. YF is classified as a BSL-3 agent, and therefore live virus must be handled in a BSL-3 facility. Staff working with live virus should be vaccinated. Inactivated virus (e.g., following nucleic acid extraction) is safe and can be handled in BSL-2 facilities.

**6. Nonhuman hosts**—YFV is restricted to humans and nonhuman primates. It is maintained and transmitted between these and *Aedes* or *Haemagogus* spp. mosquitoes. Urban outbreaks involve humans and *Aedes aegypti* mosquitoes.

**7. Sample/specimen requirements**—Serum should be collected for antibody testing, including acute and convalescent samples, collected 10–14 days apart. Cerebrospinal fluid should also be collected for IgM testing and nucleic acid amplification of RNA. Samples should be stored and transported at 4°C–8°C. If testing is delayed by more than 3–4 days, samples should be frozen, preferably at or below −20°C. Tissue samples should be placed in virus transport medium (VTM) or kept moist in saline if VTM is not available or if the sample has to be divided for other tests such as histopathology or immunochemistry. Samples for culture or RNA detection should not be placed in fixatives such as formalin or alcohol. All primary containers should be shatterproof and leakproof and placed in a leakproof external container. All samples must be clearly labeled with unique identifiers and accompanied by a matching request form. Transport by air should comply with International Air Transport Association requirements.

**8. Testing requirements**—Detection of YF virus, YF RNA, or YF antigen in blood or tissues is regarded as definitive evidence of infection, provided the tests have been conducted properly. RNA is detectable from 3–10 days after onset and sometimes earlier. Nucleic acid amplification tests such as PCR are particularly at risk of false-positive results if the laboratory does not have strict measures for preventing cross-contamination. If the person has received YF vaccine within the previous 2 weeks, then the virus should be sequenced to determine whether it is wild-type or a vaccine strain. Antigen detection tests on tissues such as liver are carried out by some reference laboratories, but they are uncommon. They are less sensitive than RNA detection, though they do provide information about the location of the virus within tissues. Diagnosis is usually made by detection of IgM in serum by enzyme immunoassays or immunofluorescent antibody assays. It appears as early as 3 days after onset of illness, and persists from several weeks. IgG antibodies appear within a few days of illness and rise over 10–14 days. As for all flaviviruses, IgG and, to a lesser extent, IgM will cross-react with other flavivirus antigens. In areas where there are other potential infecting flaviviruses, such as dengue virus or West Nile virus, cross-reacting IgM can occur, and testing for IgM to these other viruses should be undertaken to exclude that. The specificity of IgG is determined by neutralization assays, requiring the YFV titer to be at least 4-fold higher than that of other flaviviruses that may have infected the person. Antibody formed within the early convalescent period may not be specific, as the antibody response may not have matured sufficiently. Repeat testing at least a month after onset may be needed. Patients who have had previous flavivirus infections may have attenuated IgM responses and a rapid rise in IgG, with the initial response being to the previously infecting virus, the so-called original antigenic sin. Convalescent serum should show a rise in specific antibody to the recently infecting virus. YF vaccination will produce detectable IgG and if received within the preceding 4 weeks will also produce detectable IgM.

All results should be interpreted in the context of the clinical findings and the history of exposure or vaccination. Reports for serological testing should include comments that indicate the possibility of cross-reacting antibodies due to current or prior infection or vaccination and include recommendations for further testing to confirm specificity and for convalescent serum samples as appropriate.

Laboratories should participate in quality assurance activities for any testing they undertake. Preferably this should be part of a recognized external quality assurance program, such as the European Network for the Diagnostics of "Imported" Viral Diseases-Collaborative Laboratory Response Network and the Royal College of Pathologists of Australasia Quality Assurance Program. Both are distributed internationally. Other programs may be available locally or supplied by reference laboratories. Where there is no external quality assurance program available, alternatives such as specimen exchanges should be undertaken.

**9. Reporting requirements**—YF is a notifiable disease in most countries. It is of particular concern where the person has entered an area with potential vector mosquito species, in which case public health authorities should be notified immediately.

**10. Referral network**—Samples for testing and/or confirmation can be sent to state or national reference laboratories or to a WHO regional reference laboratory.

**11. Special considerations**—YFV infections require reporting to local public health authorities. They must be assessed as a possible public health emergency of international concern against WHO International Health Regulation (IHR) criteria and, if necessary, reported as such to the IHR representative.

[D. W. Smith, J. S. Mackenzie]

# YERSINIOSIS

| DISEASE | ICD-10 CODE |
|---|---|
| INTESTINAL YERSINIOSIS | ICD-10 A04.6 |
| EXTRAINTESTINAL YERSINIOSIS | ICD-10 A28.2 |

**1. Clinical features**—Typically manifested by acute febrile diarrhea with abdominal pain (especially in young children). Other manifestations include acute mesenteric lymphadenitis mimicking appendicitis (especially in older children and adults), exudative pharyngitis, and systemic infection. The most common postinfectious complications are erythema nodosum and reactive arthritis. Bloody diarrhea can also occur in patients with *Yersinia* enteritis; diarrhea may be absent in up to a third of *Yersinia enterocolitica* infections. Ileitis is the characteristic lesion induced by *Y. enterocolitica. Yersinia pseudotuberculosis* causes acute mesenteric lymphadenitis, characterized by an appendicitis-like syndrome, sometimes with diarrhea. Because infections in older children and adolescents can mimic acute appendicitis, outbreaks can sometimes be recognized by a local increase in appendectomies.

**2. Causative agents**—Gram-negative bacilli. Globally, *Y. enterocolitica* is the spp. most commonly associated with human infection, causing up to 1%–3% of acute enteritis in some areas. *Y. enterocolitica* has more than 60 serotypes and 6 biotypes, many are nonpathogenic. *Y. pseudotuberculosis* has 6 serotypes with 4 subtypes. Most human and animal infections are caused by O-group I.

**3. Laboratory diagnosis**—Usually made through stool culture. Cefsulodin irgasan novobiocin (CIN) medium is highly selective and should be used if infection with *Yersinia* is suspected; at 28°C (78.4°F), it permits identification in 24 hours. The organisms may be recovered on usual enteric media if precautions are taken to prevent overgrowth of fecal flora. Cold enrichment in buffered saline at 4°C (39°F) for 2–3 weeks can be used, but this procedure usually enhances the isolation of nonpathogenic species. *Yersinia* can be isolated from blood with standard commercial blood culture media. Serological diagnosis by agglutination test or enzyme-linked immunosorbent assay is possible, but availability is generally limited to research settings.

**4. Laboratory capability**—Access to the laboratory should be restricted to authorized persons. Bench surfaces must be impervious to water, easy to clean, and resistant to acids, alkalis, solvents and disinfectants. There must be access to an autoclave for the disposal of infectious biological material. The laboratory should contain a biosafety cabinet (BSC), and a wash basin should be located near the laboratory exit. Laboratory personnel must have specific training in handling pathogenic agents and be directed by scientists with advanced training.

**5. Safety requirements**—Biosafety level 2 is required for work involving *Y. enterocolitica* and *Y. pseudotuberculosis*, both agents of moderate potential hazard to personnel and the environment. Laboratory procedures that give rise to infectious aerosols must be conducted in a BSC, isolator, or be otherwise suitably contained. Personal protective equipment requirements include laboratory coats or gowns, which should be side- or back-fastening. At some institutions gloves and safety glasses are also required at this level. When undertaking procedures that are likely to give rise to infectious aerosols, a class I BSC (BS 5726, or unit with equivalent protection factor or performance) should be used. Some other types of equipment may provide adequate containment in their own right, but this should be verified. Hands should be decontaminated immediately when contamination is suspected after handling infective materials and before leaving the laboratory.

**6. Nonhuman hosts—***Y. enterocolitica* and *Y. pseudotuberculosis* are found in warm-blooded animals including domestic animals such as swine, goats, cattle and horses, rodents, and household pets such as dogs and cats. Pigs are the major reservoirs for human pathogenic strains of *Yersinia*, while nonporcine *Yersinia* are generally nonpathogenic. It has been found in the intestinal tracts of pigs, dogs, and cats without any clinical manifestations. In addition, *Y. enterolitica* has been isolated from birds and, occasionally, reptiles, fish, and shellfish. *Y. pseudotuberculosis* also resides in a number of avian species, including pigeons, turkeys, ducks, geese, and canaries.

**7. Sample/specimen requirements—***Y. enterocolitica* and *Y. pseudotuberculosis* can be isolated from faecal specimens, body fluids (e.g., cerebrospinal or peritoneal fluid), or tissue specimens (e.g., mesenteric lymph nodes or liver aspirates).

**8. Testing requirements—**

1) Screening: *Y. enterocolitica* and *Y. pseudotuberculosis* can be isolated using routine blood culture media and from enclosed body fluids (e.g., cerebrospinal or peritoneal fluid) or tissue specimens (e.g., mesenteric lymph nodes or liver aspirates) uncontaminated by other microorganisms. Cultural isolation of *Yersinia* from stool is hampered by slow growth and by overgrowth of other fecal flora. After 24-hour incubation at 37°C, colonies of *Y. enterocolitica* are pinpoint and barely perceptible against a background of more rapidly growing colonies of other enteric bacterial species present in fecal samples. Incubation temperatures of 22–29°C have been shown to be optimal. Cold enrichment in buffered saline at 25°C or 4°C for 2–3 weeks can optimize cultural recovery of *Yersinia* from stool specimens.
2) Diagnosis: *Y. enterocolitica* ferments lactose slowly, and colonies are colorless on media such as MacConkey agar, which incorporates lactose as a fermentable indicator substrate. Selective CIN or Congo Red agar can be used to differentiate pathogenic from nonpathogenic strains of *Yersinia*. CIN agar dramatically inhibits normal flora organisms, while *Y. enterocolitica* gives rise to distinctive

colonies with deep-red centers and a sharp border surrounded by a translucent zone. The red pigmentation is a result of mannitol fermentation.

Serological diagnosis of yersiniosis is performed in certain laboratories by enzyme immunoassay agglutination and immunoblotting techniques or by detection of specific immunoglobulin class G and immunoglobulin class A antibodies to *Yersinia* outer membrane proteins. Although not very widely available commercially, antibody testing may be useful in diagnosing the postinfectious, extraintestinal sequelae of yersiniosis where cultures of stool, blood, and other specimens are characteristically negative. In practice, cross-reactive antibodies can be seen with *Salmonella, Brucella, Escherichia coli*, and *Vibrio*, and false-positive serological results can occur.

3) Confirmatory tests: biochemical tests such as fermentation of salicin, hydrolysis of esculin, and pyrazinamidase positivity can be helpful in differentiating pathogenic from nonpathogenic strains of *Yersinia*. Polymerase chain reaction targeting species-specific regions of the 16S rRNA gene and the *inv* gene can be used for the identification of *Yersinia* isolates at the species level. Presence or absence of the *ail* and *ystB* genes can be used to differentiate between virulent (biotypes 1B and 2–5) and nonvirulent (biotype 1A) *Y. enterocolitica* strains, respectively.

**9. Reporting requirements**—All positive results from laboratory tests at clinical laboratories for *Y. enterocolitica* and *Y. pseudotuberculosis* should be reported to the national public health body. Data collated by the national reference laboratories are used for surveillance purposes. CDC monitors the frequency of *Y. enterocolitica* infections through the Foodborne Diseases Active Surveillance Network. Yersiniosis surveillance data for Europe is available at: http://ecdc.europa.eu/en/healthtopics/yersiniosis/annual-surveillance-data/pages/epidemiological_data.aspx.

**10. Referral network**—Local and regional diagnostic microbiology laboratories are required to submit cultures to national reference facilities for confirmation of the species identification, serotyping, and virulence and antimicrobial resistance profiling. Serotype is one of the main characteristics of *Y. enterocolitica* useful for epidemiological, diagnostic, and phylogenetic purposes, as strains enteropathogenic for humans are limited to a few serotypes. The classification in serotypes of *Y. enterocolitica* is determined by the O-antigen (O-ag) moiety of the cell surface lipopolysaccharide. Recently, whole genome sequencing has been used to genotype *Y. enterocolitica* and *Y. pseudotuberculosis*. A Loci index for genome *Y. enterocolitica* and Loci index for genome *Y. pseudotuberculosis* are available from GenBank (see: https://www.ncbi.nlm.nih.gov/genbank).

**11. Special considerations**—Key investigations for public health response include investigation of food (especially pork), water, and milk supplies for source of infection or cross-contamination. Collection of implicated food/water samples for testing should be performed by public health inspectors or environmental health officers. Potential occupational exposures (e.g., animal carcass handling/processing) and histories of animal contact including pets should be investigated. Individuals who have been identified as confirmed cases should be excluded from food handling and from direct care of infants, the elderly, and immunocompromised patients until 48 hours after the last symptoms. Education on personal and food hygiene should be provided (e.g., proper hand washing). Outbreaks should be investigated to identify a common source of infection and prevent further exposure to that source. The extent of outbreak investigations will depend upon the number of cases and the likely source of contamination.

[C. Jenkins]

# ZIKA

(Zika virus disease, Zika virus infection, congenital Zika syndrome)

| DISEASE | ICD-10 CODE |
|---|---|
| ZIKA | ICD-10 A92.8 |

**1. Clinical features**—Zika virus infection is thought to be asymptomatic or unrecognized in up to 80% of cases, based on seroepidemiology studies in Polynesia. It is not clear if this holds true for people when Zika infection is their first flavivirus infection or in other populations. Accurate serology assays are needed to resolve these questions, but they are not currently available. Illness due to Zika infection most commonly presents as a rash and fever following an incubation period of 3–14 days. Infection most frequently follows the bite of an infectious *Aedes* mosquito, but sexual transmission is increasingly recognized. The clinical presentation is mixed, and case series from Brazil show involvement of a maculopapular rash (>90% of cases), headache and fever (65%), myalgia and arthralgia (48%–65%), and less frequently pruritus, non-purulent conjunctivitis, and joint swelling. WHO and many national authorities have published case definitions while recognizing that these have a low specificity because distinguishing Zika infection clinically from a range of other infections including dengue and chikungunya, other causes of rash and fever (measles, parvovirus, rubella, and enterovirus) is difficult.

Neurological complications of Zika infection including Guillain-Barre syndrome (GBS), encephalitis, myelitis, and acute disseminated encephalomyelitis have been reported. These appear to be unusual complications of Zika infection. A published study estimated a GBS rate of 0.24/1,000 Zika cases in Polynesia, but this needs confirmation.

Zika virus is teratogenic, and Zika infection acquired during pregnancy can lead to congenital infection. Microcephaly has been the most commonly reported presentation. It is most frequently linked with maternal infection acquired in the first trimester, but the result of infection later in pregnancy and risk factors are not well defined. A congenital Zika syndrome with a wider range of more subtle neurological complications such as arthrogryposis and ocular signs is increasingly recognized. Some infections lead to foetal loss.

**2. Causative agents**—The virus was first isolated in 1947 from Rhesus monkeys living in the Zika forest in Uganda. Subsequently Zika virus was found in *Aedes* spp. and in humans causing a mild self-limiting infection. From 1947–2007, only limited studies of Zika infection were reported; 14 human cases confirmed by virus isolation or by serology were reported from Asia and Africa. Limited seroepidemiological studies showed a low prevalence of antibody. The first outbreak outside of Africa and Asia occurred in 2007 on Yap Island in the Federated States of Micronesia. The outbreak had 49 confirmed cases, and 73% of residents aged 3 years or older infected by immunoglobulin class M (IgM) seropositivity were reported. Recently a huge expansion in the geographic range of Zika occurred with the virus spreading through Polynesia to reach the Americas in 2013.

Zika virus belongs to the Spondweni virus serogroup of mosquito-borne flaviviruses (genus Flavivirus, Flaviviridae family). The virus particles are enveloped and spherical, 40–60 nm in diameter. Flaviviruses have a positive-sense, single-strand ribonucleic acid (RNA) genome of approximately 11 kilobases. As a flavivirus, it contains structural (E, C, prM) and nonstructural proteins (NS1–NS5) involved in virus replication. Zika virus exhibits extensive antigenic cross-reactivity with other Flaviviruses including yellow fever, dengue, and West Nile virus. The E and NS1 proteins contain a mixture of Zika-specific and cross-reactive epitopes. Phylogenetic analysis of Zika virus sequences has revealed the existence of 2 main lineages, the African lineage and the Asian lineage. All recently disseminated strains from the Americas belong to the Asian lineage. Zika virus genomes from patients infected in Brazil and Suriname in 2015 are close to strains that circulated in French Polynesia in 2013 with more than 99.7% and 99.9% level of nucleotide and amino acid identities, respectively.

**3. Laboratory diagnosis**—The laboratory diagnosis of Zika infection is necessary because clinical diagnosis is not reliable. Laboratory diagnostics for Zika virus are rapidly evolving in response to the emergence of the infection in the Americas. The first-line test for accurate diagnosis of Zika infection is the detection of viral RNA by reverse transcription polymerase chain reaction (RT-PCR). A range of different clinical specimens—serum, EDTA plasma, urine, saliva, cerebrospinal fluid (CSF), and semen—can be used. The level of virus in blood is low, and virus is only reliably detectible during the acute phase of illness, generally within 7 days of onset. In urine samples, the virus is detectible at a higher titer and for a longer period. Testing of serum and urine samples is recommended for up to 14 days after onset. The relatively short period of virus shedding means that a negative result does not rule out infection when the investigation is late in this window period. There are reports that Zika virus RNA can be detected consistently for longer in whole blood samples (≤ 2 months), and it can be detected by RT-PCR for longer in urine samples collected during pregnancy. Zika virus RNA has been detected in semen for up to 188 days after onset of illness and is reliably detected for 21 days. Sexual transmission of Zika virus as late as 41 days after onset of a partner's symptoms has been described. In cases infected in Latin America and Southeast Asia, the diagnostic challenge is compounded by the co-circulation of both dengue and chikungunya viruses together with Zika. These infections cannot be reliably distinguished on clinical grounds, and this necessitates testing for all 3 viral targets together. Triplex PCR assays are becoming available for this purpose.

Zika virus NS1 protein is secreted during infection in a similar way to dengue infection. Commercial NS1 assays, either as enzyme immunoassays or point-of-care assays, are used in the diagnosis of acute dengue infection and have a sensitivity of approximately 70%. Similar assays are in development for the diagnosis of Zika infection. NS1 is secreted in lower quantities in Zika infection and this is likely to affect sensitivity, but no commercial tests are available yet. A sample collected from an acute Zika infection giving a false-positive dengue NS1 result has been reported.

Zika infection can be diagnosed by the detection of virus-specific IgM, which develops during the first week of illness and generally persists for up to 12 weeks, although IgM persistence for longer is not uncommon. IgM assays are used to complement RT-PCR and are recommended for use in PCR-negative cases investigated after 14 days. The serological diagnosis of acute Zika infection by IgM detection is only considered presumptive even in endemic areas, due to the extensive antigenic cross-reactivity between flavivirus antibodies induced by dengue infection and yellow fever vaccination.

Current USA recommendations for serological diagnosis are to test for both Zika and dengue IgM in parallel, and if the sera reacts in both to perform a plaque reduction neutralization assay (PRNT) to resolve the cause of the illness. In pregnant travelers without symptoms returning from risk areas, IgM tests are no longer recommended because of the low predictive value of a positive result. Management is based on risk and careful assessment of the developing fetus. In Europe, indirect Zika NS1 IgM and IgG assays are more widely used and seem to be sufficiently accurate to use in travelers returning with infection.

Serological diagnosis is challenging in Latin America and other endemic areas, where all 4 dengue serotypes have circulated at times over the last

30 years and yellow fever vaccination is widespread. Thus, patients in the current Zika virus outbreak areas are likely to have a high background exposure to other flaviviruses, whereas European travelers returning from the same areas may not. A proportion of Zika virus infections in the outbreak region will mount a secondary flavivirus immune response with low IgM, and this further complicates the interpretation.

A limited number of Zika virus IgG serological tests have been described in the literature. One Indirect EIA for Zika IgG is widely available (Euroimmun); it is based on a Zika NS1 antigen. Published studies suggest it is sensitive and specific in populations with no prior exposure to other flavivirus antigens, but it has low specificity in Latin American populations. The PRNT and virus neutralization test also give nonspecific results in these populations due to cross-reactivity with other flaviviruses. Recent studies suggest that these cross-reactions are mostly at a low titer, and by using an appropriate cutoff specific results can be achieved. Published studies are needed. PRNT is performed in the USA, but these assays are technically demanding, laborious to perform, and expensive and so are not a practical option for most countries. A range of new Zika IgG assays are in development using recombinant type specific proteins (NS1, ED3) and competitor homologus dengue proteins, which hold promise for more specific serological diagnosis.

Laboratory diagnosis of the neurological complications of Zika infection uses a similar testing strategy. Since neurological symptoms may develop late after the acute illness, RT-PCR tests are often negative, serum Zika IgM gives a presumptive result, and reliable IgG tests are not widely available. CSF samples are sometimes available, and diagnosis by testing CSF by RT-PCR and Zika-specific IgM can confirm the diagnosis.

The diagnosis of congenital infection presents additional challenges. Mothers who present with an acute rash and fever are investigated using RT-PCR and IgM/IgG serology. The risk posed by subclinical infection in pregnancy is not fully understood, but services have been established in many countries to monitor returning pregnant travelers or pregnant women following sexual contact with travelers from endemic areas. Women are tested by RT-PCR if within 14 days of exposure and monitored by ultrasound for evidence of congenital abnormalities. Accurate Zika IgG assays are urgently needed to help manage these cases.

A small number of fatal cases of acute Zika infection have been reported in which virus is detectible by RT-PCR. However, it seems that in many cases of congenital infection, the virus may be cleared before birth, so diagnostic approaches are based on testing newborns by RT-PCR and for Zika IgM. In 1 microcephaly case series from Recife in Brazil, Zika virus IgM was reliably detected in CSF samples from the babies. By analogy with congenital rubella cases, it is likely that persisting Zika IgG will be the most reliable marker of congenital infection if detected between 6–12 months of age, although there are reports that neonatal IgG can be undetectible despite PCR-confirmed maternal or fetal infection. The accuracy of this approach depends on the rate of decline in passive maternal antibody, the incidence of Zika infection in the first year of life, and the availability of an accurate IgG assay. Studies are needed.

**4. Laboratory capability**—Laboratories should be accredited to perform diagnostic testing. Biosafety level 2 (BSL-2) facilities are required for work with clinical samples suspected to contain Zika virus. National authorities are responsible for licensing these facilities, and descriptions of the required design of laboratories, staff training, and competencies are available within many countries. Although Zika virus is a level 2 pathogen, laboratories also need to assess the additional risks for pregnant laboratory personnel. Some procedures using high-titer virus culture or animal experiments may pose a greater hazard to workers, and the proposed activity should be risk-assessed before work commences. They may be more appropriately conducted at BSL-3 containment.

**5. Safety requirements**—Regulators in the EU and the USA have classified Zika virus as a BSL-2 pathogen. This determines the facilities required for work with clinical samples suspected of containing the virus. No specific inactivation data is available for Zika virus. However, Zika virus is a flavivirus, which are labile RNA viruses, and Zika is likely to have similar properties to other flaviviruses. It will be inactivated if exposed to temperatures above 56°C for at least 30 minutes by ultraviolet light and by gamma-irradiation. Flaviviruses are susceptible to disinfectants such as 1% sodium hypochlorite, 2% glutaraldehyde, 70% ethanol, 3%–6% hydrogen peroxide and 3%–8% formaldehyde. During the sample preparation steps for RT-PCR assays, virus-inactivating reagents such as phenol guanidine isothiocyanate or chaotropic salts are added. These reagents inactivate flaviviruses, and therefore extracted samples can be handled in the laboratory with standard safety levels.

**6. Nonhuman hosts**—Zika virus is a mosquito-borne infection. In Africa, it has been identified in *Aedes*, *Anopheles*, and *Mansonia* mosquitoes, and in *Aedes* in Southeast Asia. *Aedes aegypti* is the key species linked to the explosive transmission seen in Latin America. The virus was first isolated from a monkey, and antibodies have been detected in sheep, goats, horses, cows, ducks, bats, and rodents, although since serology tests for Zika are not specific, the importance of these species in transmission is not established. Since 2007, the vast expansion in geographic range and numbers of cases is due to direct human-Aedes-human transmission.

**7. Sample/specimen requirements**—Serum, urine, whole blood, semen, CSF, and saliva samples are used in different contexts for virus detection by RT-PCR and to attempt virus isolation. Virus is detectible for a relatively short period, and so testing of blood and urine samples is recommended for up to 14 days after onset. The relatively short period of virus shedding means that a negative result does not rule out infection when the investigation is late in this window period. All specimens should be collected and shipped to the testing laboratory in appropriate biosafety containers within 24 hours using a 2°C–8°C cold chain. On receipt in the laboratory, samples should be centrifuged and serum collected immediately; samples should be held at 4°C and tested within 72 hours. Freeze-thawing should be avoided as it can lower the titer of virus in the sample. Long-term storage of samples for virus detection should be at −70°C. Zika IgM testing is recommended in cases investigated after 14 days. Serum samples for antibody testing are collected by venipuncture and transported to the laboratory for testing using a cold chain (2°C–8°C). On receipt in the laboratory, the clot should be allowed to separate and serum transferred to a suitable sealed vial for testing and storage. Serum samples can be stored long term at −20°C if required for antibody testing.

**8. Testing requirements**—At the time of this writing, many laboratories are running in-house PCR assays based on a published Zika real-time PCR assay.[1] False-positive results have been reported, so a cycle threshold value of 35–38 is generally used. Depending on the run conditions used, sensitivity of the assay has been reported between 50 and 500 copies. This is a rapidly developing field with new commercial tests becoming available in different regions. WHO has developed an emergency use assessment and listing (EUAL) procedure to expedite the availability of in vitro diagnostics (IVDs) needed. The EUAL procedure assesses the safety, quality, and performance of the IVD. Two assays have currently been assessed: AccuPower ZIKV (DENV, CHIKV) multiplex real-time RT-PCR Kit (Bioneer, Daejeon, South Korea) and RealStar Zika Virus RT-PCR Kit 1.0 (Altona Diagnostics GmbH, Hamburg, Germany). The sensitivity of both assays is in the range of 100 IU/ml (CI). FDA has a similar emergency use assessment process, and, as of mid-2018, 14 assays with appropriate sensitivity and specificity are now available:

- Trioplex rRT-PCR (CDC, Atlanta, GA)
- Zika virus RNA qualitative real-time RT-PCR (Quest Diagnostics, Secaucus, NJ)
- RealStar Zika virus RT-PCR kit (Altona Diagnostics, GmbH, Hamburg, Germany)
- Aptima Zika virus assay (Hologic, San Diego, CA)
- Zika virus real-time RT-PCR test (Viracor Eurofins, Viracor Eurofins, Lee's Summit, MO)
- Versant Zika RNA 1.0 assay (kPCR) (Siemens Healthcare Diagnostics, Berkeley, CA)
- xMAP MultiFLEX Zika RNA assay (Luminex, Austin, TX)
- Sentosa SA ZIKV RT-PCR test (Vela Diagnostics, Fairfield, NJ)
- Zika virus detection by RT-PCR (ARUP Laboratories, Salt Lake City, UT)
- Abbott RealTime Zika (Abbott Molecular, Des Plaines, IL)

- Zika ELITe MGB kit U.S. (ELITechGroup, Bothell, WA)
- Gene-RADAR Zika virus test (Nanobiosym Diagnostics, Cambridge, MA)
- CII-ArboViroPlex rRT-PCR (Columbia University, New York, NY)
- TaqPath Zika virus kit (Thermo Fisher Scientific, Pleasanton, CA)

RT-PCR has high specificity and, when positive, is considered a definitive diagnosis. The sensitivity depends on timing of sample collection and is poorly defined for the diagnosis of neurological complications and congenital infection (see Laboratory diagnosis). RT-PCR is used for screening semen samples used in IVF.

The most widely used Zika IgM capture assay (CDC) is based on a viral lysate, is sensitive (50%–90%, depending on population and sample timing) but gives positive results in both Zika and dengue infections and so has a low specificity, as does the equivalent dengue IgM assay with sera collected following Zika infection. A similar commercial assay is now available (InBios). More recently, an indirect assay and capture IgM assays using the Zika NS1 protein have become available. These are less sensitive but specific for the detection of Zika IgM antibody than the viral lysate assays, which has led to algorithms screening with a viral lysate assay and confirmation with an NS1-based test.

Testing must be conducted in fully accredited diagnostic laboratories. Quality assurance panels to support testing services are available through commercial sources and through WHO networks. FDA EUA commercial IgM assays available include the following:

- ZIKV MAC-ELISA (CDC, Atlanta, GA)
- ZIKV Detect IgM capture ELISA (InBios International, Seattle, WA)
- Liaison XL Zika capture IgM assay (DiaSorin Incorporated, Stillwater, MN)
- ADVIA Centaur Zika test (Siemens Healthcare Diagnostics, Berkeley, CA)
- DPP Zika IgM system (Chembio Diagnostic Systems, Medford, NY)

**9. Reporting requirements**—Most countries have clinical and laboratory surveillance schemes to monitor trends in Zika infection. Reporting of all confirmed cases by state and private laboratories is required in many public health systems to support these. In addition, Zika pregnancy registries and birth defect surveillance schemes are run in many countries, which may involve laboratory reporting.

**10. Referral network**—Most countries have established central or disseminated testing services, depending on demand. There may be a need to refer samples for specific tests such as PRNT, which is provided in only a few centers in the USA. There are no formal referral schemes for virus isolates.

**11. Special considerations**—In response to the emerging Zika epidemic, WHO declared a public health emergency of international concern in February 2016. This was in place until February 2017. WHO consolidates national surveillance reports of clinical and laboratory confirmed cases. Under the International Health Regulations (2005), international reporting of Zika infection is only required if it is the first report of infection in a new geographical region or if infection is associated with a changed disease profile.

## References

1. Lanciotti RS, Kosov OL, Laven JJ, et al. Genetic and serologic properties of Zika virus associated with an epidemic, Yap State, Micronesia, 2007. *Emerg Infect Dis.* 2008;14(8):1232-1239.

[D. W. Brown]

# INDEX

APHA

AMERICAN PUBLIC HEALTH ASSOCIATION

*For science. For action. For health.*

The American Public Health Association (APHA) champions the health of all people and communities. Our members represent all public health disciplines and more than 40 countries. APHA is the only organization that combines 140-plus years of perspective, a broad-based constituency, and the ability to influence federal policy to advocate for and improve the public's health.

APHA builds a collective voice for public health, working to ensure access to health care, protect funding for core public health services, and eliminate health disparities, among a myriad of other issues. Through its strong flagship publishing program that produces *Control of Communicable Diseases Manual,* the peer-reviewed *American Journal of Public Health,* the award-winning newspaper *The Nation's Health,* along with its e-newsletter Inside Public Health. APHA also leads public health awareness through its Get Ready campaigns and National Public Health Week. Together, we are creating the Healthiest Nation in One Generation.

To join APHA, visit www.apha.org or contact Membership Services at membership.mail@apha.org.